AF528791

Microbial Biotechnology and Ecology

Volume-1

Microbial Biotechnology and Ecology
Volume-1

Deepak Vyas
G.S. Paliwal
P.K. Khare
R.K. Gupta

2024
Daya Publishing House®
A Division of
Astral International Pvt. Ltd.
New Delhi – 110 002

First Published, 2011

Reprinted, 2024

ISBN: 978-81-7035-694-3 (HB)

Disclaimer:

Every possible effort has been made to ensure that the information contained in this book is accurate at the time of going to press, and the publisher and author cannot accept responsibility for any errors or omissions, however caused. No responsibility for loss or damage occasioned to any person acting, or refraining from action, as a result of the material in this publication can be accepted by the editor, the publisher or the author. The Publisher is not associated with any product or vendor mentioned in the book. The contents of this work are intended to further general scientific research, understanding and discussion only. Readers should consult with a specialist where appropriate.

Every effort has been made to trace the owners of copyright material used in this book, if any. The author and the publisher will be grateful for any omission brought to their notice for acknowledgment in the future editions of the book.

Published by : **Daya Publishing House®**
A Division of
Astral International Pvt. Ltd.
– ISO 9001:2015 Certified Company –
4736/23, Ansari Road, Darya Ganj,
New Delhi-110 002
Ph. 011-43549197, 23278134
E-mail: info@astralint.com
Website: www.astralint.com

Printed at : Replika Press Pvt. Ltd.

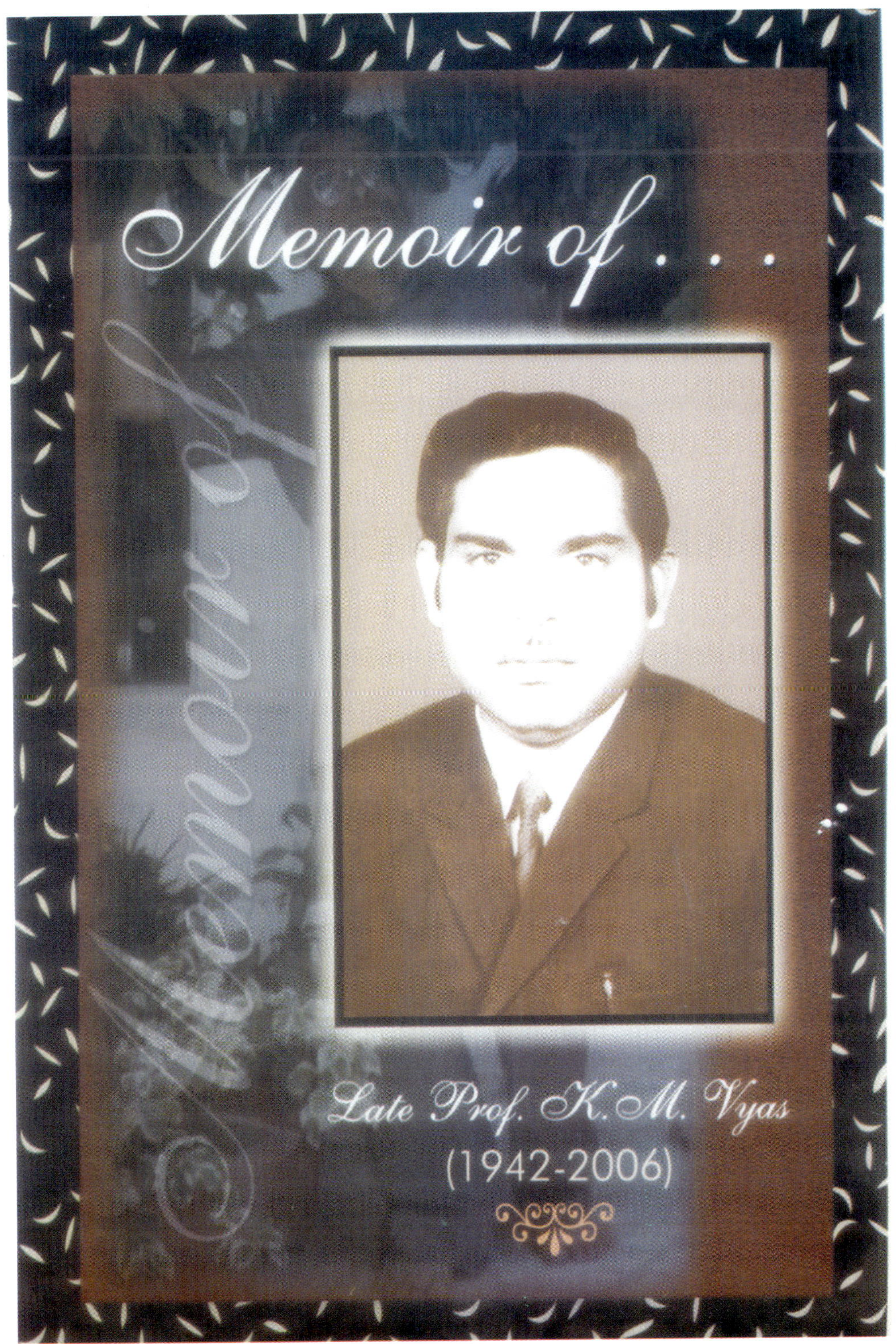

Date of Birth: 19-09-1942 to 07-09-2006

– Biography –
Late Prof. K.M. Vyas

Born on 19th September, 1942 in village Dharoan then in district Hamirpur and presently in district Mahoba (UP) in the family of Smt Radhika Rani and Sri Rooplal Vyas. Krishna Murari had his primary education in village and for the secondary education he moved to a Tehsil place in Charkhari. He obtained BSc from Maharaja College, Chhatarpur and MSc (Botany) degree from Sagour University, Sagar in 1963. Young Krishna Murari joined as a lecturer in the Botany Department then Sagour University, Sagour now Dr. H.S.G. V.V., Sagar (M.P.). Simultaneously joined PhD programme under the supervision of Prof SB Saksena (FNA), a renowned mycologist of that time. He did his PhD on *"Studies on the Ecology and Physiology of Soil Microorganisms in Relation to Soil Borne Plant Diseases"*. For post doctoral work (1973-74), he went to Department of Biochemistry, University of Hull, England (UK). He worked on *"Production and Activity of Cell Wall Degrading Enzymes by Late Blight Fungus–Phytopthora infestens"* with Prof J Friend.

Foreign Visits

Visited and delivered lectures at various important Research Institutions and Universities of England, Scotland, Belgium and Holland, Imperial College of Science and Technology, London, Long Ashton Research Station, Bristol, University of Glasgow, International Agriculture Institute, Wageninghe, Phytopathologic Research Institute Baarn, Holland.

Outstanding Research Contributions

1. Successful control of *Phytophthora* diseases of pan by streptomycin and other antibiotics.
2. Antibiotics as a new group of plant growth regulators.
3. Control of mosquitoes by certain isolates of bacteria and fungi.
4. Fungal pathogenesis of plants with special reference of cell wall degrading enzymes and phenolics in fungal pathogenesis.

5. *Alectra parasitica*: a traditional drug for the treatment of leprosy and other skin diseases.
6. Fungal respiration with special reference to mycelial respiration of plant pathogenic fungi.
7. Rhizosphere, rhizoplane, phyllosphere and phylloplane microflora and their role in plant diseases.

Professor and Head

In August 1984 he became a professor and in the month of October he became Head of the Department. As soon as he assumed the duty of HOD he brought DRS programme from UGC to strengthen the teaching and research facilities. During the period of 17 years of headship he also brought DSA phase I and II, and laid a stone for Cosist (Assistant programme) under SAP programme of UGC.

Prof Vyas established a strong centre of research in Mycology and Microbiology at Sagar. Where he undertook and successfully completed various research projects funding by UGC, CSIR, ICMR etc. He has published his work in various journals of National and International repute. He has edited book "*Recent Advances in Microbiology*". More than 40 students have obtained PhD under his supervision. Many of his students are actively engaged in research work and are occupying prestigious position in country and abroad.

During his tenure department grow, and many learned people from country and abroad visited the department and deliver their talks. He organized many seminars/ symposia/ workshops and refresher courses. Beside his scientific tamper and aptitude he has got administrative skills and proved himself an administrator in various capacities.

Administrative Experiences

1. As Head of the Botany Department. Dr. H.S.G. V.V., Sagar: 17 years (November 1984 to October 2001).
2. As Dean Faculty of Life Science: 4 years (two terms: 1988-90 and 1996-98).
3. As University Proctor: 6 Years (1986-1982).
4. As Chairman Board of Studies in Botany: 6 years (two terms: 1984-87 and 1994-97).
5. As Chief Coordinator of University Examinations: (three terms: 1985-86, 1988-89, and 1994-1995).
6. As Coordinator UGC NET- Exam, December 1996, June 1997, December 1997 and June 1998.
7. As Member of Academic Council Dr. H.S. G. V.V., Sagar: 10 years.
8. As Member of Executive Council; As Dean Faculty of Life Science (1988-90) and as Senior Professor (1996-99).
9. As Member of Central Board of Studies in Botany, Bhopal (MP): 10 years.
10. As Vice Chancellor of Dr. H.S.G. V.V., Sagar on various occasions/ day (during short term leave vacancy).
11. As Programme Coordinator of DRS/ DSA phase I and II programme of UGC in Botany Dr. H.S.G. V.V., Sagar.
12. As Member, Board of Studies, RDC and Selection Committees of various Universities and Colleges: 14 years.
13. As Professor Incharge of Development, Dr. H.S.G. V.V., Sagar: 3 years.

14. As Chairman, Organizing Committee of various symposia and seminars.
15. As Coordinator of Refresher Course in Botany: (1995-1998).
16. As Director Development in Botany: 1 October 2001–30 April 2004.

He was retired on 30th April 2004. He was an amazing personality with strong will power. His fight against Hepatitis B was amazing. After obtaining superannuation from the university he joined as a Principal at Pt. Vasudev Prasad Tiwari Degree College, Jhansi. He worked for the welfare of humanity under the umbrella of Bundelkhand Janseva Samiti, Jhansi.

Prof. Vyas was a great source of inspiration for his students, family members. His untimely death created a vacuum not only in scientific community but also in the family. It is said that there is a woman behind every great man. In this case it is Mrs Urmila Vyas, since 1958 when she was married to Prof KM Vyas. She has sacrificed all her comforts and has taken over all the household responsibilities so that Prof KM Vyas could be free to devote all his time to academics. Any visitor to their home was deeply impressed by their modesty, simplicity and warmth of their hospitability.

The Vyas are a well knit family. They have well educated children. One son and three daughters. Son is Dr Deepak Vyas presently serving in the same Department (Botany), Dr. H.S.G. V.V., Sagar married with Mrs. Nisha Vyas who is lecturer in college and have two sons Siddhant and Vedant studying in school. Among the daughters, elder daughter is Dr Jyoti married with with Dr Sanjay Chaubey, having their own hospital at Jhansi and having two sons Rohan and Kartik, then Mrs Arti married with Sunil Sharma who is working as an area manager in private firm. Arti is lecturer in private college at Bhopal have two kids Shivani and Shreyansh. Younger daughter Mrs Bharti is married with Dr Anand Sharma. Who is working at Cambridge Hospital, London, England.

List of Publications

1. Vyas, A. D. Vyas and K.M. Vyas (2006). Microbial cellulases for Industrial application. Every man's Science XL (6) 411-416.
2. Sharma, C.D., A.N. Rai and K.M. Vyas (2006). An undescribed fungal genus of the forest flora of Madhya Pradesh J. Bot. Soc. Univ. Sagar, 41 : 94-98.
3. Vyas, A., A. Jain, D. Vyas and K. M. Vyas (2005). Production and partial characterization of cellulases by two *Aspergillus* spp. on pretreated low value ligno-cellulases. Proc. Natl. Acad. Sci. India, 75(B) p. 1-7.
4. Vyas, Ashish, D. Vyas and K.M. Vyas (2005). Biodiversity conservation through integrated participatory management J. Bot. Soc. Univ. Sagar, 40 : 178-189.
5. Dwivedi, O. P., R. K. Yadav, D. Vyas and K. M. Vyas (2004). Role of Potassium in the occurrence of VAM spores in the rhizosphre soils of Lantana species. In: Microbiology and Biotechnology for sustainable development. Ed. P.C. Jain, Pp. 248–253. CBS Publishers, New Delhi.
6. Yadav, R.K., O.P.Dwivedi, D. Vyas and K. M. Vyas (2004). Antifungal effect of *Microcystis* against Beetalvine *Phytophthora*. J. Basic and applied Myco. 3(1+2) : 105–107.
7. Vyas Ashish, Vyas Deepak and Vyas K.M. (2004). Production and optimization of cellulases on pretreated groundnut shell by *Aspergillus tenuis* AV49. Journal of Scientific and Industrial Research Vol. 64, Pp. 281-286.
8. Vyas, A., D. Vyas and K.M. Vyas (2004). Cellulolytic strains of *Aspergillu* and *Penicillium*. J. Bot.Soc.Univ. Sagar 39 66-71.

9. Yadav, R.K., O.P. Dwivedi, D. Vyas and K.M. Vyas (2003). Management of *Phytophthora* disease of betel vine by plant extracts J. Basic and Applied Mycol. 2 (1) : 79-82.

10. Agrawal, R., A.N. Rai and K.M. Vyas (2003). A new species of *Tretospora* from India. J. Basic and Applied Mycol. 2 (1) 48-49.

11. Soni, Anuradha, D. Vyas and K.M. Vyas (2003). Effect of VAM fungi on the growth and productivity of Soybean (*Glycine max.*) J. Basic and Applied Mycol. 2 (1) : 40-41.

12. Vyas, Ashish, D. Vyas and K.M. Vyas (2003). Screening of extra-cellular cellulase producing fungi from different lignocellulosic wastes. J. Basic and Applied Mycol. 2 (1) : 14-16.

13. Khare, N. and Vyas K.M. (2003). Effect of nitrogen sources on the production of pectolytic and cellulytic enzymes by *Rhizopus nodosus* and *Phytophthora nicotiana* J. Bot Soc. Univ. Sagar 36 : 87-94.

14. Dwivedi, O.P., R.K. Yadav, D. Vyas and K.M. Vyas (2002). Distribution of VAM fungi in the rhizosphere soils of Betel vine J. Phytopathol. 56 (2) : 228-229.

15. Dwivedi, O.P., Yadav, R.K., Vyas, D. and Vyas, K.M. (2002). Vesicular-Arbuscular Mycorrhizal Association with *Lantana* sp. In Sagar University Campus; in Different Disordered Systems INDIAS 2000. (eds) K. Fukawa, J.T. Watson, S.N. Saxena and S.K. Shrivastava, pp. 154-157. INDIAS Publication, Allahabad.

16. Vyas, D., O.P. Dwevedi, R.K. Yadav and K.M. Vyas (2002). Arbuscular Diversity of VAM Fungi. In frontiers of fungal diversity in India. (Eds.) G.P. Rao, C. Manoharachari, D.J. Bhat, R.C. Rajak and T.N. Lakhanpal pp. 873-889. International Book Distributing Company Lucknow, India.

17. Singh, N., Vyas, D., Gupta, U.S. and Vyas, K.M (1999). Physico-chemical properties of Sagar lake with special reference to *Microcystis* bloom in the proceeding of the New Millenium Conference on Retrospect of Indian Research on Environmental Pollution : Focus 21st Century, 38.

18. Sharma, C.D., Gadpandey, K.K., Firdousi, S.A., Rai, A.N. and Vyas, K.M. (1998). Three New species of *Cladosporium* from Madhya Pradesh, India. Indian Phytopath. 51 (2): 152-160.

19. Chaursia, J.P., Chaurasia, P. and Vyas, K.M. (1997). Effect of *Ocimum sanctum* leaf extract on betelvine *Phytophthora* disease; An ecofriendly new approach. Environment pollution in 21 Century (Ed). V.S. Bais. Narendra Publishing House, Delhi, p. 46-51.

20. Chaurasia, J.P. and Vyas, K.M (1997). *In vivo* evaluation of some homoeopathic drugs against betelvine *Phytophthora* disease, Indian Phytopath. 4:148-153.

21. Vyas, K.M., Chaurasia, J.P. and Mishra, A.S. (1996). Effect of hepar sulphate on betelvine *Phytopathora* disease. Madhya Bharti Journal, Dr HS Gour Vishwavidyalaya, Sagar, India 36A 40B: 65-71.

22. Vyas, K.M. and Firdousi, S.A. (1996). Leaf blight of *Terminalia tomentosa.* Indian Phytopathology (Accepted).

23. Vyas, K.M., Gadpandey, K.K., Sharma, C.D., Firdousi, S.A. and Rai, A.N. (1996). Two new Hyphomycetes from India. Mycological Research (Accepted).

24. Vyas, K.M., Sharma, C.D., Gadpandey, K.K., Rai, A.N. and Firdousi, S.A. (1996). Three new species of *Cladosporium* from Madhya Pradesh. Indian Phytopathological Society IARI, New Delhi (In press).

25. Vyas KM, Dubey MP and Sharma RS (1995). Low cost agronomic practice for soybean (*Glycine max*) cultivation in Madhya Pradesh. Indian Journal of Agriculture Sciences 65(10):743-745.
26. Vyas KM, Kumar R and Rai AN (1995). Two new *Alternaria* species from Uttar Pradesh. Acta Botanica Indica 23 (1): 151-153.
27. Vyas KM and Firdousi SA (1994). A new leaf spot disease of *Casearia tomentosa* caused by *Asteromella* species. Acta Botanica Indica 20: 120-121.
28. Vyas KM and Saxena AP (1993). Antimicrobial activity of *Alectra parasitica,* A rice var. *chitrakutensis* rau. Journal of Economic and Taxonomic Botany 17 (1) 55-59.
29. Vyas KM, Firdousi SA and Rai AN (1993). A new species of *Stenella* from India. Acta Botanica Indica 25: 131-132.
30. Vyas KM and Firdousi SA (1993). A new spot of *Miliusa tomentosa* Roxb. Acta Botanica Indica 21 (1): 124.
31. Vyas KM and Mehta A (1992). Degradation of plant tissues by fungal enzymes. In: Dubey NK and Sharma PD, Rastogi Publications, Meerut, India.
32. Vyas KM, Firdousi SA and Rai AN (1992). A new species of *Pseudocercospora* from India. Indian Phytopathology 45(4): 449-451.
33. Vyas KM, Firdousi SA and Rai AN (1992). A new species of *Pseudocercospora* from India. Acta Botanica Indica.
34. Vyas KM, Firdousi SA and Rai AN (1992). *Mycovellosiella adinae* Sp nov. from India. Indian Phytopathology 45(4): 451-452.
35. Vyas KM (1990). A new leaf spot disease of *Ficus begalensis* caused by *Coniothyrium olivaceum* from India. Acta Botanica Indica 1: 150.
36. Vyas KM, Firdousi SA and Rai NA (1990). *Pseudocercospora gymnosporinae* sp. nov. India. Mycological Research (UK in press).
37. Vyas KM, Firdousi SA and Rai NA (1990). A new host record of *Thielvia appendiculata* from India. Indian Phytopath 43(1): 124.
38. Vyas KM, Firdousi SA and Rai NA (1990). A new leaf spot disease of *Eleodendron glaucum* from India. Indian Phytopath 43(1): 122.
39. Vyas KM and Gupta DK (1989). Efficacy of *Bacillus subtilis* against Mosquito larvae (*Anophelis culicifacies*). Zeitschrift Fur Angewandte Zoologie (German Journal for Applied Zoology) 85-91.
40. Vyas KM and Chile SK (1989). Metabolism of ascorbic acid and *Piper betle* leaves under *Phytopathora* pathogenesis. Perspective in Mycological Research 1: 143-150.
41. Vyas KM and Tripathi HSS (1986). Production of toxin by *Xanthomaonas compestris* pv *betticola* causing leaf spot disease of *Piper betle* L. Acta Botanica Indica 14: 220-225.
42. Vyas KM and Saxena NK (1986). Microbial synthesis of 11-deoxy corticosteron from progesterone by a nutant of *Rhizophus nodosus* (Abst.) XIV International Congress of Microbiology: Menchester, England 7-13 September.
43. Vyas KM and Chile SK (1985). Electrolyte leakage from *Piper betle* leaves after infection with *Phytopathora parasitica* var *piperina*. Indian Phytopathology 38 (3): 529-530.

44. Vyas KM and Tripathi HSS (1985). Production of cellulolytic enzymes by *Xanthomonas compestris* pv *betticola: in vivo* and *in vitro*. Bull Bot. Soc. 33.
45. Vyas KM, Tripathi HSS, Saxena NK and Sadique Y (1985). Efficacy of hydroxyl stilbamidine isethionate USP against *Phytopathora parasitica* var *piperina*. Phytopathora Newsletters 13: 32-33.
46. Vyas KM, Saxena NK, Tripathi HSS and Sadique Y (1985). Complete control of *Phytopathora parasitica* var *piperina* by S-flurocytosine. Phytopathora News Letters 13: 30-31.
47. Vyas KM, Dubey GL and Dubey O (1985). Physico-chemical properties of linseed oil as affected by various seed borne fungi. Phytopath. z. 113: 66-70.
48. Vyas KM and Chile SK (1984). Efficacy of *Vinca rosea* extracts against protease from human pathogenic strain of *Trichophytom rubrum* sab. Hindustan Antibiotics Bull. 26: 114-116.
49. Vyas KM, Kher AK and Saxena SB (1984). Persistence of various fungicides in soil. Indian Phytopath 27(3): 574-576.
50. Vyas KM and Shrivastava A (1984). Effect of cholesterol on the toxicity of certain antibiotics against betelvine *Phytopathora*. Phytopathora News Letter 12 pp. 33.
51. Vyas KM, Soni, Saxena NK and Tripathi HSS (1984). Decline in the total reducing sugar content during the postharvest infection of *Lycopersicon lycopersicum* L. Karsgen fruits by *Bacillus fructodrestruens*. Bull Bot. Soc. 30-31: 69-71.
52. Vyas KM, Saxena NK and Tripathi HSS (1984). Cationic degradation of Streptomycine and Kanemycine by *Aspergillus niger* in broth cultures during fragmentation in shade flask. Hindustan Antibiotics Bulletin 26 (3 and 4) pp. 96-101.
53. Chile SK, Vyas KM and Singh R (1984). Induced resistance in *Piper betle* leaves in relation to *Phytopathora parasitica* var. *piperina*. Indian Phytopath. 37: 719-721.
54. Chile SK and Vyas KM (1984). Inhibitors of certain enzymes of *Botrydiplodia theobromae* in *Piper betle* leaf extract. Hindustan Antibiotics Bull. 26: 27-32.
55. Vyas KM and Chile SK (1984). Respiratory response of betlevine *Phytopathora* induced by various volatile oils. Jr Mycology Plant Path.
56. Vyas KM, Saxena NK and Tripathi HSS (1984). Accumulation of D.L. 3,4 dihydroxy-phenyalanine during the soft rot of *Lycopersicon esculentum* fruits caused by *Bacillus fructodestruens*. Abst. 36th Ann. Meeting Indian Phytopath (Hissar) 37: 401.
57. Vyas KM, Saxena NK and Tripathi HSS (1984). Postharvest accumulation of vitamin C induced by *Bacillus fructodestruens* in the *Lycopersicon esculentum* fruits. Abst. 36th Ann. Meeting Indian Phytopath, Hissar and paper published in Nat. Acad. Sci. Letters 7(4): 109-110.
58. Vyas KM and Shrivastava A (1984). Chemical control of betelvine *Phytopathora*. Abst. Symp. Chemical Control of Plant Disease. Indian Phytopath, Hissar.
59. Vyas KM and Singh R (1984). Nitrogen nutrition of *Phytopathora parasitica* var *piperina* (Dast) causing foot and leaf rot disease of *Piper betle* Linn. Proc. 71st Ind. Sci. Cong. Part III Abstract, 57: 26.
60. Vyas KM and Atri DC (1983). Pectolytic and cellulolytic activity during pathogenesis caused by *Botryodiplodia theobromae* Pat. In *Pyrus pyrifolia* Burm. fruits. Abst National Acad. Sci. (Biol.) Abst. No. 257 pp. 94.

61. Vyas KM and Chile SK (1983). Free amino acids in relation to *Phytopthora* leaf rot pathogenesis of Pan. Indian Phytopath 36(4): 626-628.

62. Vyas KM and Chile SK (1983). Dehydrogenase activity in *Piper betle* L. leaves infected with *Phytopathora parasitica* var. *piperina*. Indian Phytopath 36(4): 613-617.

63. Vyas KM and Sxena N (1983). Effect of antibiotics on certain cell wall degrading enzymes of *Rhizopus nodosus* and *Phytopathora nitotianae*. Hindustan Antibiotics Bulletin 25 (1 and 2) pp. 21-24.

64. Vyas KM and Shrivastava A (1983). In vitro efficacy of tetracycline against betelvine *Phytopathora*. Hindustan Antibiotics Bulletin 25 (1 and 2) pp. 15-17.

65. Vyas KM and Saxena AP (1983). Ethnobotany of Dhasan valley. Jr. of Econ. Tax. Bot., Jodhpur.

66. Vyas KM and Saxena AP (1983). Traditional treatment of leprosy and leucoderma by tribals from Bundelkhand UP. Bull. of Medico Ethn. Bot. Res. CCRAS, New Delhi.

67. Vyas KM and Thakur MS (1983). Production of plant growth regulators by some *Fusarium* species. Folia Microbial. 28: 124-129.

68. Vyas KM, Gupta DK and Shrivastava A (1983). In vitro antibacterial properties of some fixed oils. Proc 70th Ind. Sci Cong. Assoc 29.

69. Vyas, Chile SK and Shrivastava A (1982). Efficacy of some growth hormones on sporulation of betelvine *Phytopathora*. Bull. Bot. Soc. Univ. Saugar 29: 25-27.

70. Chile SK and Vyas KM (1982). Efficiency of carboxin in relation to *Phytopathora* leaf rot of *Piper betle*. Abstract 1st National Symposium of Synthetic Fungicides in Plant Disease Control in IARI, June 1982.

71. Chile SK, Vyas KM and Vyas RS (1982). Effect of culture filtrate of various fungi on sporulation of betelvine *Phytopathora*. Hind. Ant. Bull. 23: 25-26.

72. Chile SK and Vyas KM (1982). Effect of culture filtrate of various fungi on acidative enzymes of betelvine *Phytopathora*. Hind. Ant. Bull. 24: 26-28.

73. Vyas KM, Gupta DK and Chile SK (1982). A fruit rot disease of Momardiaca. Indian Phytopath 35(2): 351.

74. Vyas KM and Gupta DK (1982). Biological control of mosquito. IX Annual Conference of Indian Society of Human Genetics, Bhopal 58.

75. Vyas KM and Gupta DK (1982). Effect of *Aspergillus* mycotoxin on *Culex* larvae. Proc 69th Ind. Sci. Cong. Asso. Abstract 61.

76. Vyas KM and Thomas T (1982). On the abundance of *Trichoderma* species in the soil of Andaman and Nicobar Islands. Proc 69th Ind. Sci. Cong. Asso. Abstract 59.

77. Vyas KM and Saxena N (1982). Pectolytic enzymes of *Rhizopus nodosus* and *Phytopathora nictianae* in relation to electrolyte leakage and tissue maceration. Proc 69th Ind. Sci. Cong. Asso. Abstract 44.

78. Vyas KM and Saxena AP (1982). In vitro antimicrobial activity of some medicinal plants against human pathogens. Proc 69th Ind. Sci. Cong. Asso. Pt. III: 43-44.

79. Vyas KM, Singh R and Chile SK (1982). Nitrogen nutrition of *Phytopathora parasitica* var *piperina* (Dast) Causing foot rot and leaf rot diseases of *Piper betle* Linn. Jur. Biol. Res.

80. Vyas KM (1982). Peroxiodase and catalases in relation to betelvine. Phytopathora News Letters, USA 10: 8.

81. Vyas KM and Chile SK (1982). Breakdown of disease resistance in betelvine *Phytopathora* system by vitamin C. Phytopathora News Letters, USA 10: 6-7.

82. Vyas KM and Thakur MS (1982). Plant growth regulatory metabolites produced by fungi. Abstract Symp. Fermented Foods, Food Contaminants, Biofertlizers and Bioenergy pp. 54.

83. Vyas KM and Thoimas T (1982). *Gliocladium virens*- A new report from India. Geobios News reports 1: 45.

84. Vyas KM and Saxena AP (1981). *Martynia annua* Linn. A drug for Asthma, Itch and Eczema. Bull of Medico. Ethno Bot. Res. CCRAS, New Delhi II (3): 427- 429.

85. Vyas KM (1981). Problem and progress in *Phytopathora* diseases of Pan group discussion on improvement of betelvine cultivation. NBRI, Lucknow p 92-93.

86. Vyas KM, Thomas T and Gupta DK (1981). *Gilmaniella subornate*: A new report from India. Bull. Bot. Soc. Univ. of Saugar 28: 38.

87. Vyas KM, Thomas T and Gupta DK (1981). *Trichoderma pseudo-konningii* Rifai: A new report from India. Bull. Bot. Soc. Univ. of Saugar 28: 28.

88. Vyas KM (1981). Effect of culture filtrates of various fungi on sporulation of betelvine *Phytopathora*. Hind. Antibiot. Bot. 23: 25-26.

89. Vyas KM, Chourasia SC and Saxena SB (1981). Management of *Phytopathora* diseases of Pan (*Piper betle*). Abst. 3rd International Symposium on Plant Pathology (IPS) pp. 253.

90. Chile SK and Vyas KM (1981). Polyphenol oxidase in relation to betelvine *Phytopathora* pathogenesis of Pan. Phytopathora News Letters, USA 9: 40-41.

91. Vyas KM and Saxena AP (1981). Medicinal plants of Bundelkhand I.P preliminary ethnobotanical survey of Banda district UP. Proc. 68th Ind. Sci. Cong. Pt III (Abst): 147.

92. Vyas KM and Saxena AP (1981). Flora of Bundelkhand II. Hydrophytic tract of Ken-Baghain tract (Banda district UP). Ind. Soc. Weed. Sci. Abst: 40-41.

93. Vyas KM and Saxena AP (1981). Ethnobotanical records on infectious diseases from tribals of Banda district (UP). Ind. Soc. Weed. Sci. Abst: 40-41.

94. Vyas KM and Gupta DK (1981). Biological control of mosquitoes: I Effect of culture filtrate of certain *Aspergilli* on Anopheles larvae. Proc. 51 Session Nat. Acad. Sci.: 51.

95. Vyas KM and Chile SK (1981). Effect of the age of betel vine leaves on phenolics and *Phytopathora* rot. Ind. Sci. Cong.

96. Chile SK, Chourasia and Vyas KM (1981). Role of cuttings on the growth of the betel vine *Phytopathora*. Phytopathora News Letters, USA 8: 31.

97. Vyas KM and Chile SK (1980). Role of polyphenol oxidase in disease resistance with special reference to the betel vine *Phytopathora*. Symp. Plant Disease Problem at PAU, Ludhiana (Punjab) Abstract IIX.

98. Vyas KM, Chile SK and Saraf M (1980). Effect of some fungicides on sporulation of different isolates of betel vine *Phytopathora*. Bull. Bot. Univ. of Saugar, Sagar (MP) 27 pp. 16-18.

99. Vyas KM, Chourasia SC and Chile SK (1980). Role of infested soil and cuttings on the spread of betel vine *Phytopathora*. Phytopathora News Letters, USA 8: 28.

100. Vyas KM and Chile SK (1980). Role of infested soil and cuttings on the spread of betel vine *Phytopathora*. Symp. on Phytopathora Diseases of Tropical Plants (Calicut) pp. 22.

101. Vyas KM and Chile SK (1980). Varietal reaction of *Piper betle* leaves against different isolates of betel vine *Phytopathora*. Phytopathora News Letters, USA 8: 29.

102. Vyas KM, Chile SK and Vyas RS (1980). Two new diseases of cultivated plants. Indian Phytopath. 33(3): 493-495.

103. Vyas KM and Gupta M (1979). Studies on cell wall degrading enzymes in relation to banana fruit rot. Indian Phytopath. 32: 456- 457.

104. Vyas KM, Raghvan U and Saxena SB (1979). Studies on amino acid composition of mycelia of 14 of *Botryodiplodia theobromae* Pat. Bull. Bot. Soc. Univ. Saugar, 23-24: 21-25.

105. Vyas KM and Thakur MS (1979). Production of indole auxins by *Curvularia* spp. Abst. 66th Sess. Ind. Sci. Cong. p. 38.

106. Vyas KM and Dubey GL (1979). Physico-chemical properties of linseed oil as affected by various seed borne fungi. Abst. 66th Sess. Ind. Sci. Cong. p. 15.

107. Vyas KM and Saxena AP (1979). Flora of Bundelkhand I, A contribution to grasses of Banda and Hamirpur districts (UP). Bull. Bot. Soc. Univ. of Saugar, Sagar 25-26: 73-78.

108. Vyas KM and Chourasia SC (1979). Efficacy of certain antibiotics against betel vine *Phytopathora*. Phytopathora News Letters, USA 7: 28.

109. Vyas KM and Chourasia SC (1979). Leaf spot, a new disease of bakoli (*Mimusops elengi*) in Sagar, India 63: 806.

110. Vyas KM and Chourasia SC (1979). Oxidative metabolism under *Phytopathora* leaf rot pathogenesis of Pan. Phytopathora News Letters, USA 7: 27.

111. Vyas KM (1978). Effects of fungicides on the growth of *Phytopathora parasitica* var. *piperina* causing foot rot and leaf rot diseases of Pan. Proc. Nat. Acad. Sc. (Allahabad) 47 (B) III: 141-144.

112. Vyas KM and Chourasia SC (1978). Formation of cospores in vivo by *Phytopathora parasitica* var. *piperina*. Phytopathora News Letters USA, Feb. 1978, No. 6 pp. 42-43.

113. Vyas KM and Chourasia SC (1978). Leaf surface mycoflora in relation to *Phytopathora* leaf rot on Pan (*Piper betle*). Phytopathora News Letters USA, Feb. 1978, No. 6 pp. 40-41.

114. Vyas KM and Chourasia SC (1978). Host parasite interactions in betelvine *Phytopathora* varietal response to leaf rot pathogenesis. Phytopathora News Letters USA, Feb. 1978, No. 6 pp. 38-39.

115. Vyas KM (1978). Effect of fungal metabolites on the growth ot morphogenesis of crop plants. Abst. Ibid. pp. 43.

116. Vyas KM (1978). Studies on the molds and mycotoxins with special reference to mycoflora associated with the grains of jowar. Abst. All India Symposium on Physiology of Parasitism Jabalpur. pp. 20.

117. Vyas KM, Kazmi SM and Soni NK (1978). Studies on the antifungal properties of mamalian urine. Agriculture and Agro Industries Jur.

118. Chourasia SC, Vyas KM and Pathak RK (1977). In vitro inhibitory effects of certain fungicides in the growth of *Phytopathora parasitica* var. *piperina* causing foot rot and leaf rot diseases of Pan (*Piper betel* Linn.) Proc. Nat. Acad. Sci. Ind. 47(B) III: 141-144.

119. Vyas KM and Chourasia SC (1977). Effect of fungicides on the oxidative metabolism of *Phytopathora parasitica* var. *piperina* (Dast.) causing foot rot and leaf rot diseases of Pan (*Piper*

betel) in physiology of microorganism edited by KS Bilgrami Todays and Tomorrow Printers and Publishers, New Delhi 11-16.

120. Vyas KM and Jain SK (1977). Production of auxin like plant growth regulatory metabolites by soil fungi. In: physiology of microorganisms (Edited by KS Bilgrami), Todays and Tomorrow Printers and Publishers, New Delhi 331-340.
121. Vyas KM, Thind TS and Prakash V (1977). Effect of some antibiotics on the germination of corainder seeds. Ind Jr. of Exp. Biol. Vol. 15, No. 3, March 77 pp. 247-248.
122. Vyas KM and Chourasia SC (1977). In vitro effect of some volatile oils against *Phytopathora parasitica* var. *piperina*. Jr. Res. Ind. Med. Yoga and Homoeo. 12:3. 139-142.
123. Vyas KM and Chourasia SC (1977). The influence of age and starvation on endogenous respiration of mycelium of *Phytopathora parasitica* var. *piperina*. Acta Botanica Indica 5: 54-57, 77.
124. Vyas KM (1976). Respiratory characterstics of plant pathogenic fungi, *Ibid*.
125. Vyas KM (1976). Production of cell wall degrading enzymes by *Botryodiplodia theobromae*, *Ibid*.
126. Vyas KM (1976). Microbial metabolites and plant growth promoting activity of some antifungal antibiotic compounds, *Ibid*.
127. Vyas KM (1976). Microbial metabolites and plant growth production of indole auxins by soil fungi, *Ibid*.
128. Vyas KM (1976). Effect of fungicides on the oxidative metabolism of *Phytopathora parasitica* var. *piperina* (Dast) causing foot rot and leaf rot of Pan (*Piper betle*). In: Physiology of Microorganisms (Edited by KS Bilgrami), Today and Tomorrow Publications pp. 11-16.
129. Vyas KM (1976). Interactions of soil microorganisms with *Phytopathora parasitica* var. *piperina*. Abst. Symp. on Physiology of Microorganisms held at Bhagalpur Feb. 1976.
130. Vyas KM and Chourasia SC (1976). Activity of some volatile oils against *Phytopathora parasitica* var. *piperina*. Indian Drugs Jan 9-15.
131. Vyas KM and Chourasia SC (1976). Influence of culture media on fungal respiration. Hind. Antibiot. Bull. Vol. 18: 3 and 4.
132. Vyas KM and Mehta P (1975). Effect of plat growth regulators on production and activity of cellulase. Ind. J. Exptl. Biol. Vol 14, 206-208.
133. Vyas KM and Chourasia SC (1975). Studies on leaf rot of Pan (*Piper betle*) varietal factors in relation to disease resistance. Symp. on Plant Pathlogical problems held at Udaipur 5(1): 10-11.
134. Vyas KM, Mehta P and Saxena SB (1975). Pathological studies of fruit rot diseases of tamato caused by *Alternaria solani* and *A. tenuis*. Indian Phytopath. Vol. XXVIII No 2, 247-252.
135. Vyas KM, Mehta P and Saxena SB (1975). Metabolic changes during pathogenesis of tomato fruit rot diseases. Indian Phytopath. Vol. XXVIII No 2, 253-255.
136. Vyas KM and Soni NK (1975). Effect of antibiotics and fungicides on the mycelial respiration and growth of *Rhizoctonia capsici*. Ind. Jr. Exptl. Biol. Vol. 13, pp. 216-218.
137. Vyas KM, Mehta P and Saxena SB (1975). Production of pectolytic enzymes by *Alternaria* sp. of various culture media. J. Ind. Bot. Soc. 200-206.

138. Vyas KM and Soni NK (1975). Responses of *Rhizotonia solani* Kuhn and *Colletotrichum capsici* (Syd.) Butler and Bisby to various chemical substances. Madhya Bharti Univ. Sagar, Vol. 22-23 pp. 43-48.

139. Vyas KM, Mehta P and Saxena SB (1975). Effect of native carbon sources and pH on the cellulolytic enzymes of *Alternaria solani* and *A. tenuis*. Science and Culture Vol. 41 pp. 400-402.

140. Vyas KM and Chourasia SC (1975). Effect of vitamins on the mycelial growth of *Phytopathora parasitica* var. *piperina*. Madhya Bharti, vol. 22 and 23 pp. 63-65.

141. Vyas KM and Soni NK (1975). Respiratory response of *Gleosporium papayae* induced by various substances. Proc. Ind. Sci. Acad. Vol. 41, Part B. No. 5 pp. 458-461.

142. Vyas KM, Saxena RK and Saxena SB (1974). Physiology of *Tectona grandis* leaves infected with *Uncinula tectonae*. J. Indian Bot. Soc. 53: 256-270.

143. Vyas KM, Jain SK and Raghvan P (1974). Microbial metabolites and plant growth: Plant growth regulatory activity of culture filtrates of soil microorganisms and some antibiotic compounds. Abst. Symp. on Biology of Soil Microorganisms, Sagar pp. 35-36.

144. Vyas KM, Mehta P and Saxena SB (1974). Metabolic changes during pathogenesis of fruit rot diseases of tomato. MP Vigyan Acad. Bhopal Abst. pp. 7-8.

145. Vyas KM, Saxena SB and Soni NK (1974). Effect of antibiotics and fungicides on endogenous mycelial respiration and growth of *Rhizoctonia solani* Kuhn. and *Colletotrichum capsici* (Syd.) Butler and Bisby. MP Vigyan Acad. Bhopal Abst. pp. 5-6.

146. Vyas KM, Mehta P and Saxena SB (1974). Production of pectolytic and cellulolytic enzymes by *Alternaria* sp. during pathogenesis of tomato fruits. Hind. Antibiot. Bull. Vol. 16, No. 4 pp. 20-214.

147. Vyas KM, Mehta P and Saxena SB (1974). Effect of native carbon sources and pH on the pectolytic enzymes of *Alternaria* sp. during pathogenesis of tomato fruits. Hind. Antibiot. Bull. Vol. 40 Part B, No. 4 pp. 433-439.

148. Vyas KM, Pandey P and Soni NK (1974). Effect of antibiotics on endogenous mycelial respiration and growth of some plant pathogenic fungi. Hind. Antibiot. Bull. Vol. 16: 199-201.

149. Vyas KM and Soni NK (1973). Effect of the age of culture and starvation period on mycelial respiration. Bull. Bot. Soc., Univ. Saugar, Vol. 20 pp. 17-20.

150. Vyas KM and Saxena SB (1973). Studies on mycelial respiration of *Sclerotium rolfsii*. Proc. Ind. Nat. Acad. Vol. 39 Part B No. 5 569-575.

151. Vyas KM, Raghvan P and Jain SK (1973). Auxins like activity of the antibiotic aureofungin. Hind. Antibiot. Bull. Vol. 16 No 1 pp. 29-31.

152. Vyas KM and Jain SK (1973). Production of auxins by microorganisms. Hind. Antibiot. Bull. Vol. 11, pp 217-219.

153. Vyas KM and Soni NK (1973). Respiratory and growth responses of *Fusarium oxysporum* Sacc. induced by various substances. Ind J. Exptl. Biol. Vol. 11 pp. 217-219.

154. Vyas KM, Chourasia SC and Soni NK (1973). Efficiency of certain antibiotics against *Phytopathora parasitica* var. *piperina* causing leaf rot of Pan. Hind. Antibiot. Bull. Vol. 16 No. 1 pp. 4-8.

155. Vyas KM and Soni NK (1973). Effect of antifungal antibiotics on endogenous mycelial respiration of *Rhizoctonia solani*. Hind. Antibiot. Bull. Vol. 15, pp. 160-163.

156. Vyas KM, Raghavan P and Jain SK (1973). Synergistic interaction of cloremphenicol and IAA on the growth of *Avena* coleoptile sections. Hind. Antibiot. Bull. Vol. 15, pp. 81-83.

157. Vyas KM and Mishra AS (1972). Production of P-proline by soil microorganisms. Hind. Antibiot. Bull. Vol. 15 No 1 and 2 pp. 30-33.

158. Vyas KM, Soni NK and Saxena SB (1972). Effect of culture of various fungi on the mycelial respiration of *Fusarium oxysporum* Sacc. Hind. Antibiot. Bull. Vol. 14, pp. 179-180.

159. Vyas KM, Saxena SB and Jain BK (1972). Respiratory characteristics of some soil borne plant pathogenic fungi. J. Ind. Bot. Soc. 51: 92-96.

160. Vyas KM and Mehta P (1972). Control of fruit rot of tomatoes by phenolics and fungicides. Bull. Bot. Soc., Univ. Saugar, Vol. 19 pp. 35-37.

161. Vyas KM and Dubey GL (1972). Effect of plant growth regulators on the growth of *Sclerotium rolfsii*. Bull. Bot. Soc., Univ. Saugar, Vol. 19 pp. 35-37.

162. Vyas KM, Saxena SB and Soni SK (1972). Effect of plant growth regulators on oxygen uptake and growth of *Rhizoctonia solani* Kuhn and *Colletotrihum capsici* (Syd.) Butler and Bisby. Bull. Bot. Soc., Univ. Saugar, Vol. 19 pp. 24-27.

163. Vyas KM and Mehta P (1970-71). Production of cellulose and mycelial growth of *Alternaria solani* and *A. tenuis*. Bull. Bot. Soc., Univ. Saugar, Vol. 17 and 18 pp. 71-72.

164. Vyas KM and Soni NK (1970-71). Respiratory characteristics of mycelium of *Gleosporium papaya* P. Henn. Bull. Bot. Soc., Univ. Saugar, Vol. 17 and 18 pp. 48-50.

165. Vyas KM, Soni NK and Mishra AS (1970-71). Respiratory characteristics of *Gleosporium* infected papaya fruits in relation to disease development. Bull. Bot. Soc., Univ. Saugar, Vol. 17 and 18 pp. 48-50.

166. Vyas KM, Saxena SB and Atri DC (1970-71). Production of amino acids by soil fungi. Bull. Bot. Soc., Univ. Saugar, Vol. 17 and 18 pp. 31-34.

167. Vyas KM and Saxena SB (1962-64). The wood decaying fungi of Sagar. Madhya Bharti, Vol. 11-13 pp. 15-28.

List of Ph.D. Awarded Under the Supervision of Prof. K.M. Vyas

1. Mehta, Pradeep 1974. "Biochemical Investigations of Fruit-Rot Diseases of Tomatoes."
2. Jain, Satish Kumar 1975. "Studies on the Microbial Production of Auxins".
3. Chourasia, Shiv Charan 1976. "Studies on the Foot-Rot and Leaf-Rot Diseases of Pan (*Piper betle* L.) with Special Reference to Pathogenesis and Control Measures".
4. Raghavan (alias) Srinivasan, Parvati 1976. "Physiological Studies on the Effect of Antibiotics on Plants with Special Reference to their Growth Regulatory Effects"
5. Mishra, Jayendra Kumar 1979. Biochemical Studies on Some *Botryodiplodia* Rot with Special Reference to Cell-Wall Degrading Enzymes".
6. Arti, Dinesh Chandra 1980. "Study of Fruit-Rot Disease of *Pyrus pyrifolia* Caused by *Botryodiplodia theobromae*".
7. Dubey, Guljari Lal 1980."Fungal Succession in Relation to the Bio-deterioration of Linseed".

8. Thakur, Munna Singh 1981. "Studies on the Metabolities of Some Microorganisms and their Effects on Plant Growth".
9. Jain, Maya (nee) Singhai, Maya 1982. "Studies on Plant Growth Regulatory Activities of Certain Antibiotics".
10. Saxena, Neeraj 1982. "Studies on Cell Wall Degrading Enzymes in Relation to Fungal Pathogenesis".
11. Thomas, Thankamma 1982. "Studies on the Soil Fungi of the Andaman and Nicobar Islands".
12. Chiele, Satish Kumar 1983. "Studies on Host–Parasite Relationship with Special Reference to Betel–Vine *Phytopathora*".
13. Saxena, Anand Prakash 1983. "Studies on Some Medicinal Plants of Bundelkhand Region with Special Reference to their Antimicrobial Activity".
14. Gupta, Deepak Kumar 1984. "Studies on the Microbiological Control of Mosquito, Causing Malaria".
15. Shrivastava, Anjali 1985. "Studies on the Efficacy of Certain Antibiotics Against Betel-Vine *Phytopathora*".
16. Katare, Daya Shanker 1987. "Genetic Analysis of Metric and Quality Attributes in Tomato".
17. Saxena, Nitin Kumar 1987. "Microbial Transformation of Steroids".
18. Tripathi, Hari Har Sharran 1987. "Study on the Production and Activity of Toxic Metabolites by Certain Bacterial and Fungal Pathogens of *Piper betle* L".
19. Sadiq, Yasmin 1989. "Studies on the Role of Phenolic Compounds in Disease Resistance in Plants (with special reference to Betel-vine *Phytopathora*)".
20. Shrama, Pratap Bhanu 1991. "Study on the Effect of Cultural and Chemical Control Systems of Kharif Weeds in Tawa Command Area".
21. Firdousi, Shakeel Ahamad 1992. "Studies on the Fungal Disease of Some Important Forest Plant with Special Reference to the Foliage Diseases".
22. Sediq, Roohi 1992. "Studies on the Effect of Certain Factors on the Forest Vegetation of Sagar".
23. Tewari, Prem Narayan 1992. "Studies on Yield, Oil and Protein Content of Soybean as Affected by Fertility Levels, Different Stages of Sowing and Plant Density".
24. Malaiya, Ku. Seema 1992. "Antimicrobial Evaluation of Certain Medicinal Plants of Ethnobotanical-Importance".
25. Dubey, Mahadev Prasad 1993. "Effect of Soil Tilth Seed Inoculation and Sowing Methods on Growth and Yield of Soybean".
26. Goswami, Ravi Prakash 1994. "Studies on the Effect of Volatile Fungistatic Factors on Fungal Morphogenesis".
27. Dixit, Ashwini Kumar 1995. "Ethno-medicinal, Photochemical and Anti-microbial Studies of Some Medicinal Plants of Sagar District".
28. Chourasia, J.P. 1995. "Studies on the Management of Betalvine *Phytopathora* Diseases in Sagar".
29. Sharma, C.D. 1995. "Folicolus Fungal from the Forest Flora of M.P. with Special Reference to Deuteromycotina".

30. Goswami, Sita Ram 1995. "Response of Different Levels of Phosphetic Fertilizers and their Methods of Application on Growth Parameters Productivity and Quality of Soybean".
31. Malaiya, Manju 1998. "Studies on Antimicrobial Activity of Some Indian Traditional Remedies (Ethnomedicinal plants)".
32. Mishra, Avanish 1998. "Studies on the Biology of Some Ethno-medicinal Plants of Sagar Region".
33. Kaushal, A.K. 1998. "Role of Irrigation Schedule on Productivity of Sunflower".
34. Sthapak Smt. Madhu 2000. "Studies on the Fungal Diseases of Potato Under Storage Conditions at Sagar".
35. Nema Ku. Shushma 2000. "Studies on Some *Phytopathora* Species from Central India with Special Reference to their Reproduction".
36. Dwivedi, O.P 2003. 'Studies on Soil Microorganisms with Special Reference to Vesicular-Arbuscular Mycorrhizal (VAM) Fungal Association with Wheat Crop of Sagar Region".
37. Yadav, Rajesh 2003. "Studies on Integrated Management of Betelvine *Phytopathora*".
38. Agrawal, Roop Shikha 2004. "Studies on Fungal Diseases of Forest Plants of Mandla Region".
39. Jain, Ashish 2005. "Studies on Mushroom Cultivation with Special Reference to *Pleurotus* Species and their Marketing Potential in Sagar Region".
40. Vyas, Ashish 2005. "Studies on Microbial Biodiversity with Special Reference to their Cellulolytic Activity".
41. Soni Anuradha 2006. Studies on occurrence of VAM Fungi in leguminous crops of sagar.

Acknowledgements

A journey into unknown territory, this is how I felt at the onset of this task. The work undertaken has made me experience many ups and downs throughout the duration of compilation. Although I had been living with it days and nights but there are many people who have knowingly or unknowingly figured a major role in its completion. Although words are not sufficient to express my feelings but still I shall try to comprehend as far as I can and the feelings behind are really heartfelt.

This book is presented with obligation to the under mentioned with full acceptance of its limitations.

I thanks my Shredye Guru Ji Pt Omkar Dev Ji, whose wishes enabled me to reach this mile stone who showed me path to reach the destination and responsible for how to thank god.

I note down here with humility and pride that I am fortunate enough in having support of esteemed personalities like Prof. H.D. Kumar (FNA), BHU, Varanasi, Prof. D.P. Tiwari, Ex Head, Department of Botany, Govt. Science P.G. College, Jabalpur, Prof. C. Manoharachari (Emeritus Prof.), Department of Botany, Osmania University, Hyderabad, Prof. Anupam Dixit, Department of Botany, Allahabad University, Prof. S.P. Adhikari, Department of Biotechnology, Visva Bharti University, Shantiniketan (West Bengal), Prof K.L. Tiwari, Ex Head, Department of Biotechnology, Pt R.S. University, Raipur, Prof G.S. Paliwal (Emeritus Prof.) Senior Consultant National Afforestation and Eco-development Board, New Delhi, Prof H.K. Goswami, Ex Head, Department of Genetics, Barkatullah University, Bhopal and Prof. H.C. Lakshman, Head, Department of Botany, Karnataka University, Dharwad.

I am happy to remember my teachers who happened to be students of my father late Prof. K.M. Vyas, therefore I gratefully acknowledges Prof A.D. Adoni, Prof. T.R. Sahu, Prof. N.K. Soni, Prof. D.C. Atri, Prof. A.K. Kandya, Prof. P. Mehta, Prof. P.K. Khare, Prof. A.N. Rai, Prof. (Smt.) J. Dubey, Dr. A.S. Mishra, Dr. S.K. Yadav, Dr. N.P. Bhalla and my colleague Dr. A. Mehta, Dr. A. Biswas, Miss Poonam Dehariya and Dr. Ashok Shukla for their necessary help whenever I was in need.

I express sincere gratitude to all the authors who have contributed for this volume.

It gives me immense pleasure in acknowledging with sincere gratitude, the enthusiastic co-operation received from my students Dr. O.P. Dwivedi, Dr. Rajesh Yadav, Dr. Ashish Vyas, Dr. Anuradha Soni, Dr. Ashish Jain, Dr. Archana Dubey, Dr. Mahendra Mishra, Dr. Pradeep Singh, Dr. Prashant Soni, Dr. H.C. Gena, Pramod Richhariya, Meenakshi Mishra, Anjuli Chaubey, Javed Ahmad Wagay and Mrs. Anuradha Shukla.

I express a deep valuation to all the non-teaching staff especially Dr. Pradeep Tiwari, K.K. Dixit, J.P. Chaubey, P. Gujre and Shailesh Katare of the department for their time to time help and co-operations.

It is beyond the capacity of all the words to express my respect and profound affection for my mother Mrs. Urmila Vyas. Today whatever I am that is only by virtue of her love, care, affection and blessings. At this juncture I can not forget my wife Mrs. Nisha and children Sidhhant and Vedant and pain taken and sacrifices made by them can not be summed up. They remained as a source of constant inspiration; I bow down before their love and affection towards me. The love and affection extended by my sisters Dr. Jyoti, Arti and Bharti, and their family is memorable.

Last, but certainly not the least, I must thanks to Mr. Nafees of Perfect Computers for designing this cover page in a careful and elegant manner, which is miraculous. I also thank Mr. Anil Mittal of Daya Publishing House for publishing the volume a scientific tribute to my father.

Deepak Vyas

H.D. Kumar

Ph.D. (London). FASc. FNASc, FNA

Formerly Professor of Botany,
Dean, Faculty of Science, and Coordinator,
Biotechnology Programme
Banaras Hindu University

Phone (Res.): (0542) 2315180

214, Saketnagar, Naria,
VARANASi – 221 005

Foreword

Microbes, the real masters of life on Earth, are both a boon and bane for the planet. Our microbial friends live within our body, protecting us from disease, aiding digestion, and preserving immunity. On the other side, some of the deadliest diseases are caused by viruses and pathogenic bacteria. Whereas beneficial fungi are an asset to the industrialist and the environment, pathogenic fungi cause havoc and can devastate cereal crops and fruit trees.

The present volume is a Festschrift in honour of my long-term friend, late Prof. K.M. Vyas, a reputed mycologist with strong interest in microbiology. This volume includes some 50 chapters including 23 on microbiology, 13 on biotechnology and 14 on ecology. These chapters are authored by senior professors and younger scientists. The editors are practising researchers and I have pleasure in commending this Festschrift to all those interested in the exciting fields of mycology, microbiology and general biology.

H.D. Kumar

Preface

With the advent of new technologies, the knowledge of science is expanding in new dimensions every day. The frequent review of the state of our knowledge not only to keep ourselves up to date but also to provide over the various strategies ought to be adopted for further revolution of science in all its sphere.

As one know that presently existing life form are evolve from the microorganisms during the course of evolution. These microorganisms can adapt to virtually any physio-chemical environment and are found everywhere.

Despite their huge importance, the fact is that much of what we know about and microbial processes is based on the work done on only a harmful of species-weed like species which can be readily grown in laboratory culture. The vast majority of microorganisms found in nature (Perhaps over 95 per cent) have not so far been cultured but earnest attempts are under ways to grow as many of them as possible in culture.

One most striking property of many microorganisms is the highly promiscuous mode of gene transfer among unrelated or remotely related taxa. Such horizontal (lateral) gene transfers have been the subject of intense research activity in the past few years, in view their strong bearing on the applicability of the biological species concept and the Linnaean system of binominal nomenclature to prokaryotes.

Technological advancement has revolutionized and transform microbiology with biotechnology and created exciting opportunities for agriculture, medicine, industry and environment remediation the organism involved in these mechanisms mostly belongs to bacteria, fungi, cyanobacteria etc.

To keep pace with the growing knowledge in every field of science, our agenda for the coming few years should be to identify the key organizational and genetic principles underlying various morphogenetic processes in both prokaryotes and eukaryotes, while also pursuing the laborious elucidation of the molecular network that control the organizational of living matter.

Considering the importance of microorganism and their biotechnological processes are the major contents of the monograph. Beside microbiology and biotechnology few chapters on ecology are included.

Editors

Contents

Biography: Late Prof. K.M. Vyas *vii*

Acknowledgements *xxi*

Foreword *xxiii*

Preface *xxv*

List of Editors & Contributors *xxxiii*

— Volume 1 —

— MICROBIOLOGY —

1. *Rhizobium* Biofertilizer: Retrospect and Prospects 3
S.K. Sethi and S.P. Adhikary

2. Microbial Diversity: Its Role in Ecosystem Maintenance 29
Jamaluddin

3. Thermophilic Cyanobacteria: The Wonder Organisms 34
Vidhi Verma and Meenakshi Banerjee

4. Cyanobacteria: Phenotypic to the Genotypic Diversity 41
A. Srivastava, P. Singh, A. Singh, S.S. Singh and A.K. Mishra

5. Hydrogen Production by Cyanobacteria 60
Deepak Vyas and Rajan Kumar Gupta

6. **Cyanobacterial Toxins** 94
U.S. Gupta, Deepak Vyas and Rajan Kumar Gupta

7. **The Toxins of Cyanobacteria** 150
Mukesh Kumar

8. **Antibacterial Potential of Diazotrophic Cyanobacteria: A Natural Strategy to Maintain Nitrogen Budget in Tropical Lowlands** 162
Usha Pandey

9. **Histochemical Studies on Some Petro-Plants Infected with AM Fungus (*Glomus fasciculatum*)** 168
H.C. Lakshman

10. **Biodiversity of VAM Fungi Associated with Some Common Medicinal Plants of Bihar** 189
A.K. Roy and A.N. Singh

11. **Association of Vesicular Arbuscular Mycorrhizal Fungi with Ornamental Plants** 201
Bhaskar Chaurasia and P.K. Khare

12. **Perspective of AM Fungi in Agroforestry Systems** 209
Ashok Shukla, A. Kumar, D. Vyas, A. Jha, M. Kamalvanshi and N. Chakravarty

13. **Arbuscular Mycorrhizal Fungi: The Hidden Heroes of the Soil** 225
Deepak Vyas, Meenakshi Mishra, Pradeep Singh, Ashok Shukla and R.K. Gupta

14. **Cumulative Effect of VAM Fungi** 256
O.P. Dwivedi, Meenakshi Mishra, Pradeep K. Singh, Pramod Kumar Richhariya, Prashant Soni and Deepak Vyas

15. **Some Additions to the Foliicolous Fungi from the Forest Flora of Madhya Pradesh, India** 268
P. Chauksay, A.N. Rai and Naveen Verma

16. **Current Status of Sesame and Niger Diseases and Their Management** 275
Sushma Nema, T.S. Rajpurohit and M.N. Khare

17. **Integrated Disease Management of *Piper betle*** 293
Deepak Vyas and Rajesh Yadav

18. **Thermophilic Fungi: Occurrence, Characteristics and Enzymatic Potential** 303
Naveen Kango

19. **Biodiversity and Conservation of Mushroom in Chhattisgarh Region** 320
M.P. Thakur, C.S. Shukla and V.K. Yadav

20. **Mushrooms: A Nutritive Food for Human Beings** 344
Poonam Dehariya, Anjuli Chaubey and Deepak Vyas

21. Mushroom: The Beneficial Fungi 353
Anjuli Choubey, Deepak Vyas, Poonam Dehariya, A.K. Pandey and D.C. Atri

22. *Trichoderma* Species: The History and Evolution of Current Concepts of Biological Control 377
Pradeep Kumar Singh and Deepak Vyas

— Volume 2 —

— BIOTECHNOLOGY —

23. Fungitoxic Potential of Essential oil and Extracts from Higher Plants in the Management of Postharvest Deterioration: A Review 393
Anupam Dikshit, Ravindra Kumar Pandey, Rohit Kumar Mishra, Piyush Mishra and Ahsan Kamran

24. Carbonic Anhydrase: An Ancient Enzyme with Multidimensional Roles 439
Anjana Sharma, Rajesh Pujari and Abhishek Bhattacharya

25. Pharmacological Potential of Mushrooms 452
Alka Karwa and Mahendra Rai

26. Significance of GM Crops in Modern Agriculture 472
Shweta J. Sabannavar, H.C. Lakshman, Mahesh B. Byatanal and C. Maya

27. Plant DNA Banking for Biodiversity Assessment and Conservation Research 484
D. Thangadurai, M.A.A. Pinheirho De Car Valho, D.P. Biradar, Hemanth K.N. Vasathaiah, B. Suresh and Ganesh R. Hegde

28. Progress in Biotechnology of Guava (*Psidium guajava* L.) 501
Nasim Akhtar

29. Hepatoprotective Medicinal Plants: A Review 520
Siddhartha Singh, A. Mehta and P. Mehta

30. Cyanobacterial Exploitation in Biotechnology 525
B.D. Kaushik

31. Effect of Herbicides on Mitosis, Nucleic Acids and Protein Contents in *Corchorus* and Soybean Plants 544
A.K.S. Chouhan and S.K. Yadav

32. Biotechnological Potential of Cyanobacteria 553
Surendra Singh

33. Plants and Rhizobium Techniques 571
Pooja Agrawal

34. **Quest for a Novel Tuberculosis Vaccine: A Global Endeavor** 577
Umesh Dutta Gupta, Vijender Singh and Pushpa Gupta

35. **Silver Nanoparticles: A New Generation of Antimicrobial Agents** 591
Mukesh K. Upadhyay, Devendra Jain, Abhijeet Singh, Sushma Rishi and Narayan Rishi

36. **Phenolic Quantification and Anti-Aging Activity of *Morchella esculenta*** 606
Javed Ahmad Wagay , Ashok Shukla, Anjuli Choubey, Poonam Dehairya and Deepak Vyas

37. **Antibacterial Potential of *Morchella esculenta* Against Some Human Pathogenic Bacteria** 616
Javed Ahmad Wagay, Poonam Dehariya, Anjali C. and Deepak Vyas

38. **Production and Partial Characterization of Fungal and Bacterial Cellulases on CMC and Cellulose Powder** 624
Deepak Vyas and Ashish Vyas

— ECOLOGY —

39. **Lichen Bioindicator Communities in Achanakmar: Amarkantak Biosphere Reserve, Madhya Pradesh and Chhattisgarh** 669
Satya and D.K. Upreti

40. **Silvipastoral Systems: The Solution for the Sustainable Production in Semi Arid Tropics** 683
R.K. Bhatt, A.K. Mishra and H.S. Tiwari

41. **Agroforestry: Conservation of Natural Resources, Biomass Production and Climate Moderations** 708
Ashok Shukla and V.D. Tripathi

42. **Soil Mycoflora of Forest Field at Jagdalpur Region** 724
K.L. Tiwari, S.K. Jadhav and S. Kunjam

43. **Study of Life-Forms and Biological Spectrum of Forest of Sagar District, Madhya Pradesh** 729
A.S. Thakur and P.K. Khare

44. **Environmental Impact of Fly Ash on Soil Health, Yield and Nutrient Uptake by Rice** 741
T. Thomas, Ram Bharose, Arun A. David, H. Thomas and R.K. Tamphasana

45. **Eutrophication: Causes, Consequences and Control Measures** 766
Ashu and Mukesh Kumar

46. **Aquatic Biodiversity Assessment should Trigger Freshwater Body Monitoring and Conservation** 773
S.D. Guru and H.K. Goswami

47. **Eco-Physiological Effects of Red Mud Waste of an Aluminium Industry on the Seed Biology of a Crop Plant** 780

Alka Sahu, Anita R. Patnaik, R.K. Behera and A.K. Panigrahi

48. **Effect of Pollution in Groundwater Quality and Soil Health of Naini Area at Allahabad City** 827

Saurabh Upadhyay, Arun A. David, T. Thomas, H. Thomas, R.K. Tamphasana and Ram Bharose

49. **Modifying Influence of Woody Perennials on Atmospheric Deposition of Nutrient Ions in a Dry Tropical Region of India** 837

J. Pandey

50. **Trends and Determinants of Health Practices Profile Among the Baigas** 846

Arun K. Jain and A.N. Sharma

Author Index 859

Subject Index 861

List of Editors & Contributors

Editors

Dr. Deepak Vyas
Assistant Professor, Department of Botany, Dr. H.S.G. University, Sagar – 470 003, M.P.

Prof. G.S. Paliwal
Senior Consultant, Regional Centre of the National Afforestation and Eco-development Board, Ministry of Environment and Forests, Government of India, New Delhi

P.K. Khare
Professor, Department of Botany, Dr. H.S.G. University, Sagar – 470 003, M.P.

Dr. R. K Gupta
Assistant Professor, Department of Botany, Govt. P.G. College, Rhishikesh

Associate Editors

Prof. A.K. Pandey
Chairman, M.P. Govt. Private University Commission, Bhopal, M.P.

Dr. Jamaludin
Emeritus Prof. Department of Biological Sciences, R.D. University Jabalpur, M.P.

Dr. Neeraj Khare
Department of Botany, Dr. H.S.G. University, Sagar – 470 003, M.P.

Contributors

Adhikary, S.P.
Department of Biotechnology, Vishwa-Bharti University, Shantiniketan, West Bengal

Agrawal, Pooja
Department of Applied Microbiology and Biotechnology, Dr. H.S.G. University, Sagar – 470 003, M.P.

Akhtar, Nasim
Department of Biotechnology, GITAM University, Gandhi Nagar Campus, Rushikonda, Vishakapatnam – 530 045

Ashu
Department of Botany, Sahu Jain PG College, Najibabad – 246 763, U.P.

Atri, D.C.
Department of Botany, Dr. H.S.G. University, Sagar – 470 003, M.P.

Banerjee, Meenakshi
Laboratory of Algal Biotechnology, Department of Bioscience, Barkatullah University, Bhopal, M.P.

Behera, R.K.
Department of Botany, Berhampur University, Berhampur – 760 007, Orissa

Bharose, Ram
School of Forestry and Environment, SHIATS-Deemed University, Allahabad

Bhatt, R.K.
Indian Grassland and Fodder Research Institute, Jhansi – 284 003, U.P.

Bhattacharya, Abhishek
Bacteriology Lab, Department of Biological Sciences, Rani Durgavati University, Jabalpur, M.P.

Biradar, D.P.
Department of Agronomy, UAS, Dharwad – 580 005

Byatanal, Mahesh B.
Post Graduate Department and Research in Botany (Microbiology Lab), Karnataka University, Dharwad – 580 003

Chakravarty, Neha
National Research Centre for Agroforestry, Jhansi – 284 003, U.P.

Chaubey, Anjuli
Lab of Microbial Technology and Plant Pathology, Department of Botany, Dr. H.S.G. University, Sagar – 470 003, M.P.

Chauksay, P.
Department of Botany, Dr. H.S.G. University, Sagar – 470 003, M.P.

Chaurasia, Bhaskar
Department of Botany, Dr. H.S.G. University, Sagar – 470 003, M.P.

Chouhan, A.K.S.
Department of Botany, Dr. H.S.G. University, Sagar – 470 003, M.P.

David, Arun A.
School of Forestry and Environment, SHIATS-Deemed University, Allahabad

Dehariya, Poonam
Lab of Microbial Technology and Plant Pathology, Department of Botany, Dr. H.S.G. University, Sagar – 470 003, M.P.

Dikshit, Anupam
Biological Product Laboratory, Department of Botany, University of Allahabad, Allahabad –211 002

Diwedi, O.P.
Lab of Microbial Technology and Plant Pathology, Department of Botany, Dr. H.S.G. University, Sagar – 470 003, M.P.

Goswami, H.K.
24, Kaushalnagar, PO Misrod, Bhopal – 462 047, M.P.

Gupta, Pushpa
National JALMA Institute for Leprosy and Other Mycobacterial Diseases, Agra – 282 001

Gupta, Rajan Kumar
Department of Botany, Govt. P.G. College, Rishikesh, Uttarakhand

Gupta, U.S.
Department of Zoology, Dr. H.S.G. University, Sagar – 470 003, M.P.

Gupta, Umesh Dutta
National JALMA Institute for Leprosy and Other Mycobacterial Diseases, Agra – 282 001

Guru, S.D.
Department of Botany, Ranchi Women's College, Ranchi, Jharkhand

Hegde, Ganesh R.
Department of Botany, Sri Krishnadevaraya University, Anantapur – 515 0003

Jadhav, S.K.
School of Studies in Biotechnology, Pt. Ravishankar Shukla University, Raipur – 492 010,

Jain, Arun K.
Department of Anthropology and Tribal Development, GG University, Bilaspur, C.G.

Jain, Devendra
School of Life Sciences, Jaipur National University, Jaipur – 302 025, Rajasthan

Jamaluddin
Ex Group Coordinator and Director, Tropical Forest Research Institute, Jabalpur, M.P.

Jha, Anuradha
National Research Centre for Agroforestry, Jhansi – 284 003, U.P.

Kamalvanshi, Madhavi
National Research Centre for Agroforestry, Jhansi – 284 003, U.P.

Kamran, A.
Biological Product Laboratory, Department of Botany, University of Allahabad, Allahabad –211 002

Kango, Naveen
Department of Applied Microbiology and Biotechnology, Dr. H.S.G. University, Sagar – 470 003, M.P.

Karwa, Alka
Department of Biotechnology, S.G.B. Amravati University, Amravati – 444 602

Kaushik, B.D.
Division of Biotechnology, Netaji Subash Institute of Technology, Sector 3, Dwarka, New Delhi – 110 078

Khare, M.N.
Agricultural Research Station, Mandor, Jodhpur, Rajasthan (Ex. Dean and Professor Emeritus, Plant Pathology)

Khare, P.K.
Department of Botany, Dr. H.S.G. University, Sagar – 470 003, M.P.

Kumar, Anil
Principal Scientist (Plant Pathologist), National Research Centre for Agroforestry, Jhansi – 284 003, U.P.

Kumar, Mukesh
Department of Botany, Sahu Jain PG College, Najibabad – 246 763, U.P.

Kunjam, S.
School of Studies in Biotechnology, Pt. Ravishankar Shukla University, Raipur – 492 010,

Lakshman, H.C.
Department of Botany, Microbiology Laboratory, Karnataka University, Dharwad – 580 003, Karnataka

Maya, C.
Department of Botany, Bangalore University, J.B. Campus, Bangalore – 560 056

Mehta, A.
Department of Botany, Dr. H.S.G. University, Sagar – 470 003, M.P.

Mehta, P.
Department of Botany, Dr. H.S.G. University, Sagar – 470 003, M.P.

Mishra, A.K.
Indian Grassland and Fodder Research Institute, Jhansi – 284 003, U.P.

Mishra, P.
Biological Product Laboratory, Department of Botany, University of Allahabad, Allahabad –211 002

Mishra, Arun Kumar
Laboratory of Microbial Genetics, Department of Botany, Banaras Hindu University, Varanasi – 221 005

Mishra, R.K.
Biological Product Laboratory, Department of Botany, University of Allahabad, Allahabad –211 002

Nema, Sushma
Senior Scientist, Plant Pathology, AICRP (S&N) J.N.K.V.V., Jabalpur

Pandey, A.K.
Chairman, M.P. Council Pvt University Ltd., Bhopal

Pandey, J.
Department of Botany, Banaras Hindu University, Varanasi – 221 005, U.P.

Pandey, R.K.
Biological Product Laboratory, Department of Botany, University of Allahabad, Allahabad – 211 002

Pandey, Usha
Faculty of Science and Technology, MG Kashividya Pith, Varanasi – 221 005, U.P.

Panigrahi, A.K.
Department of Botany, Berhampur University, Berhampur – 760 007, Orissa

Pataik, Anita R.
Department of Botany, Berhampur University, Berhampur – 760 007, Orissa

Pujari, Rajesh
Bacteriology Lab, Department of Biological Sciences, Rani Durgavati University, Jabalpur, M.P.

Rai, A.N.
Department of Botany, Dr. H.S.G. University, Sagar – 470 003, M.P.

Rai, Mahendra
Department of Biotechnology, S.G.B. Amravati University, Amravati – 444 602

Rajpurohit, T.S.
Pathologist, Oilseeds (Rajasthan Agricultural University)

Richhariya, Pramod K.
Lab of Microbial Technology and Plant Pathology, Department of Botany, Dr. H.S.G. University, Sagar – 470 003, M.P.

Rishi, Narayan
School of Virology, Amity University, Noida, U.P.

Rishi, Sushma
School of Virology, Amity University, Noida, U.P.

Roy, A.K.
Department of Botany, T.M. Bhagalpur University, Bhagalpur – 812 007

Sabannavar, Shweta J.
Post Graduate Department and Research in Botany (Microbiology Lab), Karnataka University, Dharwad – 580 003

Sahu, Alka
Department of Botany, Berhampur University, Berhampur – 760 007, Orissa

Satya
Lichenology Laboratory, National Botanical Research Institute (CSIR), Rana Pratap Marg, Lucknow – 226 001, U.P.

Sethi, S.K.
PG Department of Biotechnology, Utkal University, Bhubaneswar – 751 004, Orissa

Sharma, A.N.
Department of Anthropology, Dr. H.S.G. University, Sagar – 470 003, M.P.

Sharma, Anjana
Bacteriology Lab, Department of Biological Sciences, Rani Durgavati University, Jabalpur, M.P.

Shukla, Ashok
Lab of Microbial Technology and Plant Pathology, Department of Botany, Dr. H.S.G. University, Sagar – 470 003, M.P.

Shukla, C.S.
Department of Plant Pathology, Indira Gandhi Agricultural University, Raipur – 492 006, Chhattisgarh

Singh, A.
Laboratory of Microbial Genetics, Department of Botany, Banaras Hindu University, Varanasi – 221 005

Singh, A.N.
Department of Botany, T.M. Bhagalpur University, Bhagalpur – 812 007

Singh, Abhijeet
School of Life Sciences, Jaipur National University, Jaipur – 302 025, Rajasthan

Singh, P.
Laboratory of Microbial Genetics, Department of Botany, Banaras Hindu University, Varanasi – 221 005

Singh, P.K.
Department of Botany, Dr. H.S.G. University, Sagar – 470 003, M.P.

Singh, Siddhartha
Department of Botany, Dr. H.S.G. University, Sagar – 470 003, M.P.

Singh, Surendra
Centre of Advanced Study in Botany, Banaras Hindu University, Varanasi – 221 005, U.P.

Singh, Vijendra
Institute of Microbial Technology, Chandigrah – 160 036

Singh. S.S.
Laboratory of Microbial Genetics, Department of Botany, Banaras Hindu University, Varanasi – 221 005

Soni, Prashant
Department of Botany, Dr. H.S.G. University, Sagar – 470 003, M.P.

Srivastava, A.
Laboratory of Microbial Genetics, Department of Botany, Banaras Hindu University, Varanasi – 221 005

Suresh, B.
Department of Applied Genetics, Karnatak University, Dharwad – 580 003

Tamphasana, R.K.
Department of Applied Geology, Dr. H.S.G. University, Sagar – 470 003, M.P.

Thakur, A.S.
Department of Botany, Govt College, Khurai, Sagar – 470 117, M.P.

Thakur, M.P.
Department of Plant Pathology, Indira Gandhi Agricultural University, Raipur – 492 006, Chhattisgarh

Thangadurai, D.
Department of Botany, Karnatak University, Dharwad – 580 003

Thomas, H.
Department of Applied Geology, Dr. H.S.G. University, Sagar – 470 003, M.P.

Thomas, T.
School of Forestry and Environment, SHIATS-Deemed University, Allahabad

Tiwari, H.S.
Indian Grassland and Fodder Research Institute, Jhansi – 284 003, U.P.

Tiwari, K.L.
School of Studies in Biotechnology, Pt. Ravishankar Shukla University, Raipur – 492 010, C.G.

Tripathi, V.D.
National Research Centre for Agroforestry, Jhansi – 284 003, U.P.

Upadhyay, Mukesh K.
School of Life Sciences, Jaipur National University, Jaipur – 302 025, Rajasthan

Upadhyay, Saurabh
School of Forestry and Environment, SHIATS-Deemed University, Allahabad

Upreti, D.K.
Lichenology Laboratory, National Botanical Research Institute (CSIR), Rana Pratap Marg, Lucknow – 226 001, U.P.

Valho, MAA Pinheirho De Car
ISO Plexis Germplasm Bank, Department of Biology, University of Madeira, Funchal 9000-390, Portugal

Vasathaiah, Hemanth K.N.
Center for Viticulture and Small Fruit Research, Florida A and M University, 6505 Mahan Drive, Tallahassee, Florida 32317, USA

Verma, Naveen
Department of Botany, Dr. H.S.G. University, Sagar – 470 003, M.P.

Verma, Vidhi
Laboratory of Algal Biotechnology, Department of Bioscience, Barkatullah University, Bhopal, M.P.

Vyas, Ashish
Division of Biotechnology, Lovely Professional University, Ludhiana (Punjab)

Vyas, Deepak
Lab of Microbial Technology and Plant Pathology, Department of Botany, Dr. H.S.G. University, Sagar – 470 003, M.P.

Wagay, Javed Ahmad
Lab of Microbial Technology and Plant Pathology, Department of Botany, Dr. H.S.G. University, Sagar – 470 003, M.P.

Yadav, Rajesh
ABR PG College, Anpra, Sonbadhra, U.P.

Yadav, S.K.
Department of Botany, Dr. H.S.G. University, Sagar – 470 003, M.P.

Yadav, V.K.
Department of Plant Pathology, Indira Gandhi Agricultural University, Raipur – 492 006, Chhattisgarh

Microbiology

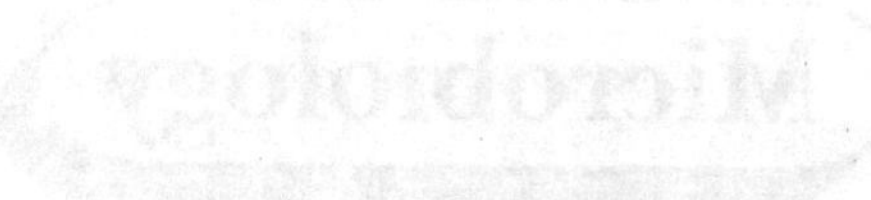

Microbial Biotechnology and Ecology (2011) *Pages* **1–28**
Editors: Deepak Vyas, G.S. Paliwal, P.K.Khare and R.K Gupta
Published by: DAYA PUBLISHING HOUSE, NEW DELHI

Chapter 1

Rhizobium Biofertilizer: Retrospect and Prospects

☆ *S.K. Sethi*[1] *and S.P. Adhikary*[2]

[1]*P.G. Department of Biotechnology, Utkal University, Bhubaneswar – 751 004*
[2]*Department of Biotechnology, Vishwa-Bharti University, Shantiniketan, West Bengal*

ABSTRACT

Basically nitrogen fixation is related to legume nodulation by the symbiotic association with rhizobia, which have the role to fix the atmospheric nitrogen and thus attain nitrogen in nitrogen deficient soils. Thus technology was developed for making rhizobial biofertilizers for nitrogen fixing plants, evaluate the growth promoting substances secreted by these bacteria and also educating about their unique benefits to the users, technique for mass multiplication and practicing the integrated nitrogen managements. The use of molecular genetic techniques could help in improvement the pathways and signal cascades involved in efficient and effective nodulation in legumes as well as non-leguminous plants. Details of the *Rhizobium* biofertilizer technology and its future prospects is reviewed in this chapter.

Introduction

India is an agricultural country. Nearly 70 per cent of the populations in rural areas are engaged in agriculture, cropping in low fertility soils, especially those poor in nitrogen contributing lower yield. Thus in modern agriculture use of chemical fertilizers has become indispensable. However, excessive use of chemical fertilizers and pesticides has generated several environmental problems including the green house effect, Ozone layer depletion and acidification of water. In some regions crop production has stagnated or even declined due to depletion in bioavailability of nitrogen. These problems can be tackled by use of biofertilizers and biopesticides, which are natural, ecologically sustainable and user friendly. Reports have shown that utilization of biological nitrogen fixation technology can decrease the use of urea-N and reduce the environmental problems to a considerable extent. About 80 per cent of stable biologically fixed nitrogen are a direct result of symbiotic interaction of diazotroph like rhizobia and some actinomycetes with the nitrogen as well as non-nitrogen fixing plants respectively (Bruijin *et al.*, 1995).

Rhizobia are gram negative, rod shaped, non-sporulating important soil microorganisms form symbiotic association with leguminous crops and contribute significant amount of fixed nitrogen. Bacteria of six genera namely *Rhizobium*, *Bradyrhizobium*, *Azorhizobium*, *Sinorhizobium* (recently changed to *Ensifer*), *Mesorhizobium* and *Allorhizobium* are of major agricultural importance because of their ability to form N_2- fixing nodules on the roots of leguminous plants.

Rhizobium and Nitrogen Fixation

Rhizobia-legume symbiosis has attracted world wide attention as it implies lesser dependence on expensive petroleum based nitrogenous fertilizers for legumes, thus reducing the chance of causing environmental pollution. The importance of this group of bacteria is further enhanced by the fact that the legumes nodulated by rhizobia include some of the most important crop plants of the world. Symbiotic nitrogen fixation is a complicated process involving reciprocal exchange of signals between rhizobia and the legumes leading to the coordinated gene-expression (Earl and Ausubel, 1993). Effective nodules formed by effective strains of rhizobia possess pink colour due to the presence of a pigment 'leghaemoglobin'. The nodule is merely a protective structure where bacteroids are the seat of nitrogen fixation. Nitrogenase is the enzyme which mediates the reduction of N_2 to NH_3. Nitrogenase can be obtained by the disintegration of bacteroids by mechanical process. This enzyme is made up of two components with both iron and molybdenum (Mo) having molecular weight of about 200,000 and second with iron and without Mo having molecular weight of about 65,000 (Quispel, 1974). The amount of leghaemoglobin and the extent of bacteroid tissue in nodules have a direct bearing on the amount of nitrogen fixed by legumes (Subba Rao, 1967; Verma and Bal, 1976).

Use of *Rhizobium* as Bioinoculant/Biofertilizer

Both inoculation success and failures at field levels have been well reported (Subba Rao and Tilak, 1977; Subba Rao, 1977). The failure to obtain the desired response may due to:

1. The presence of native ineffective strains which could not be displaced by introduced effective strains.
2. Presence of antagonists of rhizobia which minimize the number of rhizobia in the rhizosphere.
3. Availability of soil condition which limit symbiosis caused by acidity, alkalinity and other factors related to soil structure and mineral composition of soil.

Rhizobium is found in all types of soils in India. Reports have shown that utilization of *Rhizobium* as a biofertilizer for leguminous and non-leguminous crops in different soil conditions contribute significant amount of fixed nitrogen (Subba Rao, 1977). Increasing number of reports has also shown that Rhizobia can also act as PGPR in various crops (Hossain and Mårtensson, 2008). Summary of the work so far undertaken on this aspect is summarized in Table 1.1 and also are described as follows:

Survey of Different *Rhizobium* and their Host Specificity

It is possible to differentiate rhizobia on the basis of growth on defined substrates, as fast growers and slow growers. Studies have been done on morphological and physiological characters (colonial character, vitamin, carbohydrate and nitrogen nutrition, antibiotic sensitivities and infective attributes)

Table 1.1: Summary of Work on *Rhizobium* as Biofertilizer for Different Crops

Organism	*Strain*	*Isolated from*	*Growth Condition*	*Finding*	*Reference*
Rhizobium, *Brady rhizobium* sp.		Soybean *Glycine max* Arhar (*Cajanus cajan*), Chickpea (*Cicer arietinum*, *Lens culinaris*)	YEMA at 28°C for one week	The results of experiments done on all-India level showed that soybean responds spectacularly to *Rhizobium* application. Grain yield was increased up to 50 per cent over uninoculated control. Depending upon the agroclimatic conditions significant increase in yield over control of arhar, chickpea and masur was recorded. At certain sites, simple *Rhizobium* inoculation failed, however, pelleting inoculated seeds with lime or charcoal could significantly increase yield of arhar.	Subba Rao (1977)
Rhizobium, *Brady-rhizobium* sp.		*Cajanus cajan*, *Vigna mungo*, *Glycine max*	YEMA at 28°C for one week, purity tested by with Congored	Results of all India field experiments showed that all the leguminous crops responded to *Rhizobium* treatment. *Rhizobium* significantly increased grain yield of *Cajanus cajan* up to 16.4 per cent, *Vigna mungo* 2.4 per cent, *Glycine max* 65.9 per cent over uninoculated control.	Subba Rao (1984)
Rhizobium sp. and *Azospirillum* sp.				On field experiment of groundnut single or combined inoculation of *Azospirillum brasilense* and *Rhizobium* sp. with N_4(20 kg Nha^{-1}) and N_3(15 kg Nha^{-1}). height, nodulation in plant, dry matter, dry pod yield and N content of groundnut significantly increased in the highest level N treatment *i.e.* N (25 kg Nha^{-1}). For inoculation of groundnut with *A. brasilense* and *Rhizobium* sps. alone increased the growth and yield of crop and it was proved that these strains save up to 5 to 10 kg N ha^{-1}.	Wani *et al.* (1992)
Rhizobium sp.	Ie-108, SC-109, CO-57, CI-114	Wild and cultivated legumes Indigofera sp.	YEMA	Efficacy of Rhizobial strains was tested against groundnut. Maximum nodulation occurred due to inoculation of rhizobial isolates. Shoot and root length and total N content were significantly increased over uninoculated control showing they are effective in N-fixation in groundnut.	Salve and Ganawane (1992)
Rhizobium japonicum		*Glycine max*		Growth and yield of soybean forage in relation to inoculation at various nitrogen and phosphorous levels were reported. Seed treatment with *Rhizobium* culture resulted in increased production of dry matter as compared to control. Application of nitrogen @ 25kg/ha^{-1} with *Rhizobium* culture proved superior for growth and yield of soybean.	Dahiya *et al.* (1992)

Contd...

Table 1.1–Contd...

Organism	*Strain*	*Isolated from*	*Growth Condition*	*Finding*	*Reference*
Bradyrhizobium Japonicum		*Glycine max*		Seed inoculation with *B. japonicum* along with applying nitrogen and phosphorus each @ 30, 60kg and 120kg/ha respectively was carried out. Nitrogen application reduced nodulation by *Rhizobium* while phosphorous stimulated it on 30, 45 and 60 days of crop growth. N 30kg/ha and P 120 kg/ha with *B. japonicum* inoculation increased shoot dry wt. Maximum grain yield was obtained by application of 30 kg and 60 kg N/ha and P_2O_5 120 kg/ha.	Kurundkar *et al.* (1992)
Rhizobium sp.	NGR (L) VC-1163	Green gram (*Vigna radiata*)	YEMA	Eight strains of *Rhizobium* were isolated which were further tested for their survival under acid and alkaline condition. The strain INDE-2, a slow grower, and ALVG-2, a fast grower, isolated from coastal sand dune and mesophytic plain respectively. They showed compatively better survival under both acid and alkaline condition. Growth of VRNG-8 strain remained unaffected in alkaline range.	Biswal and Mishra (1992)
Bradyrhizobium japonicum		*Glycine max* Parvani isolate	YMA culture prepared with lignite based carrier	Seed inoculation was done with *B. japonicum* plus pelleting with carrier material and gypsum. Results were significant for increase in number of nodules and nodule dry wt/plant on 45·day of crop growth and dry wt. of plant at 35 and 45 days of crop growth. Seed treatment with ten times of the recommended dose recorded having higher number of nodules/plant than control. Seed inoculation plus pelleting with carrier gypsum, seed treatment with recommended dose of *Bradyrhizobium* and soil inoculation with *Rhizobium* enriched soil had given highest nodule dry wt/plant and grain yield.	Kawale *et al.* (1992)
B. japonicum	JS-2	Soybean (*Glycine max*) Parbhani isolate	YEM broth 3-4 days at 28°C	Seeds were inoculated with 10^2, 10^3, 10^4, 10^5 and 10^6 viable cells/seed rhizobial load significantly influenced all the growth and grain yield parameters of soybean except number of leaves and branches per plant.	Kurundkar *et al.* (1992)
Rhizobium sp.		Groundnut (*Arachis hypogea*)		Rhizobial culture with 40 per cent GAS (Gum arabic solution) was most effective. For groundnut lime pelleting with gum Arabic was however superior. Clay pelleting with plain water was at par. Clay pelleting with jaggery solution and gum Arabic solution yielded 13.19 q/ha and 7.66 q/ha respectively over control.	Chitriv (1992)

Contd...

Table 1.1–Contd...

Organism	*Strain*	*Isolated from*	*Growth Condition*	*Finding*	*Reference*
Rhizobium sp.	M-1, M-3, M-5, M-7 and S-8	Mung bean in the kharif season from Marathwada region	YEMA+ Congored	Combination M-5 strains of *Rhizobium* with 25kg N per hectare produced highest dry matter and nitrogen content in S-8 variety of Mung bean. The interaction between host varieties and *Rhizobium* strains revealed that M-1, M-3, M-5 and M-7 strains were superior over control.	Kore *et al.* (1992)
Bradyrhizobium japonicum	IARI-1 IARI-3	Soybean (*Glycine max*)	YEMA	A maximum nodule dry weight was recorded at 30 and 60 days of crop growth. Higher grain yield was recorded in *Rhizobium* treated plants than the control.	Kawale *et al.* (1992)
Rhizobium		*Cicer arietinum*		Maximum increase in the grain yield (16.33 per cent) was obtained with *Rhizobium* double coating.	Chopde *et al.* (1993)
Rhizobium sp.	C-235, Ca-2-Ca534 and CV-4	Chick pea (*Cicer arietinum*), collected from three districts of Haryana state	YEMA	378 native isolates were screened, of which 42 (11.1 per cent) showed antibiosis against homologous sensitive strain of CV-4 along with a standard strain Ca-181. 16 strains produced low molecular weight bacteriocin with mol.wt. above 12 KDa. The bacteriocin producing strains suppressed the growth of the sensitive strains under co-culture. Both the wild and the sensitive strains showed high nodulation ability. Co-inoculation of sensitive strain with a bacteriocin producing strains yielded 70-90 per cent nodules in the later. Bacteriocin producing strains failed to dominate the sensitive strain under co-growth condition as well as nodule competence. Bacteriogenic activity of a strain is beneficial in nodule competence among homologous strains.	Ahlawat and Dadarwal (1996)
Bradyrhizobium sp.	ARS-39	*Cajanus cajan*	YELAA (Yeast extract, L-arabinose agar)	A wild strain of *Bradyrhizobium* sp. showed high intrinsic resistance to sodium azide. Nitrogenase activity of its spontaneous mutants showed higher resistance to NaN_3. The percentage of mutants showing hyperactivity decreased with increase in azide resistance level.	Madhubala and Gaur (1996)

Contd...

Table 1.1–Contd...

Organism	Strain	Isolated from	Growth Condition	Finding	Reference
R. leguminosarum	PDR-14, HIM-1	Root exudates of *Phaseolus vulgaris*	YEMA plates at 28°C	Out of three nod regulators tested, a pigenin and naringenin enhanced the growth of *R. leguminosarum* while 7 hydroxy coumarin was found inhibitory in initial stages. Root exudates of two strains of host cultivars also stimulated the growth of rhizobia. Chemostatic response towards these flavonoids at 10^5 M and 10^{-6} M concentration ranged from 3.4 to 4.5. But this ratio towards root exudates was low.	Pathak and Khurana (1996)
Rhizobium sp.	Sb-3, SrS 35	*Sesbania bispinosa, S. rostrata*	YEMA at 28±1°C	Cross nodulation studies using all isolates of *S. bispinosa* and from *S. rostrata* showed no host species specificity as all isolates nodulated both the species. Some of the stem nodule isolates from *S. rostrata* was found to be more effective on both the host species resulting in higher gains in plant dry wt. Selected Hup^+ and Hup^- isolates were evaluated for symbiotic performance on both host species up to 50 days of plant growth. *S. bispinosa* inoculated with (Hup^-) isolate Sb-3 and SrS 35 resulted maximum gain in plant dry wt. 2 Hup^+ strains *viz.* SrR 83 and SVR8 were better in symbiotic effectivity but were not superior to Hup^-.	Saini *et al.* (1996)
Rhizobium sp.	Ca-181	Chick pea (*Cicer arietinum*)	YEMA plates at 28±1°C for 7 days	The nodule number and grain yield of *Cicer arietinum* was higher in *Rhizobium* treated plants in comparison to control indicating improvement in nodulation by native rhizobia. *Rhizobium* was effective in wilt control and promotes nodulation.	Khot *et al.* (1996)
Rhizobium sp.	VRF-10, VRF-57	*Vigna radiata*	YEMA	Two bacteriocin producing strains of *Rhizobium* sp. were studied for their nodule competitive ability on host legume green gram when used as co-inoculants in different proportions of 2 strains. VRF57 was the effective strain and formed higher proportion of nodules. The effective strain VRF57 besides producing bacteriocin was having other factors involved in nodule competence.	Goel *et al.* (1997)

Contd...

Table 1.1–Contd...

Organism	Strain	Isolated from	Growth Condition	Finding	Reference
Rhizobium sp., *Pseudomonas* sp., *Bacillus* sp.	*Rhizobium* sp. (Ca-181, Ca-534, Ca-313) *Pseudomonas* sp. (RS-13, RS-16, RS16B1 and RS-28) isolated fromgreen gram	Chick pea (*Cicer arietinum* L.)	YEMGA (Yeast extract mannitol glutamate agar)	These rhizobacteria when used as seed inoculant for chick pea some showed initial stunting effect on root seedling followed by root growth stimulation where as a few even prevented seed germination. The root growth stimulatory bacteria showed wide range of antifungal activity against the plant pathogenic fungi. The bacteria with antifungal activity exhibited enhanced production of flavonoids/flavones like compounds in the seedling roots, indicating their role in induction of systematic resistance in the plants as well as their possible role in rhizobial attachment for nodulation.	Parmar and Dadarwal (1997)
Bradyrhizobium sp.	S-24, AC-2, CC-1021, G-20, Br-9038, Br-9038U	*Vigna radiata*, *Acacia nilotica*, *Cajanus cajan*, *Cyamopsis tetragonoloba*	YEM medium	Strain Br-9038U was constructed by random Tn5 mutagenesis. For this plasmid PCAM 111 loaded with mini Tn5 containing gus-A gene, expressed from a constitutive PTAC promoter was used. The constructed strain formed blue colonies on YEMA plates containing X-GICA. The characteristic of the strain used is that it forms brown colour nodules on the host plants. This method was developed to monitor the nodule occupancy of the GUS marked strain of *Bradyrhizobium* sp. It was quicker, accurate and economical for nodule occupancy studies of the Gus marked *Bradyrhizobium* and is therefore better for ecological studies for rhizobia.	Sharma *et al.* (1997)
Bradyrhizobium sp.	Strain: USDA-110 112,31, 76,123,94 Strains used: NC-1005, SEMIA-566, CPAC-15, 7, S-204, S-335, CB-1809		7 days at 28°C in liquid medium	Parental strain SEMIA-566 produced little mucus. 59% of these isolates showed a colony diameter larger than parental strain. SEMIA-566 and S-340 showed resistance to the levels of antibiotics and only two (S-204 and S-335) were able to grow in presence of all antibiotics. Local strains showed a pattern closer to *B. elkanii*. In contrast to *B. elkanii* reference strain, *B. japonicum* was able to nodulate the Soybean. 32 strains fell into intermediate groups between the species *B. japonicum* and *B. elkanii*. CB-1809 and CPAC-7 were classified as *B. japonicum*.	Boddey and Hungria (1997)

Contd...

Table 1.1–Contd...

Organism	*Strain*	*Isolated from*	*Growth Condition*	*Finding*	*Reference*
Bradyrhizobium japonicum	SSF-4, 5, 6,7 and 8	Silt loam black in soil from Porur, near Chennai (13 N 8° E) with pH-7.2	The bacteria grow in Glutamate mdium (Bergerson, 1961) for 5 days	The strains were inoculated individually or with the type strain USDA 110 (collected from USA) at 1:1 ratio. Nodule occupancy determined by immunofluroscence and dot immunoblot assay revealed that *in vitro* condition SSF is more competitive than USDA 110 where as others were less competitive. In red soil both SSF-8 and USDA-110 were equally competitive where as in black soil SSF-8 competed better than USDA-110 and produced more nodules. In black soil field trial, when inoculated alone occupied the majority of the nodules and enhanced nodule dry weight and shoot biomass. SSF-8 was more competitive when the strains were co-inoculated.	Palaniappan *et al.* (1997
R. legumino-sarum	DGC-R1, R4, Hv-1, Hv-7, DGC-L1, DL2, VBBL-7,-18, 19 and VBK1	*Trifoilum repens* L.	Strains were grown in sherwoods medium	Enzymatic evidences supported that arabinose and ribose were metabolized through pentose phosphate, 2-oxoglutamate and 1-2 keto-3 deoxyarabinose pathways and mediated repression of phospho-fructo-kinase in *Rhizobium leguminosarum.*	Ghosh and Mandal (1998)
Bradyrhizo-bium sp.	S1,S2,S3, S4,S5,S6, S7,S8 and S9- S16, GB-2	*Cyamopsis tetragonoloba*	YEM medium	Strain GB-2 tolerated up to 85mM NaCl, S1-S5 all tolerant to 0.5 per cent NaCl, S6-S9 tolerant to 1.5 per cent NaCl and S10-S16 tolerant to 2.5 per cent NaCl. GB-2 showed a slow growth rate arriving at stationary phase 144 h after incubation. Salt tolerant showed rapid growth arriving at stationary phase 36 h after incubation. S2, S6, S7 and S16 showed an acid metabolic pattern. Salt tolerant strains gained resistance to chloramphenicol and Tetracyclins and significancly enhance their capacity to oxidize C-sources by increasing growth rate, exopolysaccharide production and involved in adhesion resulting in a greater adapting capacity to colonize unfavourable saline environments.	Barboza *et al.* (2000)

Contd...

Table 1.1–Contd...

Organism	*Strain*	*Isolated from*	*Growth Condition*	*Finding*	*Reference*
Rhizobium sp.	Mo6 (SM400) and PP9038 (Tc20+Cm200)	Mung bean collected from Deptt. of Microb. CCS Haryana Agri. University, HIsar		Role of proline dehydrogenase (PrfDH) in nodulation competitiveness of rhizobia infecting mung bean was examined. Tn5 mutagenesis of four *Rhizobium* strains resulted in proline prototrophs of two strains Mo6 and PP9038 (PH 9022) which were deficient in ProDH activity. ProDH deficient mutants affected different N_2 fixing parameters such as nodule number, nodule fresh wt., root dry wt., shoot dry wt. and total shoot nitrogen under sterilized condition. ProDH mutants deficient and wild type showed comparable nodule occupancy when used individually as inoculant. However ProDH deficient mutants were found to be poor competitor when co-inoculated in ratio with the wild type.	Chaudhury *et al.* (2000)
Rhizobium sp.	S-1230	Root nodules of *Acacia tortilis* grown in a Senegalese soil sample	YMA (Vincent, 1970) and Minimal mineral MB+7 medium	Growth parameters of C- limited continuous cultures were grown in presence and absence of 342 mM NaCl. Culturability subjected to the double stress of starvation and salinity was reduced and a high percentage of cells entered the viable but non culturable state. All the starved cultures were capable of re-growth when nutrients become available, thus showing that this strain can withstand long periods of nutrients deprivation in soil while maintaining the capacity for an active metabolism and a potential infectiousness towards an appropriate host.	Lippi *et al.* (2000)
Rhizobium sp.	CM-6, CC-6, BC-1	*Brassica campestris* var. toria)	CCM slants (combined carbon medium) 28±2°C	Out of 50 isolates only 15 were found positive for *in vitro* nitrogenase activity Maximum activity was observed for isolates CM-6 (238.24 n moles). Only four isolates possessed the ability to excrete ammonia. Out of all strains only three benefited the crop higher than control. CM6 having high nitrogenase activity could not benefit the crop yield. In contrast to CC6, BC-1 was found to give maximum benefit to the crop. There was also significant increase in the oil content of seeds as well as total oil yield of the crop due to bacterization with diazotrophs. Most efficient strains were found to be BC-1 in terms of increase in oil content.	Paul and Shende (2000)

Contd...

Table 1.1–Contd...

Organism	Strain	Isolated from	Growth Condition	Finding	Reference
Azorhizobium sp.		*Pterocarpus santalinus* L.		The effect of (IBA) Indole-3-butyric acid treatment at 50, 250, 500 and 1000μg ml^{-1} and the rhizobial inoculation on red sanders increased nodulation and biomass production. The stumps treated with 250μg IBA ml^{-1} showed higher growth, nodulation, biomass and nitrogen content over the other treatments. The combination of IBA at 250 μgml^{-1} and the rhizobial inoculation at 30 and 40 d, growth of root stumps gave maximum nodulation, biomass and 'N' content in plants.	Rajsekhar and Reddy (2000)
Rhizobium and *Bradyrhizobium*		*Acacia auriculiformis*	YEMA slants grown at 28°C and stored at 4°C	Of the 17 strains from different sources tested 10 were able to produce visible nodules and their nodulation frequency was also different. Strains isolated from other species of *Acacia* were not compatible with *A. auriculiformis*. Nodule number appeared to be a poor indicator of the nitrogen fixing potential of strains.	Sharma and Ramamurthy (2000)
Rhizobium meliloti	M-15	*Cicer arietinum*	M-15 strain grown for 24 h. Culture diluted to 1: 50-1: 100 in RMM with out N-sources. RMM at 5-10mM, Naringenin (100mM) was the inducer.	Different sources of combined N were added at a concentration of 5-100mM to *Rhizobium* minimal medium (RMM). All the N sources except KNO_3 and KNO_2 inhibited the expression of *nod* genes. Sodium glutamate was the most potent inhibitor, followed by NH_4NO_3, Urea, NH_4Cl and $(NH_4)_2SO_4$. Sodium glutamate at 25 mM repressed the expression of *nod* ABC by 85 per cent as compared to 93, 29, 54 and 49 per cent at 100mM of NH_4No_3, NH_4Cl, $(NH_4)_2$ HPO_4 respectively. KNO_3 and KNO_2 did not affect the expression of *nod* genes even at higher concentration. These results indicate that combined N affects the nodulation process by inhibiting the expression of *nod* genes.	Sharma *et al.* (2000)
Rhizobia		*Acacia sp.*	YEMA all strains stored in 50% (v/v) glycerol at (–4°C)	The rhizobia were very diverse with respect to their cross-nodulation patterns as well as their physiological and biochemical properties. Phenotypic characteristics showed that isolates could fit into four clusters below boundary level of 0.85. Some strains grew at pH ranging from 4 to 9, tolerated a high salt concentration (3 per cent NaCl) and grew at a maximum temperature between 35 and 40°C.	Zerhari *et al.* (2000)

Contd...

Table 1.1–Contd...

Organism	*Strain*	*Isolated from*	*Growth Condition*	*Finding*	*Reference*
Sinorhizobium sp.		*Sesbania cannabina*	Nodules immersed in 95 per cent ethanol for 10 sec, sterilized in 0.1% (w/v) $HgCl_2$ for 5 min, crushed and streaked on YEMA with 0.0025 per cent Congored at 28°C for 3 days.	Eighteen rhizobial isolates nodulating *S. cannabina* were isolated from sugar cane rotation fields in southern Taiwan. The taxonomy of these isolates was investigated using polyphasic approach, including phenotypic characteristics, banding pattern of total proteins from SDS-PAGE, genomic fingerprint patterns from pulse field gel electrophoresis, amplified 16s rDNA restriction analysis (ARDRA), 16s rRNA gene sequencing and Nif H gene sequencing based on results of Protein-banding patterns, ARDRA and phenotypic characters. Seven isolates belonging to *Sinorhizobium* lineage based on phylogenetic analysis, and 11 isolates belong to *Agrobacterium-Rhizobium galegae* were more closely related to *R. huautlense*.	Chen and Lee (2001)
Bradyrhizobium sp.	SEMIA-566 SEMIA-5079, 5080, 587, 5019	Soybean (*Glycine max* L. *Merril*)	YEMA containing cycloheximide (50µg/ml) at 28°C	Fifty eight isolates showed slow growth rates and alkali reaction in medium containing mannitol as C source. Twenty had fast growth rates and an acid reaction in medium containing mannitol as C source. Most isolates did not tolerate pH-4.5 or high temperature (40°C). Very few isolates shared similar protein and lipopolysaccharides profiles. Therefore high level of diversity was detected. Some of isolates showed outstanding symbiotic performance.	Chen *et al.* (2002)
Sinorhizobium and *R. leguminosarum*		*Medicago sativa* L. and *Trifolium alexandrium*	YEMA for 3 days suspended in 10% sucrose solution and inoculated seed by submerging them for 30 min.	From 125 locations represented by 14 major soil types and agroclimates in country, *S. meliloti* occurred in almost all the soils while *R. leguminosarum* bv. *trifolii* occurred in very few soils. These nodule bacteria able to survive under extremes of the environment. Inoculation of these two legumes with their respective nodule bacteria improved the yield.	Gaur *et al.* (2002)

Contd...

Table 1.1–Contd...

Organism	Strain	Isolated from	Growth Condition	Finding	Reference
Rhizobium sp.	ICC4948 and ICC 5003	Chick pea, soils of CCS Haryana Agri. University, Hissar	YEMA	Out of 350 cultures, in 110 rhizobial isolates, both from HN (high nodulation) and LN (low nodulation) plant variants, proteins of more than 45kDa were present and slight variation in the presence of proteins of lower mol.wt. in different isolates was observed. In HN selection all the 13 major bands were present while in case of LN selection varieties two major bands (8th and 9th) were absent. All the isolates from the HN and LN selections were able to nodulate plants of their respective host. Isolates selected from HN or LN selections when cross infected to LN or HN plants also formed nodules.	Chaudhary *et al.* (2002)
Bradyrhizo-bium sp.	MR125S2-SMr8	*Vigna aconitifolia*	YEMA	Fifty strains isolated were tested both for swarm size and nodulation. Majority of the isolates (74 per cent) showed large stable swarm when compared to the parent 26 isolates with lost nodulation ability. The mutants whose swarm size was larger produced pinkish nodules. In culture medium the parent and mutants preferred KNO_3 as sole N source over yeast extract and did not grow on media containing glucose or maltose. When co-inoculated with the parent, the mutant had generally higher nodule occupancy.	Chakraborty *et al.* (2003)
Bradyrhizobium japonicum	R-25B, IRJ-2180 A	Soybean (*Glycine max*) from moist Savanna of Northern nigeria		R25B indigenous strain and mixture of R-25B+IrJ2180A were experimented. About 34 per cent of nodules were formed by mixture of introduced strains and only about 24 per cent nodule was observed in R25B which did not influence biomass and grain yield. The grain yield was not higher from the uninoculated soybean showing the of competitiveness among the introduced *Rhizobium* strains and native rhizobial population.	Okogus and Sanginga (2003)
Rhizobium sp.		Soil from *Pennisetum glaucum Sorghum bicolor, Vigna uniculata, Arachis hypogea* grown fields		Soils from these legume rotation crops were collected and analyzed for microbial diversity in rhizoplane communities. Total numbers of bacterial species were observed maximum at 14 days than at 7 days after sowing.	Alvey *et al.* (2003)

Contd...

Table 1.1–Contd...

Organism	Strain	Isolated from	Growth Condition	Finding	Reference
R. tropici	CIAT-899 PRF-81 H-20, H-12	Soil of Parana state, Brazil		Nodule occupancy increased from an average of 28% in the first experiment with inoculation of rhizobia, and 56 per cent after four inoculations. The strain H-12 and H-20 showed an increase of 437 and 465 kg ha^{-1}. Inoculations with superior strains also resulted in yield increases. DGGE analysis of soil extracts showed that the massive inoculation apparently did not affect the composition of bacterial community.	Hungria *et al.* (2003)
R. leguminosarum	LX1-LX57 and 175 P4	*Pisum sativum* cv. tapper	YEM broth and growing on a gyratory shaker (150 rev/min.) at 28°C for 72h	The yield and N nutrition of pea inoculated with a superior *Rhizobium* strain was significantly enhanced by an apparently compatible AMF species. Compared to *Rhizobium* treatment, an apparently incompatible AMF sp. reduced the performance of an effective *Rhizobium* strain. In general co-inoculation treatments with effective *Rhizobium* strains and a compatible AMF species produced the best results. Total shoot dry matter, P-content and yield was enhanced.	Xavier and Germida (2003)
Rhizobium sp.	S1-S5 and P1-P5	Wild legumes of Shawara and Padubidri, Karnataka coast	YEMA	The strains isolated from four different cultivated legumes like cow pea, green gram, black gram and horse gram. Inoculation of S5 resulted in the highest increase of shoot biomass in cowpea while inoculation of P1-P5 induced the highest shoot biomass; P2 alone induced higher shoot biomass against uninoculated controls of horse gram, green gram and black gram.	Arun and Sridhar (2004)
Sinorhizobium fredii	USDA-205	*Glycine max* CV.	YEMA at 28°C	Twenty five soybean rhizobia were isolated from the soil above an altitude of 1500 m and all identified to be *S. fredii.* Their genetic diversity was characterized by 16S-23S rDNA, RFLP and RAPD analysis. All tested strains produced 2.1 kb 16S-23S rDNA ITS fragment. Tested strain could be differentiated into 11 ITS genotypes.	Chen *et al.* (2004)
Bradyrhizobium sp.	S6-1, 2, 3	Soybean	YEM broth medium	Effect of *Bradyrhizobium* strains on dry matter yield, nodulation and seed yield of soybean varieties was studied. A significant positive effect on growth, nodule number and yield of soybean was obtained. Strains S62 and S63 were more effective than strains S61. The protein content of seeds also increased after inoculation.	Egamberdiyeva *et al.* (2004)

Contd...

Table 1.1–Contd...

Organism	*Strain*	*Isolated from*	*Growth Condition*	*Finding*	*Reference*
Rhizobium sp.		From different soils	YEMA at 28°C for 4-5 days thermal shock: 45-55° C, pH-4.5-6.5, NaCl: 10000-100000 ppm	Out of 62 samples 9 showed thermal tolerance (55°C), 8 showed acidity tolerance (pH-4.5) and 11 showed tolerant to 40000 ppm NaCl. Some strains isolated from *Sesbania formosa*, *A. farnesiana* and also *D. sissoo* were adapted to grow on pH 12. Some strains tolerated salt concentration up to 5 (50,000 ppm).	Gupta *et al.* (2004)
Rhizobium, *Bradyrhizobium* and *Agrobacterium*	CA-18	Chick pea, mung bean, Pea and Sirato	YEMA Supplemented with Bromothymol blue and Congo red 28±2°C	Preliminary characterization of these isolates was done on the basis of plant infectivity test, acetylene reduction assay, C-source utilization, Phosphate solubilization, phytohormones and polysaccharide production. The plant infectivity test and acetylene reduction assay showed effective root nodule formation by all isolates on their respective hosts. All strains showed homology.	Hameed *et al.* (2004)
Rhizobium sp.		(*Trifolium ambiguum* M.B) perennial rhizomatous forage legumes	YM agar at 24°C for 4 days. Fresh YMA broth mixed with 80% glycerol solution (1:1) and preserved at –70°C for long time.	All 128 rhizobia strains were isolated from 4 sites from Kura clover. White colour clover rhizobia were finger printed using repetitive extragenic palinodromic PCR. The nodulation specificity and phenotypic diversity of a subset of 13 isolates was determined. Percentage of similarity among 13 isolates ranged between 28 and 92 per cent. Three strains formed effective nodules on both Kura clover and White clover.	Beaure-gard *et al.* (2004)
B. japonicum and *B. elkani*	CPAC-7, 15	Soybean	YEMA, broth cultures applied to sterilized peat (pH raised previously with $CaCo_3$) to reach about 50% moisture, the mixture allowed to mature at room temperature for 30 days reaching 1.8×10^8 to 2.0×10^9 cells per gram	Maximum nodule number and dry weight of nodules observed in treatments CPAC-15, CPAC-7. Grain yield also increased in treated ones. All the strains inoculated in the first year presented a successful establishment in soybean nodules with occurrence of 100 per cent. In second year formed 90-97 per cent without inoculation, 45, 30, 19 and 2 per cent of the nodule occupancy observed in un-inoculated plots.	Mendes *et al.* (2004)

Contd...

Table 1.1–Contd...

Organism	*Strain*	*Isolated from*	*Growth Condition*	*Finding*	*Reference*
Rhizobium sp.		*Acacia* plant from 14 locations, 4 sites represent semi arid, sub-moist, moist and sub humid	YEMA plates 28°C for 2-14 days	Twenty four isolates were recovered from the root nodules of trap host species and from excavated nodules. Isolates were differentiated by growth rate and colony morphology. 68.5 per cent were fast growing acid producing rhizobia. 25.3 per cent were slow growing alkali producing rhizobia and fast growing, alkali producing (2.9 per cent) and slow growing acid producing strains (3.3 per cent). All isolates showed four types of colonies *e.g.* watery translucent, white translucent, dull glistening and milky (curdled) type.	Wolde-meskel *et al.* (2004)
Rhizobium sp.				During winter seeds (pea, green gram) treated with the liquid broth of *Rhizobium* containing 1.3×10^7 rhizobia/ml showed 71.4 per cent and 78.8 per cent increase in dry shoot wt. and grain yield of pea over control. In green gram grain yield was found to be increased to 60.8 per cent higher.	Barik and Talukdar (2004)
Rhizobium sp.	LR-1, BR-12, BR-8 and AR-10, PR-16, AR-1, GR-12, WR-10, GM-16	Green gram and black gram form six districts of Assam		Experimental result showed that AR-1 was most effective in terms of nitrogenase activity and PR-16 was the poorest nitrogen fixer. Among two crops green gram was more responsive to rhizobial inoculation than black gram and among seasons Kharif season was found to be most suitable for the cultivation of the pulses over Rabi season. Maximum yield was obtained with the strain AR-1, increased the grain yield by 35.16 per cent in black gram and 31.41 per cent in green gram in Kharif and 33.89 per cent and 32.43 per cent in black gram and green gram in Rabi season respectively.	Azad, (2004)
Rhizobium sp., PSM (*Bacillus polymyxa*)	TAL 1000	Groundnut from Manipur		*Rhizobium* and PSM inoculation increased the pod yield over control (992kg/ha) by 11.9 per cent individually and by 30 per cent in dual combination. When inoculated with lime @2.5 t/ha the percent increase in pod yield was less compared to inoculated plots. The results suggest that liming was not effective in increasing the efficiency of either the rhizobial strain TAL 1000 or the PSM strain. *Bacillus* inoculated alone increased pod yield 39 per cent by increase in pH of the soil which increased the available P content and exchangeable calcium content of the soil.	Raychaudhri *et al.* (2004)

Contd...

Table 1.1–Contd...

Organism	*Strain*	*Isolated from*	*Growth Condition*	*Finding*	*Reference*
Rhizobium sp.		Groundnut from Manipur		The yield attributes, number of pods, seed wt., number of nodules and nodule mass were found highest under *Rhizobium* + FYM treatment followed by FYM+15kg N. Yield attributes under *Rhizobium* treatment was also superior to control.	Singh *et al.* (2004)
Rhizobium sp.	NC-92	Groundnut from Manipur		Result revealed that the native rhizobial population was not much effective in comparison to the applied strain which enhanced the growth and pod yield. The pod yield showed 8.8 per cent increase over control. *Rhizobium* and PSM in combination can save 10 kg of nitrogen and and 10 Kg of P_2O_5 per hectare and increase the yield to maximum by 37.5 per cent over the recommended dose of N, P, K (20 kg N, 40 kg P_2O_5 and 30 kg K_2O).	Ngachan *et al.* (2004)
Rhizobium sp.	NC-92	Groundnut acid hill utisol of Manipur		NC-92 strain was found effective in increasing the pod yield of groundnut by a maximum 27.5 per cent in an acid hill soil of Manipur. The efficiency of the strain increased by liming in furrows @500 kg and 1000kg/ha and increase the pod yield by 88 and 126 per cent respectively over control.	Raychaudhri *et al.* (2004)
Sinorhizobium meliloti	L5-30 (Φ L54)	*Medicago sativa*		Using Tn5 mutagenesis of lysogenic *Sinorhizobium meliloti strain* L5-30 three neomycin resistatant transconjugants differing in phage resistant profiles were isolated. Two of them increased the dry wt. of plants and were capable of establishing root nodules. Where as the third one was effective. The bacterium phage interaction did not have observable consequences in *Medicago sativa* and *S. meliloti* symbiosis because it did not affect the number of nodules on *M. sativa* or plant dry wt.	Kowalski *et al.* (2004)
R. japonicum	SB-16	Soybean	YEM broth at 30±2°C	*Rhizobium* inoculant as seed treatment was found to be much more effective than seed inoculation. It increased the nodule number by 74.40 per cent, pod number by 110.18 per cent, dry matter by 67.48 per cent and the grain yield by 124.8 per cent over similar soil implant at 2.5 cm (along with the seed).	Chakradhar and Jauhri (2004)

Contd...

Table 1.1–Contd...

Organism	*Strain*	*Isolated from*	*Growth Condition*	*Finding*	*Reference*
Rhizobium sp.	CRM-8, CRM-11, CRM-15, CRM-9	Collected from greengram of different locations of Tamil nadu		Sixteen isolates were obtained from green gram. Growing the isolates on osmotic substrates PEG (polyethylene glycol) the osmotic pressure level was enhanced in the cells. Out of sixteen CRM-11 and CRM-15 tolerated higher OP levels and the ability of these isolates to grow under soil moisture levels of even 5 per cent was observed. Hence such isolates which are able to survive under high OP levels may tolerate less water potentials of soils.	Kumutha *et al.* (2004)
Rhizobium sp.	CRR-6, NIT, FACT, UAS-Bangalore	Redgram (Vamban-1)		Field expt. was conducted to study the influence of commercially available carrier based rhizobial inoculants and liquid rhizobial inoculant on nodulation and grain yield. Carrier based rhizobial culture (RR-6) had given maximum nodules (14 nodules/plant), plant dry wt. and grain yield (875 kg/ha) which was 28.48 per cent higher over uninoculated control (681kg/ha). The inoculant had given a grain yield of 763kg/ha and but other commercially available culture where as liquid inoculant had recorded a grain yield of 735kg/ha only.	Gunasekarn *et al.* (2004a)
Rhizobium+ PGPR+ PSB	COC-10	Blackgram		A field trial was conducted to study sites synersism between *Rhizobium*, PGPR (*Pseudomonas*) PSB (*Bacillus megaterium*) on nodulation and yield of black gram. Inoculation of *Rhizobium* alone had given a grain yielded of 655kg/ha whereas control (uninoculated) had recorded 472 kg only. Combination of all three organisms (*Rhizobium*+ PGPR+PSB) had recorded the maximum nodules, plant biomass and grain yield (760 kg/ha) which was 61% higher than individual inoculation of *Rhizobium* alone.	Gunasekarn *et al.* (2004b)
Rhizobium sp.		Soil samples from Bhiwani and Hissar in Haryana	YMA supplemented with 25µg/ml congored	Amplified and cloned PCR products from total DNA isolated from the soil samples, the total diversity within the resulting clone libraries was higher than that recovered from trap plants but differed depending on the PCR protocols and primer used. However some plant of selected genotype could not be obtained using the community approach, probably due to variable detection limits and limited clone library.	Sarita *et al.* (2005)

Contd...

Table 1.1–Contd...

Organism	Strain	Isolated from	Growth Condition	Finding	Reference
Mesorhzobium sp.	UPM-Ca 36+	Chickpea (*Cicer arietinum* L.) alkaline soil	Maintained on Tryptone yeast agar (TYA) slants 20-37°C and preserved 4°C	Tolerance to stress (temperature and pH) was evaluated at pH-5 to 9, heat shock-46°C and 60°C. SDS-PAGE analysis revealed qualitative and quantitative differences when isolates were submitted to temperature stress. A 60 kDa protein was over produced by all isolates were more tolerant to 20°C than to 37°C. The isolates more tolerant to temperature stress showed lower symbiotic efficiency.	Rodrigues *et al.* (2006)
Mesorhizobium sp.	Ca-181	*Cicer arietinum*	YEMA medium	The symbiotic effectiveness of *Mesorhizobium* sp. *cicer* strain was further improved at 80 d of plant growth on co-inoculation with 6 *Bacillus* strains. The shoot dry wt. ratio varied from 1.62 to 1.74 times those of *Mesorhizobium* inoculated treatments. Nitrogenase activity was increased in *Mesorhizobium* treated plant than that of control.	Sivaramaiah *et al.* (2007)
Rhizobium sp.	R-39, E-11 obtained from Elosmestari Ltd, Finland		YM agar medium	The potential use of legume bacteria in non-legumes by inoculating different rhizobial strains on to mixture of six botanically different non-nitrogen fixing plant species was analyzed. Inoculation with certain rhizobial strains increased biomass. A concentration of level 10^4 c.f.u (colony forming units) ml^{-1} proved to be the best for successful growth. *In vitro* study investigating some rhizobial strains have a capability to dissolve the fungal mycelium at the initial stage.	Hossain and Martensson (2008)
Bradyrhizo-bium sp.	C-145		Grown in YEM medium for 4-6 days at 28°C	In field experiments, only 9 per cent of total nodules were formed by bacteria inoculated by direct coating of seed, whereas 78 per cent of nodules were formed by bacteria inoculated in the furrow at seeding. In each case, the other nodules were formed by indigenous strains or by both strains indicating a positional advantage of native rhizobia or in-furrow inoculated rhizobia for nodulation in plant.	Bogino *et al.* (2008)

of rhizobia. Rhizobia are able to produce acid or alkali on YEMA plates. Based on this criterion, the fast growing are acid producers while the slow growing are grouped as non acid producers. The results have shown that fast growing pea and bean rhizobia come under a common species name *Rhizobium*. *Rhizobium* is host specific and their role varies for plant to plant. Induction of nodule formation by rhizobia involves interactions between two symbiotic partners including multiple regulatory signals between the bacterium and plant to coordinate expression of gene sets in both partners (Peters and Verma, 1990). These signals include plant factors that induce rhizobial nodulation (*nod*) genes, rhizobial nod factors that induce further reactions and are essential for development of nodules, hormones and other regulatory factors involved in symbiotic nitrogen fixation. For nodulation in plant the first step is secretion of flavonoid (a class of phenolic compounds), chalcone and conjugated isoflavonoid signals by host. Induction of the nod gene operon depends upon the structure of the phenolic compounds.

N_2 Fixation Mechanism and the *nif* Genes

The genes responsible for nitrogen fixation called *nif* genes include *nod* genes (for nodulation) responsible for nod factor synthesis, nodule development and also synthesis of nitrogen fixing apparatus called as *nif* and *fix* genes. The expression of nitrogen fixation genes is controlled by cascades of organized regulatory genes. Their role of action enables bacteria to sense optimal environmental conditions required for nitrogen fixation and to transmit this information to the level of gene expression.

Molecular Protocols for Increasing Nodulation and Productivity

Present era holds the crown of numerous discoveries regarding the molecular genetics of non-legumes and the extension of legume-*Rhizobium* symbiosis to leguminous as well as non-leguminous crops. Plazinski *et al.* (1985) successfully transferred gene associated with root hair curling (*hac* genes) from *R. trifolii* into a derivative of *R. trifolii* on plasmids pKT 230 and pRK 290. The root hair curling character could then be expressed on infection of rice seedlings. Okon, (1985) suggested that genetic modification of diazotrophs helps them to acquire the genes for the synthesis of pectin degrading enzyme that could facilitate the root invasion. Rolfe and Bender (1990) described further developments to evolve rhizobia for nodulation of non-legume. Kenedy *et al.* (1997) reported that an effective associative system of cereals could be assisted by the development of genetic tools based on the application of the *lacZ* and *gusA* fusion with the promoters of genes associated with the nitrogen fixation for leguminous and non-leguminous plants.

Mass Production Methods of *Rhizobium* Biofertilizer and Field Application Protocols

Thirty days old of selected legume plants were uprooted washed in distilled water and the well-formed, healthy pinkish nodule on the tap roots were carefully cut out. The nodules were immersed in 95 per cent ethanol for 10 sec, sterilized for 5 minutes in 0.1 per cent acidified mercuric chloride ($HgCl_2$$^{-1}$g L^{-1}, Conc. HCl- 5ml.L^{-1}) and washed six times with sterile distilled water to get rid of the chemical (Chen and Lee, 2001). Each nodule was crushed using a sterile glass rod in a aliquot of sterile distilled water. Serial dilutions of the suspension were made and an aliquot of appropriate dilution was plated on Yeast-Extract Mannitol Agar medium (YEMA) and incubated at 28±2°C for 4-7 days (Bogino *et al.*, 2008). Distinct colonies were picked up and transferred to agar slants for further purification. Confirmation of the Rhizobia was ascertained by streaking on YEMA medium supplemented with congored 0.025 per cent (w/v) (Hameed *et al.*, 2004). The *Rhizobia* stand out as white, translucent colonies (Subba Rao, 1977). One week old Rhizobial colonies kept on YEM agar media (1.5 per cent agar) were used for preparation as inoculants. For this purpose loops of the respective colonies were inoculated in sterile YEMA medium containing K_2HPO_4-0.5g/l, $MgSO_4.7H_2O$-0.2g/l, NaCl-0.1g/l, Yeast Extract-0.4g/l, Mannitol-10.0g/l and pH 7.8, and the concentration of rhizobial suspension was 10^5 C.F.U/ml. Strains were routinely maintained on YEMA slants and kept at 4°C (Castro *et al.*, 1997).

For field experiments, healthy seeds of selected plants were surface sterilized with 95 per cent ethanol for 3-5 minutes followed by rinsing six times with sterile water. The seeds were then steeped in the respective rhizobial suspension. Seeds treated with distilled water were used as the control. All seeds were mixed gently in shade to bring the seeds and bacteria into close contact for 30 min.

Inoculation vs. Yield of Crops

In field demonstrations, the increases in yield of leguminous crops due to *Rhizobium* inoculation were as follows:

In India–20.36 per cent chickpea, 19.22 per cent pegion pea, 18.5 per cent mungbean, 14.29 per cent blackgram and 11.78 per cent lentil (Khurana *et al.*, 1997).

In Bangladesh–Lentil- 10-99 per cent, groundnut-8-41 per cent, soybean-18-71 per cent, chickpea-11-70 per cent, cowpea-21-26 per cent (Sattar *et al.*, 1997).

In Myanmar–chickpea (31-46 per cent), groundnut 29-44 per cent, blackgram-27-40 per cent, and butter bean-48 per cent (Thein and Hein, 1997).

In Nepal–lentil-10-80 per cent (Bhattarai *et al.*, 1997).

In Thailand–legume crops 43.5-12.6 per cent; In Vietnam- ground nut 3-47 per cent (Kongngoen *et al.*, 1997).

Future Prospective

Quantitative understanding of the ecological factors that control the future and performance of BNF systems in crop fields is essential for promotion and successful adoption of these technologies. More information about molecular genetic bases of rhizobial nodule symbiosis will improve understanding of root behavior towards microbes and provide information about the evolutionary relationships between plants process. Research in plant genes and molecules involved in *Rhizobium* is still not fully known. The interactions between host plants cells and micro-symbionts that lead to the expression of the various nodulin genes are a front line area of research today.

To induce most of the nodulins essential for functional symbiosis or signal exchanges between plant cells and bacteroids is required. Thus nodulation symbiosis and constantly evolving molecular biology techniques are now opening the way to identifying plant molecules that play an essential role in mechanisms involved in symbiotic interactions during root colonization by bacteria resources, such as rhizobial mutants are particularly valuable for such study, including search of signals and molecular approaches of the genes essential for the symbiosis. Research for the coming decades is to elucidate the various signals and signal transduction pathways operating during the nodule organogenesis and the regulation of expression of *nif* gene and *nod* gene cascades and their host specificity. Many aspects of the molecular signaling between rhizobia and leguminous plant have been already reported. Rhizobial lipochitin oligosaccharides (LCOs) that have been shown as the major determinant of the host specificity of the nodulation. It is also needed to understand the mechanisms of N gains and losses, and to identify and refine appropriate soil and crop management practices to maximize soil N and legume BNF in crop fields.

Conclusion

Biological nitrogen fixation is an important process in legume farming systems because it is an inexpensive source of nitrogen for increasing the productivity of crops. The nitrogen fixing biological systems such as *Rhizobium* were not able to adapt well in different ecological systems. So region specificity is important for development of rhizobia in addition to ecologically compatibility as well as fixing considerable amount of nitrogen. Besides nitrogen fixation, the *Rhizobium* biofertilizer also contribute the growth promoting substances. It is evidently clear now that the application of biological fertilizers were greatly involved in the accumulation of soil enzymes, which directly reflects on the soil fertility index. Thus use of biofertilizers in general, in consortia or even singly for specific crops, would reduce the cost of chemical fertilizers involved in crop production. The effective utilization of biological fertilizers for crops will not only provide economic benefits to the farmers but also improve and maintain the soil fertility and sustainability in the natural soil ecosystem.

References

Ahlawat, O. P. and Dadarwal, K. R. (1996). Bacteriocin production by *Rhizobium* sp. *cicer* and its role in nodule competence. *Indian Journal of Microbiology*, 36: 17-24.

Alvey, S., Yang, C. H., Buerkert, A. and Crowley, D. E. (2003). Cereal/legume rotation effects on Rhizosphere bacterial community structure in West African solis. *Biology and Fertility Soils*, 37: 73-82.

Arun, A. B. and Sridhar, K. R. (2004). Symbiotic performance of fast growing rhizobia isolated from the coastal sand dune legumes of west coast of India. *Biology and Fertility Soils*, 40: 435-439.

Azad, P. (2004). Screening of native *Rhizobium* strains for sustainable crop production in pulse-rice cropping system. In *Biotechnology in Sustainable and Organic Farming* (Eds. A. K. Yadav, S. R. Chaudhary and N. C. Talukdar) pp-244-248. Shree Publishers and Distributors, New Delhi.

Barboza, F., Correa, N. S. and Rosas, S. B. (2000). Metaboilc and physiological characteristics of salt-tolerant strains of *Bradyrhizobium* spp. *Biology and Fertility Soils*, 32: 368-373.

Barik, J. and Talukdar, N. C. (2004). Seasonal variation in response of pea (*Pisum sativum*) and Green gram (*Vigna radiata*) to *Rhizobium* inoculation in Assam. In *Biotechnology in Sustainable and Organic Farming* (Eds. A. K. Yadav, S. R. Chaudhary and N. C. Talukdar) pp-240-243. Shree Publishers and Distributors, New Delhi.

Bhattarai, S., Maskey, S. L., and Karna, R. L. (1997). On-farm experiments on rhizobial inoculants in Nepal. *In Extending Nitrogen Fixation Research to Farmers fields. Proceeding of an international workshop on Managing Nitrogen Fixation in the cropping systems of Asia.* 20-24 August 1996. ICRISAT Asia Centre, India. (Eds. O. P. Rupela, C. Johensen and D. F. Herridge. ICRISAT, Pantencheru, India). pp. 235-242.

Biswal, A. K. and Mishra, A. (1992). Selection of *Rhizobium* as biofertilizer for Greengram cultivation under acid and alkaline conditions. In *Biofertilizer Technology Transfer* (Ed. L. V. Gangawane) pp-121-126. Associated Publishing Co. New Delhi.

Beauregard, M.–S., Zheng, W. and Seguin, P. (2004). Diversity of *Trifolium ambiguum*-nodulating rhizobia from the lower Caucasus. *Biology and Fertility Soils*, 40: 128-135.

Boddey, L. H. and Hungria, M. (1997). Phenotypic grouping of Brazilian *Bradyrhizobum* Strains which nodulate Soybean. *Biology and Fertility Soils*, 25: 407-415.

Bogino, P. Banchio, E., Bonfiglio, C. and Giordano, W. (2008). Competitiveness of a *Bradyrhizobium* sp. strains in soils containing indigenous Rhizobia. *Current Microbiology* 56: 66-72.

Chakraborty, M., Khan, H. and Ramkrishna, K. (2003). Symbiotic properties of hypermotile mutants of *Bradyrhizobium* sp. (*Vigna aconitifolia*). *Indian Journal of Microbiology*, 43: 101-105.

Chakradhar, T. and Jauhri, K. S. (2004). Soil implant inoculants for increased crop production. In *Biotechnology in Sustainable and Organic Farming* (Eds. A. K. Yadav, S. R. Chaudhary and N. C. Talukdar) pp-214-217. Shree Publishers and Distributors, New Delhi.

Chaudhary, S., Dudeja, S. S., Sharma, H. R. and Khurana, A. L. (2000). Competitiveness of proline dehydrogenase of mungbean Rhizobia. *Indian Journal of Microbiology*, 40: 199-202.

Chaudhury, P., Khurana, A. L. and Dudeja, S. S. (2002). Heterogenecity of Rhizobia isolated from Chickpea nodulation variants. *Indian Journal of Microbiology*, 42: 195-200.

Chen, W., Huang, Q. and Xiong, X. (2004). Distribution and biodiversity of soybean rhizobia in the soils of Shennongjia forest reserve, China. *Biology and Fertility Soils*, 40: 306-312.

Chen, L. S., Figueredo, A., Villani, H., Michajluk, J. and Hungria, M. (2002). Diveristy and symbiotic effectiveness of rhizobia isolated from field-grown soybean nodules in paraguay. *Biology and Fertility Soils*, 35: 448-457.

Chitriv, A. J. and Chavan, O. G. (1992). Efficacy of different methods of inoculating Groundnut seed with *Rhizobium*. In *Biofertilizer Technology Transfer* (Ed. L. V. Gangawane) pp- 127-132. Associated Publishing Co. New Delhi.

Chen, W. M. and Lee, T. M. (2001). Genetic and phenotypic diversity of rhizobial isolates from sugarcane-*Sesbania cannabina*- rotation fields. *Biology and Fertility Soils*, 34: 14-20.

Chopde, S. T., Kolte, S. O. and Khan, Y. D. (1993). Effect of BGA and *Rhizobium* inoculation on wilt sensitive and resistant varieties of chickpea (*Cicer arietinum*). *Phykos*, 32:115-120.

Dahiya, D. R.., Hooda, R. S. and Hooda, I. S. (1992). Effect of inoculation, nitrogen and phosphorus levels on summer soybean forage. In *Biofertilizer Technology Transfer* (Ed. L. V. Gangawane) pp-101-105. Associated Publishing Co. New Delhi.

De Bruijin, F., Jing, Y. and Dazzo, F. (1995); Potential and pitfalls of trying to extend symbiotic interactions of nitrogen fixing organisms to presently non-nodulated plants such as rice. *Plant and Soil*, 174: 225-240.

Earl, C. D. and Ausubel, F. M. (1993). The genetic engineering of nitrogen fixation. *Nutrition Review*, 41: 1-6.

Egamberdiyeva, D., Quarshieva, D. and Davranov, K. (2004). Growth and yield of soybean varieties inoculated with *Bradyrhizobium* spp. in N-deficient calcareous soils. *Biology and Fertility Soils*, 40: 144-146.

Ghosh, A. C. and Mandal, N. C. (1998). Metabolism of pentose sugars in *Rhizobium leguminosarum bv. trifolii*. *Indian Journal of Experimental Biology*, 36: 1056-1057.

Gour, Y. D., Rewari, R. B., Bhatnagar, R. S., Narayan, K. P. and Sen, A. N. (2002). *Sinorhizobium meliloti* and *Rhizobium leguminosarum bv. trifoliii* in Indian soils and their inoculation response. *Indian Journal of Microbiology*, 42: 23-28.

Goel, A. K., Sindhu, S. S. and Dadarwal, K. R. (1997). Nodule competence between bacteriocin producing effective and in effective *Rhizobium* strains of *Vigna. Indian Journal of Microbiology*, 37, 51-52.

Gunasekaran, S., Balachandar, D. and Mohanasundaram, K. (2004) (a). Field evaluation of liquid and carrier based Rhizobial inoculants in Redgram. In *Biofertilizer Technology*. (Eds. S. Kannaiyan, K. Kumar and K. Gobindarajan) pp. 265-268. Scientific Publishers, Jodhpur, Rajasthan.

Gunasekaran, S., Balachandar, D. and Mohanasundaram, K. (2004) (b). Studies on synergism between *Rhizobium*, plant growth promoting rhizobacteria (PGPR) and phosphate solubilizing bacteria in blackgram. In *Biofertilizer Technology*. (Eds. S. Kannaiyan, K. Kumar and K. Gobindarajan) pp. 268-272. Scientific Publishers, Jodhpur, Rajasthan, India.

Gupta, S. B., Tedia, K., Singh, A., Anurag, Lakpale, N., Pal, A. and Chhonkar, P. K. (2004). Formulation of stress tolerant bioinoculants for rainfed cropping system. In *Biofertilizer Technology*. (Eds. S. Kannaiyan, K. Kumar and K. Gobindarajan) pp. 256-264. Scientific Publishers, Jodhpur, Rajasthan.

Hameed, S., Yasmin, S., Malik, K. A., Zafar, Y. and Hafeez, F. Y. (2004). *Rhizobium*, *Bradyrhizobium* and *Agrobacterium* strains isolated from cultivated legumes. *Biology and Fertility Soils*, 39: 179-185.

Hossain, M.S. and Mårtensson, A. (2008). Potential use of *Rhizobium* spp. to improve fitness of non-nitrogen-fixing plants. *Soil and Plant Science*, I: 1-7.

Hungria, M., Campo, R. J. and Mendes, I.C. (2003). Benefits of inoculation of the common bean (*Phaseolus vulgaris*) crop with efficient and competitive *Rhizobium tropici* strains. *Biology and Fertility Soils*, 39: 88-93.

Kawale, B. R., Thombre, P. A., Kurundkar, B. P. and Mayee, C. D. (1992). Efficacy of *Bradyrhizobium japonicum* inoculation methods in soybean under rainfed condition. In *Biofertilizer Technology* Transfer (Ed. L. V. Gangawane) pp. 107-110. Associated Publishing Co. New Delhi.

Kawale, B. R., Thombre, P. A., Kurundkar, B. P. and Mayee, C. D. (1992). Evaluation of the efficiency of the *Rhizobium* cultures for soybean varieties under rainfed condition. In *Biofertilizer Technology* Transfer (Ed. L. V. Gangawane) pp. 149-154. Associated Publishing Co. New Delhi.

Kennedy, I. R., Pereg, Gerk, L. L., Wood, C., Deaker, R., Gilchrest, K. and Katupitiya, S. (1997); Biological nitrogen fixation in non-leguminous field crops: facilitating the evolution of an effective association between *Azospirillum* and wheat. *Plant and Soil*, 194: 65-79.

Khurana, A. L., Namdeo, S. L., Patel, B. J. and Dudeja, S. S. (1997); On-farm experiments on Rhizobial inoculants–problems and possible solutions. In *Extending Nitrogen Fixation Research to Farmers Fields. Proceedings of an International workshop on Managing Nitrogen Fixation in the cropping Systems of Asia*. 20-24 August 1996. ICRISAT Asea Centre, India. (Eds. O. P. Rupela, C. Johensen and D. F. Herridge. ICRISAT, Pantencheru, India). pp. 217-226.

Khot, G. G., Tauro, P. and Dadarwal, K. R. (1996). Rhizobacteria from Chickpea (*Cicer arietinum* L.) Rhizosphere effective in wilt control and promote Nodulation. *Indian Journal of Microbiology*, 36, 217-222.

Kowalski, M., Malek, W., Czopska-Dolecka, J. and Szlachetka, M. (2004). The effect of rhizobiophases on *Sinorhizobum meliloti–Medicago sativa* symbiosis. *Biology and Fertility Soils*, 39: 292-294.

Kongngoen, S., Charoensaksiri, A., Kongngoen, R. and Chanaseni, C. (1997). On-farm experiments on Rhizobial inoculants in Thailand: Problems and likely solutions. In *Extending Nitrogen Fixation Research to Farmers Fields. Proceedings of an International workshop on Managing Nitrogen Fixation in the cropping Systems of Asia*. 20-24 August 1996. ICRISAT Asea Centre, India. (Eds. O. P. Rupela, C. Johensen and D. F. Herridge. ICRISAT, Pantencheru, India). pp. 243-248.

Kore, S. S., Deshmukh, G. V. and Jadav, V. T. (1992). Green house evaluation of *Rhizobium* strains of Mungbean. In *Biofertilizer Technology Transfer* (Ed. L. V. Gangawane) pp. 141-147. Associated Publishing Co. New Delhi.

Kurundkar, B. P., Kawale, B. R., Thombre, P. A., Mayee, C. D. and Chandrawanshi, R. D. (1992). Effect of nitrogen and phosphorus application on Rhizobial symbiosis in soybean. In *Biofertilizer Technology Transfer* (Ed. L. V. Gangawane) pp. 111-116. Associated Publishing Co. New Delhi.

Kurundkar, B. P., Thombre, P. A., Kawale, B. R., Mayee, C. D. and Chandrawanshi, R. D. (1992). Effect of Rhizobial load/seed on nodulation, vegetative growth and yield of soybean. In *Biofertilizer Technology Transfer* (Ed. L. V. Gangawane) pp. 117-120. Associated Publishing Co. New Delhi.

Kumutha, K., Sempavalan, J. and Vijila, K. (2004). Induction of Desiccation tolerance in greengram rhizobia. In *Biofertilizer Technology*. (Eds. S. Kannaiyan, K. Kumar and K. Gobindarajan) pp. 253-255. Scientific Publishers, Jodhpur, Rajasthan.

Lippi, D., Depaolis, M. R., DiMattia, E., Grego, S., Pietrosanti, T. and Cacciari, I. (2000). Effect of salinity on growth and starvation-survival of a tropical *Rhizobium* strain. *Biology and Fertility Soils*, 30: 276-283.

Madhuwala and Gaur, Y. D. (1996). Ex-planta Nitrogenase Activity of Bradyrhizobium sp. (Cajanus) and its Azide Resistant Mutants. *Indian Journal of Microbiology*, 36: 73-74.

Mendes, C. J., Hungria, M. and Vargas, M. A. T. (2004). Establishment of *Bradyrhizobium japonicum* and *B. elkanii* strains in a Brazilian Cerrado Oxisol. *Biology and Fertility Soils*, 40: 28-35.

Ngachan, S. V., Yadav, A. K., Raychaudhuri, S., Lokeswarsingh, K., Ingobisingh, L., Raghumanisingh, Th. and Sharma, B. K. (2004). *Rhizobium* application in groundnut in the farmers field. In *Biotechnology in Sustainable and Organic Farming* (Eds. A. K. Yadav, S. R. Chaudhary and N. C. Talukdar) pp. 229-231. Shree Publishers and Distributors, New Delhi.

Okon, Y. P. G. (1985); *Azospirillum* as a potential inoculant for agriculture. *TIB Technology*, 3: 223-228.

Okogun, J. A. and Sanginga, N. (2003). Can introduced and indigenous rhizobial strains compete for nodule formation by promiscuous soybean in the moist savanna agroecological zone of Nigeria?. *Biology and Fertility Soils*, 38: 26-31.

Pathak, D. V. and Khurana, A. L. (1996). Effect of Nod Gene Regulators on Growth and Chemotaxis of *Rhizobium leguminosarum bv. Phaseoli*. *Indian Journal of Microbiology*, 36: 89-92.

Peters, N. K. and Verma, D. P. S. (1990). Phenolics compounds as regulators of gene expression in plant-microbe interactions. *Molecular Plant Microbe Interactions*, 3: 4-8.

Palaniappan, S. P., Sudhisreedhar, P., Loganathan, P. and Thomas, J. (1997). Competitiveness of native *Bradyrhizobium japonicum* strains in two different soil types. *Biology and Fertility Soil*, 25: 279-284.

Paul, S., and Shende, R. (2000). Influence of ammonia excreting diazotrophs on growth and yield of rape seed. *Indian Journal of Microbiology*, 40: 255-258.

Parmar, N. and Dadarwal, K. R. (1997). Rhizobacteria from rhizosphere and rhizoplane of Chickpea (*Cicer arietinum* L.). *Indian Journal of Microbiology*, 37: 205-210.

Plazinski, J. Innes, R. and Rolfe, B. (1985). Expression of *Rhizobium trifolii* early nodulation genes on maize and rice plants. *Journal of Bacteriology*, 163: 812-815.

Raghuchaudhuri, M., Ngachan, C. V., Raychaudhuri, S. and Singh, A. L. (2004). Yield responses of groundnut to dual inoculation and liming in an acid hill ultisol of Manipur. In *Biotechnology in Sustainable and Organic Farming* (Eds. A. K. Yadav, S. R. Chaudhary and N. C. Talukdar) pp. 235-239. Shree Publishers and Distributors, New Delhi.

Rajsekhar, A. and Reddy, T. K. K. (2000). Effect of Indole-3-Butyric Acid (IBA) and *Rhizobium* on Red Sanders (*Pterocarpus santalinus* L.) *Indian Journal of Microbiology*, 40: 137-140.

Raychaudhuri, M., Kumar, K., Raychaudhuri, S. and Sanjeev Kumar. (2004). Efficiency of *Rhizobium* with liming in furrows in groundnut. In *Biotechnology in Sustainable and Organic Farming* (Eds. A. K. Yadav, S. R. Chaudhary and N. C. Talukdar) pp. 224-228. Shree Publishers and Distributors, New Delhi.

Rodrigues, C. S., Laranjo, M. and Oliveira, S. (2006). Effect of heat and pH stress in the growth of Chickpea Mesorhizobia. *Current Microbiology* 53: 1-7.

Rolfe, B. G. and Bender, G. L. (1990); Evolving a *Rhizobium* for non-legume nodulation. In: *Nitrogen Fixation: Achievements and Objectives* (Eds. P.M. Gresshoff, L. E. Roth, G. Stacey and W. E. Newton). Chapman and Hall, New York, pp. 829.

Sharma, P. K., Kambhoj, D. V., Rustagi, N. and Dogra, R. C. (1997). A Simple Method to study nodule occupancy of *Bradyrhizobium* sp. marked with *gus*A gene. *Indian Journal of Microbiology*, 37: 91-94.

Sharma, P.K., Srivastava, P., Upadhyay, K. K., Pathak, D. V., Dogra, R. C. and Kundu, B. S. (2000). Effect of Combined Nitrogen on the expression of nod genes in *Rhizobium* sp. (*Cicer*). *Indian Journal of Microbiology*, 40: 125-130.

Sattar, M. A., Khanam, D., Ahmad, S., Haider, M. R., Podder, A. K. and Bhuiyan, M. A. (1997). On-farm experiments on rhizobial inoculants in Bangladesh: Results, problems and possible solutions. In *Extending Nitrogen Fixation Research to Farmers Fields. Proceedings of an International workshop on Managing Nitrogen Fixation in the cropping Systems of Asia.* 20-24 August 1996. ICRISAT Asea Centre, India. (Eds. O. P. Rupela, C. Johensen and D. F. Herridge. ICRISAT, Pantencheru, India). pp. 201-216.

Sarita, S., Sharma, P. K., Priefer, U. B. and Prell, J. (2005). Direct amplification of rhizobial *nodC* sequences from soil total DNA and comparison to *nodC* diversity of root nodule isolates. *FEMS Mcrobiol Ecology*, 54: 1-11.

Saini, I., Sindhu, S. S. and Dadarwal, K. R. (1996). Uptake hydrogenase, nitrate respiration, *Explanta* Nitrogenase Expression and symbiotic effectivity of *Sesbania Rhizobia*. *Indian Journal of Microbiology*, 36: 93-98.

Sivaramaiah, N., Malik, D. K. and Sindhu, S. S. (2007). Improvement in symbiotic efficiency of chickpea (*Cicer arietinum*) by co-inoculation of *Bacillus* strains with *Mesorhizobium* sp. *Cicer*. *Indian Journal of Microbiology*, 47:51-56.

Subba Rao, N. (1977). Rhizobium and legume root nodulation. In *Soil Microbiology* (Eds. N. S. SubbaRao) pp. 166-228. Oxford and IBH Publishing Co. New Delhi.

Singh, K. P., Raychaudhuri, M. and Munda, G. C. (2004). Nitrogen economy in groundnut through *Rhizobium* in an acid hill soils of Manipur. In *Biotechnology in Sustainable and Organic Farming*

(Eds. A. K. Yadav, S. R. Chaudhary and N. C. Talukdar) pp. 232-234. Shree Publishers and Distributors, New Delhi.

Sharma, R. S. and Ramamurthy, V. (2000). Nodulation compatibility and growth promoting ability of *Rhizobium* and *Bradyrhizobium* strains for *Acacia auriculiformis*. *Indian Journal of Microbiology*, 40: 131-136.

Salve, P. B. and Gangawane, L. V. (1992). *Rhizobium* from wild legumes and nitrogen fixation in Groundnut. In *Biofertilizer Technology* Transfer (Ed. L. V. Gangawane) pp. 95-100. Associated Publishing Co. New Delhi.

Subba Rao, N. (1984). Rhizobium inoculant. In *Biofertilizer in Agriculture* (Eds. N. S. SubbaRao) pp-17-73. Oxford and IBH Publishing Co. New Delhi.

Thein, M. M. and Hein, M. (1997). Rhizobial inoculants production and their on-farm use in Myanmar. In *Extending Nitrogen Fixation Research to Farmers Fields. Proceedings of an International workshop on Managing Nitrogen Fixation in the cropping Systems of Asia*. 20-24 August 1996. ICRISAT Asea Centre, India. (Eds. O. P. Rupela, C. Johensen and D. F. Herridge. ICRISAT, Pantencheru, India). pp. 227-234.

Wani, P. V., Bambarse, L. B., Konde, B. K. and Indi, D. V. (1992). Effect of single and combined inoculation of *Azospirillum* and *Rhizobium* on the yield of Groundnut under different levels of nitrogen in field conditions. In *Biofertilizer Technology Transfer* (Ed. L. V. Gangawane) pp. 60-64. Associated Publishing Co. New Delhi.

Wolde-meskel, E., Berg, T., Peters, N. K. and Frostegård, Å. (2004). Nodulation status of native woody legumes and phenotypic characteristics of associated rhizobia in soils of southern Ethiopia. *Biology and Fertility Soils*, 40: 55-66.

Xavier, L. J. C. and Germida, J. J. (2003). Selective interactions between arbuscular mycorrhizal fungi and *Rhizobium leguminosarum bv. viceae* enhance pea yield and nutrition. *Biology and Fertility Soils*, 37: 261-267.

Zerhari, K., Aurag, J., Khabaya, B., Kharchaf, D. and Filali-Maltouf, A. (2000). Phenotypic characteristics of rhizobia isolates nodulating *Acacia* species in the arid and Saharan regions of Morocco. *Letter of Applied Microbiology*; 30: 351-357.

Microbial Biotechnology and Ecology (2011)
Editors: **Deepak Vyas, G.S. Paliwal, P.K.Khare and R.K Gupta**
Published by: **DAYA PUBLISHING HOUSE, NEW DELHI**

Pages **29–33**

Chapter 2

Microbial Diversity: Its Role in Ecosystem Maintenance

☆ *Jamaluddin**

Emeritus Scientist,
Department Bioscience, R.D. University, Jabalpur, M.P.

ABSTRACT

Microorganisms are responsible for maintenance of nitrogen cycle. They have a unique role in the cycling of elements essential to plant life on the earth. They also serve as early warming system in biomonitoring global ecology, climate change, pollutants and habitat disturbance. They are the primary producers, and dominate the biogeochemical cycles in extreme environments and stresses and counteract them.

Microorganisms constituting the major part of biodiversity on earth are a major source of useful bioactive compounds and therefore emphasize the need for their *in situ* conservation cannot be overemphasized. Because of the uncertainty of long term security of this strategy and the isolation from nature of many microorganisms being problematic, *ex situ* collections alone can ensure conservation of microbial diversity for future investigations and use by man. Microbial diversity of the world is widely covered at an IUBS/IUMS Workshop in 1991.

Biodiversity has played a major role in the evolution and diversification of macroorganisms. As mutualists, mycorrhizae are either involved in nutrient supply or perform other biochemical processes on which they depend. Bacteria, fungi and protozoa in the guts of insects and herbivores performs crucial role in their digestive processes particularly in the breakdown of cellulose and lignin.

Formation of soil biomass through biodegradation of residue, breakdown of rock and nutrient cyling is performed mainly through fungi. In monitoring microorganisms with reference to

* Ex Group Coordinator and Director Tropical Forest Research Institute, Jabalpur, M.P.....

conservation of biodiversity in macroorganisms, the maintenance of functional group rather than individual species can be presumed to be limiting except where a particular microorganisms if keystone species. Microorganisms also contribute to the maintenance of ecosystem structures through natural biocontrol. Plant pathogenic microorganisms can limit plant population. Similarly entomophagus fungi (microorganisms) can limit population of insects that otherwise become major pests.

Microorganisms play a major role in the maintenance of the global ecology through various biogeochemical cycles. Some of the bacteria produces oxygen and thereby reduce the CO_2. Supply other elements like carbon, nitrogen, sulphur and minerals are also maintained in the biosphere by microorganisms.

Microorganisms are beneficial in sustainable development particularly by increasing productivity of forest and agricultural lands through: (i) efficacious nitrogen-fixing strains into legume crops, (ii) enhancement of natural nitrogen fixation by application of cyanobacterial inocula, (iii) role of mutualists (mycorrhizas) in nutrient cycling in higher plants, (iv) the use of bacteria and fungi as biocontrol agents, (v) role of microbes in genetic manipulation, (vi) biotechnological aspects and (vii) CO_2 fixation, etc.

The forest ecosystems in Madhya Pradesh are highly rich in biological diversity. Though there are many variability of biological resources in M.P. yet the studies on microbial diversity are very few and peripheral. Variability in microbes occurring in sal, teak and miscellaneous forests are well as in mine disturbed ecosystem requires systematic study and documentation of effective beneficial microbial populations for biological rejuvenation of such disturbed areas. Fire and grazing in the forest not only disturb the forest and its regeneration but also affect the microbial population occurring in different habitat, which plays a key role in the maintenance of above ground biodiversity. The documentation and listing of such important functional groups is very essential for increasing the productivity of forests.

Introduction

Variability of microbes occurs in the global resources of microorganisms. As habitat destruction and species extinction rates accelerate, biotechnology is identifying new ways to use information and product from biota Management of microbial diversity is a serious task as there is little baseline information about the amount and distribution of microbes. In majority of case–microorganisms remain either on the fringes of biodiversity programmes or left out entirely. Microbial biodiversity provides the foundation for biotechnology, *i.e.* the basis for new product discovery, bioremediation and genetic manipulation of organisms for new commercial products and processes. Thus, retention and conservation of microbial genomic variation for future applications is not only an obligation of highest order but also of great importance for global economy.

Microorganisms constituting the major part of biodiversity on earth are a major source of useful biotic bioactive compounds and therefore, emphasize the need for their *in situ* conservation cannot be overemphasized. Because of the uncertainty of long term security of this strategy and the isolation from nature of many microorganisms being problematic, *ex situ* collections alone can ensure conservation of microbial diversity for future investigations and use by man. Microbial diversity of the world is widely covered at an IUBS/IUMS Workshop in 1991 (Hawksworth, 1991a,b; Hawksworth and Colwell, 1992).

Significance of Microbial Diversity

1. Microbial 'diversity must be treated as a global resource, to be indexed, used and preserved.
2. As habitat destruction and species extinction rates accelerate, biotechnology is identifying new ways to use information and products from the microbiota.
   - ☆ Basis for new product discovery
   - ☆ Bioremediation
   - ☆ Genetic manipulation organisms for new commercial products and processed.
3. Retention and conservation of microbial genomic variations for future applications.
4. Inventory of microbial species.

Species Diversity

Comparisons of species numbers between microorganisms reflected into several variations in species concept. This difficulty arises because sexual processes are either absent or *difficult* to detect in many microorganism groups. In practice micro biologists tend to be pragmatic and recognize species or strains on the basis of morphological, biochemical or molecular similarity. The process of assimilation, substrate utilization and cultural attributes are extensively used as the taxonomic criteria more in bacteria and yeasts than filamentous fungi and protozoa.

Genetic Diversity

The genetic diversity exhibited by microorganism group is very vast. The extent of genetic diversity now demonstrated between the higher ranks of microorganisms is also reflected at the species level.

Ecosystem Habitat Diversity

The variety of ecological niches exploited by the major groups of macro and microorganisms is directly related to their geological age. The greatest niche breadth is seen in the bacteria with declining sequence in the algae, protozoa and fungi. There is every reason to believe that regions and habitats with a maximum diversity of macroorganisms will also be rich in genetic base of microorganisms. A sequence of the larger number of host-specific parasites, mutualists and saprobes is considered for the conservation of macroorganisms diversity. Extreme environment also continues to be a rich source of previously unknown microorganisms, belonging to divers groups. Studies on the number of species of particular families and general of fungi in different geographic regions can particularly lead to the recognition of centres of diversity. Various edaphic and biotic factors also contribute towards change in species and genera.

Biodiversity Maintenance

Biodiversity has played a major role in the evolution and diversification of macroorganisms. As mutualists, mycorrhizae are either involved in nutrient supply or perform other biochemical processes on which they depend. Bacteria, fungi and protozoa in the guts of insects and herbivores performs crucial role in their digestive processes particularly in the breakdown of cellulose and lignin.

About 85 per cent of the earths vascular plants form mycorrhizas.:This association in life cycle of symbionts often obligate in nature, the mycorrhizas being crucial to the absorption of growth limiting *nutrients.* The very existence of many macroorganisms is consequently dependent on the continued availability of the requisite mutalistic microorganisms: In the absence of mutualistic microorganisms (crustess cerallinelgae), coral reef ecosystems simply cannot exist. Formation of soil biomass through biodegradation of residue, breakdown of rock and nutrient cycling is performed mainly through fungi. In monitoring microorganisms with reference to conservation of biodiversity in macroorganisms, the maintenance of functional group rather than individual species can be presumed to be limiting except where a particular microorganisms is keystone species. Microorganisms also contribute to the maintenance of ecosystem structures through natural biocontrol. Plant pathogenic microorganisms can limit plant population. Similarly entomophagus fungi (microorganisms) can limit population of insects that would otherwise become major pests.

Microorganisms in Biosphere Function

Microorganisms play a major role in the maintenance of the global ecology through various biogeochemical cycles. Some of the bacteria produces oxygen and thereby reduce the CO_2. Supply other elements like carbon, nitrogen, sulphur and minerals are also maintained in the biosphere by microorganisms.

Microorganisms are beneficial in sustainable development particularly by increasing productivity of forest and agricultural lands through: (i) efficacious nitrogen-fixing strains into legume crops, (ii) enhancement of natural nitrogen fixation by application of cyanobacterial inocula, (iii) role of mutualists (mycorrhizas) in nutrient cycling in higher plants, (iv) the use of bacteria and fungi as biocontrol agents, (v) role of microbes in genetic manipulation, (vi) biotechnological aspects and (vii) CO_2 fixation, etc.

Microbial Diversity in Madhya Pradesh

The biodiversity in Madhya Pradesh is very rich. The forest cover comprising sal forest, teak forest and miscellaneous forest, cover the vast area of the state. Due to rich diversity in the macro-organisms, microbial diversity is equally very high. The microbes belonging to different groups particularly fungi, bacteria, actinomycetes etc. live closely with the macro organisms in diverse habitat. Some of these organisms are causing diseases particularly fungal and bacterial diseases and they belong to different taxonomic groups. These microbes are capable of damaging leaf, stem roots, stored woods, flower and seeds etc.

The microbes are also capable of decomposing the forest litter and the major group of the microbes belongs to thermophilic or thermotolerant bacteria and fungi. The decomposition of and organic acid etc. (Satyanarayana *et al.*, 1992). The enzyme produced by this group of fungi are thermostable.

Scope of Microbial Diversity

The studies on microbial diversity are very scant, there is need to investigate and list out the fungi and bacteria and actinomycete from the soil and different habitat in forest ecosystem. There is need to identify the major functional groups of microorganisms responsible for biological diversity of macro-organisms particularly the mycorrhizae, N-fixers, phosphate solubilizing bacteria and many other biocontrol agents.

The microbes specifically involved in the biochemical process like bio-remediation, bio-indication as well as synthesis of important chemicals need identification and documentation. *Ex-situ* conservation of the microbes by making the life cultu Teherbaria is very essential to exploit their potential. *In situ* maintenance and marking of the potentially important microbes is also equally important.

Since there is no any specific account listing out the microbial diversity of M.P., therefore it is necessary to prepare a project, to document the relevant literature on microbial diversity and also to list out the significance microbe in different habitats.

References

Hawksworth, D.L. (1991a). The fungal dimension of biodiversity magnitude, significance and conservation. *Mycological Research*, 95 : 641-655.

Hawksworth, D.L. (1991b). *The biodiversity of microorganisms and Invertebrates: Its Role in sustainable Agriculture*, Wallingford: CAB International.

Hawksworth, D.L. and Colwell, RR (1992). Microbial diversity and biodiversity amongst microorganisms and its relevance. *Biodiversity and Conservation*, 1: 221–226.

Jamaluddin and Chandra, KK. (1999). Application of VAM technology in bamboo cultivation in mine soils. In: *Modern Approaches and Innovation in Soil Management*. Editors: D.I. Bagyaraj, Ajit Verma, K.K. Khanna and H.I. Kehri, Rastogi Publications, Meerut.

Microbial Biotechnology and Ecology (2011) *Pages* **34–40**
Editors: **Deepak Vyas, G.S. Paliwal, P.K.Khare and R.K Gupta**
Published by: **DAYA PUBLISHING HOUSE, NEW DELHI**

Chapter 3

Thermophilic Cyanobacteria: The Wonder Organisms

☆ *Vidhi Verma and Meenakshi Banerjee*

Laboratory of Algal Biotechnology,
Department of Bioscience, Barkatullah University, Bhopal, M.P

Introduction

After the evolution of life on Earth over 3 billion years ago several life forms have evolved since then. Living systems have to continuously interact with an environment that is not always kind to them. As a result they encounter various stresses at the organism and cellular level. Lazcano and Miller (1996); Ward and Castenholz (2000).

Such common niches that encompass a number of extreme physical stresses are found in the endolithic rock environment of hot and cold deserts with regard to temperature as well as marine environments and hot springs that are highly haline in nature. Bhaya *et al.* (2000); Norris and Castenholz (2006); Fleming and Castenholz (2007); Roeselers *et al.* (2007). In such environment microorganism must endure extremes of temperature, desiccation, low nutrient supply and low photon flux. Geothermal springs of temperature between 45-100°C are almost exclusively inhabited by thermophilic prokaryotic microorganisms, photosynthetic flexi bacteria and certain non-photosynthetic autotrophic and heterotrophic bacteria (Pentecost 2003, Banerjee and Castenholz 2007 (In Press), Norris and Castenholz 2007). In most extreme habitats the microbial communities which dominate are composed primarily of photosynthetic microorganism mainly the cyanobacteria.

Cyanobacteria, are a group of Gram-negative phototrophic prokaryotes which carryout oxygenic photosynthesis as well as nitrogen fixation. These blue green algae are ubiquitous in nature and have very simple nutrient requirement that allow these organisms to occupy highly diverse ecological niches. Maeda and Omata (2004); Banerjee and Verma (2007).

The hot water source contains most of the essential nutrients and permits a steady growth of cyanobacteria throughout the year. As the effluent moves away from the source of the spring the water cools, thus setting up a temperature gradient (Banerjee *et al.*, 2001; Banerjee and Sharma 2004). It is accompanied by concentration gradient of sulphides (decreasing) due to oxidation, oxygen (increasing) and pH (increasing) with concomitant gradual changes in the composition of the micro flora. Downstream as the temperature gradually decreases from 73°C to about 53°C, populations of unicellular and filamentous heterocystous cyanobacteria, forms deep green to reddish brown mats. These algae withstand 'or' tolerate a very high temperature. Castenholz (1969); (1977); Norris and Castenholz (2007) Banerjee and Sharma (2005). Thermophilic cyanobacteria have become an experimental system for the basic and applied research due to their unique properties. These include growth and temperature optima, habitat relationship, enzymatic abilities, and the study of pigments and the role in detecting evolution (Maheshwari *et al.*, 1987; Tomitani *et al.*, 1999; Whitton and Potts 2000).

Thermophilic Cyanobacteria

Temperature is an important environmental factor, which can create a series of challenges. A thermophile is an organism capable of living at temperature at 'or' near the maximum for the taxonomic group of which it is a part (Brock 1978; 1986; Ward and Castenholz 2000; Norris and Castenholz 2006). The blue-green algae are considered to be thermophilic when part or all of their optimal growth temperature range is above 45 °C (Castenholz 1969; Castenholz and Pierson 1995).

Thermophilic cyanobacteria have adopted themselves to wide range of ecological niches such as, thermal waters, geothermal hot spring, hot spring, volcano etc. (Madigan and Brock 1976). The thermal area is an area where warm water ascends through fissures, cervices and volcanic crust. Cold rainwater pours down into porous bedrock, is heated from the old magma chamber and fissures and ascends to the surface, as it gets hotter. Thermophilic cyanobacteria are predominant flora of thermal waters. The cyanobacteria are considered as thermophilic when their most favorable growth temperature range is above 45°C (Castenholz 1969). Setchell suggested the upper limit of temperature for cyanobacteria as 65° to 68°C and Lammerman described it as 69°C but we do have some cyanobacteria in the Yellowstone National Park USA grow at 95°C (Brock 1978; Castenholz 1996; Pentecost 2003; Norris and Castenholz 2006; Banerjee and Castenholz 2007) (In Press).

The morphological diversity of the cyanobacteria is considerable. Both unicellular and filamentous forms of thermophilic cyanobacteria are known and considerable variations with in these morphological types occur. Unicellular form like *Synechococcus elongates* found in cylindrical or ellipsoidal shape in thermal water where the temperature is above 75°C. *S. elongates* doesn't have heterocyst Desikachary (1959; Brock 1978; Castenholz 1969; Miller and Castenholz 2001; Bird and Wyman 2003). Filamentous type, like *Mastigocladus laminosus* forms single filament with one side branching and an intercalary heterocyst but hormogones are absent (Desikachary 1959; Stewart 1970; Wickstorm 1980; Jha *et al.*, 1986 Robinson *et al.*, 2007; Miller and Castenholz 2007). *Leptolyngbya*, a polyextremophile that can survive more than one extreme habitat like high temperature as well as high salt concentration, forms thin filaments with trichomes but without heterocyst (Rippka *et al.*, 1979; Anagnostidis and Komárek 1988; Albertano and Kovácik 1994; Castenholz 2001; Komárek and Anagnostidis 2005).

Distribution of Thermophilic Cyanobacteria

The water of hot springs may discharge at temperatures somewhat higher than the common boiling temperature, although superheated waters are uncommon except in volcanic regions (Ward and Castenholz 2000; Kiyoshi *et al.*, 2004). Generally thermal habitats are aquatic, and Earth is the only source of heat, for nearly all of these. In spite of that, solar radiation adequately increases the temperature in a few situations and the self-heating of organic material may bring localized temperature to the point of ignition Castenholz (1969). Hot springs and their drain ways provide the most adequate aquatic habitats for thermophilic blue-green algae. Cyanobacteria have been reported from thermal waters all over the world.

Natural geothermal areas are widely distributed around the Earth. Springs in which the water discharges at a temperature of over 45° C occur in every continent except Antarctica. The most studied biological sites are Yellowstone National Park Plateau of North America, Japan, Iceland, and North Island of New Zealand. The large numbers of hot springs are also widely scattered over most of the United States west of the Great Plains, the line of the Andes, Italy, Algeria-Tunisia, Greece, Turkey, portions of central Africa, central Asia, Indonesia, Philippines, Kamchatka Peninsula in Siberia, Naples area in Italy, Bakereshwar, West Bengal and Rajgir Bihar in India (Castenholz, 1969; Jana, 1970; 1973). Some prominent thermophilic cyanobacteria are *Chroococcales, Calothrix* sp., *C. thermalis, Aphanocapsa thermalis, Oscillatoria terebriformis, O. animalis, Spirulina* sp., *Phormidium laminosum, Mastigocladus laminosus, Synechococcus elongates, Synechococcus lividus, S. minervae, Phormidium tenue, Oscillatoria cf. terrbriformis* and *Leptolyngbya* that grow at very high temperatures.

Adaptation for Thermal Environment

These thermophilic cyanobacteria have very altered structural and metabolic differences from their normal counterparts that enable them to survive such adverse situations. Temperatures approaching 100°C normally denature proteins and nucleic acids, and increase the fluidity of membranes to lethal levels. Chlorophyll degrades above 75 °C, excluding photosynthesis (Rothschild *et al.*, 2001). In cyanobacteria lipids, nucleic acids and proteins are generally susceptible to heat and therefore there is no single factor that enables all thermophiles to grow at extreme temperature. High temperature increases the fluidity of membranes. To maintain optimal membrane fluidity the cell must adjust the composition of the membrane including the amount and type of lipids. The lipid membranes of thermophiles have saturated and straight chain of fatty acids to provide right degree of fluidity needed for membrane function. Some species contain paracrystalline surface layer that function as external protective barrier (Norris and Castenholz 2007; Rothschild *et al.*, 2001).

Temperature also effects the structure and function of proteins (Jaenicke, 1996). Ways that proteins have evolved to cope with high temperatures include increasing ion-pair content, forming higher-order oligomers and decreasing flexibility at room temperature. Decreasing the length of surface loops is also known; in particular those loops that connect elements of secondary structure, optimize electrostatic and hydrophobic interactions, and exchange amino acids to increase internal hydrophobicity and helix tendency of residues in α-helices. Heat shock proteins, chaperons are also present and are likely to play an important role in stabilizing and refolding of proteins as they begin to denature (Kallas and Castenholz, 1982a; Ferris *et al.*, 1997; Rothschild *et al.*, 2001).

DNA at high temperatures such as above 70°C is normally denatured. The DNA of hyperthermophiles is known to be more stable *in vivo* than that of a mesophile. Monovalent and divalent salts enhance the stability of nucleic acids because these salts screen the negative charges of the phosphate groups (Peak, *et al.*, 1995; Marguet, *et al.*, 1998; Rothschild, *et al.*, 2001). Thermophiles also have, histone like protein that protects DNA, and have reverse gyrase that is responsible for positive super coiling in DNA. The Guanine and Cytosine pair of nucleic acids is more thermostable than the Adenine and Thymine or Adenine and Urasil pairs because of the additional hydrogen bond.

But elevated G and C ratios are not found among thermophilic prokaryotes because of the stability of the chromosomal DNA, although thermo stability is correlated with G and C content of their ribosomal and transfer RNAs (Galtier *et al.*, 1997; 1999; Rothschild, *et al.*, 2001).

Importance

It is generally assumed that blue-green algae evolved in the early Precambrian period and were responsible for the first significant increase in atmospheric oxygen. Microfossils of cyanophyte like filaments have recently been found in early, middle, and late Precambrian strata. Fossils of the late Precambrian (about 1 billion years ago) resemble living members of the blue green algae (Swain, 1969; Schopf, 1968). The study of cyanobacteria from extreme thermophilic environments greatly expands our understanding of the survival of these organisms at very inhospitable environments. The cyanobacteria from extreme thermophilic environments have attracted great attention in recent years because of their ability to endure extreme environmental conditions and the regulatory mechanisms involved in the process of survival because, these microbes have several biotechnological applications. We can use thermophilic cyanobacteria as biofertilizers in region of very high temperatures because it is documented that thermophilic cyanobacteria like *Mastigocladus* can fix atmospheric nitrogen (Fogg, 1951; Stewart, 1970; Banerjee and Bhattacharya, 2001).

These microorganisms therefore produce unique biocatalyst that function under extreme condition comparable to those prevailing in various industrial processes. Some of the enzymes from extremophiles have already been purified and their genes successfully cloned in mesophilic host. These organisms therefore are very important biotechnologically with potential use in food, chemical and pharmaceutical industry as well as environmental biotechnology.

References

Albertano, P. and Kovácik, L. (1994). Is the genus *Leptolyngbya* (Cyanophyte) a homogeneous taxon? *Archiv für Hydrobiologie/Algological Studies* (75): 37–51.

Anagnostidis, K. and Komárek J. (1988). Modern approach to the classification system of cyanophytes 3–*Oscillatoriales*. *Archiv für Hydrobiologie/Algological Studies* (50–53) : 327–472.

Brock, T. D. (1976). Upper pH limit for the existence of blue-green algae: evolutionary and ecological implications. *Science*. (179): 480-483.

Brock, T. D. (1986). Introduction: An overview of the thermophiles. In *Thermophiles: General, Molecular and Applied Microbiology* (ed. Brock, T. D.), John Wiley and Sons, New York.; 1–16.

Brock, T. D. (1978) *Thermophilic Microorganisms and Life at High Temperatures*. Heidelberg, New York: Springer-Verlag.

Bargagli, R. Broady, F. A. and Walton, D. W. H. (1996). Preliminary investigation of the thermal biosystem of Mount Rittmon Fumaroles Northern Victoria Land Antarctica. *Antarctica Science*. (32): 239-250.

Banerjee, M. Verma, V. (2006). Nitrogen assimilation studies of four cyanobacteria from different ecological niches. *Indian Journal of Botanical Research*. 2 (2): 157-162.

Banerjee, M. Banik, J. and Bhattacharya, S. (2001). Influence of different physiological parameters on the N_2 fixation of *Mastigocladus*. *Journal of Nat. Con.* 14 (2): 8-12.

Banerjee, M. and Sharma, D. (2004). Regulation of phosphatase activity of *Chroococcidiopsis* isolates from two diverse habitats. Effect of light pH and temperature. *Applied Ecol. Environ. Res.* 2 (1): 71-82.

Banerjee M, Sharma D. (2005). Comparative studies on growth and phosphatase activity of endolithic cyanobacterial isolate *Chroococcidiopsis* from hot and cold deserts. *Journal of Microbiology and Biotechnology*. 15 (1): 125-130.

Banerjee, M. Castenholz, R.W. (2007). Characterization of a novel thermo-halophilic clade of cyanobacteria from saline thermal springs and endolithic habitats. *Environ. Microbiol* (In Press).

Bird C, Wyman M. Nitrate/Nitrite assimilation system of the marine picoplanktonic cyanobacterium *'Synechococcus'* sp. Strain WH 8103: (2003). Effect of nitrogen source and availability on gene expression. *Applied Environ. Microbiol*. 7009-7018.

Bhaya D, Schwarz R, Grossman A R. (2000). Molecular responses to environmental stress. In: Whitton BA. and Potts M. (eds) *Ecology of cyanobacteria, their diversity in time and space*. Kluwer Academic, Dordrecht.; 397- 442.

Castenholz, R. W. (1969). Thermophilic blue-green algae and the thermal environment. *Bacteriol. Rev*. 33:476–504.

Castenholz, R. W. (1977). The effect of sulfide on the blue-green algae of hot springs. II. Yellowstone National Park. *Microbiol Ecol*. (3) : 79-105.

Castenholz, R. W. and Pierson, B. K. (1995) *Ecology of Thermophilic Anoxygenic Phototrophs*. Kluwer, Dordrecht, The Netherlands.

Castenholz, R. W. (1996). Endemism and biodiversity of thermophilic cyanobacteria. *Nova Hedwigia* (112): 33–47.

Castenholz R.W. (2001). Oxygenic photosynthetic bacteria. In: D.R. Boone and R.W. Catenholz (eds) *Bergey's Manual of Systematic Bacteriology* (2nd edition), Springer?Verlag, New York: 473–600.

Desikachary T. V. (1959). *Cyanophyta*, Indian council of Agriculture Research. New Delhi.

Fogg, G. E. (1951). Studies on nitrogen fixation by blue-green algae. II. Nitrogen fixation by *Mastigocladus laminosus* Cohn. *J. Exp. Bot*. (2): 117.

Fleming DE, Castenholz RW. (2007). Effects of periodic desiccation on the synthesis of the UV-screening compound, scytonemin in cyanobacteria. *Environ. Microbiol*.; 9(6): 1448-1455.

Ferris, M. J. Nold, S. C. Revsbech, N. P., and Ward, D. M. (1997). Population structure and physiological changes within a hot spring microbial mat community following disturbance. *Appl Environ Microbiol*. (63): 1367-1374.

Galtier, N. and Lobry, J. R. (1997). Relationships between genomic G and C content, secondary structures and optimal growth temperature in prokaryotes. *J. Mol. Evol*. (44), 632.

Galtier, N., Tourasse, N. and Gouy, M. A (1999). Non-hyperthermophilic, common ancestor to extinct life forms. *Science* 283, 220–221.

Jana, B. B. (1970). On the study of limnology and bacteriology of the thermal springs of Bakreshwar *Ph.D. Thesis* Visva Bharti University Shantiniketan, India.

Jana, B. B. (1973). The thermal springs of Bakreshwar, India-physico-chemical conditions, Flora and Fauna. *Hydrobiologia*. (41): 291-307.

Jha M Ashok Kumar and H D Kumar (1986). Stimulation of *in vivo* nitrate reductase activity in the thermal cyanobacterium *Oscillatoria princeps* under microaerobic conditions. *Current Microbiology* (14): 145-147.

Jaenicke, R. (1996). Stability and folding of ultra stable proteins: eye lens crystallins and enzymes from thermophiles. *FASEB J.* (10): 84–92.

Kallas, T., Castenholz, R. W. (1982a). Internal pH and ATP-ADP pools in cyanobacterium *Synechococcus* sp. During exposure to growth–inhibiting low pH. *J. Bacteriol* (149): 229-236.

Komárek J. and Anagnostidis K. (2005). Cyanoprokaryota–2. Teil/2nd Part: Oscillatoriales. In: B. Büdel, L. Krienitz, G. Gärtner and M. Schagerl (ed.) *Süsswasserflora von Mitteleuropa* 19/2, Elsevier/ Spektrum, Heidelberg; 759 pp.

Kiyoshi O, Megumi M, Shino I, Kazuhisa O, and Masahiro I (2004). Circadian rhythms in the thermophilic cyanobacterium *Thermosynechococcus elongatus*: Compensation of Period Length over a Wide Temperature Range. *Journal of Bacteriology* (186): 4972-4977.

Lynn J. Rothschild and Rocco L Mancinelli (2001). Life in extreme environments. *Nature* (409): 1092-1101.

Madigan, M. T. Brock, T. D. (1977). Adaptation of hot spring phototrophs to reduced light intensity. *Arch. Microbiol.* (113): 111-120.

Marguet, E. and Forterre, P (1998). Protection of DNA by salts against thermo degradation at temperatures typical for hyperthermophiles. *Extremophiles* 2, 115–122.

Maeda, S. Omata, T. (2004). A novel gene (narM) required for expression of nitrate reductase activity in the cyanobacterium *Synechococcus elongates* strain PCC 7942. *J. Bacteriol.* (186): 2107-2114.

Norris, T. B. Castenholz, R. W. (2006). Endolithic photosynthetic communities with in ancient and recent travertine deposits in Yellowstone National Park. *FEMS Microbiol. Ecol.* 57 (3): 470–483.

Norris, T. B. Castenholz, R. W. (2007). Effect of environmental stressors on photosynthetic microorganisms in geothermal springs of Yellowstone National Park: Geothermal biology and Geochemistry in Yellowstone National Park. 221-234.

Peak, M. J. Robb, F. T. and Peak, J. G. (1995). Extreme resistance to thermally induced DNA backbone breaks in the hyperthermophilic archaeon *Pyrococcus furiosus*. *J. Bacteriol.* (177): 6316–6318.

Pentecost A. (2003). Cyanobacteria associated with hot spring travertines. *Can. J. Earth Sci.* (40): 1447-1457.

Rippka R., Deruelles J., Waterbury J.B., Herdman M. and Stanier R.Y. (1979). Generic assignments, strain histories and properties of pure cultures of cyanobacteria. *Journal of General Microbiology* (111): 1–61.

Robinson W. Brad Mealor, Augustus E., S Stevens, Jr. Edward and Mark Ospeck (2007). Measuring the Force Production of the Hormogonia of *Mastigocladus laminosus*. *Biophysical Journal* (93): 699-703.

Roeselers G, Norris TB, Castenholz RW, Rygaard S, Glud RN, Kühl M, Muyzer G. (2007). Diversity of photoautotrophic bacteria in microbial mats from Arctic hot springs (Greenland) *Environ. Microbiol.* 9(1): 26-38.

Schopf, J. W. (1968). Microflora of the Bitter Springs Formation, Late Precambrian, Central Australia. *J. Paleontol.* (42): 651-688.

Scott R. Miller Richard W. Castenholz, and Deana Pederse (2007). Phylogeography of the thermophilic cyanobacterium *Mastigocladus laminosus*. *Applied and Environmental Microbiology*. (73): 4751-4759.

Swain, F. M. (1969). Paleomicrobiology. *Annual Review Microbiol*. (23): 455-472.

Stewart W D P (1970). Nitrogen fixation by blue-green algae in Yellowstone thermal areas. *Phycologia*. (9): 261-268.

Tomitani A, Okada K, Miyashita H, Mathiys H C P, Ohno T and Tonak A. (1999). Chlorophyll *b* and phycobillins in the common ancestor of cyanobacteria and chloroplast. *Nature* (400): 159-162.

Wickstorm C E (1980). Distribution and physiological determinants of blue green algal nitrogen fixation along a thermogradient. *J. Phycol* (16): 436-443.

Ward, D. M. and Castenholz, R. W. (2000). In: *The Ecology of Cyanobacteria*, Eds. Whitton, B. A. and Potts, M. (Kluwer, Dordrecht, the Netherlands), pp. 37–59.

Microbial Biotechnology and Ecology (2011) *Pages* **41–59**
Editors: **Deepak Vyas, G.S. Paliwal, P.K.Khare and R.K Gupta**
Published by: **DAYA PUBLISHING HOUSE, NEW DELHI**

Chapter 4

Cyanobacteria: Phenotypic to the Genotypic Diversity

☆ *A. Srivastava, P. Singh, A. Singh, S.S. Singh and A.K. Mishra**

Laboratory of Microbial Genetics, Department of Botany, Banaras Hindu University, Varanasi – 221 005

ABSTRACT

Cyanobacteria, the pioneer model for evolution of photosynthetic machinery, have played an important role in the process of life sustenance on the planet. Their autotrophic nature in conjunction with the nitrogen fixation capacity of some of its members makes it an indispensable link in the carbon and nitrogen economy on the globe. They are the vital colonizers in all sorts of ecosystems varying from hot deserts to polar ice caps, rocky mountains to benthic locale, exposed soils to endosymbiotic milieu etc. Their caliber of such diverse habitation lies in the variety of morphological and physiological attributes that they can exhibit. For a long period, diversity assessment of cyanobacteria has been one of the prime objectives of microbiology researchers. Initially, morphological specifications in combination with cytochemical and physiological characteristics were the prime basis for cyanobacterial characterization. Any phenotypic character when considered alone is of less utility as it is generally shared by one or the other biological groups. Currently, increasing numeric and molecular taxonomic tools have widely aided, if not replaced the traditional morphological and physiological criteria. Protein, fatty acid and pigment analysis, isozyme profiling and nucleic acid studies are some of the presently used tools of taxonomy. Any particular trait when used in isolation, may lead to misleading results for identification, further classification and diversity assessment of the group. Therefore, a polyphasic top-to-bottom approach based on information reclaimed from techniques varying from microscopic observation to genome analysis provides better resolution at taxonomic level.

* E-mail: akmishraau@rediffmail.com.

Cyanobacterial Characteristics

Cyanobacteria (also called blue green algae) are gram negative photoautotrophic prokaryotes, stand at one of the major turnouts of evolutionary history. They are characterized by possession of machinery for synthesis of chlorophyll *a* and phycobilin. Apart from their flair for utilization of water (or H_2S under certain conditions) as an electron donor, some of its members also have a capacity for nitrogen fixation (Berman-Frank *et al.*, 2003; Bergman *et al.*, 1997). The evolutionary and ecological essence of cyanobacteria lies in the two above stated facets. Apart from chlorophyll *a* and *c*-phycocyanin production, it has capacity for synthesis of carotene and *c*-phycoerythrin (Prasanna *et al.*, 2007; Six *et al.*, 2004).

Cyanobacteria enjoy a very wide distribution. Most of them are freshwater forms except for a few like *Dermocarpa* and *Trichodesmium* which thrive well in marine locale. Terrestrial habitat is common for most of the species of *Nostoc* and *Oscillatoria*. Benthic habitation is also as common as planktonic one. Endophytic and symbiotic temperament of some distinguished species of this class such as *Nostoc, Anabaena, Chroococcus, Gloeocapsa, Scytonema,* and *Stigonema* forms a very fascinating aspect (Bergman *et al.*, 2007; Usher *et al.*, 2007; Carpenter and Foster, 2002; Perkins and Peters, 1993). The presence of cyanobacteria in freshwater blooms, marine ecosystems, soils and rice fields, within limestone, salt subjugated lands, deserts, polar environments and within other living forms highlight their propensity to survive in and moreover dominate the above niches (Whitton and Potts, 2000).

Members of cyanophyceae have a prokaryotic structure with an incipient type of nucleus, thylakoids and storage products called cyanophycean starch and cyanophycin granules (Fritsch, 1945; Kylin, 1943). Non existence of sex organs, gametes and flagellated zoospores grounds the way for vegetative and asexual reproduction. Vegetative reproduction occurs by cell division, fragmentation, hormogonium formation and asexual reproduction by means of akinetes, endospores, exospores, heterocysts and nannocytes.

As per the traditional botanical taxonomic conduct based on morphological and developmental attributes, cyanobacteria are currently alienated into five orders (Castenholz, 1989; Waterbury 1989; Waterbury and Rippka, 1989) that correspond closely to the five groups used by Stanier and his collaborators (Rippka *et al.*, 1979).

Chroococcales, the first order, comprises mainly of unicellular forms that reproduce by binary fission or budding but cell aggregates are equally prevalent. The members of order Pleurocapsales range from unicellular forms to cell aggregates that give rise to unicellular structures called 'baeocytes' (Pinevich *et al.*, 2008). They harbour an explicit feature of multiple fissions. All the undifferentiated filamentous cyanobacteria have been placed in the order Oscillatoriales. Trichome fragmentation or production of undifferentiated hormogonia (specialized reproductive trichomes) is the chief mode of reproduction. Members of the order Nostocales possess a unique property of cell differentiation. Normal cells can be specialized to form (a) heterocysts (specialized cells meant for nitrogen fixation), (b) akinetes and (c) hormogonia. Many members of this order are ecologically highly valued because of their role as converters of unusable dinitrogen to ammonia. The last order Stigonematales also comprises filamentous forms that can differentiate into a number of cellular subtypes. The only difference lies in the plane of binary fission as members of stigonematales can divide in multiple planes resulting in multiseriate trichomes (Whitton and Potts, 2000).

Characters such as prokaryotic cell construction, absence of division of labor, dearth of flagella and sexuality advocate their primitive nature. Paleontological, geological and isotopic geochemical substantiations have been instrumental in documenting the antiquity of cyanobacteria to early

Precambrian period. A considerably less rRNA sequence diversity has been reported among the members of this class as compared to other taxa (Giovannoni *et al.*, 1988). The above fact gives an obvious clue of a close knit phylogenetic relationship. Within the phylogenetic tree, members of Chroococcales and Oscillatoriales are omnipresent, members of Pleurocapsales show a single lineage and members of Nostocales and Stigonematales confirm a single coherent lineage. Cyanobacteria have been on the earth for over 3.5 billion years. During the course of the evolution, they have provided the major source of the oxygen and acquired several morphological, physiological, biochemical and molecular specialization, in order to survive best in diverse ecological conditions which ultimately leads to the evolution of diversified cyanobacteria.

Cyanobacterial Diversity

Cyanobacteria are a class that illustrates an assortment of diversities *viz.* morphological, habitat and physiological miscellany. The diversity it exhibits is visible in multitude of its metabolic tactics, motility, cell division, developmental biology and other structural and functional aspects of cell morphology. Thus, its diversity is seen at various levels *viz.* morphological, physiological and genetic. Morphological and physiological diversity can be a manifestation of either genetic or environmental factors. The correlations among all the factors taken into account reveal the overall similarity and contrast and this forms the basis of systematic groupings. The foundation for such groupings is the core fact that each and every organism is related through evolutionary decent (Luuc *et al.*, 1999). The investigation for International Code of Botanical Nomenclature (ICBN) included a wide range of eukaryotic and prokaryotic organisms and blue green algae (Geitler, 1932) were considered the largest prokaryotic group of organisms.

Morphological Diversity

Cyanobacteria are characterized by different types of cellular structures. Each order is characterized by some particular cell type. Unicellular, isopolar cyanobacteria occur in the order Chroococcales; pseudoparenchymatous in the order Pleurocapsales, and unicellular, heteropolar in the order Chamaesiphonales. Members of the order Oscillatoriales are multicellular, trichal and lack heterocyst while those of the order Nostocales have similar structure as that of oscillatoriales but with an added presence of heterocyst. Cyanobacteria of the order Stigonematales are also multicellular, trichal and heterocystous just like members of Nostocales, but their trichomes show proper branching (Komarek, 1994). Unicells may occur singly or grouped in colonies as reported in *Schizothrix*. Filamentous forms are also equally prevalent. The trichomes may be straight or coiled. Uniseriate and unbranched trichomes bearing absolutely identical cells are characteristic of the order Oscillatoriales. On the contrary, orders such as Nostocales and Stigonematales have trichomes bearing heterogeneous cellular composition. The branching pattern can be categorized as true or false. In true branching, cells in a filament can divide in more than one plane (*e.g. Haplosiphon*). In the case of false branching, division in a filament with a sheath occurs in such a way so as to give rise to two separate filaments that grow separately *e.g. Tolypothrix, Scytonema.*

In filamentous forms there are two modes of growth. In some filaments showing false branching patterns, growth is apical and the cells at the base die off simultaneous with growth. As a result of the above process, persistent sheaths present in some filamentous forms develop into a mass of old sheaths under the living material (*e.g. Scytonema*). In the other form of growth, cell divisions occur at the base of a sheathed trichome and consequently the apical cells become devoid of chlorophyll, become narrow, take the appearance of multicellular hair and their thylakoids rip apart in order to form liquid filled vacuoles (*e.g. Calothrix*).

Even cultivated strains of the same species (monospecies) do not always show exact similarity. They differ in their morphological features with respects to the varying growth conditions (Zapomelova, 2008; Gupta and Agarwal, 2006a, b; Lyra *et al.*, 2001; Nalewajko and Murphy, 2001; Gugger *et al.*, 2002a,b; Anand, 1988). Cyanophyceae exhibits lavish cellular and functional polymorphism in possession of different types of cells, with each one suited to a particular function.

This class enjoys cellular division of labour aided by a variety of cells. An akinete is a thick walled dormant cell derived from the enlargement of a vegetative cell (Moore *et al.*, 2005) and is much larger compared to latter. It depicts a resistant resting stage. The process of its derivation from vegetative cell is accompanied with immense thickening of cell wall so as to acquire entire protoplast within it. It is processed only under adverse conditions and circumstances leading to its formation vary among species and also among strains of monospecies (Whitton, 1992). Their occurrence is greatly constrained to heterocystous species, but may also be found in some non-filamentous species. Another specialized structure called gas vesicles/vacuoles are found in a number of aquatic species of many different genera such as *Anabaena* and are meant for buoyancy regulations. They are cylindrical in shape, filled with gas and are highly important for planktonic species and aid in adjustment of the cyanobacterium's vertical position in the water column (Walsby, 1987). Number of gas vesicles increases with reduction in light intensity and abating growth rate. Heterocysts are specialized nitrogen fixing cells that differentiate from vegetative cells in response to deprivation of fixed nitrogen *i.e.* ammonium or nitrate. In *Anabaena* spp., Nostoc spp. and many other strains, heterocysts differentiate at semiregular intervals along vegetative filaments, forming a spacing pattern. In *Gloeotrichia* spp., *Rivularia* spp. and other strains heterocyst occupy terminal position in the filaments while lateral heterocyst has been found in *Nostochopsis* sp. (Wolk 2000). The establishment and maintenance of the heterocyst spacing pattern depends upon two factors. Firstly, interaction between diffusible substances *i.e.* glutamine that originates from the heterocyst and move along the filament and secondly, other factors, presumably proteins that interact with diffusible substances and directly or indirectly control gene expression (Wolk 2000; Golden 2000; Mishra, 2003). All the cyanobacteria that form heterocyst are assorted in the orders Stigonematales and Nostocales which are characterized by branched and simple filaments respectively. Altogether they constitute a monophyletic group which shows very petite genetic variability (Anagnostids and Komarek, 1992). They may occur as solitary structures or in pairs as in *Anabaenopis*. They originate from vegetative cells that are slightly enlarged and possess pore at one or both poles. Such pores are usually present at single pole in case of terminal heterocysts. Differentiation of a vegetative cell to a heterocyst is unidirectional and the process cannot be reverted. Nitrogenase and other proteins involved in nitrogen fixation are synthesized within the heterocyst (Ernst *et al.*, 1992; Buikema *et al.*, 1991, 1993). They synthesize three additional cell walls, including one of glycolipid that forms a hydrophobic barrier to oxygen (Fay, 1992). Latter function is particularly important so as to protect the oxygen labile nitrogenase enzyme. For further enhancement of the above process they also degrade oxygen producing photosystem II within them. In conjugation with the above process, they up regulate the synthesis of glycolytic enzymes. Since the photosystem II is dismantled, heterocysts do not photosynthesize. They are provided with carbohydrates, mainly in the form of disaccharides, by vegetative cells. Heterocysts sustain photosystem I which permits ATP generation by cyclic photophosphorylation. In certain filamentous cyanobacteria, the function of nitrogen fixation is performed in typical cells called 'diazocytes' that may be joined together to form specialized portions of trichomes (Komárek and Anagnostidis, 2005). They posses the enzyme nitrogenase and are mainly found in non-heterocystous cyanobacteria such as *Trichodesmium, Oscillatoria* etc. (Ohki, 2008; El-Shehawy, 2003; Lugomela, 2002).

Hormogonia are short, motile chains of rather uniform cells (Desikachary, 1959), but this definition does not hold true for all hormogonia. More or less, they can be considered as motile filaments formed by some cyanobacteria in the family Nostocaceae which are responsible for conducting a number of indispensable physiological processes in cyanobacteria (Tandeau de Marsac, 1994). Being the smallest unit of infection, they are generally formed for the purpose of asexual reproduction in unicellular, filamentous forms and have affluent stores of nitrogen, phosphorus and other nutrients. Hormogonia can be dispersed either through their rapid motility on surface or even with the aid of gas vacuoles. Any unexpected environmental stress or transfer to a new medium can induce the differentiation of a cyanobacterium into hormogonium. In some genera such as *Rivularia*, a number of hormogonia are required for generation of a colony while in case of others such as *Nostoc*, colony originates from a single hormogonium. According to Herdman and Rippka (1988), a hormogonium possesses a lower number of genome copies as compared to vegetative cells. Nitrogen fixing plant cyanobacteria symbiosis (especially in case of genus *Nostoc*) is largely dependent on the formation of hormogonium. Plant host releases a 'hormogonium inducing factor' (HIF) that is recognized by the cyanobacterial symbiont. In response to this particular biochemical signal, the cyanobacterium differentiates into a hormogonium and further dedifferentiates back into vegetative cells after about 96 hours. By this time they manage to reach the desired site within their host.

Hormogonium is released from the end of a heterocystous trichome with the aid of a sacrificial cell called necridium. It facilitates division of some non-heterocystous forms and also formation of two daughter trichomes (Lamont, 1969).

Physiological and Habitat Diversity

Members of Cyanophyceae are ubiquitously present in numerous habitats ranging from hot springs to polar ice caps; dry soils to salt brines; plant roots to limestone etc. Their ability to inhabit all these extreme locales demonstrates the range of physiological modifications that they can undergo for survival. Each peculiar state of its existence reveals the amendments that it has to make at all possible levels of functional organization and hence is a mark of physiological diversity.

Cyanobacteria have been linked with freshwater blooms for times immemorial. A bloom generally comprises of only one or two species and the surface blooms are dominated by cyanobacteria capable of floatation with the help of gas filled cell inclusions called gas vacuoles. Members varying in structure from small filaments to large globular colonies can form blooms, for *e.g.* filamentous forms including *Anabaena*, *Nodularia*, *Gloeotricha*, *Oscillatoria*, *Spirulina* etc. and nonfilamentous forms such as *Microcystis*, *Coelosphaeria*, *Gomphosphaeria* etc. The filamentous forms often get twisted and entangled to form secondary aggregations (Reynolds and Walsby, 1975; Lewis, 1976) that leads to immense increase in the biomass. Shallow, well mixed, eutrophic lakes are dominated by *Oscillatoria*; clear water, temperate lakes are inhabited by *Aphanizomenon flos-aquae* and *Oscillatoria agardhii*; tropical waters experience a sequential growth of different cyanobacteria such as *Dactylococcopsis* (capable of growth in water at times of high nutrient availability and mixing and low light intensity), *Aphanotheceae* (growing under moderate to low nutrient availability, lesser turbulence and better light conditions), and some other genera such as *Microcystis aeruginosa* and *M. flos-aquae* are permanent inhabitants (Oliver and Ganf, 2000). Stratification in terms of nutrients, light intensity, turbidity etc. and seasonal periodicity determine the species dominating the habitat at a particular time. Appearance of bloom is not a sudden phenomenon, as it is normally thought. It is a physiological adaptation of already existing species in response to the changing environmental conditions. On calming down of water bodies carrying dispersed population of cyanobacteria, latter develop gas vacuoles and move upwards. There are several benefits associated with the buoyancy control such as, reduction in sedimentation losses (Reynolds, 1984), ability of better light harvest (Walsby *et al.*, 1997) and capacity to utilize the available nutrients in a better way (Ganf and Oliver, 1982). Phytoplanktonic forms also show a diversion from the normal nutrient cycle as an adaptation to the current requirement. Apart from carbohydrate accumulation they exhibit a lesser cell-specific quantum yield of photosynthesis (Turpin, 1991). The amount of limiting nutrient (nitrogen, phosphorus or others depending on the water body) within the cell gets highly reduced (Riegman and Mur, 1984) and an augmentation in the specific uptake rate of the limiting nutrient (Kromkamp, 1987; Riegman and Mur, 1984) is generally observed. Inclusion of many representatives from the family Nostocaceae indicate nitrogen fixation being performed under nitrogen limiting conditions during phytoplankton growth.

The oceanic environment is generally considered unproductive or oligotrophic and short of essential nutrients. Even then, former can sustain a variety of cyanobacteria ranging from picoplanktons (<5 mm), nanoplanktons (5–20 mm) to microplanktons (>5 mm). They act as major carbon fixers (*Synechococcus, Synechocystis* and *Prochlorococcus*) and also as dinitrogen fixers (*Trichodesmium, Nodularia* etc.) when present in nitrogen deplete waters. The localizers vary from unicellular (solitary–*Synechococcus, Aphanothece* and colonial–*Merismopedia*) to filamentous forms (heterocystous–*Anabaena, Richelia* and non-heterocystous–*Lyngbya, Spirulina*). Apart from showing adaptations to tolerate nutrient deficiency, most of them are also capable of tolerating saline conditions. Though nitrogen fixation gets highly hampered under increasing salt concentrations, other metabolic processes are stabilized by synthesis of compatible osmolytes (Reed and Stewart, 1985).

Cyanobacteria dwelling on and below soils withstand a variety of stresses such as desiccation, pH alterations, ultra violet radiation, low light intensity, mineral and nutrient deficiency and presence of herbicides and pesticides. Water and salt stress tolerance is prevalent in many species but they are not abundant in soils with pH less than 6. Contrary to the above fact, they can thrive well at low pH if the temperature is considerably high as in tropical soils. There have been prior documentations of use of cyanobacteria as a biofertilizer for reclamation of saline (usar) soils in India (Singh, 1961). *Microcoleus* is perhaps the most widespread cyanobacteria in saline soils (Whitton, 1990). According to Shibata (1969), some cyanobacteria accumulate colorless UV absorbing compounds which are members of a family of mycosporine-like amino acid derivatives (MAAs) (Garcia-Pichel and Castenholz, 1993; Sinha *et al.*, 1998). Cyanobacteria living on the soil surface generate dark coloration as an adaptive strategy against short wavelength insolation. The pigment 'scytonemin' is responsible for the dark colour and is capable of absorbing UV radiation (Garcia-Pichel and Castenholz, 1991). Those species which are present under soil are skilled for photosynthesizing at low photon flux densities (van Liere and Walsby, 1982). Studies have been performed on herbicide, fungicide and pesticide resistance in cyanobacteria (Peterson *et al.*, 1997; Das and Adhikary, 1996; Tiwari *et al.*, 1991). Results have shown that *Anabaena, Nostoc* and *Oscillatoria* are found to be tolerant to Fentin derivatives and sodium dithiocarbamate (Bisiach, 1970) and in general nitrogen fixing cyanobacteria are comparatively tolerant to 2,4 D (2,4-dichlorophenoxy acetic acid) (Leganes and Fernandez-Valiente, 1992).

Cyanobacterial occupants are diversely scattered from extremely hot to cold desert ecosystems. Desert dwellers can be divided into soil crust species, *e.g. Lyngbya, Phormidium, Plectonema* (Friedmann and Galun, 1974) etc. and *Nostoc commune, Anacystis montana, Oscillatoria lutea, Schizothrix calcicola* etc. particularly in cold deserts (Cameron, 1971); epilithic species such as *Gloeocapsa* spp., *Stigonema minutum, Calothrix* spp. etc. (Broady, 1989); and endolithic species such as *Hormathonema, Gloeocapsa* (Friedmann *et al.*, 1993). They have adopted several strategies to combat typical stresses found in such environments–EPS mucilage production for adhesion to substratum (Cameron and Devaney, 1970);

absorption of snow, water vapour and sheltered growth to overcome low humidity (Vestal, 1988; Palmer and Friedmann, 1990); production of trehalose and polyols to combat desiccation (Potts, 1994); and sunscreens such as caretenoids for tolerance of high light intensity (Downes *et al.*, 1993); reallocation of carbon and nitrogen, autotrophy and symbiosis under oligotrophic conditions (Friedmann and Ocampo, 1976; Vestal, 1988) and several other sunscreens to tolerate UV radiation (Garcia-Pichel and Castenholz, 1991).

Cyanobacteria are believed to not only survive but thrive optimally in harsh conditions like high latitude, glaciers, ice shelves, streams, ponds and lakes (Vincent, 2000). Some common species found in this extreme habitat are *Calothrix parietina* (Wharton *et al.*, 1983), *Phormidium frigidum*, *Nodularia harveyana*, *Lyngbya martensiana* etc. The importance of cyanobacteria is highlighted in areas like exposed moraines after the retreat of glaciers where they act as primary colonizers. They display a high degree of resilience as the optimum temperature for their growth ranges from 15 to 30°C and they still show tolerance for temperatures around 5°C. Apart from temperature regulatory adaptations, they share same desiccation, UV, light and salinity tolerance mechanisms as present in desert inhabiting cyanobacteria.

Some strains can tolerate free sulphide much better than other eukaryotic algae (Whitton and Potts, 2000; Padan and Cohen, 1982) and further many can even utilize H_2S in place of H_2O as a hydrogen donor (Cohen *et al.*, 1975). Under some circumstances, certain cyanobacteria show well elaborated circadian rhythms (Kondo and Ishiura, 1999) to accord with the fluctuating light and temperature during the day (Whitton and Potts, 2000).

Biochemical and Molecular Diversity

Taxonomy of cyanobacteria has been a highly debatable topic and has undergone several revisions (Turner *et al.*, 1999; Turner, 1997; Wilmotte and Golubic, 1991; Komarek, 1994). Bacteriological criteria have gained more importance than botanical criteria and major consideration for taxonomic determination depends heavily on morphological and physiological attributes. Latter are the consequences of various environmental and growth conditions. Sometimes these characters can even be lost during cultivation. Such contemplations among cyanobacteria lead to inaccurate identification and classification among taxa (Nelissen *et al.*, 1992). At present, cyanobacterial diversity assessment depends reliably on chemotaxonomic parameters including whole cell protein, isozyme analysis, fatty acid profiles, carotenoids or mycosporine like amino acids (Prasanna and Kaushik, 2005). These techniques are of particular interest in case of toxic cyanobacteria as toxicity is very insignificantly related to morphology. Therefore, differentiation of toxic and non-toxic cyanobacteria on morphological basis is barely possible (Golubic *et al.*, 2009). Difference in the protein profile has been utilized in number of instances. SDS-PAGE of whole cell protein has been used to obtain heterozygosity among planktonic filamentous cyanobacteria (Lyra *et al.*, 1997). MALDI-TOF MS analysis of oligopeptides within a natural population of *Microcystis* spp. revealed possession of a particular group of peptides by individual species (Fastner *et al.*, 2001). Cluster analysis among *Azolla* isolated cyanobionts (Sood *et al.*, 2007) and among *Anabaena* (from 6 *Azolla* species), *Notoc* (from *Anthoceros* sp., *Cycas* sp. and *Gunnera monoika*) and certain free living cyanobacteria (Sood *et al.*, 2008) disclosed taxonomic relationships based on whole cell protein profiles and molecular markers. Another important criterion is based on zymogram analysis and isozyme profile is considered a tool of utility for taxonomic studies at species and genus level (Holton, 1981). Heterogeneity in band pattern was observed between two unicellular strains, *Synechococcus* sp. strain PCC 6301 and *Synechococcus elongates* strain CCAP 1497/1 (Schenk *et al.*, 1973) where no common bands were found, in marine phytoplankton (Medlin *et al.*, 2000) and among axenic *Anabaena* sp. strains where five enzymes were studied (Stulp and Stam, 1984). α-esterase isozyme pattern was earlier studied in *Phormidium* strains (Klein *et al.*, 1973) and similarity obtained in zymograms of *Phormidium ectocarpi* strain PCC 7375 and *Phormidium persicinum* strain CCAP 1462/5 was used for their assignment to the same species (Wilmotte, 1994). Utility of phycoerythrin synthesis ability (Bryant, 1982) and fatty acid profile (Kenyon *et al.*, 1972) as a taxonomic marker has been well established. Fatty acid profiling has been used as a biochemical marker in various studies such as diversity assessment in 66 cyanobacetrial strains (Kenyon, 1972; Kenyon *et al.*, 1972), among free living strains of *Nostoc* and *Anabaena* (Caudales *et al.*, 1992) and marine picoplankton (Merritt *et al.*, 1992). A valuable unknown highly polar glycolipid was reported (Sallal *et al.*, 1990) which was found only in three heterocystous strains (namely *Anabaena Cylindrica*, *Nostoc canina* and *Nostoc muscorum*) studied (Wilmotte, 1994).

Still, analyses of photosynthetic pigment content, isoenzyme variation or differentiated cell culture may also be misleading because of the variable expression of cyanobacterial gene products in culture (Kato *et al.*, 1991; Rippka *et al.*, 1979). Morphological changes are based on factors such as cell dimensions and ecology which are not very reliable for distinct separation as per the species definition (Nubel *et al.*, 1997). This creates a vacuum in taxonomic studies which can be fulfilled by speculations based on molecular and genetic data. An appropriate blend of phylogenetic, phenotypic and genotypic analysis forms the basis of an unwavering form of taxonomy known as 'polyphasic taxonomy' (Luuc *et al.*, 1999; Vandamme *et al.*, 1996). A combination of genetic and phenotypic strategies aid in enhancement of methodology for complex natural community analysis (Rudi *et al.*, 2000; Nubel *et al.*, 1999). There are several examples of contradictions between phylogenetic results obtained on the basis of morphological and molecular data. For example, *Nostoc* PCC 7120 was formerly regarded as *Anabaena* species and *Nostoc* PCC 6720 was at one time described as *Anabaenopsis* (Henson *et al.*, 2002). On the basis of morphological characteristics and life cycle differences, *Nostoc* and *Anabaena* were traditionally placed in different groups (Turner *et al.*, 1999; Turner, 1997; Wilmotte, 1994). But now, 16S rRNA studies have shown that *Nostoc* and *Anabaena* are closely related. *Fischerella* spp. and *Chlorogloeopsis* spp. are placed in stigonematales order based on true branching; however, the two genera are clearly distinguished on the basis of 16S rRNA sequences (Wilmotte, 1994). From the above discussion it can made out that due to environmental influences on morphological characteristics, the use of morphological or physiological data or even biochemical data is insufficient. Under such circumstances, analysis of molecular data becomes the most effective and valued method of determining genetic variability and evolutionary relationships among cyanobacteria. Genotypic characters such as DNA-RNA hybridization and DNA base composition are a direct indication of relatedness of various organisms that can serve as taxonomic markers for phylogenetic purpose (Wood and Townsend, 1990; Lachance, 1981; Herdman *et al.*, 1979). Among molecular parameters, amplification and sequence analysis of hypervariable and conserved region of 16S rRNA, *nifH*, *nifD* and PC-IGS regions are most widely used to detect genetic relatedness and molecular phylogeny within the cyanobacteria. The 16S rRNA molecule contains variable regions (Woese, 1987); it is very highly conserved and can be instrumental in studying species identity (Fox *et al.*, 1992) or intra-species variation. *NifH* and *nifD* genes possess a highly conserved region as well as a great divergence in other regions. The molecular analysis of highly variable and conserved sequence of 16S rRNA and nitrogenase (*nifH* and *nifD*) genes (*i.e.* highly conserved throughout the evolution) will not only provide a stable genetic marker but will also serve to infer the phylogenetic relationship among the heterocystous cyanobacteria. DNA sequences of a fragment *nifH* and *nifD* from about diverse cyanobacterial strains were amplified, cloned and sequenced to determine the evolutionary relationship within cyanobacteria as a group

(Henson *et al.*, 2004; Zehr *et al.*, 1995). Studies examining the 16S rRNA have indicated that morphological characters may not coincide with molecular data in cyanobacteria.

PCR/RFLPs/RAPDs are among the most popular techniques employed by cyanobacteriologists to obtain more precise and genuine data about the cyanobacterial diversity and their phylogenetic relationship. PCR-amplified fragments can be used as substrate for RFLP or sequence analysis.

RAPD is a type of PCR reaction in which DNA segments are randomly amplified. Short arbitrary primers are used for binding to their specific sequence in a large template of genomic DNA (Bardakci, 2001). Its advantage lies in the fact that no prior knowledge of the entire genome is required for its operation. This technique allows random identification of polymorphisms at genetic level and aids in deducing phylogenetic relationships. This method has certain drawbacks which limit its application. From the band pattern obtained as a result of RAPD-PCR, it is difficult to make out whether a DNA segment is amplified from a heterozygous or a homozygous locus. The interpretation of RAPD results becomes difficult at times because of mismatching between the primer and the template resulting in total absence of PCR products. Apart from these technical downsides, it is cumbersome, non-reproducible at times and varies with handling due to involvement of various components as have been reported by number of workers (Hansen *et al.*, 1998; Newbury and Ford-Lloyd, 1993). A slightly modified and highly precise method of genomic fingerprinting involves the use of DNA primers corresponding to naturally occurring interspersed repetitive elements such as REP (Repetitive Extragenic Palindromic) and ERIC (Enterobacterial Repetitive Intergenic Consensus) sequences. PCR conducted by using both of these as primers is highly reproducible and comparatively simple for distinguishing closely related strains, inferring phylogenetic relationships and their diversity consideration in a variety of habitats (Lyra *et al.*, 2001; Rasmussen and Svenning, 1998).

RFLP analysis of DNA can be also used for genetic and phyletic analysis. This tool is of great help in identifying even minor variations in sequences if they are present in restriction sites. Another modification of this technique is 'Terminal Restriction Fragment Length Polymorphism (TRFLP). This technique was earlier used for characterization of bacterial communities in mixed-species samples, and is now used for other rhizoforms (Jin-Book *et al.*, 2004; Frias-Lopez *et al.*, 2003). Here, the primer pairs are labeled with fluorescent tags. After amplification with these specially tagged primers, PCR products are digested with restriction enzymes and the resulting sequences are visualized with a DNA sequencer.

Differentially, PCR products can also be analyzed through Denaturing Gradient Gel Electrophoresis (DGGE) (Boutte *et al.*, 2006). Here, non-descriptive similar sized PCR products can be differentiated as they move through increasingly higher concentrations of chemical denaturant. The weaker melting domains get fixed earlier as their threshold denaturant concentration is encountered earlier. This results in a pattern of bands in which each band represents a specific population.

RAPD has been used in identification of several organisms to strain level (Hadrys *et al.*, 1992). Neilan *et al.* (1995) performed RFLP of PCR products with a range of 4-base pair recognizing restriction endonucleases. 40 toxigenic strains of freshwater cyanobacteria belonging to genera *Anabaena*, *Microcystis*, *Aphanizomenon*, *Nodularia*, *Nostoc*, *Oscillatoria*, *Pseudomonas* and *Synechococcus* were analyzed; 28 equally parsimonious trees were obtained by using the DOLLOP programme from the PHYLIP package and the strains were clustered into two distinct groups. PCR fingerprinting using short tandemly repeated repetitive (STRR) sequence was performed by Zheng *et al.* (1999) to determine genetic diversity in cyanobacteria residing in different species of *Azolla*. The banding pattern depicted that cyanobacteria from *Euazolla* section showed similarity and this pattern was precisely different from that of *Rhizosperma* section. The occurrence of similar sized four clustered bands in cyanobacterial isolates from all *Azolla* species shows a common monophyletic origin. Costa *et al.* (2001) used RAPD with primers specific for the tRNA^{leu} gene in *Nostoc* species present in symbiotic relationship with two species of thalloid bryophytes, *Anthoceros fusiformis* and *Blasia pusilla*. Results confirmed that several different strains of *Nostoc* are involved in symbiosis but single bryophyte thalli never contained colonies with a mixture of different intron sequences. RAPD analysis of 17 different cyanobacterial cultures derived from 6 different decamer primers (Jeberlin Prabina *et al.*, 2005) provide diagnostic fingerprints for each culture and their genetic distance (Perumal *et al.*, 2009). RAPD of genomic DNA using 7 different primers was used for identification and phylogenetic analysis of 12 cyanobacterial strains belonging to genera *Oscillatoria* and *Lyngbya* by Perumal *et al.* (2009). Some of the strains showed close genetic relationship while two *Lyngbya* strains were grouped separately.

16S rRNA/rDNA cloning, sequencing and further analytic reconstruction is one of the most popular bases for phylogenetic grouping and biodiversity assessment of cyanobacteria (Robertson, 2001; Turner *et al.*, 1999; Schmidt *et al.*, 1991; Giovannoni *et al.*, 1990; Giovannoni *et al.*, 1988). Comparative analysis with the aid of 16S rRNA gene sequence is a proper way to explore the discrepancy between strain collections and natural communities (Garcia-Pichel *et al.*, 1998, 1996). Application of DNA array hybridization using nonspecific labeling of the nucleic acid to 16S rDNA and 16S rRNA (Guschin *et al.*, 1997) is a powerful cyanobacterial appraisal tool. Rudi *et al.* (2000) investigated the presence and abundance of cyanobacteria in natural habitats using sequence specific labeled 16S rRNA gene probe. A good correlation was observed among the cyanobacterial groups *i.e.* *Nostoc*, *Microcystis* and *Planktothrix* spp. in the selected mesotrophic and eutrophic lakes. West and Adams (1997) did PCR amplification using either short arbitrary primers or primers specific for the regions flanking the 16S-23S rRNA internal transcriber spacer to evaluate the diversity of cyanobacterial symbionts from the hornwort *Phaeoceros laevis*. Even a single bryophyte thallus showed diverse populations of *Nostoc* strains but a single strain never occurred at more than one field site. *Anabaena* and *Aphanizomenon* were considered to be distinct on the basis of morphological characters (Gugger *et al.*, 2002a, b) but were shown to be highly similar on the basis of 16S rDNA profile (Gugger *et al.*, 2002; Lyra *et al.*, 2001). Thacker and Paul (2004) tried to use taxonomic relationships among several collections of *Lyngbya* spp. and *Symploca* spp. One of the various parameters taken into consideration was 16S rDNA sequence. A pair wise sequence divergence of 10 to 14 per cent was observed across 605 bp of 16S rDNA among the collected species (Thacker and Paul, 2004). Phylogenetic deduction on the basis of 16S rDNA sequences clearly voiced the reciprocal monophyly of *Lyngbya* and *Symploca*. Owing to the complexity of the 16S rDNA and 16S rRNA analysis, it is not suited for large-scale screening. Apart from 16S rRNA analysis, nitrogenase genes can also be employed for diversity estimation. Genes for nitrogenase enzyme complex are highly conserved and contain valuable taxonomic information (Ben-Porath and Zehr, 1994). Phylogenetic analysis of nucleotide sequence of *nifD* was used by Henson *et al.* (2004) to verify the distribution of heterocystous cyanobacteria belonging to subsections IV and V. Heterocystous cyanobacteria can be considered monophyletic but none of the subsections can be said to be monophyletic. Members of both subsections show intermixing in two sister clades and hence there is no meaning of two isolated subsections (Henson *et al.*, 2004). *NifH* analysis has been done to evaluate genetic diversity analysis of diazotrophs in the rice rhizosphere (Wartiainen *et al.*, 2008). Haande *et al.* (2008) characterized new isolates of *Cylinrospermopsis raciborskii* from Europe and Africa by sequencing *nifH* along with ITS1, PC-IGS and *rpoC1*. Within the African isolates and the European isolates, the amplified *nifH* gene showed 100 per cent sequence similarity while the similarity between the isolates from the two different continents was >93.3 per cent. All the parameters produced similar tree topology (Haande *et al.*, 2008). However 16S rRNA/rDNA and *nif* gene data show contamination with bacterial samples. To overcome this hindrance, study of phycocyanin gene has proved to be an influential tool. The PC operon consists of genes coding for 2 bilin subunits and 3 linker polypeptides (BelKnap and Hazelkorn, 1987). The intergeneric spacer (IGS) between the two bilin subunits–β (cpcB) and α (cpcA) is a highly variable region of DNA sequence and therefore serves prominently for cyanobacterial identification at strain level. Neilan *et al.* (1995) amplified the PC-IGS region of 44 cyanobacterial strains with specifically designed primers. The strains were distinctly grouped according to the results of RFLP data. In an attempt to validate the assumption that isolates able to grow in laboratory culture are representative of the entire diversity within the natural population, Hayes and Barker (1997) amplified the PC-IGS region of *Nodularia* strains taken from clonal cultures as well as natural populations. More variation was found among the culture isolates as compared to specimens from natural population. Bittencourt-Oliveira *et al.* (2001) used PC-IGS region amplification as a means to determine the genetic variability among 15 Brazilian strains of *Microcystis aeruginosa* and compare it with reference strains of *Microcystis aeruginosa*, *M. viridis*, and *M. wesenbergii*. Nucleotide sequences of the *cpc*BA IGS and flanking regions unambiguously stated that Brazilian strains classified as *M. aeruginosa* are phylogenetically diverse from the reference strains of *M. aeruginosa*. Phylogenetic analysis of *Anabaenopsis abijatae* and *Anabaenopsis elenkinii* from tropical inland water bodies of Kenya and Mexico showed low similarity value in PC-IGS sequences and thus the two clusters indicated two separate genera (Ballot *et al.*, 2008). Sequence analysis of ITS and *cpc*BA-IGS showed high level of differentiation between *Pseudoanabaena* isolates demonstrated considerable microdiversity (Acinas *et al.*, 2009).

Conclusion

Cyanobacteria are a diverse and cosmopolitan group possessing a number of unique properties. Their pliability for divergent atmospheric and vicinity situations is the major reason for their widespread existence. Members of this group are deemed as pioneers of life on earth. Their importance as primary producers, nitrogen fixers, and source of antibiotics, antifungal agents, restriction enzymes and pharmaceutically important products highlight the importance of their existence in biosphere. Their taxonomic classification has been based on morphological and physiological attributes that are prone to variations because of environmental and culture conditions. With this view, it has become important to analyze the characters and phylogeny of cyanobacteria on a larger canvas. Latter demands data analyses made on the basis of molecular parameters such DNA/RNA sequence of 16S ribosomal RNA, *nif* genes, phycocyanin genes etc. Advancements made in last two decades have enlightened the subject of cyanophycean description to a great extent. It is expected that an appropriate amalgamation of phenotypic, physiological and molecular surveillance will floor the way for cyanobacterial study to infinitesimal details.

Acknowledgement

Authors are thankful to the CSIR and DST, New Delhi for their financial support. Head, Department of Botany, BHU, Varanasi is gratefully acknowledged for their help and support.

References

Acinas, S.G., Haverkamp, H.A., Huisman, J. and Stal, L.J. (2009). Phenotypic and genetic diversification of *Pseudoanabaena* spp. (cyanobacteria). *The ISME J.* 3: 31-46.

Anagnostidis, K. and J. Komarek (1989). Modern approach to the classification system of Cyanophytes. 4–Nostocales. *Algological Studies* 56: 247–345.

Anand, N. (1988). Culture studies and taxonomy of blue-green algae–certain identification problems. *Arch. Hydrobiol. Suppl.* 80: 141–147.

Bardakci, F. (2001). Random amplified polymorphic DNA (RAPD) markers. *Turk J Biol.* 25: 185-196.

Bellknap, W.R. and Haselcorn, R. (1987). Cloning and light regulation of expression of the phycocyanin operon of the cyanobacterium *Anabaena. EMBO J.* 6: 871-884.

Ben-Porathj, Zehr J. (1994). Detection and characterization of cyanobacterial *nif*H genes. *Appl. Environ. Microbiol.* 60: 880-887.

Bergman, B. Gallon, J.R., Rai, A.N. and Stal, L.J. (1997). N_2 fixation by non-heterocystous cyanobacteria. *FEMS Microbiol Rev.* 19: 139-185.

Bergman, B., Rasmussen, U. and Rai, A.N. (2007). Cyanobacterial associations. In: Associative and Endophytic Nitrogen-Fixing Bacteria and Cyanobacterial Associations. Elmerich, C. and Newton, W.E. (ed) 5: 257–301. Dordrecht: Kluwer Acad.

Berman-Frank, I., Lundgren, P. and Falkowski, P. (2003). Nitrogen fixation and photosynthetic oxygen evolution in cyanobacteria. *Res Microbiol.* 154: 157-164.

Bisiach, M. (1970). Primi dati sulle infestazioni algali da cianoficee nelle risiae italiane. *Riso.* 19: 129-134.

Bittencourt-Oliveira, M.C., Oliveira, M. and Bolch, C.J.S. (2001). Genetic variability of brazilian strains of the *Microcystis aeruginosa* complex (Cyanobacteria/Cyanophyceae) using the phycocyanin intergenic spacer and flanking regions (*cpc*BA). *J. Phycol* 37: 810–818.

Broady, P.A. (1989). Survey of algae and other terrestrial biota at Edward VII peninsula, Marie Byrd Land. *Antarct Sci.* 1: 215-224.

Bryant, D.A. (1982). Phycoerythrocyanin and phycoerythrin: properties and occurrence in cyanobacteria. *J Gen Microbiol* 128: 835–844.

Boutte C., Grubisic, S. Balthasart, P. and Wilmotte, A. (2006). Testing of primers for the study of cyanobacterial molecular diversity by DGGE. *J. Microbiol Methods.* 65(3): 542-550.

Buikema, W.J and Haselkorn, R. (1991). Characterization of a gene controlling heterocyst differentiation in the cyanobacterium Anabaena 7120. *Genes Devel* 5: 321–330.

Cameron, R.E. and Devaney, J.R. (1970). Antarctic soil algal crusts. A scanning electron and microscope study. *Trans Am Microsc Soc.* 80: 264-273.

Carpenter, E.J and Foster, R.A. (2002). Marine Cyanobacterial Symbioses. In: Rai, A.N., Bergman, B. and Rasmussen, U. (eds) *Cyanobacteria in symbiosis.* pp. 11-17, Kluwer Academic Publishers, The Netherlands.

Castenholz, R.W. and Waterbury, J.B. (1989). Cyanobacteria (eds.) Staley, J.T., Bryant, M.P., Pfennig, N., and Holt, J.H. *Bergey's Manual of Systematic Bacteriology,* Vol. 3. Section 19: Oxygenic photosynthetic bacteria. Williams and Wilkins, Baltimore.

Caudales, R., Wells, J.M. andAntoine, A.D. (1992). Cellular fatty acid composition of symbiotic cyanobacteria isolated from the aquatic fern *Azolla. J Gen Microbiol* 138: 1489–1494.

Cohen, Y.J., Padan, E. and Shilo, M. (1975). Facultative anoxygenic photosynthesis in the cyanobacterium *Oscillatoria limnetica. J. Bacteriol.* 123: 855-863.

Costa, J.L., Paulsrud, P., Rikkinen, J. and Lindblad, P. (2001). Genetic Diversity of *Nostoc* Symbionts Endophytically Associated with Two Bryophyte Species. *Appl Env Microbiol.* 67(9): 4393-4396.

Das, M.K. and Adhikary, S.P. (1996). Toxicity of three pesticides to several rice-field cyanobacteria. *Tropical Agriculture* 73: 155-157.

Desikachary, T.V., (1959). Cyanophyta. Indian Council of Agricultural Research, New Delhi. 686 pp.

Downes, M.T., Hrstich, L. and Vincent, W.F. (1993). Extraction of chlorophyll and caretenoid pigments from Antarctic benthic mats for analysis by HPLC. *J. Appl Phycol.* 5;623-628.

El-Shehawy, R., Lugomela, C., Ernst, A. and Bergman, B. (2003). Diurnal expression of *hetR* and diazocyte development in the filamentous non-heterocystous cyanobacterium *Trichodesmium erythraeum*. *Microbiol* 149: 1139-1146.

Ernst, A., Black, T., Cai, Y., Panoff, J.M., Tiwari, D.N. and Wolk, C.P. (1992). Synthesis of nitrogenase in mutants of the cyanobacterium *Anabaena* sp. strain PCC 7120 affected in heterocyst development or metabolism. *J Bacteriol* 174: 6025–6032.

Fastern, J., Erhard, M. and Von Dohren, H. (2001). Determination of Oligopeptide Diversity within a Natural Population of *Microcystis* spp. (Cyanobacteria) by Typing Single Colonies by Matrix-Assisted Laser Desorption Ionization–Time of Flight Mass Spectrometry. *Appl Env Microbiol.* 67(11): 5069-5076.

Fay, P. (1992): Oxygen relations of nitrogen fixation in cyanobacteria. *Microbiol. Rev.* 56: 340-373.

Fox, G.E., Wisotzkey, J.D. and Jurtshuk. P. Jr. (1992). How close is close: 16S rRNA sequence identity may not be sufficient to guarantee species identity. *Int. J. System. Bacteriol.* 42: 166–170.

Frias-Lopez, J., Bonheyo, G.T., Jin, Q. and Fouke, B.W. (2003). Cyanobacteria associated with coral black band disease in Caribbean and Indo-Pacific reefs. *Appl Env Microbiol.* 69(4): 2409-2413.

Friedmann, E.I., Kappen, L., Meyer, M.A. and Nienow, J.A. (1993). Long-term productivity in the cryptoendolithic microbial community of the Ross desert, Antarctica. *Microb Ecol.* 25: 51-69.

Friedmann, E.I. and Ocampo, R. (1976). Endolithic blue-green algae in the dry valleys. Primary producers in the Antarctic desert ecosystem. *Sci.* 193: 1247-1249.

Fritsch, F.E. (1945). Structure and function of the algae, Vol II, Cambridge University Press.

Ganf, G.G. and Oliver, R.L. (1982). Vertical separation of light and available nutrients as a factor causing replacement of green algae by blue-green algae in the plankton of a stratified lake. *J. Ecol.* 70: 829-844.

Garcia-Pichel, F. and Castenholz, R.W. (1991). Characterization and biological impliations of scytonemin, a cyanobacterial sheath pigments. *J. Phycol.* 27: 395-409.

Garcia-Pichel, F. and Castenholz, R.W. (1993). Occurrence of UV-absorbing, mycosporine-like compounds among cyanobacterial isolates and an estimate of their screening capacity. *Appl Env Microbiol.* 59: 163-169.

Geitler, L. (1932). Cyanophyceae. In: Rabenhorst's Kryptogamenflora von Deutschland, Österreich und der Schweiz, Leipzig, Akad. Verslagsges. 1932. Reprinted 1971, New York, Johnson, pp. 1-1196.

Giovannoni, S.J., Turner, S., Olsen, G.J., Barns, S., Lane, D.J. and Pace, N.R. (1988). Evolutionary relationships among cyanobacteria and green chloroplasts. *J. Bacteriol* 170: 3584-3592.

Giovannoni, S.J., Britschgi, T.B., Moyer, C.L. and Field, K.G. (1990). Genetic diversity in Sargasso Sea bacterioplankton. *Nature.* 345: 60-63.

Golden, J.W., Whorff, L.L. and Wiest, D.R. (1991). Independent regulation of *nifHDK* operon transcription and DNA rearrangement during heterocyst differentiation in the cyanobacterium *Anabaena* sp. strain PCC 7120. *J. Bacteriol*. 173: 7098-7105.

Golubic, S., Abedb, R.M.M., Palinskac, K., Pauillacd, S., Chinaine, M. and Laurent, D. (2009). Marine toxic cyanobacteria: Diversity, environmental responses and hazards. *Toxicon* (in press).

Gugger, M., Lyra, C., Suominen, I., Tsitko, I., Humbert, J.F., Salkonoja-Salonen, M.S. and Sivonen, K. (2002a). Cellular fatty acids as chemotaxonomic markers of the genera *Anabaena, Aphanizomenon, Microcystis, Nostoc* and *Planktothrix* (cyanobacteria). *Int J Syst Evol Microbiol* 52: 1007–1015.

Gugger, M., Lyra, C., Henriksen, P., Coute, A., Humbert, J.F. and Sivonen, K., (2002b). Phylogenetic comparison of the cyanobacterial genera *Anabaena* nad *Aphanizomenon*. *Int J Syst Evol Microbiol*. 52: 1867-1880.

Gupta, S. and Agrawal, S.C. (2006a). Survival of blue-green and green algae under stress conditions. *Folia Microbiol*. 51: 121–128.

Gupta, S. and Agrawal, S.C. (2006b). Motility in Oscillatoria salina as affected by different factors. *Folia Microbiol*. 51 565–572.

Haande, S., Rhorlack, T., Ballot, K., Skulberg, R., Martin, B. and Wiedner, C. (2008). Genetic characterization of *Cylindrospermopsis raciborskii* (Nostocales, Cyanobacteria) isolates from Africa and Europe. *Harmful Algae*. 7(5): 692-701.

Hadrys, H., Balick, M. and Schierwater, B. (1992). Applications of random amplified polymorphic DNA (RAPD) in molecular ecology. *Mol. Ecol*. 1(1): 55-63.

Hayes, P.K. and Barker, G.L.A. (1997): Genetic diversity within Baltic Sea populations of *Nodularia* (Cyanobacteria). *J. Phycol*. 33: 919-923.

Henson, M., Hallden, C. and Sall, T. (1998): Error Rates and Polymorphism Frequencies for Three RAPD Protocols. Pl Mol Biol Reporter. 16(2): 139.

Henson, B.J., Watson, L.E. and Barnum, S.R. (2002). Molecular differentiation of the heterocystous cyanobacteria, *Nostoc* and *Anabaena*, based on complete *nifD* sequences. *Curr Microbiol* 45: 161–164.

Henson, B.J., Hesselbrock, S.M., Watson, L.E. and Barnum, S.R. (2004). Molecular phylogeny of the heterocystous cyanobacteria (subsections IV and V) based on *nifD Int. J. System. Evol. Microbio.*, 54: 493-497.

Herdman, M. and Rippka, R. (1988). Cellular differentiation: Hormogonia and baeocytes. *Methods Enzymol*. 167: 232-242.

Herdman, M., Janvier, M., Waterbuyr, J.B., Rippka, R. and Stanier, R.Y. (1979). DNA base composition of cyanobacteria. *J. Gen. Microbiol*. 111: 63–71.

Jeberlin Prabina, B., Kumar, K. and Kannaiyan, K. (2005). DNA amplification fingerprinting as a tool for checking genetic purity of strains in the cyanobacterial inoculum. World J. Microbiol. Biotechnol. 21: 629-634.

Jin-Book, K., Mi-Sook, M., Dong-Hun, L., Sung-Taik, L., Marco, B. and Chi-Kyung, K. (2004). Comparative analysis of cyanobacterial communities from polluted reservoirs in Korea. *J. Microbiol*. 42(3): 181-187.

Kato, T., Watanabe, M.F. and Watanabe, M. (1991). Allozyme divergence in microcystis and its taxonomic inference. *Arch. Hydrobiol*, 64: 129-140.

Kenyon, C.N. (1972). Fatty acid composition of unicellular strains of blue-green algae. *J Bacteriol* 109: 827–834.

Kenyon, C.N., Rippka, R. and Stanier, R.Y. (1972). Fatty acid composition and physiological properties of some filamentous blue-green algae. *Arch Mikrobiol* 83: 216–236.

Klein, S. Chapman, D.J. and Garber, E.D. (1973). Chemotaxonomy of the *Oscillatoria-Phormidium* complex. *Biochem Syst* 1: 173–177.

Komarek, J. (1994). Current trends and species delimitation in the cyanoprokaryote taxonomy. In: , Cyanobacteria, Morphology, Taxonomy, Ecology, Toxicology: Proceedings of the 12th Symposium of the International Association for Cyanophyte Research (IAC), (eds. Cronberg, G., O.M. Skulberg, and T. Willen), Sjoarp (Sweeden) 1992. *Algological Studies* 75: 11-29.

Komarek, J. and Anagnostidis, K. (2005). Cyanoprokaryota, 2. Teil: Oscillatoriales. Heidelberg: Elsevier/ Spektrum.

Kondo, T. and Ishiura, M. (1999). The circadian clocks of plants and cyanobacteria. *Trends in Pl Sci.* 4(5): 171-175.

Kromkamp, J. (1987). Formation and functional significance of storage products in cyanobacteria. *N Z J Mar Freshwater Res* 21: 457-465.

Kylin, H. (1943). Zur biochemie der rhodophyceen. Forh. Kgl. Fysiograf. Sallsk. I Lund 13b: 1-13.

Lachance, M.A. (1981). Genetic relatedness of heterocystous cyanobacteria by deoxyribonucleic acid-deoxyribonucleic acid reassociation. *Int. J. Syst. Bacteriol.* 31: 139–147.

Lamont, H.C. (1969): Sacrificial cell death and trichome breakage in an Oscillatorean Blue-Green Alga: the role of murein. *Arch Microbiol.* 69: 237-259.

Leganes, F.and Fernandez-Valiente, E. (1992). Effects of phenoxy acetic herbicides on growth, photosynthesis, and nitrogenase activity in cyanobacteria from rice fields. *Archives of Environmental Contamination and Toxicology*. 22: 130–134.

Lewis, W.M. (1976). Surface/Volume Ratio: implications for phytoplankton morphology. *Science*. 192: 885-887.

Lugomela, C., Lyimo, T., Bryceson, I., Semesi, A.K. and Bergman, B. (2002). *Trichodesmium* in coastal waters of Tanzania: diversity, seasonality, nitrogen and carbon fixation. *Hydrobiologia* 477: 1–13.

Luuc, Mur R., Skulberg, O.M. and Utkilen, H. (1999). Cyanobacteria in the environment. In: Chorus, I. and Bartram, J. (eds) Toxic cyanobacteria in water; A guide to their public health consequences, monitoring and management, WHO.

Lyra, C., Hantula, J., Vainio, E., Rapala, J., Rouhiainen, L. and Sivonen, K. (1997). Characterization of cyanobacteria by SDS-PAGE of whole-cell proteins and PCR/RFLP of the 16S rRNA gene. *Arch Microbiol.* 168: 176-184.

Lyra, C., Suomalainen, S., Gugger, M., Vezie, C., Sundman, P., Paulin, L. and Sivonen, K. (2001). Molecular characterization of planktic cyanobacteria of *Anabaena, Aphanizomenon, Microcystis,* and *Planktothrix* genera. *Int. J. Syst. Evol. Microbial.* 51: 513-526.

Medlin, L.K., Lange, M. and Nothig, E. (2000). Genetic diversity in the marine phytoplankton: a review and a consideration of Antarctic phytoplankton. *Antarctic Sci.* 12(3): 325-333.

Mishra, A.K. (2003): Fox- and Fix-mutants of Anabaena 7120 defective in heterocyst development and nitrogen fixation. *Algol Stud.* 108, pp. 75-85.

Moore, D., O'Donohue, M., Garnett, C., Critchley, C. and Shaw, G. (2005). Factors affecting akinete differentiation in *Cylindrospermopsis raciborskii* (Nostocales, Cyanobacteria), *Freshwater Biol.* 50(2), pp. 345–352.

Nalewajko, C. and Murphy, T.P. (2001). Effects of temperature, and availability of nitrogen and phosphorus on the abundance of Anabaena and Microcystis in Lake Biwa, Japan: an experimental approach. *Limnology* 2: 45–48.

Neilan, B.A., Jacobs, D. and Goodman, A.E. (1995). Genetic diversity and phylogeny of toxic cyanobacteria determined by DNA polymorphism within the phycocyanin locus. *Appl Environ Microbiol* 61: 3875-3883.

Nelissen, B., Wilmotte, R., De Baere, R., Haes, F., Van de Peer, Y., Neefs, J.M. and R. de Wachter (1992). Phylogenetic study of cyanobacteria on the basis of 16S ribosomal RNA sequences, *Belg. Journ. Bot.* 125: 210-213.

Newbury, J.H. and Ford-Lloyd, B.V. (1993). The use of RAPD for assessing variation in plants. *Pl Growth Reg.* 12(1-2): 43-51.

Nubel, U., Garcia-Pichel, F. and Muyzer, G. (1997). PCR primers to amplify 16S rRNA genes from cyanobacteria. *Applied and Environmental Microbiology.* 63: 3327-3332.

Nubel, U., Garcia-Pichel, F., Kuhl, M. and Muyzer, G. (1999). Quantifying microbial diversity: morphotypes, 16S rRNA genes, and carotenoids of oxygenic phototrophs in microbial mats. *Appl. Environ. Microbiol.* 65: 422-430.

Ohki, K. (2008). Intercellular localization of nitrogenase in a non-heterocystous cyanobacterium (cyanophyte) *Trichodesmium* sp. NIBB1067. *J Oceanography.* 64(2);211-216.

Oliver, R.L. and Ganf, G.G. (2000). Freshwater blooms. In: Whitton, B. A. and Potts, M. (eds) The Ecology of Cyanobacteria, pp. 149–194. Kluwer Academic Publishers.

Padan, E. and Cohne, Y. (1982). Anoxygenic photosynthesis. In: Carr, NG and Whitton, BA (eds) *The biology of cyanobacteria*.pp 215-235. Blackwell, Oxford and University of California Press, Berkeley.

Palmer, R.J.J. and Friedmann, E.I. (1990). Water relations and photosynthesis in the cryptoendolithic microbial habitat of hot and cold deserts. *Microb Ecol.* 19: 111-118.

Perumal, G.M., Ganesan, V. and Anand, N. (2009). Identification and phylogenetic analysis of filamentous Cyanobacteria using random amplified polymorphic DNA (RAPD) fingerprinting. *African J Biotech.* 8(6): 974-978.

Perkins, S.K. and Peters, G.A. (1993). The *Azolla-Anabaena* symbiosis: endophyte continuity in the *Azolla* life-cycle is facilitated by epidermal trichomes. I. Partitioning of the endophytic *Anabaena* into developing sporocarps. *New Phytol.* 123: 53-64.

Peterson, H.G., Boutin, C., Freemark, K.E. and Martin, P.A. (1997). Toxicity of hexazinone and diquat to green algae, diatoms, cyanobacteria and duckweed. *Aquatic Toxicol.* 39: 111-134.

Pinevich, A.V., Averina, S.G., Gavrilova, O.V. and Migunova, A.V. (2008). Baeocytes in the cyanobacterium Pleurocapsa sp.: Characterization of the differentiated cells produced by multiple fission. *Microbiol.* 77(1): 62-68.

Potts, M. (1994). Dessication resistance of prokaryotes. *Microbiol Revs.* 58: 755-805.

Prasanna, A. and Kaushik, B.D. (2005). Algal diversity- from morphology to molecules. In: Satyanarayana, T. and Johri, B.N. (eds) Microbial diversity: current perspectives and potential applications. pp. 323-344. International Publishing House Pvt. Ltd., New Delhi.

Prasanna, R., Sood, A., Suresh, A., Nayak, S. and Kaushik, B.D. (2007). Potentials and applications of algal pigments in biology and industry. *Act Biol Hungarica.* 49(1-2): 131-156.

Rasmussen, U. and Svenning, M.M. (1998). Fingerprinting of Cyanobacteria Based on PCR with Primers Derived from Short and Long Tandemly Repeated Repetitive Sequences.*Appl Env Microbiol.* 64(1): 265-272.

Reed, R.H. and Stewart, W.D.P. (1985). Osmotic adjustment and organic solute accumulation in unicellular cyanobacteria from planktonic and marine habitats. *Mar Biol.* 88: 1-9.

Reynolds, C.S. and Walsby, A.E. (1975). Water blooms. *Biol. Rev.*, 50: 437–481.

Riegman, R. and Mur, L.C. (1984). Regulation of phosphate uptake kinetics in *Oscillatoria agardhii. Arch Microbiol.* 139: 28-32.

Rippka, R., Deruelles, J., Waterbury, J.B., Herdman, M. and Stanier, R.Y. (1979). Genetic assignments, strain histories and properties of pure culture of cyanobacteria. *J.Gen. Microbiol.*, 111: 1-61.

Robertson, B.R., Tezuka, N.R. and Watanabe, M.M. (2001). Phylogenetic analyses of Synechococcus strains (cyanobacteria) using sequences of 16S rDNA and part of the phycocyanin operon reveal multiple evolutionary lines and reflect phycobilin content. *Int J Systm Evol Microbiol.* 51: 861-871.

Rudi, K., Skulberg, O.M., Skulberg, R. and Jacobsen, K.S. (2000). Application of Sequence-Specific Labeled 16S rRNA Gene Oligonucleotide Probes for Genetic Profiling of Cyanobacterial Abundance and Diversity by Array Hybridization. *Appl Env Microbiol.* 66(9): 4004-4011.

Sallal, A.K., Nimer, N.A. and Radwan, S.S. (1990). Lipid and fatty acid composition of freshwater cyanobacteria. *J Gen Microbiol* 136: 2043–2048.

Schenk, H.E.A., Hofer, I. and Metzner, H. (1973). Malat-Dehydrogenase Isoenzymbanden als potentielles chemotaxonomisches Kriterium für Cyanophyceen-Species. *Biochem System* 1: 179–184.

Schmidt, T.M., Delong, E.F. and Pace, N.R. (1991). Analysis of a marine picoplankton community by 16S rRNA gene cloning and sequencing. *J. Bacteriol.* 173(14): 4371-4378.

Shibata, K. (1969). Pigments and a UV-absorbing substance in corals and a blue green alga living in the Great Barrier Reef. *Plant Cell Physiol.* 10: 325-335.

Sinha, R.P., Klisch, M., Groniger, A. and Hader, D.P. (1998). Ultraviolet-absorbing/screening substances in cyanobacteria, phytoplankton and macroalgae. *J. Photochem. Photobiol. B: Biol.* 47: 83-94.

Six, C., Thomas, J.C., Brahmsha, B., Lemoine, Y. and Partensky, F. (2004). Photophysiology of the marine cyanobacterium *Synechococcus* sp. WH8102, a new model organism. *Aqua Microbiol Ecol.* 35: 17-29.

Sood, A., Prasanna, R. and Singh, P.K. (2007). Fingerprinting of freshly separated and cultured cyanobionts from different *Azolla* species using morphological and molecular markers. *Aqua Bot.* 2: 142-147.

Sood, A., Prasanna, R., Prasanna, B.M. and Singh, P.K. (2008). Genetic diversity among and within cultured cyanobionts of diverse species of *Azolla*. *Folia Microbiol.* 53(1): 35-43.

Stulp, B.K. and Stam, W.T. (1984). Genotypic relationships between strains of *Anabaena* (Cyanophyceae) and their correlation with morphological affinities. *Br Phycol J* 19: 287–301.

Tandeau de Marsac, N. (1994). Differentiation of hormogonia and relationships with other biological processes. In: Bryant, DA (ed) The molecular biology of cyanobacteria, pp. 825-842. Kluwer Academic Publishers, Dordrecht, The Netherlands.

Tiwari, D.N., Kumar, A. and Mishra, A.K. (1991). Use of cyanobacterial diazotrophic technology in rice agriculture. *Appl Biochem Biotechnol.* 28/29: 387-396.

Thacker, R.W. and Paul, V.J. (2004). Morphological, chemical and genetic diversity of tropical marine cyanobacteria *Lyngbya* spp. And *Symploca* spp. (Oscillatoriales). *Appl and Env Microbiol.* 70(6): 3305-3312.

Turner, S. (1997). Molecular systematics of oxygenic photosynthetic bacteria. *Plant syst Evol.* 11: 13-52.

Turner, S., Pryer, K., Miao, V. and Palmer, J. (1999). Investigating deep phylogenetic relationships among cyanobacteria and plastids by small subunit rRNA sequence analysis. *J. Eukaryote Microbiol.* 46: 327-338.

Turpin, D.H. (1991): Effect of inorganic N availability on algal photosynthesis and carbon metabolism. *J. Phycol* 27: 14-20.

Usher, K.M., Bergman, B. and Raven, J.A. (2007). Exploring cyanobacterial mutualisms. *Ann Rev Ecol Evol Systm.* 38: 255-273.

Vestal, J.R. (1988). Carbon metabolism in the cryptoendolithic microbiota in the Antarctic desert. *Appl Env Microbiol.* 54: 960-965.

Van Liere, L. and Walsby, A.E. (1982). Interactions of cyanobacteria with light. In: Carr, NG and Whitton BA (eds) The biology of Cyanobacteria, pp. 9-45. Blackwell Scientific Publications, Oxford.

Vandamme, P., Pot, B., Gillis, M., De Vos, P., Kersters, K. and Swings, J. 1996. Polyphasic taxonomy, a consensus approach to bacterial systematics. *Microbiol. Rev.* 60: 407-438.

Vincent, W.F. (2000). Cyanobacterial fominance in the polar regions. In: Whitton, BA and Potts, M (eds) The ecology of cyanobacteria. pp. 321-340. Kluwer Academic Publishers, The Netherlands.

Walsby, A.E., Hayes, P.K., Boje, R. and Stal, L.J. (1997). The selective advantage of buoyancy provided by gas vesicles for planktonic cyanobacteria in the Baltic Sea. *New Phytol.*, 136, 407–417.

Wartiainen, I., Eriksson, T., Zheng, W. and Rasmussen, U. (2008). Variation in the active diazotrophic community in rice paddy-*nif*H PCR-DGGE analysis of rhizosphere and bulk soil. *Appl Soil Ecol.* 39(1): 65-75.

Waterbury, J.B. (1989). Subsection II, order Pleurocapsales Geitler 1925, emend. Waterbury and Stanier 1978. In: Staley JT, Bryant MP, Pfennig N and Holt JG (eds) *Bergey's Manual of Systematic Bacteriology*, Vol 3, pp. 1746–1770. Williams and Wilkins Co., Baltimore.

Waterbury, J.B. and Rippka, R. (1989). Subsection I, order Chroococcales Wettstein 1924, emend. Rippka *et al.*, 1979. In: Staley JT, Bryant MP, Pfennig N and Holt JG (eds) Bergey's Manual of Systematic Bacteriology, Vol 3, pp. 1728–1746. Williams and Wilkins Co, Baltimore.

West, N.J. and Adams, D.G. (1997). Phenotypic and genotypic comparison of symbiotic and free-living cyanobacteria from a single field site. *Appl. Environ. Microbiol.* 63: 4479-4484.

Wharton, R.A., Parker, B.C. and Simmons, G.M. (1983). Distribution, species composition and morphological algal mats (stromatolites) in Antarctic dry valley lakes. *Phycologia.* 22: 355-365.

Whitton, B.A. (1990). *Microcoleus.* In: Kumar HD (ed) Phycotalk, pp. 173-182. Rastogi Publications, Meerut, India.

Whitton, B.A. (1992). Diversity, ecology, and taxonomy of the cyanobacteria. In: Mann NH and Carr NG (eds) Photosynthetic Prokaryots, pp. 1-51. Plenum, New York.

Whitton, B.A. and Potts, M. (2000). The ecology of cyanobacteria. Kluwer Academic Publishers, The Netherlands.

Wilmotte, A. (1994). Molecular evolution and taxonomy of cyanobacteria. In: Bryant D (ed) The molecular biolgy of cyanobacteria. Netherlands: Kluwer Academic Publishers, pp, 1-25.

Wilmotte, A. and Golubic, S. (1991). Morphological and genetic criteria in the taxonomy of cyanophyta/ cyanobacteria. *Arch. Hydribio.* Suppl. 64: 1-24.

Wilmotte, A. (1994). Molecular Evolution and Taxonomy of the Cyanobacteria. In: Bryant, A. (ed) The molecular biology of cyanobacteria, pp. 1-25. Kluwer Academic Publishers, The Netherlands.

Woese, C.R. (1987). Bacterial evolution. *Microbiol Rev.* 51(2): 221-271.

Wolk, C.P. (2000). Heterocyst formation in *Anabaena.* In: Brun, YV, Shimkets, LJ (eds) Prokaryotic development. American Society of Microbiology, pp 83-104, Washington, D.C.

Wood, A.M. and Townsend, D. (1990). DNA polymorphisms within the WH7803 serogroup of marine *Synechococcus* spp. (cyanobacteria). *J. Phycol.* 26: 576–585.

Zapomelova, E., Hrouzek, P., Rehakova, K., Sabacka, M., Stibal M., Caisova, L., Komarkova, J. and Lukesova, A. (2008). Morphological variability in selected heterocystous cyanobacterial strains as a response to varied temperature, light intensity and medium composition. *Folia Microbiol.* 53(4): 333-341.

Zehr, J. P., Mellon, M.T., Braun, S., Litaker, W., Steppe, T. and Paerl, H.W. (1995). Diversity of heterotrophic nitrogen Fixation genes in a marine cyanobacterial mat. *Appl Environ Microbiol* 61: 2527-2532.

Zehng, W.W., Nilsson, M., Bergman, B. and Rasmussen, U. (1999). Genetic diversity and classification of cyanobacteria in different Azolla species by the use of PCR fingerprinting. TAG Theor Appl Gen. 99(7-8): 1187-1193.

Microbial Biotechnology and Ecology (2011) *Pages* **60–93**
Editors: **Deepak Vyas, G.S. Paliwal, P.K.Khare and R.K Gupta**
Published by: **DAYA PUBLISHING HOUSE, NEW DELHI**

Chapter 5

Hydrogen Production by Cyanobacteria

☆ *Deepak Vyas*[1]* *and Rajan Kumar Gupta*[2]

[1]*Department of Botany, Dr. H.S. G. University, Sagar – 470 003, M.P.*
[2]*Government P.G. College, Rishikesh, Uttranchal*

Introduction

First of all Jackson and Ellms (1896) reported that *Anabaena* species from a massachusetts reservoir immediately produced H_2 when placed in a sealed bottle. Whether H_2 production was by algae or by contaminationg bacteria is still unclear. There was a considerable gap in this area of research since the first report appeared. It was in 1942, that gaffron and Rubin demonstrated H_2 production by anaerobically incubated *Secnedesmus obliquus*, a green alga, and since then this alge has become a major focus of research for H_2 metabolism. Blue-green algae again came into focus when the occurrence of a reversible hydrogenase was demonstrated in a unicellular blue green alga *synechococcus elongatus* obviously after several hours of anaerobic preincubation (Frenkel *et al.*, 1950). Studies on H_2 metabolism by blue-green algae restarted only after the unequivocal report of N_2 fixation by this group of algae. The real H_2 production mediated by the nitrogenase enzyme complex was first of all reported in *Anabaena cylindrical* under in vitro conditions by Haystead *et al.* (1970). Subsequently H_2 production by intact filaments of *A. cylindrica* in the light under an atmosphere of argon and CO_2 was reported by Benemann and Weare (1974a,b). In the same year H_2 production by other cyanobacteria was independently reported by Russian worklers (Oshchepkov *et al.*, 1974). Since then extensive work has been done on various aspects of H_2 metabolism employing a variety of blue-green algal strains (Tamagnini *et al.*, 2002; Vyas and Kumar, 1995; Vyas and Gupta, 2003; Vyas, 2004) (Table 5.1).

---

* E-mail: dvyas64@yahoo.co.in

Enzymes Involved in H_2 Metabolism

Nitrogenase

Nitrogenase, a typical enzyme present in all the N_2–fixing microorganisms, forms H_2 both under in vivo and in vitro conditions with normal growth at the expense of dinitrogen, nitrogenase reduces N_2 to ammonia under consumption of electrons, protons, and ATP. Some of the reduced protons are evolved as H_2. H_2 formation by a blue-green algal nitrogenase was first of all demonstrated in vitro by Haystead and coworkers (1970). Nitrogenase has been isolated and purified by a number of workers (see Stewart, 1980; Lambert and Smith, 1981; fay and Van baalen, 1987).

Table 5.1: Important Reviews on H_2 Metabolism of Blue-green Algae (Cyanobacteria)

1.	Benemann 1977
2.	Benemann and Hallenbeck 1978
3.	Bothe *et al.*, 1978
4.	Schlegel and Schneider 1978
5.	Hallenbeck and Benemann 1979
6.	Benemann *et al.*, 1980
7.	Bothe *et al.*, 1980
8.	Lambert and Smith 1981
9.	Bothe 1982
10.	Kerfin and Boger 1982
11.	Kumazawa ans Mitsui 1982
12.	Houchins 1984
13.	Robinson *et al.*, 1986
14.	Calvin and Taylor 1989
15.	Tamagnini *et al.*, 2002
16.	Vyas and Kumar 1995
17.	Vyas and Gupta 2003
18.	Vyas, 2004

Hydrogenases

Nitrogenase/Hydrogenase

When nitrogenase specifically produces H_2 in an ATP-dependent reaction, such nitrogenase is preferably called as hydrogenase. This hydrogenase is basically a nitrogenase enzyme and shares all the properties of a typical nitrogenase.

Reversible Hydrogenase/Soluble Hydrogenase/Bidirectional Hydrogenase

This enzyme may catalyze either uptake or evolution of H_2 and is called reversible hydrogenase. Reversible hydrogenase couples to a low potential electron carrier (with Emnear- O.4.V). This is easily solubilized, evolves hydrogen from reduced methyl viologen, and catalyzes the reduction of phenazine methanosulfate, methylene blue, and dichloropheno lindophenol with PMS being the most effective electron acceptor.

Uptake Hydrogenase/Unidirectional Hydrogenase

This enzyme is membrane bound, saturated by low H_2 tension, and is capable of reducing methylene blue but not low-potential acceptors. In the heterocystous, nitrogen-fixing cyanobacteria, possession of a unidirectional hydrogenase enables them to catalyze the H_2 consumption reactions typical of anaerobically adapted algae, and at the same time, probably increases the efficiency of H_2 fixation in these organisms. This enzyme also takes part in the oxy-hydrogen reaction in a number of blue-green algae (Lambert and Smith, 1981b). Evidence has been presented that this hydrogenase is capable of recycling some of the energy lost as hydrogen by supplying nitrogenase with some form of reductant (Benemann and Weare, 1974a; Lambert and Smith, 1981b). This uptake "hydrogenase" enzyme is particularly active in heterocysts and is weakly or not at all expressed in NH^+_2–grown and heterocyst-free filaments of cyanobacteria (Lambert and Smith, 1981b).

The Capacity to Metabolize H_2 Species Distribution

Table 5.2 lists the names of blue-green algal species capable of metabolizing H_2. Earlier there was a belief that only heterocystous cyanobacteria fix N_2. But with the discovery that non-heterocystous forms fix N_2 under aerobic and/or anaerobic conditions, the number of N_2–fixer species has increased drastically. So far all the N_2-fixing species tested have shown the capacity of evolve H_2. Thus hydrogenase has now been reported from all sections of blue-green algae, *viz.*, unicellular, non-heterocystous filamentous and heterocystous-filamentous species. Nevertheless, the number of hydrogenases present in different species shows considerable differences. Thus it is possible for an organism to possess methylviologen- dependent hydrogen formation only under the specified growth conditions, nitrogenase and uptake hydrogenase only, nitrogenase only, uptake hydrogenase only or none of these activities under the conditions tested. Species like *Anabaena cylindrica* possess all three activities *viz.*, nitrogenase, uptake hydrogenase and reversible hydrogenase under N_2–fixing conditions, but methylviologen dependent H_2 formation, when grown in ammonium salts. Figure 5.1 outlines the general scheme showing the inter-relationship between vegetative cell and heterocyst.

Table 5.2: Occurrence of Hydrogenase in Blue-green Algae (Cyanobacteria)

Species	References
A. Unicellular	
Anacystis nidulans	Eisbrenner *et al.*, 1981 Peschek 1979a
Aphanothece holophytica	Belkin and Padan 1978
Cyanothece sp. 7822	Van der Oost *et al.*, 1987
Gloeocapsa species	Gallon *et al.*, 1974
Gloeothece sps.6909	Van der Oost *et al.*, 1987
Cyanophora paradoxa	Eisbrenner *et al.*, 1981
Microcystis aeruginosa	Asada and Kawamura 1985
Synechococcus elongatus	Frenkel *et al.*, 1950
Synechococcus sp. strain Miami Bg043511	Arai and Mitsui 1987
Synechococcus cedorum	Gerasimenko and Zavarzin 1981
Synechococcus sp.7425	Van der Oost *et al.*, 1987
Synechococcus sp.	Frenkel and Rieger 1951
B. Non heterocystous filamentous	
Lyngbya sp. 108	Kuwada and Ohta 1987
Myxosarcina chroococcoides	Lambert and Smith 1980
Oscillatoria limnetice	Belkin and Padan 1978
Oscillatoria brevis	Lambert and Smith 1980
Oscillatoria thiebautii	Scranton *et al.*, 1987
Oscillatoria sp. Miami BG–7	Kumazawa and Mitsui 1981
Plectonema boryanum	Pàdan and Schneider 1978
Phormidium angustissimum	Gerasimenko and Zavarzin 1981
Phormidium laminosum	Smith *et al.*, 1982
Spirulina sp.	Liama *et al.*, 1979
Schizothrix calciola	Lambert and Smith 1980

Contd...

Table 5.2–Contd...

Species	References
C. Heterocystous-filamentous forms	
Anabaena cylindrica	Hattori 1963
Anabaena sp. N-7363	Asada *et al.*, 1985
Anabaena variabilis	Eisbrenner and Bothe 1979 Almon and Boger 1984
Anabaena azollae	Peters *et al.*, 1977 Chen Ven *et al.*, 1983
Anabaena sp.	Jones *et al.*, 1976
Anabaena 7120	Peterson and Burris 1978
Anabaena cycadeac	Perraju *et al.*, 1986
Anabaena sp. strain CA	Xiankong *et al.*, 1984
Anabaena sp. strain 1F	Xiankong *et al.*, 1984
Anabaena oscillaroides	Paerl 1980
Anabaena variabilis	Vyas 1992; Vyas and Kumar 1995; Vyas, 2004
Anabaena sp.	Srivastava *et al.*, 1989
Anabaena sp.	Chen *et al.*, 1989
Aphanizomenon sp.	Paerl 1982
Cylindrospermum licheniforme	Hirosawa and Wolk 1979
Cylindrospermum sp.	Srivastava *et al.*, 1989
Fischerella muscicola	Lambert and Smith 1980
Fischerella sp.	Srivastava *et al.*, 1989
Hapalosiphon sp.	Chen *et al.*, 1989
Macrozamia communis	Daday and Smith 1987
Mastigocladus laminosus	Ernst *et al.*, 1979 Singh and Kashyap 1988
Nostoc spongifermae	Vyas 1992; Vyas and Kumar 1995; Vyas, 2004
Nostoc sp.	Srivastava *et al.*, 1989
Scytonema hofmanii	Srivastava *et al.*, 1989

Isolation, Purification and Characterization of Different Hydrogenases

Excepting nitrogenase, very little work has been done on the biochemical characterization of hydrogenase from cyanobacteria (Lambert and Smith, 1981b; Houchins, 1984; Rao and Hall, 1988). This has been mainly due to oxygen sensitivity of hydrogenase which ultimately creates problem during isolation (Houchins, 1984). However, now methods have been developed which yield good preparation of hydrogenase from a selected cyanobacteria (Rao and Hall, 1988). Due to limited investigations on hydrogenase, especially reversible hydrogenase, there still exists confusion about the exact number and localization of hydrogenase among cyanobacteria (Houchins, 1984; Rao and Hall, 1988). Extensive work is needed to obtain clearer picture about the hydrogenases in cyanobacteria. In this section a brief account is given for all types of hydrogenase including nitrogenase separately.

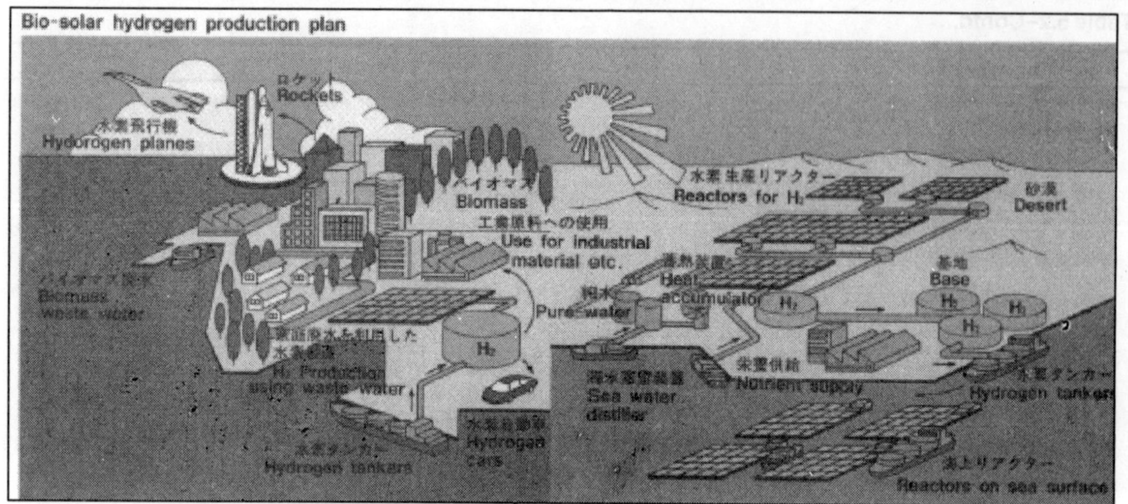

Figure 5.1: Use Cyanobacteria Combine Photosynthesis with Hydrogen Evolution Catalysed by Hydrogenases (Linblad, 2002)

Nitrogenase (ATP-Dependent Hydrogen Formation)

Nitrogenases from all organisms are very similar in their physical and chemical properties (Adams *et al.*, 1980; Bothe, 1982; Fay and Van Baalen, 1987; Mortenson, 1978; Mortenson and Chen, 1974; Mortenson and Thorneley, 1979; Stewart, 1980). The nitrogenase complex is comprised of two protein components. The larger component dinitrogenase (also called MoFe protein or component I) is responsible for reduction of substrate molecules. The MoFe component of *A. cylindrica* is an acidic tetramer (216,000 mol wt) with nonidentical subunits (52,600 and 55,000 mol wt); its isoelectric point lies between pH 4.72–4.99, and the Mo: Fe: s per mole ratio is 2.2:20.4:20 per cent in amino acid composition relatedness it resembles MoFe components from other N_2 fixers, particularly *Rhodospirillum rubrum* (Stewart, 1980; Fay and Van Baalen, 1987). The second coponent, dinitrogenase reductase, accepts electrons from donors such as ferredoxin, flavodoxin of dithionite and transfers these electrons to dinitrogenase with the concomitant hydrolysis of two molecules of ATP per electron transferred. The Fe protein (component II) is a highly labile dimer (60,000 mol wt; two identical subunits). The MoFe and Fe proteins of *A. cylindrica* and *P. boryanum* cross react with 65-90 per cent of the efficiency of homologous crosses (Stewart, 1980).

The six electron reduction of N_2 to 2 NH_3, therefore requires a minimum of 12 ATP molecules, making N_2 fixation an energetically expensive process. In addition to reducing N_2 to NH_3, dinitrogenase can reduce a number of other substrates including H^+ and acetylene.

The six electron reduction of N_2 to 2 NH_3, therefore requires a minimum of 12 ATP molecules, making N_2 fixation an energetically expensive process. In addition to reducing N_2 to NH_3, dinitrogenase can reduce a number of other substrates including H^+ and acetylene.

Both components of nitrogenase are repidly and irreversibly inactivated by O_2 (Mortenson, 1978; Mortenson and Thorneley, 1979). Organisms that fix N_2 in aerobic environments, therefore, must provide some means of protecting nitrogenase from oxygen. Cyanobacteria are the only organisms capable of simultaneous O_2 evolution and N_2 fixation, demonstrating that these processes can be compatible under suitable conditions.

Like the reduction of N_2, reduction of protons by nitrogenase requires ATP and a strong reductant. Reductant can be provided as reduced ferredoxin, flavodoxin or, as commonly employed in laboratory experiments, dithionite (Asada and Kawamura, 1985, 1986; Yu and Wolin, 1969). The evolution of H_2 by nitrogenase always occurs during N_2 fixation and a minimum of 25 per cent of total electron flux through nitrogenase is diverted to the reduction of H^+ even at very high partial pressures of N_2 and optimal levels of ATP and reductant (Houchins, 1984). If the rate of dinitrogenase turnover is slowed owing to limitation in the supply of ATP or reductant, the relative proportion of electrons diverted to H^+ reduction increases (Bothe, 1982). The evolution of H_2 by nitrogenase, therefore, consumes a substantial amount of the reductant and ATP utilized by nitrogenase.

Reversible Hydrogenase

Unlike "uptake" hydrogenase, reversible hydrogenase has been demonstrated in representatives of nearly every major cyanobacterial group (Houchins, 1984; Tables 5.3–5.8). Reactions catalyzed by reversible hydrogenase have been demonstrated in the unicellular organisms, *Synechococcus, Synechocystis* and *Aphanocapsa* (Asada and Kawamura, 1985; Asada *et al.*, 1987; Belkin and Padan, 1978; Mitsui *et al.*, 1979, 1985, 1987; Peschek, 1979a). in filamentous non-heterocystous strains such as *Spirulina, Lyngbya* and *Oscillatoria* (Belkin) and Padan, 1978; Kumazawa and Mitsui, 1982; Kuwada and Ohta, 1987, 1988, 1989, Llama *et al.*, 1979; Mitsui, 1978, 1979, 1981; Phlips and Mitsui, 1983a, b; Ramchandran and Mitsui, 1984; Scranton *et al.*, 1987; Smith *et al.*, 1982); and in heterocystous organisms including several strains of *Anabaena, Nostoc* and *Mastigocladus* (Almon and Boger, 1984; Asasda *et al.*, 1979; Benemann and Weare, 1974; Benemann *et al.*, 1982; Benemann and Weare, 1974; Benemann *et al.*, 1982; Chen *et al.*, 1989; Eisbrenner and Bothe,1979; Ernst *et al.*, 1979; Ewart and Smith, 1989; Houchins and Burris, 1981a, b,d; Laczko, 1980; Laczko and Brabas, 1981; Miura *et al.*, 1982; Miyamoto

Table 5.3: Profiles of Hydrogenase Activities in Different Cyanobacteria

Organism	*Growth Conditions*	*Nitrogenase Activity*	*H_2- Consumption*	*MV- Dependent H_2 Formation*	*References*
Anmacystis nidulans	Various	-	+	+[b]	Peschek (1979a,b,c)
Myxosarcina chrococcoides	NH^+_4-grown	-	-	-	Lambert and Smith (1980)
Oscillatoria brevis	NH^+_4-grown	-	-	+	Lambert and Smith (1980)
Plectonema boryanum	Air-grown	-	-	+	Weare and Benemann (1974)
	Anaerobic induction	+	-	-	Lambert and Smith (1980)
Schizothrix calcicola	NH^+_4-grown	-	-	-	Lambert and Smith (1980)
Anabaena cylindrica	N_2- grown	+	+	+	Bothe *et al.* (1977) Lambert and Smith (1980b)
	NH^+_4-grown	-	-	+	Lambert and Smith (1980)
Fischerella musciola	N_2–grown	+	+	+	Lambert and Smith (1980)

a: Modified from Lambert and Smith (1981b).

b: Activity was demonstrated to be membrane bound.

Table 5.4: Purification of Hydrogenase from *Spirulina maxima**

Step	*Total Protein (mg)*	*Total Activity (units)*[a]	*Specific Activity (units/mg protein)*	*Purification (–fold)*	*Yield (Per cent)*
Lysate	12,800	12,860	1.0	1.0	100.0
40,000 g supernatant	1,207	6,265	5.2	5.2	48.7
100,000 g supernatant	800	6,027	7.5	7.5	46.8
DE-52 eluate	107	3,750	35.0	35.0	29.0
Sephacryl S-200	6.6	1,453	112.4	112.4	11.3

* Modified from Llama *et al.* (1979).

[a]Activity expressed as mol H_2 evolved/hr.

Table 5.5: Partial Purification of *Oscillatoria limnetica* Hydrogenases*

Step	*Total Protein (mg)*	*Total Activity (units)*[a]	*Specific Activity (units/mg protein)*	*Purification (–fold)*	*Recovery (Per cent)*
Crude sonicate	5,190	4,418	0.85	1.0	100.0
35,000 g Supernatant	1,875	3,225	1.72	2.0	75.0
77,000 g supernatant	1,540	3,004	1.95	2.3	68.0
75 per cent $(NH_4)_2$ SO_4	311	928	2.98	3.5	21.0
First DEAT-Sephacel					
Form I	41	353	8.7	10.2	8.0
Form II	43	530	10.5	12.4	12.0
Second DEAT-Sephacel					
Form I	15	191	13.0	15.3	4.3
Form II	19	295	15.6	18.4	6.7
Sephacryl S-200					
Form I	6	106	17.6	20.7	2.3
Form II	6	158	25.8	30.3	3.6

* Modified from Belkin *et al.* (1981)

[a] Activity expressed as/mol H_2 evolved/hr.

et al., 1979, 1984; Spiller *et al.*, 1983; Tel-Or *et al.*, 1977, 1978; Weare *et al.*, 1980. In most cases, reversible hydrogenase was based on elution from a Sephacryl S-200 column for the enzyme from *Spirulina maxima*. The enzyme from *Anabaena* 7120 eluted in two peaks of molecular weight 113,000 and 165,000 (Houchins and Burris, 1981a,b). If this enzyme was first heated at 70°C for 1 h, an additional peak of 55,000 appeared suggesting that the larger forms might be multimers of a single polypeptide. Hallenbeck and Benemann (1978) have reported a molecular weight of 230,000 for the enzyme from *A. cylindrica*. Multiple forms of reversible hydrogenase which may or may not correspond to different for hydrogenase activity are invariably observed on polyacrylamide gels (Ward, 1970; Ewart and Smith, 1989, Kentemick *et al.*, 1989). Some of the characteristics of reversible hydrogenase are represented in Table 5.6.

Table 5.6: Properties of Reversible and Uptake Hydrogenases from *Anabaena* sp. Strain 7120*

	Uptake Hydrogenase	*Reversible Hydrogenase*
Cellular localization	heterocysts	both cell types
Subcellular localization	membrane-bound	cytoplasmic
Effect of NH_3 during growth	repressed	no effect
Response to anaerobic conditions during growth	increased activity	• large increase in activity
Effect of H_2	increased activity	no effect
Stability to atmospheric O_2 labels	irreversible inactivation	stable
Acceptor specificity	positive Em only	both positive and negative Em
Km for H_2	0.9/um	2.3/um
Molecular weight	56,000	55,000-230,000
Ki for CO	0.039 atm	0.0095 atm
Stability to 70°C heat treatment	$T_1/2$ = 12 min	stable
pH optimum for H_2 uptake	6.0, 8.5	9.0

*After Houchins (1984).

Table 5.7: Localization of the Reversible Hydrogenase in Aerobically and Microaerobically Grown *Anacystis nidulans* by the Immuno-Gold Labelling Technique*

	Cells Grown Aerobically	*Microaerobically*
Specific H_2- evolution activity[a]	269	408
Gold label associated with the cytoplasmic membrane	65±11	108±9
Gold label associated with the cytoplasm	26±11	28±8

* After Kenemich *et al.* (1989).

[a] The specific activity is given in nmol H_2 evolved/mg protein/h.

Partially purified preparations of reversible hydrogenase are usually quite resistant to irreversible inactivation by O_2. Samples of the enzyme from *Oscillatoria limnetica* (Belkin *et al.*, 1981) exposed to air for 50 days at 20 or –196°C retained about 80 per cent of the activity of an anaerobic control sample. Contrary to this result, the enzyme from *Mastigocladus* was considerably more O_2–sensitive and lost about 75 per cent of its activity relative to a control after 8 days under air (Riedar and Hall, 1981).

Two soluble hydrogenase activities were obtainable from cell extracts of the cyanobacterium *A. cylindrica*, one detectable by the tritium exchange assay, the other having a relatively low tritium exchange activity but catalyzing methylviologen dependent hydrogen formation. Their molecular weights by gel filtration chromatography, were 42,000 and 100,000 respectively (Ewart and Smith, 1989). Ewart and Smith (1989c) have futher raised antibodies in mice against the 42 Kd subunit of the soluble hydrogenase purified from *A. cylindrica*. The antibody did not cross-react with the 50 Kd protein, which appears to be necessary to confer methyl viologen-dependent reductive hydrogenase activity. Using western blotting procedures they found no evidence for the 42 Kd protein in heterocyst cells (Ewart and Smith, 1989a). Furthermore, although the protein was found only in the soluble fraction of vegetative cells from cultures grown in air/CO_2, antibody reactivity was also obtained with

Table 5.8: Purification of the Reversible Hydrogenase from *Anabaena nidulans**

Purification Step	*Specific Activity*[a]	*Enrichment*	*Total Activity (X 10^3 U)*[b]	*Yield (Per cent)*
Crude extract	855	1.0	329	100
Supernatant after 20 per cent $(NH^-)_2$ SO_4 addition	929	1.1	2.54	77
Linear KCL gradient on DEAE-cellulose fraction No. 10	2631	3.0	69	21
No. 11	3993	4.6	110	33
No. 12	2170	2.5	24	7
Octyl–sepharose CL-4B chromatography Fraction No. 4	16136	18.9	53	16
No. 5	214408	250.7	85	26

*After Kentemich *et al.* (1989).

a: The specific activity is given in nmol H_2/mg protein/h in the $Na_2S_2O_4$ and methyl viologen dependent evolution assay. The total activity refers to a 91 culture which was concentrated to 90 ml crude extract.

b. 1 U corresponds to 1 nmol H_2 evolved/h.

(Peschek, 1979a). A comparative account of reversible and uptake hydrogenase for Anabaena 7120 is presented in Table 5.6.

the particulate fraction when cultures were grown in nitrogen/4 per cent H_2/0.3 per cent CO_2. They have also developed an activity stain for the detection of cyanobacterial hydrogenase in polyacrylamide gels (Ewart and Smith, 1989b). In another study on *Anacystis nidulans*, Kentemich *et al.*, 1989 have reported isolation and purification of reversible hydrogenase (250-fold) by classical methods. Activity staining on gels obtained by native PAGE allowed to identify two bands. Antibodies were raised against the electrophoretically homogeneous protein. Crude extracts from the unicellular *Anacystis* and from heterocysts and vegetative cells of *Anabaena variabilis* showed precipitation bands of 56 and 17 Kd. From their study it appears that *Anacystis* has two different hydrogenases; the reversible or bidirectional hydrogenase which is located exclusively at the cytoplasmic membrane of the cells and thylakoid-bound enzyme which catalyzes only the uptake of H_2. The activity as per different purification steps is represented in Tables 5.6–5.8.

Inspite of many new reports appearing on reversible hydrogenase, the ambiguity still persists about the number and localization of this bidirectional enzyme. A systematic investigation is needed to reveal the exact nature and types of reversible hydrogenase in cyanobacteria.

Uptake Hydrogenase

Uptake hydrogenase has been demonstrated in all heterocystous cyanobacteria so far examined (Lambert and Smith, 1981b; Houchins, 1984; Rao and Hall, 1988). There exists great variations in activity with growth conditions and in some strains of *A. cylindrica*, activity is nearly undetectable under certain growth conditions (Bothe *et al.*, 1978; Jones and Bishop, 1976; Lambert and Smith, 1980). So far uptake hydrogenase has not been detected in any non-heterocystous N_2- fixers. The only non-heterocystous organism so far shown to possess uptake hydrogenase is the non–N_2–fixers unicell, *Anacystic nidulans* (Peschek, 1979a,b,c,).

The properties of cyanobacterial uptake hydrogenase in vitro are similar to those from other bacteria. Houchins and Burris (1981 a,b) have shown that when isolated heterocysts were broken with a French press, about 70 per cent of the recovered activity was membrane-bound and could be solubilized by detergent treatments or by prolonged sonication. The remaining 30 per cent of the activity that was released into the soluble fraction during the French press treatment resembled the membrane-bound uptake hydrogenase in physical and catalytic properties and is probably the same enzyme. The solubilized enzyme from Anabaena 7120 eluted from Sephadex G-100 with a molecular weight of 56,000. Co inhibition was competitive versus H_2 with a Ki of 0.039 atm. Exposure to O_2 results in both reversible inhibition and irreversible inactivation, the sensitivity to O_2 increasing with increasing disruption of the system (Houchins and Burris, 1981a,b; Lambert and Smith, 1981b). Irreversible inactivation of solubilized uptake hydrogenase displays biphasic kinetics with half-times of 2 and 14 min. Optimal O_2 levels for oxyhydrogen activity were 20 per cent for whole filaments, 10 per cent for isolated heterocysts and 2.5 per cent for heterocyst membranes (Houchins and Burris 1981d). In *Ancystis nidulans*, the oxyhydrogen reaction in isolated membranes was completely resistant to an O_2 concentration of 30 per cent.

Nitrogenase-Mediated H_2 Formation

Extensive studies have been conducted on H_2 production employing a number of N_2-fixing cyanobacteria including both heterocystous and non-heterocystous forms. A number of factors have been reported to affect H_2 formation (Lambert and Smith, 1981; Houchins, 1984). Excepting a few species, when cultures are grown in air, net H_2 formation is almost zero (Lambert and Smith, 1981; Xiankong *et al.*, 1983, 1984). This is mainly due to recycling of H_2 formed via "uptake" hydrogenase (Adams *et al.*, 1980; Bothe 1982; Bothe *et al.*, 1980; Peterson and Burris 1987a,b; Spiller *et al.*, 1978; Xiankong *et al.*, 1974; Vyas and Kumar, 1995). The basic strategy to obtain net H_2 formation is either to remove H_2 from the gas phase or to prevent H_2 incorporation, so that the assimilating power or to prevent N_2 incorporation, so that the assimilating power available to nitrogenase is all channelled into H_2 formation. A number of methods have been employed to optimize H_2 formation, and these allow the proper conditions for optimal gas production to be deduced.

Selection of Species and Strains

Studies of H_2 formation have focussed largely on the filamentous heterocystous cyanobacteria (Lambert and Smith, 1981b). *Anabaena cylindrica* has been consistently used as model organism for H_2 formation by a number of workers (Hallenbeck and Benemann, 1979; Lambert *et al.*, 1979). The rate of H_2 formation particularly in *A. cylindrica* obtained by various workers shows close similarity and reported differences if any, may be due to differences in culture and/or incubation conditions (Bothe *et al.*, 1978; Lambert and Smnith, 1981b; Tel-Or *et al.*, 1978). In general, the capacity to photoproduce H_2 varies widely depending on the levels of nitrogenase and hydrogenase activities of the cyanobacterium used. Although, any strain showing highest nitrogenase activity may or may not show the highest rate of H_2 formation. Anabaena CA, the fastest growing cyanobacterium, is reported to have the highest nitrogeanase activity amoongst all the cyanobacteria so for tested but it does not show the highest rate of H_2 formation (Xiankong *et al.*, 1983, 1984). On the other hand a few marine non-heterocystous cyanobacteria though having moderate level of nitrogenase activity show a very high rate of H_2 formation (Kumazawa and Mitsui, 1981, 1982, 1985; Mitsui *et al.*, 1977, 1979, 1985). Thus it is evident that rates of H_2 formation can vary widely with different species (Table 5.9). Therefore screening of many cyanobacteria isolated from diverse ecosystems may provide more suitable H_2 producers or strains for investigation. Non-heterocystous strains may be useful for biochemical studies on H_2

formation as well as H_2 formation may be enhanced as all the cells may contain nitrogenase unlike in heterocystous cyanobacteria.

Table 5.9: Rates of H_2 Production in Different Cyanobacteria[a]

Species	μmoles H_2 Produced per Hour		Method	References
	mg dry wt	mg Chl a		
Anabaena cylindrica	1.4	320	GLC[b]	Weissman and Benemann 1977
	0.17	0.7	GLC	Bothe *et al.*, 1977
	0.58	11.0	GLC	Daday *et al.*, 1977
	0.10	6.7	GLC	Jeffries *et al.*, 1978
				Lambert and Smith 1977
Anabaena Strain CA	40 u1			
Anabaena ambigua	-	8.5	GLC	Srivastava 1990
Anabaena cycadeae	-	1.56	GLC	Srivastava *et al.*, 1989
Anabaena (N–7363)	-	72	GLC	Asada *et al.*, 1979
Anabaena flosaquae	0.025/u1 pcv[d]		AMP[c]	Jones and Bishop 1976
Anabaena doliolum	-	1.90	GLC	Srivastava *et al.*, 1989
Calothrix membranacea	0.108		GLC	Lambert and Smith 1977
Calothrix scopulorum	0.128		GLC	Lambert and Smith 1977
Cylindrospermum majus	-	3.25	GLC	Srivastava 1990
Fischerella musciola	-	9.10	GLC	Srivastava 1990
Mastigocladus laminosus	8.5 ul	70 nmol	GLC	Benemann *et al.*, 1982
Nostoc muscorum	20mg	Chl a/h	GLC	Weisshaar and Boger 1983
Oscillatoria brevis	0.168	-	GLC	Lambert and Smith 1977
Oscillatoria sp.	0.26	260	GLC	Mitsui and Kumazaw 1977
Oscillatoria BG-7	0.183	-	GLC	Kumazawa and Mitsui 1985
Scytonema hofmanni	-	9.36	GLC	Srivastava *et al.*, 1989

a. Incubation conditions are not similar in all the cases.

b. GLC–Gas Liquid Chromatography

c. AMP–Amperometric

d. Pcv: Packed cell volume.

Factors Affecting Hydrogen Formation

As stated earlier a number of factors have been reported to affect nitrogenase-mediated H_2 formation. In this section a brief account is given for all those factors affecting the rate and duration of H_2 formation.

Growth Conditions Affecting H_2 Production

Gas Atmosphere for Growth

The most commonly used gas atmosphere for the growth of N_2 firming cultures is air supplemented with CO_2, growth is drastically slowed (Fay and Van Baalen, 1987; Stewart, 1980) and the characteristic blue-green coloration due to phycocyanin is reduced (Lambert *et al.*, 1979b). It has been demonstrated that cultures grown under limiting CO_2 conditions have H_2 photoproduction rates proportional to their growth rates (Jones and Bishop, 1976). The concentration of CO_2 also affects the rate of H_2 formation. A concentration below 5 per cent CO_2 is most suitable for growth as well as H_2 production (Benemann and Weare, 1974a; Lambert *et al.*, 1979b; Tel-Or *et al.*, 1978). It has been observed that both tested (Ernst *et al.*, 1979). It has been observed that both acetylene reduction and H_2 formation increased slighly. Azolla fronds when incubated in air + CO_2 showed higher H_2 formation than those growing on air alone (Banerjee *et al.*, 1989; Peters *et al.*, 1976). Tel-Or *et al.*, 1977 have also reported the induction of hydrogenases by $N_2/H_2/CO_2$ (75:20:5) enhanced nitrogenase and hydrogenase activities between days 4 and 8 growth of *A. cylindrica* and *Nostoc muscorum* (Tel–Or *et al.*, 1977). The maximum enhancement of nitrogenase activity was 3- to 5- fold and H_2 consumption and methyl viologen-dependent H_2 formation, 5 to 50-fold. This induction of hydrogenase has been observed in a number of other cyanobacteria (Eisbrenner *et al.*, 1979; 1981; Howarth and Codd, 1985) on the contrary increase in H_2 Production has also been observed following CO_2 deprivation in *A. cylindrica* (Jeffries *et al.*, 1978). Furthermore, obligated requirement of CO_2 at least in aged cultures for prolonged H_2 production has been demonstrated in a number of cyanobacteria (see Lambert and Smith, 1981b). In summary it seems that CO_2 is essential for continued H_2 production and this effect seems to be mediated via net CO_2 fixation.

Culture Medium

Culture medium used for growth of various cyanobacteria plays an important role in regulating the evolution of H_2 (Lambert and Smith, 1981; Stewart, 1980). The most commonly employed medium has been that of Allen and Arnon (1955). However, this medium does not constitute the minimal nutritional requirement for cyanobacteria and some of the trace elements are possibly unnecessary. However, *Azolla* fronds when incubated with different and Arnon's medium (Banerjee *et al.*, 1989; Kumar *et al.*, 1990). A number of other media have been used for various cyanobacteria; howerver BG–11 seems to be most suitable medium for growth and H_2 formation for a variety of cyanobacterial strains (Lambert and Smith, 1981b).

Many other constituents and added chemicals have been demonstrated to affect subsequent H_2 formation. Almost all the combined nitrogen sources *viz.*, NH_2^+, NO_3^-, NO_2^- and a few amino acids like glutamine, asparagine, arginine and glutamic acid inhibit H_2 formation. The inhibition of H_2 formation is solely due to loss of heterocyst and/or nitrogenase activity (Banerjee *et al.*, 1989; Bothe, 1982; Ernst *et al.*, 1979; Hounchins, 1984; Lambert *et al.*, 1979c; Srivastava, 1990; Stewart, 1980). Addition of exogenous NaH CO_3 to culture medium has been reported to stimulate H_2 formation in a number of cyanobacteria (Srivastava *et al.*, 1989). Similarly supplementation of a few metal ions and their concentration had been demonstrated to affect H_2 evolution Jeffries *et al.* (1978) showed that cultures grown with 5.0 mg of Fe^{3+}/litre produced H_2 at a rate about twice the rate of cultures with 0.5 mg Fe^{3+}/ litre. Nickel addition significantly affects up.

Light

Light quality and intensity both affect H_2 formation in a number of cyanobacteria. This effect is indirect and mainly through photosynthesis and nitrogenase activity (Stewart, 1980). A number of studies have demonstrated that pigment content of cyanobacteria can vary according to the vavelength characteristics of the light source used (Fay and Van Baalen, 1987; Frenkel *et al.*, 1950; Greenbaum, 1977; Kerfin and Boger, 1992; Lambert and Smith, 1980; Phlips and Mitsui, 1983b; Stewart, 1980). Chan Van *et al.* (1983) have demonstrated a close correlation between wavelength of light and photosynthesis together with H_2 production. Gogotov *et al.*, 1976 demonstrated that light of low intensity (2.5,10^{3}erg/cm^2/s) stimulates H_2 production by cell suspensions of *A. variabilis* in the presence of glucose, pyruvate and formate. The maximum rate of H_2 production in the presence of these substrates was observed at light intensities of 650, 1400 and 2250 erg cm^{-2} s^{-1} respectively. In another study it has been demonstrated that *A. cylindrica* sparged with argon gas produced H_2 continuously for 20 days under limited light conditions (6.0 W m^{-2}) and for 180 days under elevated light conditions (32 W m^{-2}) in the absence of exogenous nitrogen. Kumar and Kumar (1988) have observed that low light intensity favours H_2 production in *Anabaena* CA. In *Oscillatoria* sp. strain Miami BG-7, the rate of H_2 production saturates at low light intensity (*i.e.* 15–30 uE m^{-2} s^{-1}). Although so far no systematic studies on the effect of light intensity during growth on subsequent H_2 formation have been performed but studies so far conducted suggest that lower light intensity favours H_2 production.

Under dark, rate of H_2 production remains only about 10 per cent of the light incubated cultures. As yet, not a single species has been found to show sustained H_2 production shows almost similar trend in terms of duration as observed with nitrogenase activity.

Temperature

Excepting the thermophilic cyanobacterium *Mastigocladus laminosus*, in all the mesophilic cyanobacteria H_2 formation follows the pattern of growth and temperature (Lambert and Smith, 1981b). In marine *Oscillatoria* sp. strain Miami BG-7, the upper temperature limit for H_2 production has been found at 46°C.

H_2 evolution by the thermophilic cyanobacterium *Mastigocladus laminosus* has been studied by a few worker (Benemann *et al.*, 1982; Miura *et al.*, 1980, 1981, 1982; Miyamoto *et al.*, 197, 1984; Smith *et al.*, 1982). The optimal temperature for H_2 production was 44-49°C (Miura *et al.*, 1980).

Age of Culture

It has been realized lately that the age of cultures used for H_2 measurements is an important factor (Lambert and Smith, 1981). First of all Benemann and Weare (1974a) showed that H_2 formation in *A. cylindrica* is optimal when harvested at about 0.3 mg dry wt/ml of cyanobacterial concentration, after which a sharp decline is observed. This decline in H_2 formation is more pronounced than the observed decline in nitrogenase activity suggesting that hydrogen recycling capacity remains relatively constant. Similar finding was later on reported by Daday *et al.*, 1977. In *Nostoc muscorum* a similar optimum H_2 production in logarithmic growth was observed which correlated with changes in heterocyst frequency (Ernst *et al.*, 1979). The decline of H_2 evolution in aged cultures seems mainly due to gradual loss of nitrogenase activity and also the pigments of PS II (Lambert and Smith, 1981; Stewart, 1980).

Concentration of Culture

Concentration of culture has been implicated in regulating the net H_2 formation. H_2 formation has been shown to increase linearly with algal concentration to about 1.5 mg dry wt/ml suspension for *A. cylindrica* (Daday *et al.*, 1977). Subsequent decrease in H_2 formation is probably due to self shading of the culture.

Factors Employed to Enhance Nitrogenase-Catalyzed H_2 Production

Choice of Gas Atmosphere During Assay

Argon/CO_2

As most of the N_2-fixing cyanobacteria lack the capacity to produce H_2 under aerobic conditions, cultures are frequently incubated in argon in the absence of CO_2 to avoid generation of O_2 through photosynthesis during the experimental incubations (Lambert and Smith, 1981b). However, these conditions are not optimal for H_2 formation and generally result in lower rate of H_2 formation. It has been also demonstrated that the longer the incubation, the greater the requirement for CO_2 for prolonged H_2 formation (Chen *et al.*, 1989; Daday *et al.*, 1977; Ernst *et al.*, 1979; Kuwada and Ohta, 1989; Laczko, 1980; Lambert *et al.*, 1979; Lambert and Smith, 1980, 1981a,b). The reason for lower rate of H_2 formation under argon alone is primarily due to depletion of stored reductant (Lambert and Smith, 1981b). With argon alone there is no CO_2 fixation and hence stored reductant is gradually consumed in all other metabolic reactions including nitrogenase (Ernst *et al.*, 1979; Lambert *et al.*, 1979a).

To improve the efficiency of H_2 production, use of 99 per cent argon + 1 per cent CO_2 has been demonstrated to be the best alternative (Asada *et al.*, 1985; Banerjee *et al.*, 1989; Bothe *et al.*, 1978; Kerfin and Boger, 1982; Kosyak *et al.*, 1978; Kumazawa and Mitsui 1981; Scherer *et al.*, 1980; Tel-Or *et al.*, 1977, 1978). Preincubation under 99 per cent argon + 1 per cent CO_2 leads to multifold stimulation of H_2 production rate although depending upon the strains used (Lambert and Smith, 1981b). However, prolonged incubation under nitrogen starvation leading to the death and decay of cultures. Thus, this treatment has been found suitable for short term H_2 evolution study (Lambert and Smith, 1981b). However, investigators have shown that continued production of H_2 may be attained in the same culture if a very low concentration of NH^+_4 is added to the cultures so as to keep them under growing condition (Lambert *et al.*, 1979; Lambert and Smith, 1980; Mitsui, 1987; Mitsui *et al.*, 1985; Weaver *et al.*, 1980).

Dinitrogen (N_2)

To attain anaerobic condition, a number of workers have used N_2 gas in place of argon (see Lambert and Smith, 1981b), furthermore the effect of N_2 along with argon has also been tested. In either condition, N_2 inhibits H_2 formation due to competition of N_2 reduction with proton reduction (Houchins, 1984). N_2 at 4 per cent of the gas phase has been found to inhibit H_2 formation in argon by about 50 per cent, with complete inhibition occurring at 25 per cent N_2 for *A. cylindrica* (Jones and Bishop, 1979).

Oxygen

The effect of O_2 in argon or N_2 atmosphere has also been tested (Ernst *et al.*, 1979; Spiller *et al.*, 1978). Added oxygen inhibits H_2 formation in all the cyanobacteria (Asada and Kumazawa, 1986; Banerjee *et al.*, 1989; Daday *et al.*, 1977; Kumar and Kumar, 1990b,c; Lambert *et al.*, 1979c; Smith *et al.*, 1983, 1984). In an *Anabaena* sp., it was found that 5 per cent O_2 with argon stimulated H_2 production but this very concentration was inhibitory under N_2 (Asada *et al.*, 19790. The inhibition of H_2 formation by O_2 seems to be due to O_2 sensitivity of nitrogenase or by the facilitation of an oxyhydrogen reaction in heterocyst which diminishes net H_2 production (Ernst *et al.*, 1979; Spiller *et al.*, 1978; Xiankong *et al.*, 1983, 1984).

Carbon Monoxide/Acetylene

Carbon monoxide has been extensively employed in H_2 formation studies because it specifically inhibits N_2 fixation and C_2H_2 reduction but does not inhibit the nitrogenase mediated H_2 formation reaction (Bradbeer and Wilson, 1963). Similarly, C_2H_2, an inhibitor of hydrogenase in many bacteria, has been frequently used (Smith *et al.*, 1976). Stimulation of H_2 formation by the addition of CO and C_2H_2 in an argon gas phase was first of all shown in *A. cylindrica* by Bothe *et al.* (1977a). Subsequently, H_2 formation was obtained even in air with the use of CO + C_2H_2 for *A. cylindrica* (Daday *et al.*, 1977) and also in marine cyanobacteria (Lambert and Smith, 1981b). At optimal concentrations of CO and C_2H_2, H_2 formation occurred at the same rate in air after a lag phase of 2-3 has in argon gas phase (Lambert *et al.*, 1979c). A number of other workers have shown the same effect of CO + C_2H_2 on H_2 formation in various cyanobacteria (Miura *et al.*, 1981, 1982; Miyamoto *et al.*, 1984; Srivastava, 1990; Xiankong *et al.*, 1984; Figure 5.4). Increase of H_2 formation by CO + C_2H_2 seems to be mediated by number of ways. Bothe (1982) provided evidence that C_2H_2 inhibits by H_2 recycling and that this inhibition is increased somewhat by CO. There is also a report that pre-incubation with C_2H_2 alters the conformation of the nitrogenase complex. Still other workers have suggested that the effect of C_2H_2 is to alter the H_2 tension than C_2H_2 itself that causes a conformational activation of the enzyme (Scherer *et al.*, 1980).

Metabolic Inhibitors

DCMU (3-(3,4 dichlorophenyl) -1, 1-dimethylurea)

Out of various metabolic inhibitors, DCMU, an inhibitor of PS II, has been frequently used to optimize H_2 production (Lambert and Smith, 1981b). The possible effect of DCMU may be: (a) a reduction in H_2 formation by decreasing reductant supply to PS I from PS II, or (b) an increase in H_2 formation due to elimination of an oxyhydrogen reaction that uses photosynthetically generated O_2 and nitrogenase-mediated H_2. Both these effects have been observed in some cyanobacteria (Houchins, 1984). That a loss of reductant does take place by DCMU treatment was first of all proved by Benemann and Weare (1974b) was demonstrated H_2-dependent acetylene reduction in the presence of DCMU. Gogotov *et al.* (1976) have reported that H_2 evolution is not inhibited by DCMU in the presence of pyruvate or formate in *Anabaena variabilis*. Working with isolated heterocysts fo *Anabaena* sp. strain CA, it has been demonstrated that DCMU has no effect on H_2 formation (Kumar and Kumar, 1990b). Xiankong *et al.* (1983) have reported that DCMU addition immediately inhibits H_2 production in *Anabaena* CA. It seems that the effect of DCMU depends on the particular cyanobacterium used; those that produce little H_2 in the absence of DCMU and exhibit a vigorous oxyhydrogen reaction might be stimulated in H_2 formation by DCMU, whereas those in which H_2 and O_2 are not re-utilized until significant tensions accumulate in the environment, such as in the case of *A. cylindrica* will show no benefit from DCMU addition (Lambert and Smith, 1981b). As a whole if DCMU results in stimulation of H_2 formation, the effect is temporary. Furthermore, the effect of DCMU also depends on the level of endogenous reductant present in a particular alga.

Metronidazole (2-methyl-5-nitroimidazole-1-ethanol)

Tetley and Bishop (1979) first of all showed that metronidazole at 1-2 mM levels was a selective inhibitor of nitrogenase activity in *Anabaena* sp. Hydrogenases are insensitive to metronidazole. Although this chemical does not stimulate H_2 production but it offers a model system to distinguish between hydrogenase and nitrogenase activity.

MSO (L-Methionine-DL-Sulforimine)

MSO, an inhibitor of glutamine synthetase which depresses nitrogenase activity, has been found to increase H_2 production for shorter duration (Lambert and Smith, 1981b; Stewart, 1980; Srivastava, 1990). Lambert *et al.* (1979b) found stimulation of H_2 production by treatment of MSO (2μM) in *A. cylindrica* B 629. Use of MSO is important especially where cultures are grown at lower concentration of NH_4Cl for longer duration of H_2 production. MSO drepresses nitrogenase even in the presence of NH_4Cl and thus continued production of H_2 occurs.

Organic Carbon Sources

Cyanobacteria are obligate photoautotrophs and as such do not require any organic carbon sources for normal growth (Stewart, 1980). However, there are certain species which show stimulation of growth in light and a few show growth in dark in the presence of certain organic carbon sources. As most of the cyanobacteria show little or no H_2 formation in dark, the role of exogenous organic carbon sources seems important. Chan Van *et al.* (1983) have reported that pyruvate and glucose stimulate photohydrogen production in *Anabaena azollae*. Kumar and Kumar (1990a) did not observe stimulation of H_2 evolution by addition of fructose and erythrose in *Anabaena* CA. Srivastava *et al.* (1989) have reported significant stimulation of H_2 production in a number of N_2-fixing cyanobacteria. They have demonstrated stimulation of H_2 production by exogenously added carbon sources in the dark (Srivastava, 1990; Srivastava *et al.*, 1989). So far no attempt has been made to study the response of added organic carbon sources on H_2 production in any typical heterotrophic cyanobacteria. Differential response of organic carbon sources on H_2 formation seems to be related with transport of carbon sources by specific cyanobacterial species.

Nickel

Nickel has been demonstrated to be an essential metal for uptake hydrogenase activity (Almon and Boger, 1984; Daday and Smith, 1983; Daday *et al.*, 1985; Srivastava, 1990; Xiankong *et al.*, 1984; Vyas, 2004). In almost all the cyanobacteria tested, nickel addition stimulates uptake of H_2 and thus inhibition of H_2 formation takes place. Attempts are being made to isolate nickel-resistant mutant which might be uptake hydrogenase negative (Hup-) and therefore may prove better strain in terms of H_2 production.

Na_2S, Thiosulfate and Other Reducing Agents

A number of workers have tested the effect of a variety of reducing agents on H_2 production in a few cyanobacteria. It was found that Na_2S addition showed stimulation of H_2 production in *Nostoc muscorum* (Fry *et al.*, 1984). The results obtained by various workers are variable and as such no definite conclusion can be drawn on the role of these substances on H_2 production.

H_2 Production by Hydrogenase (Reversible Hydrogenase)

In comparison to nitrogenase-mediated H_2 formation, little work has been done on H_2- formation by hydrogenase (Houchins, 1984; Lambert and Smith, 1981b). Whereas nitrogenase catalyzed H_2 formation takes place solely in N_2 fixing forms, hydrogenase is present both in N_2-fixer and non-N_2 fixer forms. There is a lot of confusion about the exact found in vegetative cells even when grown in the absence of heterocysts it is unlikely that its function relates to nitrogen fixation. Furthermore there is still ambiguity about the exact number of reversible hydrogenases in cyanobacteria. However, now it is believed that two pools of hydrogenase exist, an oxygen-sensitive activity in vegetative cells and an oxygen-resistant activity in heterocysts.

Reversible hydrogenase activities are usually present in aerobically grown cyanobacteria prior to a dark, anaerobic adaptation period (Daday and Smith, 1979; Houchins and Burris, 1981a,b; Tel-Or *et al.*, 1978). Demonstration of activity requires reductive activation of the enzyme or removal of a tightly bound O_2 molecule. This activation can be achieved in intact cells by addition of dithionite and methyl viologen. The methyl viologen-dependent H_2 evolution activity in cyanobacteria usually increases 2-fold during a dark anaerobic adaptation period (Houchins and Burris, 1981a,b; Spiller *et al.*, 1983).

Little reversible hydrogenase activity develops in the presence of molecular oxygen. By far the most dramatic and sustained increase in activity can be obtained by removal of O_2 during continuous illumination. Increases in activity of one to three orders of magnitude occur over a period of hours to days when cultures are sparged with an anaerobic gas mixture during growth (Houchinc, 1984; Tel-Or *et al.*, 1977; Lambert and Smith, 1981b). The enzyme is not catalytically functional in vivo under these conditions but is maintained in an inactive state by photosynthetically produced O_2 (Houchins and Burris, 1981a,b; Houchins, 1984).

The presence of combined nitrogen in the growth medium has little effect on the level of reversible hydrogenase activity, but an indirect effect is observed in heterocystous organisms (Houchins, 1984). Though reversible hydrogenase occurs in both heterocysts and vegetative cells, the specific activity in heterocyst during aerobic growth is about 4-times that in vegetative cells (Houchins and Burris, 1981a, b). The microaerobic environment within the heterocyst probably leads to additional reversible hydrogenase synthesis.

Reversible hydrogenase also shows oxyhydrogen reaction in *Anabaena* 7120 when traces of O_2 are added although the reaction is repidly inactivated by O_2 levels as low as 0.1 per cent in contrast to the reaction catalyzed by uptake hydrogenase (Houchins and Burris, 1981a,b). CO_2-dependent H_2 uptake occurs at low light intensity, and higher light intensities leads to deadaptation and reversion to normal O_2-evolving photosynthesis. This reaction has been shown to be strictly light-dependent and is completely inhibited by the uncoupler CCCP, demonstrating a requirement for photophosphorylation.

Hydrogenase dependent H_2 evolution has been demonstrated in a number of species of cyanobacteria (Adams *et al.*, 1980; Asada and Kawamura, 1985; Asada *et al.*, 1987a,b,c; Belkin and Padan, 1978; Benemann *et al.*, 1982; Daday *et al.*, 1979; Daday and Smith, 1987; Ewart and Smith, 1989a,b,c; Houchins, 1984; Houchins, 1981d; Howarth and Codd, 1985; Laczko, 1980; Laczko and Barabas, 1981; Llama *et al.*, 1979; Mitsui, 1979b; Miyamoto *et al.*, 1982, 1984; Peschek, 1979a,b,c,d; Spiller *et al.*, 1983; Tel-Or *et al.*, 1977; Yagi, 1976). A few organic carbon sources have been reported to enhance reversible hydrogenase activity.

H_2 Metabolism in Symbiotic Cyanobacteria

Symbiotic cyanobacteria have not been widely employed for studies on H_2 production or uptake. However, a few workers have made attempts to screen the capacity of H_2 production/uptake in *Anabaena azollae*, *Anabaena cycadeae* and *Nostoc* sp. (from lichen) (Newton, 1976; Peters, *et al.*, many N_2 -fixing organisms, there was no short term effect of nitrate on H_2 production. H_2 production was observed with *Azolla* fronds grown for even 1 to 9 months on nitrate supplemented medium. H_2 production was found almost comparable in experiments where *Azolla* was grown under 1 per cent CO_2 in air or under 1 per cent CO_2, 20 per cent O_2 in argon.

Increase of light intensity showed parallel increase in the rate of H_2 production. Thus incubation of Azolla under 1200 ft-C showed the highest production of H_2. There was almost insignificant level of H_2 production under dark. Experiments done with O_2 under dark showed no production of H_2 suggesting the presence of an "uptake hydrogenase". *Anabaena azollae* freshly isolated from Azolla also showed active formation of H_2. A rate of 50.4 nmoles H_2/mg Chl. a/min was routinely obtained under Ar + CO_2. Addition of C_2H_2 and CO greatly stimulated H_2 formation. Overall studies conducted by Peters *et al.* (1976) are indicative of nitrogenase-mediated H_2 formation by *Azolla* plants or isolated *A. azollae*. Effects of a number of other factors on H_2 production have also been reported (Newton, 1976; Peters *et al.*, 1987).

Another water fern Azolla pinnata has been employed for studies on H_2 production by Banerjee *et al.*, 1989. With this water fern, highest H_2 evolution (5.40 nmol H_2/mg fresh wt at 24 h) was observed if the fronds were incubated in allen and Arnon's medium devoid of combined nitrogen sources. H_2 evolution was 4-5 times higher under light-anaerobic medium. Addition of NH_4Cl or KNO_3 (10mM) did not inhibit H_2 production. H_2 evolution was significantly stimulated by the exogenous addition of phosphate. 60 PPm phosphate addition elicited 6-8 times higher H_2 formation than the control. Furthermore, there were significant differences in the rate of H_2 production between pink and green fronds of *Azolla*. Pink frond always showed higher rate of H_2 formation than the green one. Although considerable activity (H_2 formation) was detected in the dark but addition of PS-II inhibitor completely suppressed H_2 formation. Possible presence of a soluble hydrogenase has been suggested though mainly based on the data of dark and NO^-_3- grown *Azolla* fronds. A number of workers have recently studied H_2 evolution by immobilized *A. azollae* (Brouers and Hall, 1986; Shi *et al.*, 1987; Srivastava, 1990). Immobilization elicited multifold stimulation of H_2 production.

Perraju *et al.*, 1986 have studied H_2 evolution and uptake in cycas *Anabaena* cycadeae association. They demonstrated that H_2 evolution was undetectable in free-living H_2 fixing cultures of *A. cycadeae* but intact coralloid roots showed a rate of 4umol H_2/mg Chl. a/h. Furthermore, it was found that H_2 uptake was absent in the coralloid root but free-living *A. cycadeae* showed an H_2 uptake rate of 28 umol formation (1.56 nmol H_2/ug Chl a/h) in *A. cycadeae* has this rate is almost 2-3 fold lower than the intact coralloid roots.

Other than Azolla and Cycasc, H_2 evolution and uptake studies have been performed with three N_2 fixing lichens *viz.*, *Peltigera membranacea*, *P. polydactyla* and *Lobaria pulmonaria* (Millbvank, 1981). It was found that H_2 evolved concomitant with N_2 fixation was recycled by means of an uptake hydrogenase, and in general the net evolution was zero or small at 5 and 15°C. At 25°C there was appreciable net evolution of H_2 in the *Peltigera* sp. but *Lobaria* showed no net evolution. Extensive study is essential to understand the mode of H_2 metabolism in symbiotic cyanobacteria in general.

H_2 Production by Immobilized Cyanobacteria

Immobilization is a method of conversion of enzyme or whole cells from a water soluble mobile state to a water insoluble immobile state, by trapping them in an insert, insoluble, solid support. In recent years immobilizing action of enzymes, microbial cells and other living systems is being used extensively for the large-scale production of drugs and other compounds (Brodelius, 1985). A number of matrixes are used for immobilization *viz.*, glass beads, agar-agar, alginate etc. although the use of particular system depends upon the nature of investigation. The most common procedure for immobilizing microbes is cell entrapment in natural polymers, in particular agar, shaped into blocks, layers or beads.

Immobilization of cyanobacteria for H_2 production is preferred over liquid culture mainly due to two reasons. First cyanobacteria require continuous agitation in liquid culture to keep cultures uniformaly suspended, since without it the organisms settle out and form clumps which exhibit no H_2 formation (Weissman and Benemann, 1977). Second, agitation causes filament breakage and structural degeneration of vegetative cells, both of which are associated with cessation of biophotolysis in liquid cultures.

H_2 production by immobilized cells of cyanobacteria has been studied by a few workers (Weissaman and Benemann, 1977; Lambert *et al.*, 1979; Kayanlo *et al.*, 1981; Ocjhiai *et al.*, 1983; Brouers and Hall, 1986; Robinson *et al.*, 1986; Kuwada and Ohta, 1987; Shi *et al.*, 1987). In almost all the studies so far conducted, immobilization of cultures showed significant stimulation of H_2 production (Table 5.10). The duration of H_2 evolution was also prolonged significantly. The immobilizing conditions have been found to vary from strains to strains. Similarly types of matrix used also show significant differences in rate as well as duration of H_2 production. For example, *Anabaena* N-7363 showed maximum hydrogen production 90.53 umole H_2 h^{-1} b^{-1} (wet gel) with 2 per cent agar gel at 30°C and 3000 lux light intensity (Kayano *et al.*, 1981). This rate was three times higher than that of free algae. On the other hand *Lyngbya* sp. strain 108 showed optimum H_2 production when immobilized on 4 per cent alginate; 0.5 M $CaCl^2$ and 0.11 mg dry microbial cells ml^{-1} gel (Kuwada and Ohta, 1987). The pH temperature, and light intensity were kept at 9.0, 30°C and 1000 lux. On the other hand *A. azollae* showed maximum yield of H_2 production when immobilized on polyvinyl (Brouers and Hall, 1986; Shi *et al.*, 1987). Higher yield with polyvinyl has been shown to be partly related to changes in membranes permeability induced by the immobilization process itself. A similar increase in yield of H_2 production was observed when membrane permeability of alginate immobilized *A. azollae* was increased by an acetone pretreatment (Brouers and Hall, 1986).

Table 5.10: H_2 Production by Immobilized Cyanobacteria

Test Organism	*Matrix Used*	*Increase % of Fold*	*Duration of H_2 Production*	*References*
Anabena cylindrica	Alginate	two-fold		Weissman and Benemann 1977
A. cylindrica B-629	Glass beads	5 per cent	upto 57 days	Lambert *et al.*, 1979a
Anabaena N-7363	Agar-agar	3-fold	upto 7 days	Kayano *et al.*, 1981
Phormidium sp.	SnO_2 OTE Calcium alginate	ND*	ND	Ochiai *et al.*, 1983
Anabaena azollae	Polyvinyl polyurethane and alginate	2-fold		Brouers and Hall 1986
Mastigocladus laminosus				
Lyngbya sp. strain 108	Calcium alginated	3.4 fold	5 days	Kuwada and Ohta 1987
Anabaena azollae	Polyurethane, polyvinyl and alginate	2-fold	ND	Shi *et al.*, 1987

* ND–not determined; –: Measurement of photocurrent.

The exact reasons pertaining to the enhancement of H_2 formation following immobilization are as yet not clearly known (Robinson *et al.*, 1986). However, unlike free-living cultures, immobilized cyanobacteria do not settle out and form clump. Moreover, cyanobacteria are protected from filament breakage and structural degeneration which occurs as a result of agitation. Furthermore, increase of heterocyst frequency in immobilized cyanobacteria may also account for the increased rate of H_2 production. Increase in heterocyst frequency has been reported in the cyanobacterium immobilized on calcium alginate beads (Kerby *et al.*, 1986).

The prolonged duration of H_2 formation following immobilization has been demonstrated to be a phenomenon related with growth (Srivastava, 1990). The non-growth period is prolonged especially in agar-agar and thus results in sustained H_2 production for a longer period. A potential limitation of immobilization for an organism is the problem of light penetration through the supporting matrix. However, as cyanobacteria themselves stick to the cubes or beads, the large surface area provided would thus ensure a uniform distribution of organisms and thus light penetration. Even if lesser light intensity favours H_2 production (Lambert and Smith, 1981b; Kuwada and Ohta, 1987). Stimulation of H_2 production following immobilization has also been claimed to be due to oxygen tolerance. Although immobilization does not prevent the inhibitory effects of O_2 but most probably it does not production by cyanobacterial system.

Immobilization and Development of Photochemical Fuel Cell

One of the first biological fuel cells designed to use H_2 was developed by Rohrback *et al.* (1962), who reported on the production of hydrogen from glucose by *Clostridium butyricum*. In this biological fuel cell, glucose was used as a nutrient; however, it is expensive as an energy resource. Solar energy is very attractive for energy production and Berk and Canfield (1964) reported one of the first photochemical fuel cells utilizing microorganisms. In the presence of light, *R. rubrum* produced hydrogen, which was oxidized on the surface of the anode. Later on, coupling of immobilized chloroplasts with *Clostridium butyricum* made possible water-splitting hydrogen evolution (Kayano *et al.*, 1981) and the hydrogen prduced was applied to a hydrogen oxygen fuel cell. A photo-current of 0.4–1.5 mA was obtained for 4 h from the photochemical fuel cell system using immobilized chloroplasts and *C. butyricum*.

Using the cyanobacterium *Anabaena* No. 7363, a photochemical fuel cell system was first developed by Kayano *et al.*, 1981. In this system the alga *Anabaena* No. 7363 was immobilized in 2 per cent agar gel and thus produced 3-fold higher H_2 in light (10,000 lux). The oxygen evolved was removed by reactor containing aerobic bacterium *Bacillus subtilis*. The H_2 evolved was passed through soda lime and the flow was regulated by a flow meter before reaching the anode chamber of the fuel cell. The hydrogen-oxygen fuel cell consisted of platnized platinum anode (10 x 50 cm), a porous active carbon cathode (7.5 x 8.0 x 2.5 cm) and the electrolyte (0.1 M phosphate buffer solution, pH 8.0). The anode and cathode were separated by an anion exchange membrane. The current, the anode potential and the cell voltage were measured by a millivolt-millimeter and displayed on a recorder. A photo-current of 15-30 mA was continuously produced for 7 days by the photochemical fuel cell consisting of the immobilized *Anabaena* reactor, the O_2-removing reactor and the hydrogen-oxygen fuel cell. The conversion ration of hydrogen to current was from 80 to 100 per cent.

Ochiai *et al.*, 1983 have developed semiconducter electrodes coated with living films of cyanobacteria. They have demonstrated that the intact *Phormidium* sp. cells immobilized on SnO_2 semiconductor electrode are capable of transferring electrons to SnO_2 in a light-dependent reaction. They have also demonstrated that the drying of a "wet" algal electrode at 50ºC for 60 min increases photocurrent output capacity by 100-fold.

Hydrogen Uptake

Uptake of H_2 occurs via uptake hydrogenase and/or reversible hydrogenase in all the cyanobacteria. Hydrogen functions as an electron donor for both respiratory and light dependent photosynthetic electron flow, the precise nature of which appears to vary from species to species. The characteristics of enzymes involved in uptake of H_2 are described elsewhere (Figures 5.1, 5.2 and Tables 5.6–5.8).

Like nitrogenase-mediated H_2 formation, uptake of H_2 is affected by gas atmospheres, culture medium, light intensity and quality, and age of the culture (Lambert and Smith, 1981b; Vyas and Kumar, 1995). Furthermore, the uptake is influenced by incubation conditions (Houchins, 1984). Combined nitrogen sources *viz.*, NO^-_3 NH^+_4 and amino acids completely inhibit uptake hydrogenase activity. Nickel has been demonstrated to be involved in regulating uptake hydrogenase activity (Smith *et al.*, 1985; Xinankong *et al.*, 1984; Vyas, 2004) Friedrich *et al.*, 1982 have reported that nickel is a constituent of soluble and particulate hydrogenase of *Alcaligenes eutrophus*. However, till now, nickel as a prosthetic group or co-factor of cyanobacterial hydrogenases has not been demonstrated by any workers (Houchins, 1984; Lambert and Smith, 1981b; Xiankong *et al.*, 1984). However, it has been suggested that nickel may be required for activation of an uptake hydrogenase, or for hydrogenase synthesis, or for synthesis of another protein which is involved in H_2 uptake (Almon and Boger, 1984; Daday and Smith, 1983; Daday *et al.*, 1985; Pederson *et al.*, 1986; Srivastava, 1990; Xiankong *et al.*, 1985; Pederson *et al.*, 1984; Srivastava, 1990; Xiankong *et al.*, 1984). For cyanobacteria uptake of H_2 has many possible functions, *viz.* (a) as a scavenger of O_2; (b) as a mechanism that prevents H_2 inhibition of nitrogenase; (c) in the production of ATP via H_2 oxidation (Knallgas reaction). Physiological function

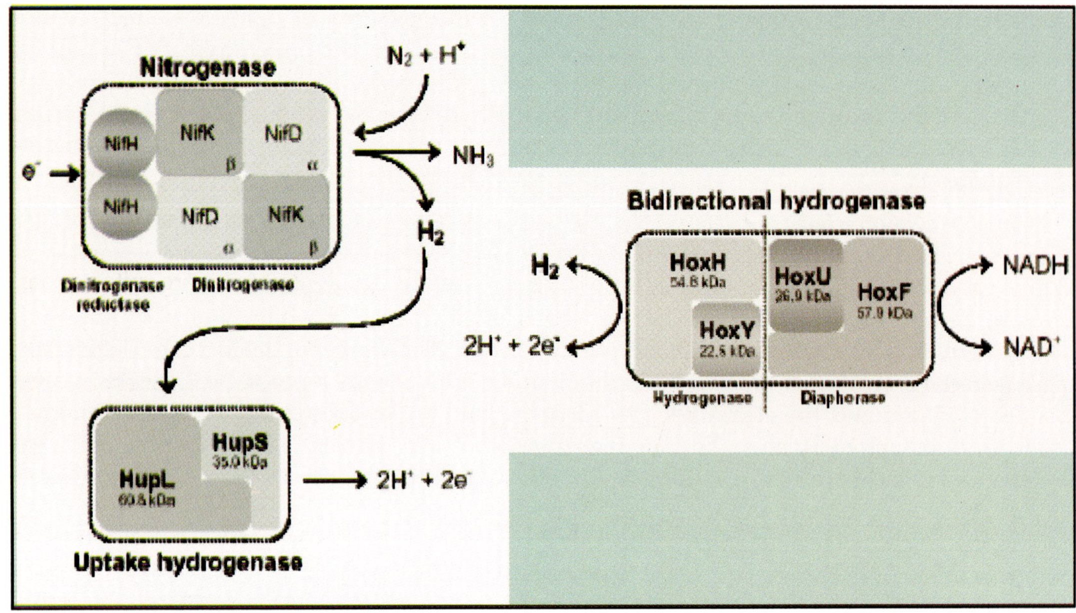

Figure 5.2: Cyanobacterial Enzymes Directly Involved in H_2 Metabolism

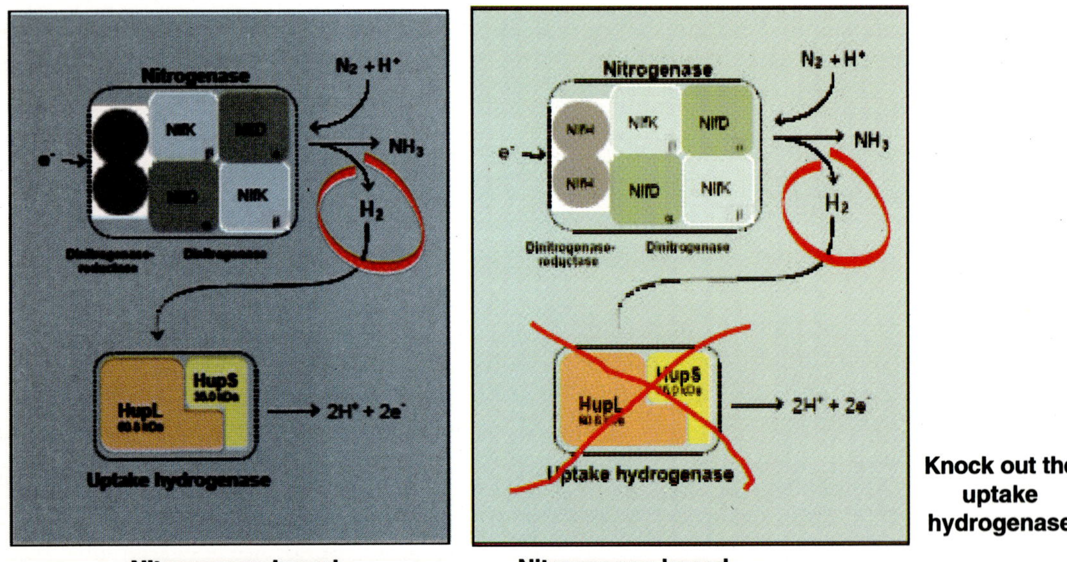

Figure 5.3: Two Different Approaches for Cyanobacterial Biohydrogen

of the uptake hydrogenase in cyanobacteria is to catalyse the consumption of hydrogen produced by nitrogenase (Happe *et al.*, 2000; Lindberg *et al.*, 2002). All these function have been demonstrated in one or another cyanobacteria (Houchins, 1984). Though uptake hydrogenase does increase the efficiency of nitrogenase, it adversely affects H_2 evolution activity.

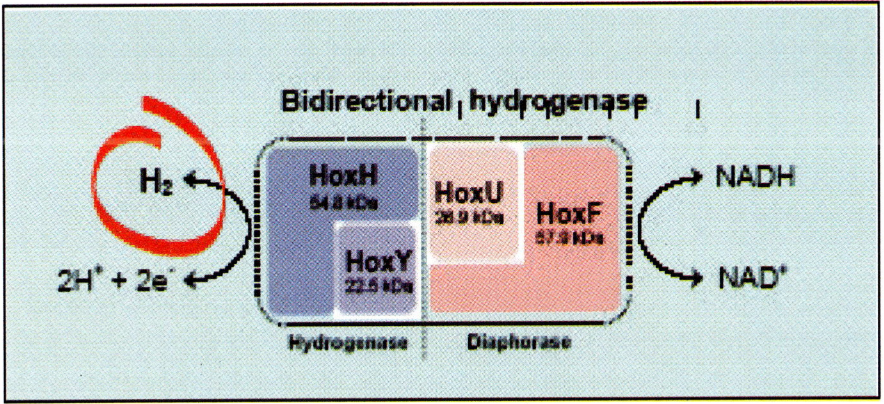

Figure 5.4: Hydrogenase Based + Fermentation (Linblad, 2002)

Cyanobacterial uptake hydrogenases consist of two subunits, encoded by hupS and hupL respectively the small subunit. HupS contains the iron-sulphur (Fe-S) cluster necessary for electron transfer to active site, which is located in the large subunit HupL. HupL contains two putatine binding sites (RXCGXC) necessary for the coordination as the nickel in the activity site (Happe *et al.,* 2000). Recently Vyas and Gupta (2007) reviewed transcriptional regulation of hydrogenases.

Bioengineering Aspects of H_2 Production

The proposal to produce hydrogen from water using solar energy and a biological catalyst has been the major impetus behind most recent research in the hydrogen metabolism of algae. On the basis of present knowledge of algal physiology two basic concepts have been considered: two stage systems and single-stage systems. In a two stage system photosynthetic CO_2 fixation would lead to O_2 evolution and bring about the accumulation of stable reduced carbon compounds which would then be transferred by pumping to an anaerobic chamber where a hydrogen fermentation would take place. In single stage systems hydrogen and oxygen would be released under a transparent covered collector either simultaneously or alternatively.

Two stage system has not yet been demonstrated in practice. One stage system has been employed for outdoor H_2 production (Benemann *et al.,* 1978). To date one oxygen stable biophotolysis catalyst has been demonstrated–the heterocystous nitrogen–fixing cyanobacteria–in which O_2 and H_2 production are separated spatially at the microscopic level. Use of these organisms has already demonstrated a catalytic, sustained, stoichiometric production of O_2 and H_2 using sunlight in an outdoor test (Benemann *et al.,* 1978). The experimnents involved sparging the cultures with a mixture of CO_2 (0.3 per cent), N_2 (1 per cent) and argon (balance) in vertical glass tubes containing 1-liter of culture. The low N_2 -concentrations maintained the algae in a healthy condition, substituting for the periodic additions of ammonia used in the laboratory experiments. H_2- production rates followed the sunlight intensities, decreasing to zero after sunset. A rate of 24 um/mg decreased but H_2 production continued upto 19 days.

A modified single-stage system has been suggested (Benemann *et al.*, 1978; Hallenbeck and Benemann, 1979). The vertical glass tubes fused in current experiments will have to be replaced by horizontal glass tubes, where gas flows over the surface of the algal cuture. This will minimize the energy required to pump the gas phase through the system. There is utmost need to make trials of such system at larger scale for large scale production of H_2.

Conclusion and Future Strategy for Photobiological H_2 Production

Studies so far made on H_2 metabolism on cyanobacteria reveall presence of H_2 metabolizing pathways in almost all the cyanobacteria. However, N_2-fixing cyanobacteria seem more suitable than non-N_2^+ fixers due to presence of the O_2 protection mechanism in them. Much more work is needed to understand exactly the biochemistry of hydrogenase.

There are a few aspects which need to be dealt with extensively in future studies. They are:

1. Isolation of efficient aerobic H_2 producers from various habitat,
2. Isolation of Hup-mutants,
3. Screening of depressed strains which can evolve H_2 even in the presence of combined nitrogen sources,
4. Isolation of some mutant which is defective in N_2 fixation but can produce H_2,
5. Thorough study on immobilization employing various matrices.

References

Asada, Y. and Kawamura, S. (1986). Aerobic hydrogen accumulation by a nitrogen-fixing cyanobacterium, *Anabaena* sp. *Appl. Environ. Microbiol.* 51: 1063-1066.

Belkin, S. and Padan, E. (1978). Hydrogen metabolism in the facultative anoxygenic cyanobacteria (blue-green algae) Oscillatoria limnetica and *Aphonothece halphytica. Arch. Microbiol.* 116: 109-111.

Benemann, J.R. and Weare, N.M. (1974a). Hydrogen evolution by nitrogen-fixing *Anabaena cylindrica* cultures. *Science* 184: 174-175.

Benemann, J. (1977). Hydrogen and methane production through microbial photosynthesis. In: *Living Systems as Energy Converters* (eds. Buvet, R., Allen, and Massue, J.P.) PP. 285. Elsevier/North Holland Biomedical Press, Amsterdam.

Benemann, J.R. and Hallenbeck, P.C. (1978). Basic and applied studies of hydrogenase in cyanobacteria. In: *Hydrogenases: Their Catalytic Activity, Structure and Functions* (eds.) Schlegel, H.G. and Schneider, K. P. 395. Goltze. Gotingen.

Benemann, J.R. and Weare, N.M. (1974b). Nitrogen fixation by *Anabaena cylindrica*. III. Hydrogen-supported nitrogenase activity. *Arch. Microbiol.* 101: 401-408.

Benemann, J.R. Miyamoto, K, Hallenbeck, P.C. and Murray, M.A. (1982). Hydrogenase activity in the thermophile *Mastigocladus laminosus*. *Biochem. Biophys. Res. Commun..* 106: 1196–1202.

Benemann, J.R. Miyamoto, K. and Hallenbeck, P.C. (1980). Bioengineering aspects of biophotolysis. *Enzyme Microbiol. Technol.* 2: 103-111.

Benerjee, M., Kumar, A. and Kumar, H.D. (1989). Factors regulating nitrogenase activity and hydrogen evolution in *Azolla Anabaena* symbiosis. *Int. J. Hydrogen Energy* 14: 871-879.

Berk, R.S. and Canfield, J.H. (1964). Bioelectrochemical energy conversion. *Appl. Microbiol.* 12: 10-12.

Bothe, H., Neuer, G., Kalbe, I. and Eisbrenner, G. (1980). Electron donors and hydrogenase in nitrogen-fixing microorganisms. In: *Nitrogen Fixation* (Eds.) Stewart, W.D.P. and Gallon, J.R. pp. 83-112. Academic press, New york.

Bothe, H., Tennigkeit, J. and Eisbrenner, G. (1977b). The hydrogenase-nitrogenase relationship in the blue-green alga *Anabaena cylindrica*. *Planta* 133: 237-242.

Bothe, H, Distler, E. and Eisbrenner, G. (1978). Hydrogen metabolism in blue-green algae. *Biochimie* 60: 277-289.

Bothe, H. (1982). Nitrogen fixation. In: *The Biology of Cyanobacteria* (eds.) Carr, N.G. and whitton, B.A.) pp. 87-104. The University of California Press, Berkeley, Los Angeles.

Bothe, H., Tennigkeit, J. and Eisbrenner, G. (1977a). The utilization of molecular hydrogen by the blue-green alga *Anabaena cylindrica*. *Arch. Microbiol.* 114: 43-49.

Brodelius, P. (1985). The potential role of immobilization in plant cell biotechnology. *Trends Biotechnol.* 3: 280-285.

Brouers, M. and Hall, D.O. (1986). Ammonia and hydrogen production by immobilized cyanobacteria. *J. Biotechnol.* 3: 307-322.

Calvin, M. and Taylor, S.E. (1989). Fuels from algae. In: *Algal and Cyanobacterial Biotechnology* (eds.) Cresswell, R.C., Rees, T.A.V. and Shah, N. Longman Group, UK Ltd.

Chan, Van, N., Hai, C. and Gogotov, I.N. (1983). Photosynthesis and hydrogen metabolism in *Anabaena azollae*. *Mikrobiologiya* 52: 896-901.

Chen, C.P., Almon, H. and Boger, P. (1989). Physiological factors determining hydrogenase activity in nitrogen-fixing heterocystous cyanobacteria. *Plant Physiol.* 89: 1035-1038.

Daday, A. and Smith, G.D. (1983). The effect of nickel on the hydrogen metabolism of the cyanobacterium *Anabaena cylindrica*. *FEMS Microbiol. Lett.* 20: 327-330.

Daday, A. and Smith, G.D. (1987). The hydrogenase-nitrogenase relationship in a symbiotic cyanobacterium isolated from *Macrozamia communis* L. Johnson. *Aust. J. plant Physiol.* 14: 319-324.

Daday, A., Lambert, G.R. and Smith, G.D. (1979). Measurement in vivo of hydrogenase-catalysed hydrogen-evolution in the presence of nitrogenase enzyme in cyanobacteria. *Biochem. J.* 177: 139-144.

Daday, A., Mackerras, A.H. and Smith, G.D. (1985). The effect of nickel on hydrogen metabolism and nitrogen fixation in the cyanobacterium *Anabaena cylindrica*. *J. Gen. Microbiol.* 131: 231-238.

Daday, A., Platz, R.A. and Smith, G.D. (1977). Anaerobic and aerobic hydrogen gas formation by the blue-green alga *Anabaena cylindrica*. *Appl. Environ. Microbiol.* 34: 478-483.

Davis, D.D. and Stevenson, K.L. (1977). A recording gas microvolumeter. *J. Chem. Educ.* 54: 394-395.

Eisbrenner, G. and Bothe, H. (1979). Modes of electron tansfer from molecular hydrogen in *Anabaena cylindrica*. *Arch. Microbiol.* 123: 37-48.

Eisbrenner, G., Roos, P. and Bothe, H. (1981). The number of hydrogenases in cyanobacteria. *J. Gen. Microbiol.* 125: 385-390.

Ernst, A., Kerfin, W., Spiller, H. and Boger, P. (1979). External factors influencing light-induced hydrogen evolution by the blue-green alga *Nostoc muscorum*. *Z. Naturforsch.* 34: 820-825.

Ewart, G.D. and Smith, G.D. (1989a). Immunochemical analysis of the soluble hydrogenase from the cyanobacterium *Anabaena cylindrica*. *Biochim. Biophys. Acta* 997: 83-89.

Ewart, G.D. and Smith, G.D. (1989b). An activity stain for the detection of cyanobacterial hydrogenase in polyacrylamide gels. *Biochem. Intl.* (19: 89-97.

Ewart, G.D. and Smith, G.D. (1989c). Purification and properties of soluble hydrogenase from the cyanobacterium *Anabaena cylindrica*. *Arch Biochem. Biophys.* 268: 327-337.

Frenkel, A.H., Gaffron, H. and Battley, E.H. (1950). Photosynthesis and photoreduction in the blue-green alga, *Synechococcus elongatus* Nag. Biol. Bulletin. Marine Biological Laboratory, Woods Hole, Mass. 99: 157-162.

Fry, I., Robinson, A.E., Spath, S. and Packer, L. (1984). The role os sodium sulfide in anoxygenic photosynthesis and hydrogen production in the cyanobacterium *Nostoc muscorum*. *Biochem. Biophys. Res. Commun.* 123: 1138-1143.

Gerasimenko, L.M. and Zavarzin, G.A. (1981). Anabolic hydrogen uptake by cyanobacteria. *Mikrobiologiya* 50: 955-959.

Gogotov, I.N. and Kosyak, A.V. (1976). Hydrogen metabolism by *Anabaena variabilis* in the dark. *Mikrobiologiya* 45: 586-591.

Gogotov, I.V., Kosyak, A.V. and Krupenko, A.N. (1976). Hydrogen production by the cyanobacterium *Anabaena variabilis* in light. *Mikrobiologiya* 45: 941-945.

Greenbaum, E. (1977). The molecular mechanisms of photosynthetic hydrogen and oxygen production. In: *Biological Solar Energy Conversion* (Eds.) Mitsui, A., Miyachi, S., San Pietro, A. and Tamura, S. pp. 101-107. Academic Press, New York.

Hallenbeck, P.C. and Benemann, J.R. (1979). Hydrogen from algae. In: *Photosynthesis in Relation to Model Systems* (ed. Barber, J.). Elsevier/Noth-Holland Biomedical Press, Amsterdam.

Hallenbeck, P.C. Kochian, L. V. and Benemann, J.R. (1981). Hydrogen evolution catalyzed by hydrogenase in cultures of cyanobacteria. *Z. Naturforsch.* 36c: 97-92.

Happe, T., Schute, K. and Bohme, H. (2000). Transcriptional and mutational analysis of the uptake hydrogenase of the filamentous cyanobacterium *Anabaena variabilis* ATCC 29413. J. Bacteriol. 182: 1624–1631.

Hartman, H. and Krasna, A.I. (1963). Studies on the "adaptation" of hydrogenase in Scenedesmus. J. Biol. Chem. 238: 749-757.

Hattori, A. (1963). Microalgae and photosynthetic bacteria. Special Issue of plant and Cell physiology, University of Tokyo Press, pp. 485-492.

Haystead, A., Robinson, R. and Stewart, W.D.P. (1970). Nitrogenase activity in extracts of heterocystous blue-green algae. *Arch. Mikrobiol.* 82: 325-336.

Hillmer, P. and Gest, H. (1977). H_2 metabolism in the photosynthetic bacterium *Rhodopseudomonas capsulata*: H_2 production by growing cultures. *J. Bacteriol.* 129: 724-731.

Hirosawa, T. and wolk, C.P. (1979). Factors controlling the formation of akinetes adjacent to heterocyst in the cyanobacterium *Cylindrospermum licheniforme. J. Gen. Microbiol.* 114: 423-432.

Houchins, J. and Burris, R.H. (1981a). Comarative characterization of two distinct hydrogenases from *Anabaena* sp. strain 7120. *J. Bacteriol.* 146: 215-221.

Houchins, J.P. (1984). The physiology and biochemistry of hydrogen metabolism in cyanobacteria. *Biochim. Biophys. Acta* 768: 227-255.

Houchins, J.P. and Burris, R.H. (1981b). Occurrence and localization of two distinct hydrogenases in the heterocystous cyanobacterium *Anabaena* sp. strain 7120. *J. Bacteriol.* 146: 209-214.

Houchins, J.P. and Burris, R.H. (1981c). Light and dark reactions of the uptake hydrogenase from Anabaena 7120. *Plant Physiol.* 68: 712-716.

Houchins, J.P. and Burris, R.H. (1981d). Physiological reaction of the reversible hydrogenase from *Anabaena* 7120. *Plant Physiol.* 68: 717-721.

Howarth, D.D. and Codd G.A. (1985). The uptake and production of molecular hydrogen by unicellular cyanobacteria. *J. Gen. Microbiol.* 131: 1561-1570.

Jackson, D.D. and Ellms, J. W. (1886). On odors and tastes of surface waters, with special reference to *Anabaena*, a microscopical organism found in certain water supplies of Massachusetts. In the 1896

Jouanneau, Y., Kelley, B.C., Barlier, Y., Lespinat, P. A. and Vignais, P.M. (1980). Continuous monitoring by mass spectrometry of H_2 production and recycling in *Rhodopseudomonas capsulata. J. Bacteriol.* 143: 628-636.

Kayano, H., Karube, I., Matsunaga, T., Suzuki, S. and Nakayama, O. (1981). A photochemical fuel cell system using *Anabaena* N-7363. *Eur. J. Appl. Microbiol. Biotechnol.* 12: 1-5.

Kerby, N. W., Musgrave, S.C., Rowell, P., Shestakov, S.V. and Stewart, W.D.P. (1986). Photoproduction of ammonium by immobilized mutant strains of *Anabaena variabilis. Appl. Microbiol. Biotechnol.* 24: 42-46.

Kerfin, W. and Boger, P. (1982). Light-induced hydrogen evolution by blue-green algae (cyanobacteria) physiol. *Plant.* 54: 93-98.

Kerfin, W., Spiller, H., Ernst, A. and Boger, P. (1978). Properties of the hydrogen producing system in the blue-green alga Nostoc muscorum. In: Hydrogenases: Their Catalytic Activity, Structure and Function (eds.) Schlegel, H.G. and Schneider, K. pp. 381-386. E. Goltze KG. Gottingen.

Kosyak, A.V. Gogotov, I.N. and Kulakova, S.M. (1978). Photoproduction of hydrogen by the cyanobacterium *Anabaena cylindrica. Mikrobiologiya* 47: 605-610.

Krasna, A.I. (1978). Oxygen-stable hydrogenase and assay. *Methods Enzymol.* 53: 314-332.

Krasna, A.I. (1979). Hydrogenase: Properties and applications. *Enzyme Microbial Technol.* 1: 165-172.

Krasna, A.I. (1977). Catalytic and structural properties of the enzyme hydrogenase and its role in biophotolysis of water. In: *Biological Solar Energy Conversion* (eds.) Mitsui, A., Miyachi, S., San Pietro, A. and Tamura, S. P. 53. Academic Press, New York.

Kumar, D. (1986). Effects of amitrol on cyanobacterium *Nostoc linckia. J. Gen. Appl. Microbiol.* 32: 51-56.

Kumar, D. and Kumar, H.D. (1988). Light-dependent acetylene reduction and hydrogen production by the cyanobacterium, *Anabaena* sp. (strain CA). *Int. J. Hydrogen Energy* 13: 573–575.

Kumar, D. and Kumar, H.D. (1989). Effects of glucose and fructose on acetylene reduction, photosynthesis, respiration and hydrogen evolution by whole cells of the cyanobacterium *Anabaena* sp. strain CA. In *Proc. Intl. Phycotalk Symp.*, Dept. of Botany, Banaras hindu University, Varanasi.

Kumar, D. and Kumar, H.D. (1990b). Effects of some inhibitors and carbon sources on acetylene reduction and hydrogen production by isolated heterocysts of *Anabaena* sp. (strain CA). *British Phycol. J.* (Accepted).

Kumar, D. Kumar, H.D. (1990c). Protection of nitrogenase levels in dark-incubated cultures of *Anabaena* sp. strain CA by various carbon sources, and restoration of nitrogenase activity by oxygen. *Br. Phycol. J.* 25: (in press).

Kumar, D., Pandey, A.B. and Kumar, H.D. (1990a). Effect of some physiological factors on the nitrogenase and hydrogenase of the *Azolla-Anabeana azollae* association. *Int. J. Hydrogen Energy* 15: 313-317.

Kumazawa, S. and Mitsui, A. (1981). Characterization and optimization of hydrogen photoproduction by a saltwater bluegreen alga, *Oscillatoria* sp. miami BG7. I. Enhancement through limiting the supply of nitrogen nutrients. *Int. J. Hydrogen Energy* 6: 339-348.

Kumazawa, S. and Mitsui, A. (1985). Comparative reproduction activities between heterocystous cyanobacterium *Anabaena cylindrica* B 629 and non heterocystous cyanobacterium *Oscillatoria* sp. strain Miami BG 7. *Appl. Environ. Microbiol.* 50: 287-291.

Kumazawa, S. and Mitsui, A. (1982). Hydrogen metabolism of photosynthetic bacteria and algae. In: *Handbook of Biosolar Resources, Vol. I. Basic principles* (eds. Mitsui, A. and Black, C.C.O. pp. 299-316. CRC Press, Boca Raton, Florida.

Kuwada, Y. and Ohta, Y. (1987). Hydrogen production by an immobilized cyanobacterium, *Lyngbya* sp. *J. Ferment. Technol.* 65: 597-602.

Kuwada, Y. and Ohta, Y. (1989). Hydrogen production and carbohydrate consumption by *Lyngbya* sp. No. 108. *Agric. Biol. Chem.* 53: 2847-2851.

Kuwada, Y., Nakatsukasa, M. and Ohta, Y. (1988). Isolation and characterization of a non heterocystous cyanobacterium *Lyngbya* sp. isolate No. 108, for large quantity hydrogen production. *Agric. Biol. Chem.* 52: 1923-1928.

Laczko, I. (1980). Mechanism of hydrogen evolution by nitrogen starved *Anabaena cylindrica*. *Z. Pflanzenphysiol.* 100: 241-246.

Laczko, I. and Barabas, K. (1981). Hydrogen evolution by photobleached *Anabaena cylindrica*. *Planta* 153: 312-316.

Lambert, G.R. and Smith, G.D. (1977). Hydrogen formation by marine blue-green algae. *FEBS Letts.* 83: 159-162.

Lambert, G.R. and Smith, G.D. (1980). Hydrogen metabolism by filamentous cyanobacteria. *Arch. Biochem. Biophys.* 205: 36-50.

Lambert, G.R. and Smith, G.D. (1981a). Hydrogen uptake by the nitrogen-starved cyanobacterium *Anabaena cylindrica*. *Arch. Biochem. Biophys.* 211: 360-367.

Lambert, G.R. Daday, A. and Smith, G.D. (1979a). Hydrogen evolution from immobilized cultures of the cyanobacterium *Anabaena cylindrica. FEBS Letts.* 101: 125-128.

Lambert, G.R. Daday, A. and Smith, G.D. (1979b). Duration of hydrogen formation by *Anabaena cylindrica.* B 629 in atmospheres of argon, air and nitrogen. *Appl. Environ. Microbiol.* 38: 530-536.

Lambert, G.R. Smith, G.D. (1981b). The hydrogen metabolism of cyanobacteria (blue-green algae). *Biol. Rev.* 56: 589-660.

Lambert, G.R., Daday, A. and Smith, G.D. (1979c). Effects of ammonium ions, oxygen, carbon monoxide and acetylene on anaerobic and aerobic hydrogen formation by *Anabaena cylindrica.* B-629. *Appl. Environ. Microbiol.* 38: 521-529.

Liama, M.J., Serra, J.L., Rao, K.K. and Hall, D.O. (1979). Modes of reduction of nitrogenase in heterocysts isolated from *Anabaena* species. *Biochim. Biophys. Acta* 502: 298-308.

Lindberg, P., Schulz, K., Happe, T. and Lindblad, P. (2002). A hydrogen producing, hydrogenase free mutant-strain of Nostoc punetiforme ATEC 29133. *Int. J. Hydrogen Energy*, 27: 1291-1296.

Millbank, J.W. (1981). Nitrogenase and hydrogenase in cyanophilic lichens. *New Phytol.* 92: 221-228.

Mitsui, A. (1980a). Nitrogen fixation and hydrogen production by marine blue-green algae used as a source of food, feed and chemicals. In: *Proceedings of the International Symposium on Biological Application of Solar Energy* (eds.) Gnanam, A. and Kahn, J. pp. 109-115. Viking publ., New Delhi.

Mitsui, A. (1975a). Photoproduction of hydrogen via microbial and biochemical processes. In: *Symposium Proceedings of Hydrogen Energy Fundamental: Symposium Proceedings of Hydrogen Energy Fundamental* (ed.) Veziroglu, T.N. pp. 52 31-48. University of Miami Press, Miami.

Mitsui, A. (1975b). Hydrogen production via photosynthetic processes. In: Key Technologies for Hydrogen Energy Systems. (ed. Ohta, T.) pp. 75-92. Yokohama National University Press.

Mitsui, A. (1975c). Utilization of solar energy for hydrogen production by cell-free system of photosynthetic organisms. In: *Hydrogen Energy, Part A* (ed.) Veziroglu, T.N. pp. 309-316. Plenum publishing Corp., New York.

Mitsui, A. (1976). Bioconversion of solar energy in salt water photosynthetic hydrogen production system. In: *Proceedings of 1st World Hydrogen Energy Conference: Progress in World Hydrogen Energy projects and planning* (ed.) Veziroglu, T.N. pp. 4B: 77-99. University of Miami Press.

Mitsui, A. (1978a). Bio-solar hydrogen production. In: *Hydrogen Energy System*, Vol. 3 (eds.) Veziroglu, T.N. and Seifritz, W. pp. 1267-1291. Pergamon Press, Oxford, England.

Mitsui, A. (1978b). Solar energy conversion to hydrogen by bacteria and algae. In: *Bio-Energy* (ed.) Gottib Duttweiler-Institute. Zurich, pp. 205-236.

Mitsui, A. (1978c). Solar energy conversion in marine biological systems. In: An International Compendium (ed.) Veziroglu, T.N.. Hemisphere Publ. Co., Washington, 2: 1013-1017.

Mitsui, A. (1979a). Biosaline research: The use of photosynthetic marine organisms in food and feed production. In: *The Biosaline Concept* (eds.) Hollaender *et al.* pp. 177-215. Plenum Press, New York.

Mitsui, A. (1979b). Biological and biochemical hydrogen production. In: Solar Hydrogen Energy Systems (ed.) Ohta, T. pp. 171-191. Pergamon press, Oxford and New York.

Mitsui, A. (1980b). Salt water based biological solar energy conversion for fuel, chemicals, fertilizer, food and feed. In: *Proceedings of Bio-Energy* (80. World Congress and Exposition, (ed.) pp. 486-491. Bio-Energy Council, Washington, D.C.

Mitsui, A. (1981). *Hydrogen production by marine photosynthetic microorganisms.* Kitani, O. pp. 165-180. Japan Scientific Society Press, Tokyo.

Mitsui, A. (1987). Photobiological production of hydrogen from water and waste. In: *Proceedings of the Hydrogen Photoproduction workshop* (eds.) Seki, A., Morgan, B. and Takahashi, P.O. pp. 32-39.

Mitsui, A. and Black, C.C. (eds.) (1982). *CRC Handbook of Biosolar Resources. Vol. 1. Basic Principles,* Part 1, pp. 643. CRC Press, Boca Raton, Florida.

Mitsui, A. and Black, C.C. (eds.) (1982). *CRC Handbook of Biosolar Resources. Vol. 1. Basic Principles,* Part 2, CRC Press, Boca Raton, Florida, pp. 657.

Mitsui, A. and Kumazawa, S. (1978). Hydrogen production by marine photosynthetic organisms on a potential energy resource. In: *Biological Solar Energy Conversion* (eds.) Mitsui, A., Miyachi, S., San Pietro, A. and Tamura, S.. Academic Press, London and New York.

Mitsui, A. and Kumazawa, S. (1979). Solar energy biological conversion research. *J. Solar Energy* (in Japanese) 5: 55-67.

Mitsui, A. and Matsunaga, T. (1983). Hydrogen production by photosynthetic microorganisms. In: *Biomass Energy Conversion* (ed. Suzuki, S.) pp. 194-228. Kodansha Scientific Press, Tokyo.

Mitsui, A., Duerr, E. Kumazawa, S., Phlips, E. and Skjoldal, H. (1979). Biological solar energy conversion: hydrogen production and nitrogen fixation by marine blue-green algae. In: *Sun II. Proceedings of the International Solar Energy Society Silver Jubilee Congress, Vol. I* (eds.) Boer, K. and Glenn, B.H. pp. 31-35. Pergamon Press, New York and Oxford.

Mitsui, A., Kumazawa, S., Phlips, E.J., Reddy, K.J., Gill, K., Renuka, B.R. Kusumi, T., Reyes-Vasques, G., Miyazawa, K., Haynes, L., Ikemoto, h., Duerr, E., Leon, C.B. Rosner, D., Sesco, R. and Moffat, E. (1985). Mass cultivation of algae and photosynthetic bacteria: Concepts and Application. In: *Biotechnology and Bioprocess Engineering* (ed.) Ghosh, T.K. pp. 119-155. International Union of Pure and Applied Chemistry and Indian National Science Academy, United India Press, New Delhi.

Mitsui, A., Kumazawa, S., Takahashi, A., Ikemoto, H., Coa, S. and Arai, T. (1987). Relevance of the study of the strategy by which nitrogen-fixing unicellular cyanobacteria grow photoautotrophically to the hydrogen photoproduction research. *J. Hydrogen Energy Systems Society of Japan* 12: 39-49 (in Japanese).

Mitsui, A., Miyachi, S., San Pietro, A. and Tamura, S. (Eds.) (1977). *Biological Solar Energy Conversion.* Academic press, London and New York.

Mitsui, A., Philips, E.J., Kumaawa, S., Reddy, K.J., Ramachandran, S., Matsunaga, T., Haynes, L. and Ikemoto, H. (1983). Progress in research toward outdoor biological hydrogen production using solar energy, sea water and marine photosynthetic microorganisms. *Ann. NoY. Acad. Sci.* 413: 514-530.

Mitsui, A., Rosner, D., Kumazawa, S., Barciela, S., Phlips, E., Ramachandran S., Takahashi, A. and Richard, J. (1985). Hydrogen production from salt water by marine blue green algae and solar radiation. In: *Proceedings of Twenty-Second Space Congress* (ed.) Haise, F.W. pp. 11.7-11.14. Canaveral Council of Technical Societies, Revised form.

Miura, Y, Yokoyama, H., Kimura, M., Iwamoto, T. and Miyamoto, K. (1981). Effect of acetylene and carbon monoxide on hydrogen uptake and evolution by nitrogen-starved cultures of *Mastgocladus laminosus. Plant Cell Physiol.* 22:1375-1383.

Miura, Y., Yokoyama, H., Takahara, K. and Miyamoto, K. (1982). Effects of acetylene and carbon monoxide on long-term hydrogen production by *Mastgocladus laminosus*: A thermophilic blue-green alga. *J. Ferment Technol.* 60: 411-416.

Miura, Y.H., Kanaoka, K., Saito, S., Iwasa, K., Okazaki, M. and Komemushi, S. (1980). Hydrogen evolution by a thermophilic blue-green *Mastgocladus laminosus. Plant Cell Physiol.* 21: 149-156.

Miyamoto, K., Takahara- Ishikawa, K., Horie, H. and Miura, Y. (1984). Dark period nitrogen fixation by *Mastgocladus laminosus* and its application to a biophotolysis system. *J. Ferment. Technol.* 62: 13-18.

Miyamoto, K.,Hallenbeck, P.C. and Benemann, J.R. (1979). Hydrogen production by the thermophilic alga *Mastgocladus laminosus* : Effects of nitrogen, temperature and inhibitors of photosynthesis. *Appl. Environ. Microbiol.* 38: 440-446.

Mortensen, L.E. (1978). The role of dihydrogen and hydrogenase in nitrogen fixation. *Biochimie* 60: 219-223.

Mortensen, L.E. and Chen J.S. (1974). Hydrogenase. In: *Microbial Iron Metabolism, a Comprehensive Treatise* (ed.) Neilands, J.B. P. 231. Academic Press, London and New York.

Mortensen, L.E. and Thorneley, R.N.F. (1979). Structure and function of nitrogenase. *Ann. Rev. Biochem.* 48: 387-418.

Newton, J.W. (1976). Photoproduction of molecular hydrogen by a plant algal symbiotic system. *Science,* 191: 559-561.

Ochiai, H., Shibata, H., Sawa, Y., Shoga, M. and Ohta, S. (1983). Properties of semiconductor electrodes coated with living films of cyanobacteria. *Appl. Biochem. Biotechnol.* 8:289-303.

Ochial, H., Shibata, H., Sawa, Y. and Katoh, T. (1980). 'Living electrode' as a long-lived photoconverter for biophotolysis of water. *Proc. Natl. Acad. Sci.*, USA 77: 2442-2444.

Ormeland, R. (1983). Hydrogen metabolism by decomposing cyanobacterial aggregates in Bio-Soda Lake, Nevada (USA). *Appl. Environ. Microbiol.* 45: 1519-1525.

Oschchepkov,V.P., Nikitina, A. A., Gusev, M.V. and Krasnovskii A.A. (1974). Evolution of molecular hydrogen by cultures of blue-green algae. Doklady Akademii Nauk, *SSSR* 215: 557-560.

Oschchepkov,V.P., Nikitina, K.A., Gusev, MoV. and Krasnovskii A.A. (1973). Evolution of molecular hydrogen by blue-green algal cultures. Doklady Nauk *SSSR Biol.* 213: 739-742.

Padan, E. and Schuidiner, S. (1978). Energy transduction in the photosynthetic memberanes of the cyanobacterium blue-green alge *Plectonema boryanum. J. Biol. Chem.* 253: 3281-3286.

Paerl, H, W. and Bland, P.T. (1982). Localized tetrazolium reduction in relation to N_2 fixation, and CO_2 fixation, and H_2 uptake in aquatic filamentous cyanobacteria. Appl. Environ. *Microbiol.* 43: 218-226.

Paerl, H.W. (1980). Ecological rationale for hydrogen metabolism during aquatic blooms of the cyanobacterium *Anabaena*. *Oecologia* 47: 43-53.

Paerl, H.W. (1982). *In situ* hydrogen production and utilization by natural population of nitrogen-fixing blue-green algae. *Can. J. Bot.* 60: 2542-2546.

Peck, H.D. Jr. and Gest, H. (1956). A new procedure for assay of bacterial hydrogenase. *J. Bacteriol.* 71: 70-80.

Perderson, D.M. Daday, A. and Smith, G.D. (1986). The use of nickel to probe the role of hydrogen metabolism in cyanobacterial nitrogen fixation. *Biochimie* 68: 113-120.

Perraju, B.T. Rai, A.N., Kumar, A.P. and Singh, H.N. (1986). *Cycas circinalis-Anabaena cycadeae* symbiosis: Photosynthesis and the enzymes of nitrogen and hydrogen metabolism in symbiotic and cultued *Anabaena cycadeae*. *Symbiosis* 1: 239-250.

Peschek, G.A. (1978). Reduced sulfur and nitrogen compunds and molecular hydrogen as electron donors for anaerobic CO_2 photoreduction in *Anacystis nidulans*. *Arch. Microbiol.* 119: 203-215.

Peschek, G.A. (1979a). Anaerobic hydrogenase activity in *Anacystis nidulans*. Hydrogen dependent photoreduction and related reaction. *Biochim. Biophys. Acta* 548: 187-202.

Peschek, G.A. (1979b). Aerobic hydrogenase activity in *Anacystis nidulans*. The oxyhydrogen reaction. *Biochim. Biophys. Acta* 548: 203-215.

Peschek, G.A. (1979c). Evidence for functionally distinct hydrogenases in *Anacystis nidulans*. *Arch. Microbiol.* 123: 81-92.

Peschek, G.A. (1979d). Nitrate and nitrite reductase and hydrogenase in *Anacystis nidulans*. grown in Fe- and Mo-deficient media. *FEMS Microbiol. Letts.* 6: 371-374.

Peschek, G.A. (1980). Electron transport reactions in respiratory particles of hydrogenase- induced *Anacystis nidulans*. *Arch. Microbiol.* 125: 123-131.

Peters, G.A. Evans, W.R. and Toia, R.E. Jr. (1976). *Azolla anabaena* cycadeae relationship V. $^{15}N_2$ fixation, acetylene reduction and H_2 production. *Plant Physiol.* 59: 1021-1025.

Peterson, R.B. and Burris, R.H. (1978a). Hydrogen metabolism in isolated heterocysts of *Anabaena* 7120. *Arch. Microbiol.* 116: 125-132.

Peterson, R.B. and Wolk, C.P. (1978b). Localization of an uptake hydrogenase in *Anabaena*. *Plant Physiol.* 61: 688-691.

Phlips, E.J. and Mitsui, A. (1983a). Role of light intensity and temperature in the regulation of hydrogen photoproduction by the regulation of hydrogen photoproduction by the marine cyanobacterium Oscillatoria sp. strain Miami BG 7. *Appl. Environ. Microbiol.* 45: 1212-1220.

Phlips, E.J. and Mitsui, A. (1984). Development of hydrogen production activity in the marine blue-green alga *Oscillatoria* sp. Miami BG 7 under natural sunlight conditions. In: *Advances in Photosynthesis Research* (ed.) Sybesm, C. pp. 810-804 Vol. II, Martinus Nijhoff/Dr W. Junk Publishers, Hague,

Planchard, A., Mignot, L., Jouenne, T. and Junter, G. (1989). Photoproduction of molecular hydrogen by *Rhodospirillum rubrum*: immobilized in composite agar layer/microporous membrane structures. *Appl. Microbiol. Biotechnol.* 31: 49-54.

Ramachandran, S. and Mitsui, A. (1984). Effect of seawater quality on biomiass and hydrogen photoproduction by a marine blue-green alga *Oscillatoria* sp. Miami BG 7. In: *Advances in Photosynthesis Research* (ed.) Sybesma, C. Vol. II, pp. 805-808. Martinus Nijhoff/Dr W. Junk Publishers, Hague.

Ramachandran, S. and Mitsui, A. (1986). Biosystem catalyzed continuous hydrogen photoproduction from seawater using solar energy. In: *Proc. 6th International Symp. Hydrogen Energy* (ed.) Veziroglu, T.N. pp. 1371-1381.

Scherer, S., Kerfin, W. and Boger, P. (1980b). Increase of nitrogenase activity in the blue green alga *Nostoc muscorum* (cyanobacterium). *J. Bacteriol.* 144: 1017-1023.

Schlegel, H.G. and Schneider, K. (1978). Introductory report: distribution and physiological role of hydrogenases in microorganisms. In: *Hydrogenases: their Catalytic Activity Structure and Function* (eds.) Schlegel, H.G. and Schneider, K. p. 15. Goltze, Gottingen.

Scranton, M.I., Novelli, P.C. Michaels, A., Horrigan, S.G. and Carpenter, E.J. (1987). Hydrogen production and nitrogen fixation by *Oscillatoria thiebautii* during *in situ* incubations. *Limnol. Oceanogr.* 32: 998-1006.

Shi, D.J., Brouers, M., Hall, D.O. and Robins, R.J. (1987). The effects of immobilization on the biochemical, physiological and morphological features of *Anabaena azollae. Planta* 172: 298-308.

Singh, S. and Kashyap, A.K. (1988). Photoevolution of hydrogen during oxygenic photosynthesis of cyanobacterium *Nostoc muscorum. Biotech. Lett.* 10: 921-925.

Smith, R.L., Kumar, D., Xiankong, Z., Tabita, F.R. and Van Baalen, C. (1985). H_2, N_2 and O_2 metablism by isolated heterocysts from *Anabaena* sp. strain Ca. *J. Bacteriol.* 162: 565-570.

Smith, G.D., and Lambert, G.R. (1981). Outdoor biophotolytic system using the cyanobacterium, *Anabaena cylindrica* B 629. *Bioeng.* 23: 213-220.

Smith, G.D., Mualiem, A. and Hall, D.O. (1982). Hydrogenase-catalyzed photoproduction of hydrogen by photosystem I of the thermophilic blue-green algae *Mastigocladus laminosus* and *Phormidium laminosum. Photobiochem. Photobiophys.* 4: 307-320.

Spiller, H., Bookjans, G. and Shanmugam, K.T. (1983). Regulation of hydrogenase activity in vegetative cells of *Anabaena variabilis. J. Bacteriol.* 155: 129-137.

Spiller, H., Ernst, E., Kerfin, W. and Boger, P. (1978). Increase and stabilization of photoproduction of hydrogen in *Nostoc muscorum* by photosynthetic electron transport inhibitors. *Z. Naturforsch.* 33c: 541-547.

Srivastava, M. (1990). Regulation of nitrogen fixation and hydrogen production in *Anabaena* species. *Ph.D. Thesis*, Banaras Hindu University, Varanasi.

Srivastava, M., Sharma. A., Kumar, A. and Kumar, H.D. (1989). Hydrogen production by nitrogen-fixing cyanobacteria. In: *Proc. Intl. Phycotalk Symposium*, Department of Botany, Banaras Hindu University, Varanasi-221005, pp. 26-29.

Stewart, W.D.P. (1980). Some aspects of structure and function in N_2-fixing cyanobacteria. *Ann. Rev. Microbiol.* 34: 497-536.

Stuart, T.S. Herold, E.W. Jr. and Gaffron, H. (1972). A simple combination mass spectrometer inlet and oxygen electrode chamber for sampling gases dissolved in liquids. *Anal. Biochem.* 46: 91-100.

Tamagnini, P., Axelsson, R., Lindberg, P., Oxelfelt, F., Wunschiers, R. and Lindblad, P. (2002). Hydrogenases and Hydrogen Metabolism of Cyanobacteria. *Microbiology and Molecular Biology Reviews*. 66(1) : 1-20.

Tamiya, N., Kondo, Y., Kameyama, T. and Akabori, S. (1955). Determination of hydrogenase by the hydrogen evolution from reduced methyl viologen. *J. Biochem*. 42: 613-614.

Tel-Or, E., Luijk, L.W. and packer, L. (1977). An inducible hydrogenase in cyanobacteria enhances N_2 fixation. *FEBS Lett*. 78: 49- 52.

Tel-Or, E., Luijk, L.W. and Packer, L. (1978). Hydrogenase in N_2 fixing cyanobacteria. *Arch. Biochem. Biophys*. 185: 185-194.

Tetley, R.M. and Bishop, N.I. (1979). The differential action of metronidazole an nitrogen fixation, hydrogen metabolism, photosynthesis and respiration in *Anabaena* and *Scenedesmus*. *Biochim. Biophys. Acta* 546: 43-53.

Umbreit, W. W., Burris, R.H. and Stauffer, J.F. (1972). *Manometric and biochemical techniques*. 5th Edition. Burgess publ. C., Minneapolis, Minnesota, pp, 387.

Van Der Oost, J., Kanneworff, W.A. Krab, K. and Kraayenhof, R. (1987). Hydrogen metabolism of three unicellular nitrogen-fixing cyanobacteria. *FEMS Microbiol. Lett*. 48: 41-45.

Vyas, D. (2004). Cyanobacterial biodiversity and their hydrogen production potential. *J. Bot. Asoc. Univ. Sagar*. 39:55-65.

Vyas, D. and Gupta, R.K. (2003). Impact of ultraviolet B radiation on hydrogen production, and nitrogen fixation in *Cyanobacterium nostoc* sp. *J. Bot. Asoc. Univ. Sagar*. 36-38:89-97.

Vyas, D. and Kumar, H.D. (1995). Nitrogen fixation and hydrogen uptake in four cyanobacteria. *Int. J. Hydrogen Energy*. 20:163-168.

Vyas, D. and Gupta, R.K. (2007). Cynobacterial hydrogen metabolism with special reference to transcriptional regulation of hydrogenases. In: Advances in Applied Phycology. (eds.) Gupta, R.K. and Pandey, V.D. pp. 155–168. Daya Publishing House, New Delhi.

Wang, R., Healey, F.P. and Myers, J. (1971). Amperometric measurement of hydrogen evolution in *Chlamydomonas*. *Plant Physiol*. 48: 108-110.

Ward, M.A. (1970). Whole cell and cell free hydrogenases of algae. *Phytochemistry* 9: 108-266.

Weaver, P.F., Lien, S. and Seibert, M. (1980). Photobiological production of hydrogen. *Solar Energy* 24: 3-45.

Weisshaar, H. and Boger, P. (1983). Sulfide stimulation of light induced hydrogen evolution by the cyanobacterium Nostoc muscorum. *Z. Naturforsch*. 38: 237-242.

Weisshaar, H. and Boger, P. (1985). Pathways of hydrogen uptake in the cyanobacterium *Nostoc muscorum*. *Arch. Microbiol*.142: 349-353.

Weissman, J.C. and Benemann, J.R. (1977). Hydrogen production by nitrogen starved cultures of *Anabaena cylindrica*. *Appl. Environ. Microbiol*. 33: 123-131.

Xiankong, Z., Haskell, J.B., Tabita, F.R. and Van Baalen, C. (1983). Aerobic hydrogen production by the heterocystous cyanobacteria *Anabaena* spp. strains CA and 1F. *J. Bacteriol*. 156: 1118-1122.

Xiankong, Z., Tabita, F.R. and Van Baalen, C. (1984). Nickel control of hydrogen production and uptake in *Anabaena* spp. strains CA and 1F. *J. Gen. Microbiol.* 130: 1815-1818.

Yagi, T. (1976). Separation of hydrogenase-catalysed hydrogen evolution system from electron donating system by means of enzymic electric cell technique. *Proc. Natl. Acad. Sci.,* U.S.A.. 73: 2947-2949.

Yagi, T. (1977). Use of an enzymic electric cell and immobilized hydrogenase in the study of the biophotolysis of water to produce hydrogen. In: *Biological Solar Energy Conversion* (eds.) Mitsui, A., Miyachi, S., San Pietro, A. and Tamura, S. pp. 61-68. Academic Press, New York.

Yu, L. and Wolin, M.J. (1969). Hydrogenase measurement with photochemically reduced methyl viologen. *J. Bacteriol.* 98: 51-55.

Zajic, J.E., Kosaric, N. and Brosseau, J.D. (1978). Microbial production of hydrogen. *Adavances in Biochem. Engin.* 9: 57-109.

Microbial Biotechnology and Ecology (2011) *Pages* **94–149**
Editors: **Deepak Vyas, G.S. Paliwal, P.K.Khare and R.K Gupta**
Published by: **DAYA PUBLISHING HOUSE, NEW DELHI**

Chapter 6

Cyanobacterial Toxins

☆ *U.S. Gupta*[1], *Deepak Vyas*[2]* *and Rajan Kumar Gupta*[3]

[1]*Department of Zoology,* [2]*Department of Botany, Dr. H.S. Gour University, Sagar – 470 003, M.P.*
[3]*Government P.G. College, Rishikesh, Uttranchal*

Introduction

The cyanotoxins are a diverse group of natural toxins, both from the chemical and the toxicological points of view. In spite of their aquatic origin, most of the cyanotoxins that have been identified to date appear to be more hazardous to terrestrial mammals than to aquatic biota. Cyanobacteria produce a variety of unusual metabolites, the natural function of which is unclear, although some, perhaps only coincidentally, elicit effects upon other biota. Research has primarily focused on compounds that impact upon humans and livestock, either as toxins or as pharmaceutically useful substances. Further ranges of non-toxic products are also being found in cyanobacteria and the biochemical and pharmacological properties of these are totally unknown. An overview of the currently identified cyanotoxins is given and their toxicological properties are discussed. Studies on the occurrence, distribution and frequency of toxic cyanobacteria were conducted in a number of countries during the 1980s using mouse bioassay. Analytical methods suitable for quantitative toxin determination only became available in the late 1980s, but studies of specific cyanotoxins have been increasing since then. The results of both approaches indicate that neurotoxins are generally less common, except perhaps in some countries where they frequently cause lethal animal poisonings. In contrast, the cyclic peptide toxins (microcystins and nodularins) which primarily cause liver injury are more widespread and are very likely to occur if certain taxa of cyanobacteria are present. The data currently available on the occurrence of cyanotoxins is noteworthy, however, that current knowledge is clearly biased by the inconsistent distribution of research effort around the world, with studies from Asia, Africa and South

* E-mail: dvyas64@yahoo.co.in

America beginning to appear in the 1990s. Because the ecological role of the toxins is unclear, it is not possible to use a functional approach to study the factors that enhance toxicity. The relationships between environmental factors and toxin content and at the emerging understanding of genetic regulation of toxin production by cyanobacteria is increasing, and a better understanding of toxin function may provide a basis for predicting occurrence of toxicity in the future.

For assessing the health risk caused by cyanotoxins, an understanding of their persistence and degradation in aquatic environments is of crucial importance.

Classification

Mechanisms of cyanobacterial toxicity currently described and understood are very diverse and range from hepatotoxic, neurotoxic and dermatotoxic effects to general inhibition of protein synthesis. To assess the specific hazards of cyanobacterial toxins it is necessary to understand their chemical and physical properties, their occurrence in waters used by people, the regulation of their production, and their fate in the environment.

Cyanotoxins fall into three broad groups of chemical structure: cyclic peptides, alkaloids and lipopolysaccharides (LPS). An overview of the specific toxic substances within these broad groups that have been identified to date from different genera of cyanobacteria, together with their primary target organs in humans, is given in Table 6.1.

Table 6.1: General Features of the Cyanotoxins

Toxin Group	*Primary Target Organ in Mammals*	*Cyanobacterial Genera*
Cyclic peptides		
Microcystins	Liver	*Microcystis, Anabaena, Planktothrix (Oscillatoria), Nostoc, Hapalosiphon, Anabaenopsis*
Nodularin	Liver	*Nodularia*
Alkaloids		
Anatoxin-a	Nerve synapse	*Anabaena, Planktothrix (Oscillatoria), Aphanizomenon*
Anatoxin-a(S)	Nerve synapse	*Anabaena*
Aplysiatoxins	Skin	*Lyngbya, Schizothrix, Planktothrix (Oscillatoria)*
Cylindrospermopsins	Liver	*Cylindrospermopsis, Aphanizomenon, Umezakia*
Lyngbyatoxin-a	Skin, gastro-intestinal tract	*Lyngbya*
Saxitoxins	Nerve axons	*Anabaena, Aphanizomenon, Lyngbya, Cylindrospermopsis*
Lipopolysaccharides (LPS)	Potential irritant; affects any exposed tissue	All

Hepatotoxic Cyclic Peptides-Microcystins and Nodularins

Globally the most frequently found cyanobacterial toxins in blooms from fresh and brackish waters are the cyclic peptide toxins of the microcystin and nodularin family. They pose a major challenge for the production of safe drinking water from surface waters containing cyanobacteria with these toxins. In mouse bioassays, which traditionally have been used to screen toxicity of field and laboratory samples, cyanobacterial hepatotoxins (liver toxins) cause death by liver haemorrhage within a few hours of the acute doses. Microcystins have been characterised from planktonic *Anabaena*, *Microcystis*, *Oscillatoria* (*Planktothrix*), *Nostoc*, and *Anabaenopsis* species, and from terrestrial *Hapalosiphon* genera. Nodularin has been characterised only from *Nodularia spumigena*.

The cyclic peptides are comparatively large natural products, molecular weight (MW) >> 800-1,100, although small compared with many other cell oligopeptides and polypeptides (proteins) (MW > 10,000). They contain either five (nodularins) or seven (microcystins) amino acids, with the two terminal amino acids of the linear peptide being condensed (joined) to form a cyclic compound. They are water soluble and, except perhaps for a few somewhat more hydrophobic microcystins, are unable to penetrate directly the lipid membranes of animal, plant and bacterial cells. Therefore, to elicit their toxic effect, uptake into cells occurs through membrane transporters which otherwise carry essential biochemicals or nutrients, this restricts the target organ range in mammals largely to the liver. In aquatic environments, these toxins usually remain contained within the cyanobacterial cells and are only released in substantial amounts on cell lysis. Along with their high chemical stability and their water solubility, this containment has important implications for their environmental persistence and exposure to humans in surface water bodies.

The first chemical structures of cyanobacterial cyclic peptide toxins were identified in the early 1980s and the number of fully characterised toxin variants has greatly increased during the 1990s. The first such compounds found in freshwater cyanobacteria were cyclic heptapeptides. cyclo-(D-alanine^1-X^2-D-MeAsp^3-Z^4-Adda^5-D-glutamate^6-Mdha^7) in which X and Z are variable L amino acids, D-MeAsp^3 is *D*-erythro-β-methylaspartic acid, and Mdha is *N*-methyldehydroalanine (Figure 6.1). The amino acid Adda, (2S,3S,8S,9S)-3-amino-9-methoxy-2,6,8-trimethyl-10-phenyldeca-4,6-dienoic acid, is the most unusual structure in this group of cyanobacterial cyclic peptide toxins.

These compounds were first isolated from the cyanobacterium *Microcystis aeruginosa* and therefore the toxins were named microcystins (Carmichael *et al.*, 1988). Structural variations have been reported in all seven amino acids, but most frequently with substitution of L-amino acids at positions 2 and 4, and demethylation of amino acids at positions 3 and/or 7 (Figure 6.1A). About 60 structural variants of microcystins have been characterised so far from bloom samples and isolated strains of cyanobacteria (Table 6.2).

In one species of brackish water cyanobacterium, an identically acting and structurally very similar, cyclic pentapeptide occurs. It has been named as nodularin after its producer, *Nodularia spumigena*. The chemical structure of nodularin is cyclo-(D-MeAsp^1-L-arginine^2-Adda^3-D-glutamate^4-Mdhb^5), in which Mdhb is 2-(methylamino)-2-dehydrobutyric acid (Figure 6.1B). A few naturally occurring variations of nodularins have been found: two demethylated variants, one with D-Asp^1 instead of D-MeAsp^1, the other with DMAdda^3 instead of Adda^3; and the non-toxic nodularin which has the 6Z-stereoisomer of Adda^3 (Namikoshi *et al.*, 1994). The equivalent 6Z-Adda^3 stereoisomer of microcystins is also non-toxic. In the marine sponge, *Theonella swinhoei*, a nodularin analogue called motuporin has been found. It differs from nodularin only by one amino acid, having hydrophobic L-Val in place of the polar L-Arg in nodularin (de Silva *et al.*, 1992). The toxin might be cyanobacterial in origin because the sponge is known to harbour cyanobacterial symbionts.

The mammalian toxicity of microcystins and nodularins is mediated through their strong binding to key cellular enzymes called protein phosphatases. In solution, microcystins and nodularins adopt a chemical "shape" that is similar, especially in the Adda-glutamate part of the cyanotoxin molecule (Rudolph-Böhner *et al.*, 1994; Annila *et al.*, 1996). Recent studies have shown that this region is crucial for interaction with the protein phosphatase protein molecule, and hence it is crucial for the toxicity of

Figure 3.1: The Structure of Cyclic Peptide Toxins and Cylindrospermopsin

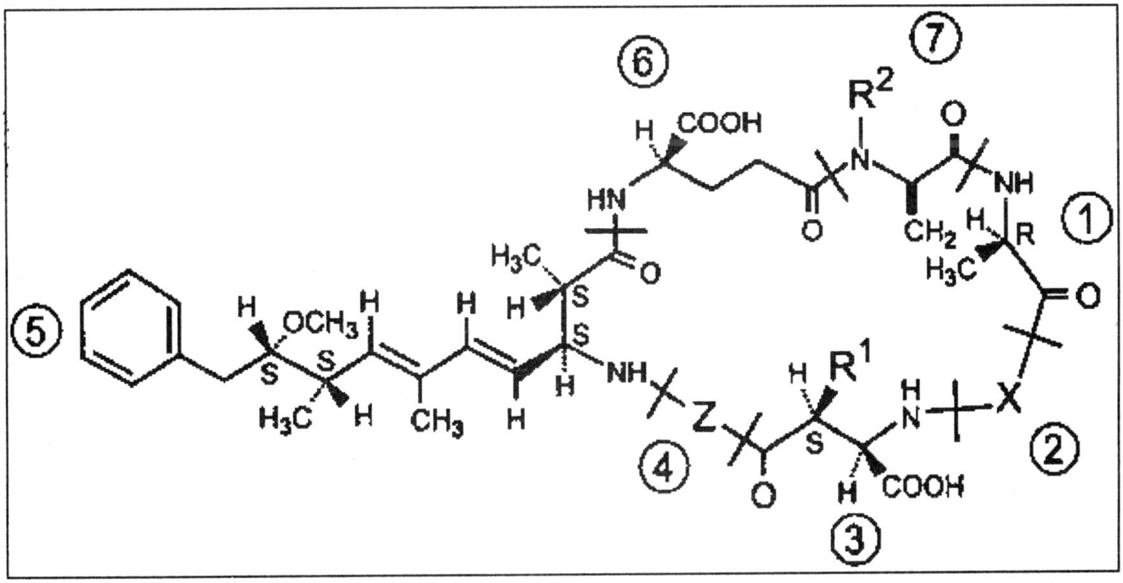

A: General structure of microcystins (MCYST), cyanobacterial heptapeptide hepatotoxins, showing the most frequently found variations. X and Z are variable L-amino acids (in MCYST-LR, X = L-Leusine (L) and Z = L-Arginine (R)); R[1] and R[2] are H (demethylmicrocystins) or CH_3; D-MeAsp is D-*erythro*-β-methylaspartic acid; Adda is (2*S*,3*S*,8*S*,9*S*)-3-amino-9-methoxy-2,6,8-trimethyl-10-phenyldeca-4,6-dienoic acid and Mdha is N-methyldehydroalanine (Dha = dehydroalanine) (see Table 3.2 for known microcystins); General structure of microcystins cyclo-(D-Ala[1]-X[2]-D-MeAsp[3]-Z[4]-Adda[5]-D-Glu[6]-Mdha[7])

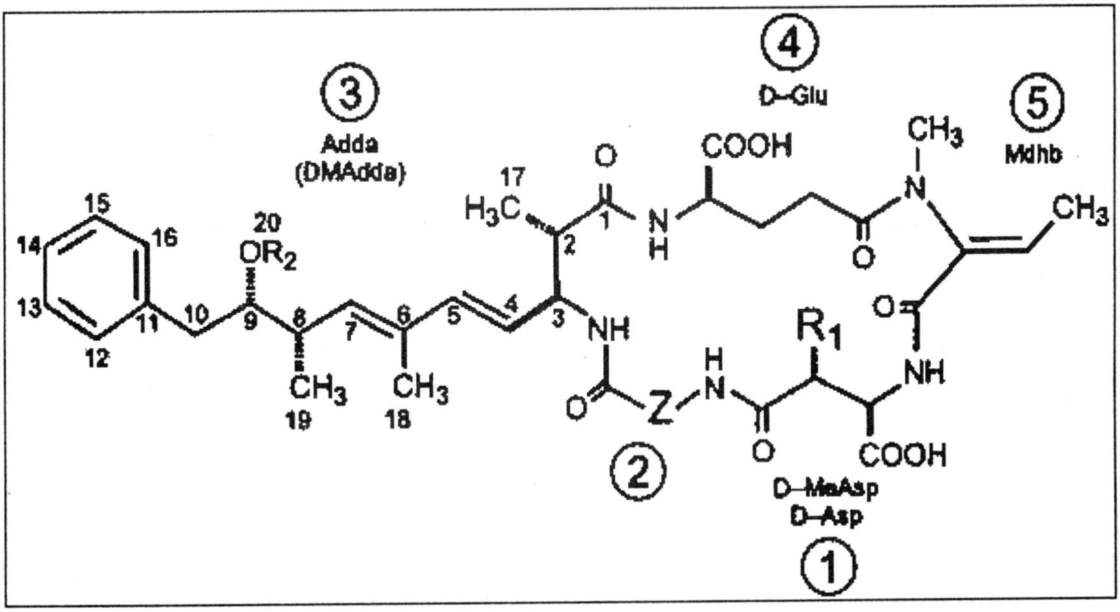

B: Structures of nodularins (Z = L-arginine) and motuporin (Z = L-Valine). Mdhb is N-methyldehydrobutyrin; Nodularin R_1,R_2 = CH_3; D-Asp[1] Nodularin R_1 = H, R_2 = CH_3; DMAdda[3] Nodularin R_1 = CH_3, R_2 = H; Structure of nodularins cyclo-(D-MeAsp[1]-Z[2]-Adda[3]-D-Glu[4]-Mdhb[5]).

Contd...

Figure 3.2–Contd...

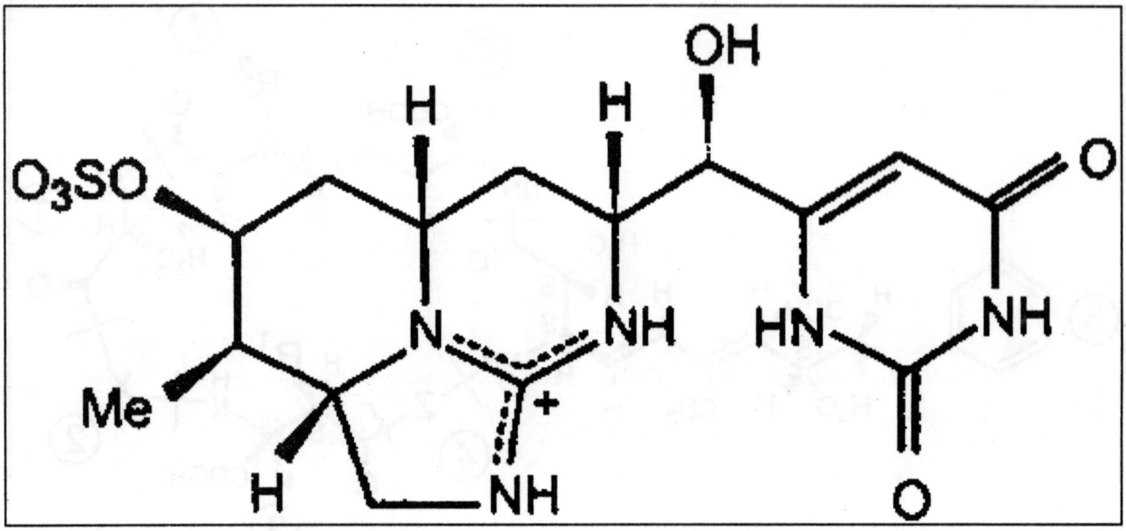

C: Structure of cylindrospermopsin; Cylindrospermopsin MW 415; $C_{15}H_{21}N_5O_7S$.

these cyanotoxins (Barford and Keller, 1994; Goldberg *et al.*, 1995). Microcystins show an additional characteristic of forming a covalent bond between the Mdha residue and the protein phosphatase molecule.

Table 6.2: The Microcystins (MCYST) Reported in the Scientific Literature

Microcystin	*Molecular Weight*	*Toxicity* LD_{50}[2]	*Organism*[3]	*Reference(s)*
MCYST-LA	909	50	*M. aeruginosa*[s], *M. viridis*[s]	Botes *et al.*, 1984; Kaya and Watanabe, 1990
MCYST-LAba	923	NR	*M. aeruginosa*[s]	Gathercole and Thiel, 1987
MCYST-LL	951	+	*M. aeruginosa*[b]	Craig *et al.*, 1993
MCYST-AR	952	250	*Microcystis* spp.[b]	Namikoshi *et al.*, 1992a
MCYST-YA	959	NR	*M. aeruginosa*[s]	Botes *et al.*, 1985
[D-Asp^3,Dha^7]MCYST-LR	966	+	*M. aeruginosa*[s], [s] *Anabaena* sp.	Harada *et al.*, 1991b; Sivonen *et al.*, 1992a
[D-Asp^3,Dha^7]MCYST-EE(OMe)	969	+	*Anabaena* sp.[s]	Namikoshi *et al.*, 1998
MCYST-VF	971	NR	*M. aeruginosa*[s]	Bateman *et al.*, 1995
(D-Asp^3]MCYST-LR	980	160-300	*A. flos-aquae*[s], *M. aeruginosa*[s], *M. viridis*[b], *O. agardhii*[b]	Krishnamurthy *et al.*, 1989; Cremer and Henning, 1991; Harada *et al.*, 1990b; 1991a; Luukkainen *et al.*, 1993
[Dha^7]MCYST-LR	980	250	*M. aeruginosa*[s], *Anabaena* sp.[s], *O. agardhii*[b]	Harada *et al.*, 1991b; Sivonen *et al.*, 1992a; Luukkainen *et al.*, 1993

Contd...

Table 6.2–Contd...

Microcystin	Molecular Weight	Toxicity LD_{50}[2]	Organism[3]	Reference(s)
[DMAdda[5]]MCYST-LR	980	90-100	*Microcystis* spp.[b,s] *Nostoc* sp.	Namikoshi *et al.*, 1992a; Sivonen *et al.*, 1992b
[Dha[7]]MCYST-EE(OMe)	983	+	*Anabaena* sp.[s]	Namikoshi *et al.*, 1998
[D-Asp[3],Dha[7]]MCYST-E(OMe)E(OMe)	983	+	*Anabaena* sp.[s]	Namikoshi *et al.*, 1998
MCYST-LF	985	+	*M. aeruginosa*[s]	Azevedo *et al.*, 1994
MCYST-LR	994	50	*M. aeruginosa*[s], *A. flos-aquae*[s] *M. viridis*[s]	Botes *et al.*, 1985; Rinehart *et al.*, 1988; Krishnamyrthy *et al.*, 1989; Watanabe *et al.*, 1988
[D-Asp[3],D-Glu(OCH_3)[6]]MCYST-LR	994	NR	*A. flos-aquae*[s]	Sivonen *et al.*, 1992d
[(6Z)-Adda[5]]MCYST-LR	994	>1,200	*M. viridis*[b]	Harada *et al.*, 1990a,b
[Dha[7]]MCYST-E(OMe)E(OMe)	997	+	*Anabaena* sp.[s]	Namikoshi *et al.*, 1998
[L-Ser[7]]MCYST-LR	998	+	*Anabaena* sp.[s]	Namikoshi *et al.*, 1992c
MCYST-LY	1,001	90	*M. aeruginosa*[s]	Stoner *et al.*, 1989
[L-Ser[7]]MCYST-EE(OMe)	1,001	+	*Anabaena* sp.[s]	Namikoshi *et al.*, 1998
[D-Asp[3],Ser[7]]MCYST-E(OMe)E(OMe)	1,001	+	*Anabaena* sp.[s]	Namikoshi *et al.*, 1998
MCYST-HilR	1,008	100	*Microcystis* spp.[b]	Namikoshi *et al.*, 1995
[D-Asp[3],ADMAdda[5]]MCYST-LR	1,008	160	*Nostoc* sp.[s]	Sivonen *et al.*, 1990a; Namikoshi *et al.*, 1990
[D-Glu(OCH_3)[6]]MCYST-LR	1,008	>1,000	*A. flos-aguae*[s], *Microcystis sp.*[s]	Sivonen *et al.*, 1992d; Bateman *et al.*, 1995; Rinehart *et al.*, 1994
[D-Asp[3],Dha[7]]MCYST-RR	1,009	+	*O. agardhii*[b], *Anabaena* sp.[s], *M. aeruginosa*[s]	Krishnamyrthy *et al.*, 1989; Sivonen *et al.*, 1992a; Luukkainen *et al.*, 1994
[D-Asp[3], ADMAdda[5], Dhb[7]]MCYST-LR	1,009	+	*Nostoc sp.*[s]	Beattie *et al.*, 1998
[L-MeSer[7]]MCYST-LR	1,012	150	*Microcystis* spp.[b]	Namikoshi *et al.*, *1992a;* 1995
[Dha[7]]MCYST-FR	1,014	NR	*Microcystis sp.*[s]	Luukkainen *et al.*, 1994
[L-Ser[7]]MCYST-E(OMe)E(OMe)	1,015	+	*Anabaena* sp.[s]	Namikoshi *et al.*, 1998
[ADMAdda[5]]MCYST-LR	1,022	60	*Nostoc* sp.[s]	Sivonen *et al.*, 1990a; Namikoshi *et al.*, 1990
[D-Asp[3],ADMAdda[5]]MCYST-LHar	1,022	+	*Nostoc* sp.[s]	Sivonen *et al.*, 1992b
[D-Asp[3]]MCYST-RR	1,023	250	*O. agardhii*[b], *Anabaena* sp.[s], *M. aeruginosa*[s]	Meriluoto *et al.*, 1989; Sivonen *et al.*, 1992a; Luukkainen *et al.*, 1994
[Dha[7]]MCYST-RR	1,023	180	*M. aeruginosa*[s], *Anabaena* sp.[s], *O. agardhii*[b]	Kiviranta *et al.*, 1992; Sivonen *et al.*, 1992a; Luukkainen *et al.*, 1993
MCYST-LW	1,024	NR	*M. aeruginosa*[s]	Bateman *et al.*, 1995
MCYST-FR	1,028	250	*Microcystis* spp.[b]	Namikoshi *et al.*, 1992a

Contd...

Table 6.2–Contd...

Microcystin	Molecular Weight	Toxicity LD_{50}[2]	Organism[3]	Reference(s)
MCYST-M(O)R	1,028	700-800	*Microcystis* spp.[b]	Namikoshi *et al.*, 1992a
[Dha[7]]MCYST-HphR	1,028	+	*Anabaena* sp.[s]	Namikoshi *et al.*, 1992b
[D-Asp[3], Dha[7]]MCYST-HtyR	1,030	+	*Anabaena* sp.[s]	Namikoshi *et al.*, 1992b
[Dha[7]]MCYST-YR	1,030	+	*M. aeruginosa*[s]	Sivonen *et al.*, 1992c
[D-Asp[3]]MCYST-YR	1,030	+	*Microcystis* spp.[b]	Namikoshi *et al.*, 1992d
MCYST-YM(O)	1,035	56	*M. aeruginosa*[b]	Botes *et al.*, 1985; Elleman *et al.*, 1978
[ADMAdda[5]]MCYST-LHar	1,036	60	*Nostoc* sp.[s]	Sivonen *et al.*, 1990a; Namikoshi *et al.*, 1990
MCYST-RR	1,037	600	*M. aeruginosa*[s], *M. viridis*[s], *Anabaena* sp.[s]	Kusumi *et al.*, 1987; Painuly *et al.*, 1988; Watanabe *et al.*, 1988; Sivonen *et al.*, 1992a
[(6Z)-Adda[5]]MCYST-RR	1,037	>1,200	*M. viridis*[b]	Harada *et al.*, 1990a,b
[D-Ser[1], ADMAdda[5]]MCYST-LR	1,038	+	*Nostoc* sp.[s]	Sivonen *et al.*, 1992b
[ADMAdda[5],MeSer[7]]MCYST-LR	1,040	+	*Nostoc* sp.[s]	Sivonen *et al.*, 1992b
[L-Ser[7]]MCYST-RR	1,041	+	*Anabaena* sp.[s], *M. aeruginosa*[s/b]	Namikoshi *et al.*, 1992c; Luukkainen *et al.*, 1994
[D-Asp[3],MeSer[7]]MCYST-RR	1,041	+	*O. agardhii*[s]	Luukkainen *et al.*, 1993
MCYST-YR	1,044	70	*M. aeruginosa*[s], *M. viridis*[s]	Botes *et al.*, 1985; Watanabe *et al.*, 1988
[D-Asp[3]]MCYST-HtyR	1,044	160-300	*A. flos-aquae*[s]	Harada *et al.*, 1991a
[Dha[7]]MCYST-HtyR	1,044	+	*Anabaena* sp.[s]	Namikoshi *et al.*, 1992b
MCYST-(H_4)YR	1,048	NR	*Microcystis* spp.[b]	Namikoshi *et al.*, 1995
[D-Glu-$OC_2H_3(CH_3)OH$[6]]MCYST-LR	1,052	>1,000	*Microcystis* spp.[b]	Namikoshi *et al.*, 1992a
[D-Asp[3],ADMAdda[5], Dhb[7]]MCYST-RR	1,052	+	*Nostoc* sp.[s]	Beattie *et al.*, 1998
MCYST-HtyR	1,058	80-100	*A. flos-aquae*[s]	Harada *et al.*, 1991a
[L-Ser[7]]MCYST-HtyR	1,062	+	*Anabaena* sp.[s]	Namikoshi *et al.*, 1992b
MCYST-WR	1,067	150-200	*Microcystis* spp.[b]	Namikoshi *et al.*, 1992a
[D-Asp[3],ADMAdda[5],Dhb[7]]MCYST-HtyR	1,073	+	*Nostoc* sp.[s]	Beattie *et al.*, 1998
[L-MeLan[7]]MCYST-LR	1,115	1,000	*Microcystis* spp.[b]	Namikoshi *et al.*, 1995

Aba: Aminoisobutyric acid; ADMAdda: *O*-Acetyl-*O*-demethylAdda; Dha: Dehydroalanine; Dhb: Dehydrobutyrine; DMAdda: *O*-DemethylAdda; E(OMe): Glutamic acid methyl ester D; (H_4)Y: 1,2,3,4,-tetrahydrotyrosine; Har: Homoarginine; Hil: Homoisoleucine; Hph: Homophenylalanine; Hty: Homotyrosine; MeLan: *N*-Methyllanthionine; M(O): Methionine-*S*-oxide; MeSer: *N*-Methylserine; (6Z)-Adda: Stereoisomer of Adda at the D^6 double bond.

1 Several partial structures of microcystins have been reported in addition to those shown in this table (see Boland *et al.*, 1993; Craig *et al.*, 1993; Jones *et al.*, 1995; Sivonen *et al.*, 1995)

2 Toxicity determined i.p. mouse (μg kg^{-1}); the LD_{50} value is the dose of toxin that kills 50 per cent of exposed animals; a '+' denotes a toxic result in a non-quantitative mouse bioassay or inhibition of protein phosphatase and 'NR' denotes 'Not reported'

3 An '*s*' denotes toxins isolated from culture samples and a '*b*' denotes toxins isolated from bloom samples

Most of the structural variants of microcystin and nodularin are highly toxic within a comparatively narrow range (intra-peritoneal (i.p.) mouse toxicities largely in the range 50-300 $\mu g\ kg^{-1}$ body weight (bw); Table 6.2). Only a few non-toxic variants have been identified. In general, any structural modifications to the Adda-glutamate region of the toxin molecule, such as a change in isomerisation of the Adda-diene (6(E) to 6(Z)) or acylation of the glutamate, renders microcystins and nodularins non-toxic (Harada *et al.*, 1990 a,b; Rinehart *et al.*, 1994). Linear microcystins and nodularin are more than 100 times less toxic than the equivalent cyclic compounds. The linear microcystins are thought to be microcystin precursors and/or bacterial breakdown products (Choi *et al.*, 1993; Rinehart *et al.*, 1994; Bourne *et al.*, 1996).

Microcystins and nodularin have been characterised from axenic cyanobacterial strains (*i.e.* strains free of contaminating bacteria) and thus the cyanobacterial origin of these compounds is clear. At the present time, it is known that microcystins are produced by bloom forming species of *Microcystis, Anabaena, Oscillatoria* (*Planktothrix*), and *Nostoc* (Table 6.2), by a species of *Anabaenopsis* and by a soil isolate of *Haphalosiphon hibernicus.* Nodularins have been found, with the exception of the marine sponge *Theonella* already mentioned, only in *Nodularia spumigena* (see section 3.2 for more details). Further species may yet be demonstrated to produce microcystin.

Neurotoxic Alkaloids-Anatoxins and Saxitoxins

Mass occurrences of neurotoxic cyanobacteria have been reported from North America, Europe and Australia, where they have caused animal poisonings. In mouse bioassays death by respiratory arrest occurs rapidly (within 2-30 minutes). Three families of cyanobacterial neurotoxins are known:

- ☆ Anatoxin-a and homoanatoxin-a, which mimic the effect of acetyl choline,
- ☆ Anatoxin-a(S), which is an anticholinesterase, and
- ☆ Saxitoxins, also known as paralytic shellfish poisons (PSPs) in the marine literature, which block nerve cell sodium channels.

Anatoxin-a has been found in *Anabaena, Oscillatoria* and *Aphanizomenon,* homoanatoxin-a from *Oscillatoria,* anatoxin-a(S) from *Anabaena,* and saxitoxins from *Aphanizomenon, Anabaena, Lyngbya* and *Cylindrospermopsis.* Sixteen confirmed saxitoxins from cyanobacterial samples have been reported, some of which (*e.g.* the decarbamoyl-gonyautoxins) may be chemical breakdown products in some species.

The alkaloid toxins are diverse, both in their chemical structures and in their mammalian toxicities. Alkaloids, in general, are a broad group of heterocyclic nitrogenous compounds (*i.e.* they contain ring structures with at least one carbon-nitrogen bond) usually of low to moderate molecular weight (< 1,000). They are produced, in particular, by plants and by some bacteria, and are invariably bioactive and commonly toxic. The non-sulphated alkaloid toxins of freshwater cyanobacteria (anatoxins and saxitoxin) are all neurotoxins. The sulphated PSPs, C-toxins and gonyautoxins (sulphated derivatives of saxitoxin) are also neurotoxins, but the sulphated alkaloid cylindrospermopsin blocks protein synthesis with a major impact on liver cells. Some marine cyanobacteria also contain alkaloids (lyngbyatoxins, aplysiatoxins) which are dermatoxins (skin irritants), but have also been associated with gastro-enteritis and more general symptoms such as fever.

Alkaloids have varying chemical stabilities, often undergoing spontaneous transformations to by-products which may have higher or lower potencies than the parent toxin. Some are also susceptible to direct photolytic degradation.

Anatoxin-a

Anatoxin-a is a low molecular weight alkaloid (MW = 165), a secondary amine, 2-acetyl-9-azabicyclo(4-2-1)non-2-ene (Figure 6.2) (Devlin *et al.*, 1977). Anatoxin-a is produced by *Anabaena flos-aquae*, *Anabaena* spp. (*flos-aquae-lemmermannii* group), *Anabaena planktonica*, *Oscillatoria*, *Aphanizomenon* and *Cylindrospermum* (see section 3.2 for details). Homoanatoxin-a (MW = 179) is an anatoxin-a homologue isolated from an *Oscillatoria formosa* (*Phormidium formosum*) strain (Figure 6.2). It has a propionyl group at C-2 instead of the acetyl group in anatoxin-a (Skulberg *et al.*, 1992). The LD_{50} (lethal dose resulting in 50 per cent deaths) of anatoxin-a and homoanatoxin-a are 200–250 µg kg^{-1} bw (Devlin *et al.*, 1977; Carmichael *et al.*, 1990; Skulberg *et al.*, 1992).

Figure 6.2: The Chemical Structures of Cyanobacterial Neurotoxins, Anatoxin-a, Homoanatoxin-a, Anatoxin-a(S), and the General Structure of Saxitoxins. Sixteen different saxitoxins have been reported from cyanobacteria (for details see Table 6.3). MW = molecular weight

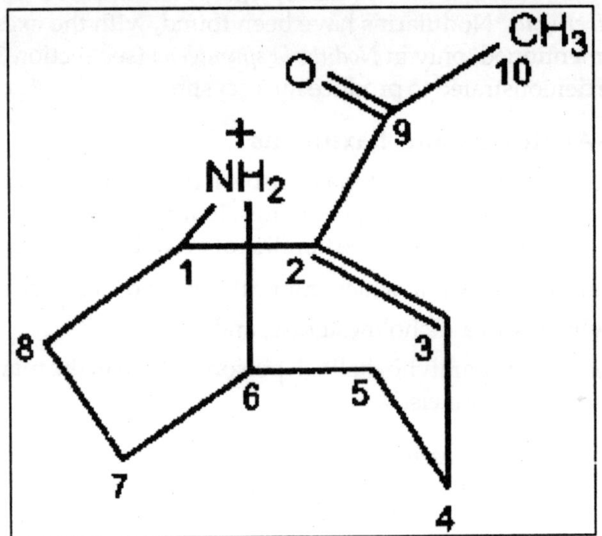

Anatoxin-a MW 165; $C_{10}H_{15}NO$

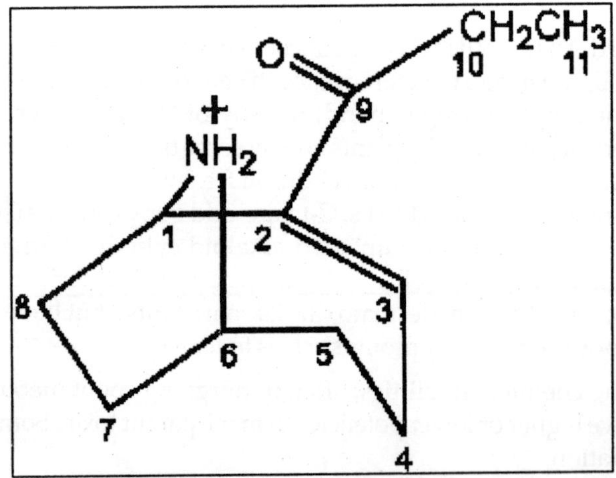

Homoanatoxin-a MW 179; $C_{11}H_{17}NO$

Contd...

Figure 6.2–Contd...

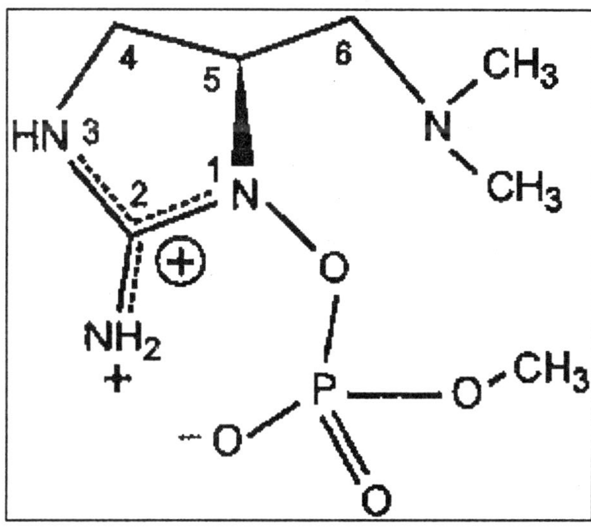

Anatoxin-a(S) MW 252; $C_7H_{17}N_4O_4P$

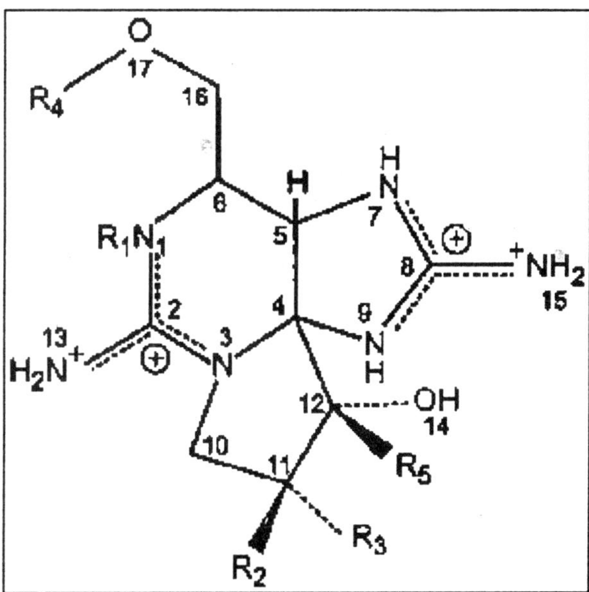

General structure of saxitoxins

Anatoxin-a(S)

Anatoxin-a(S) is a unique phosphate ester of a cyclic N-hydroxyguanine (MW = 252) (Figure 6.2) produced by *Anabaena flos-aquae* strain NRC 525-17 (Matsunaga *et al.*, 1989). It has more recently been identified in blooms and isolated strains of *Anabaena lemmermannii* (Henriksen *et al.*, 1997; Onodera *et al.*, 1997a). The LD_{50} of anatoxin-a(S) is 20 µg kg^{-1} bw (i.p. mouse) (Carmichael *et al.*, 1990). Structural variants of anatoxin-a(S) have not been detected.

Saxitoxins

Saxitoxins are a group of carbamate alkaloid neurotoxins which are either non-sulphated (saxitoxins–STX), singly sulphated (gonyautoxins–GTX) or doubly sulphated (C-toxins) (Figure 6.2 and Table 6.3). In addition, decarbamoyl variants and several new toxins have been identified in some species.

Table 6.3: Saxitoxins Reported from Cyanobacterial Strains and Bloom Samples (for the chemical structure see Figure 6.2)

Name of Toxin	*Variable Chemical Groups in Toxins*					*Cyanobacteria*			
	R_1	R_2	R_3	R_4	R_5	*Aph*[1]	*Ana*[2]	*Lyn*[3]	*Cyl*[4]
STX	H	H	H	$CONH_2$	OH	+	+		+
GTX2	H	H	OSO_3^-	$CONH_2$	OH		+		
GTX3	H	OSO_3^-	H	$CONH_2$	OH		+		
GTX5	H	H	H	$CONHSO_3^-$	OH		+		
C1	H	H	OSO_3^-	$CONHSO_3^-$	OH		+		
C2	H	OSO_3^-	H	$CONHSO_3^-$	OH		+		
NEO	OH	H	H	$CONH_2$	OH	+			+
GTX1	OH	H	OSO_3^-	$CONH_2$	OH		*		
GTX4	OH	OSO_3^-	H	$CONH_2$	OH		*		
GTX6	OH	H	H	$CONHSO_3^-$	OH		*		
dcSTX	H	H	H	H	OH		+	+	
dcGTX2	H	H	OSO_3^-	H	OH		+	+	
dcGTX3	H	OSO_3^-	H	H	OH		+	+	
LWTX1[3]	H	OSO_3^-	H	$COCH_3$	H			+	
LWTX2[3]	H	OSO_3^-	H	$COCH_3$	OH			+	
LWTX3[3]	H	H	OSO_3^-	$COCH_3$	OH			+	
LWTX4[3]	H	H	H	H	H			+	
LWTX5[3]	H	H	H	$COCH_3$	OH			+	
LWTX6[3]	H	H	H	$COCH_3$	H			+	

STX: Saxitoxin; GTX: Gonyautoxins; C: C-toxins; dcSTX: Decarbamoylsaxitoxin; LWTX: Lyngbya-wollei-toxins.

1 Toxins found in *Aphanizomenon flos-aquae,* New Hampshire, USA (Ikawa *et al.,* 1982; Mahmood and Carmichael, 1986).

2 Toxins reported in an *Anabaena circinalis* strain and bloom samples, Australia (Hump-age *et al.,* 1994; Negri *et al.,* 1995; Negri *et al.,* 1997). dcGTX2 and dcGTX3 are probably break down products of C1 and C2 in this species (Jones and Negri, 1997). An asterisk in this column denotes toxins reported by Humpage *et al.,* 1994 for *Anabaena circinalis* based on retention time data, but not confirmed by mass spectrometry, and not found in subsequent studies.

3 Toxins detected in *Lyngbya wollei,* USA (Onodera *et al.,* 1997b).

4 Toxins thus far found in *Cylindrospermopsis raciborskii,* Brazil (Lagos *et al.,* 1997).

Saxitoxins were originally isolated from shellfish where they are concentrated from marine dinoflagellates (so called "red tide" algae) and have caused deaths in humans (Anderson, 1994).

Saxitoxins have been found in the cyanobacteria *Aphanizomenon flos-aquae, Anabaena circinalis, Lyngbya wollei* and *Cylindrospermopsis raciborskii.* The North American *Aphanizomenon flos-aquae* strains NH-1 and NH-5 contain mostly neosaxitoxin and less saxitoxin (plus a few unidentified neurotoxins). *Anabaena circinalis* strains (from Australia) contain mostly C1 and C2 toxins, with lesser amounts of gonyautoxins 2 and 3. The freshwater cyanobacterium *Lyngbya wollei* produced three known and six new saxitoxin analogues. *Cylindrospermopsis raciborskii* in Brazil was found to contain mostly neosaxitoxin and a smaller amount of saxitoxin.

Other Neurotoxic Cyanobacteria

In marine *Trichodesmium* blooms from the Virgin Islands, a neurotoxic factor has been reported which was not anatoxin-a or anatoxin-a(S) but remains to be characterised (Hawser *et al.*, 1991).

Cytotoxic Alkaloids

In tropical and subtropical waters of Australia, the alkaloid hepatotoxin cylindrospermopsin with a completely different mechanism of toxicity has caused health problems in drinking water supplies. It is a cyclic guanidine alkaloid with a molecular weight of 415 (Figure 6.1C). It is produced by *Cylindrospermopsis raciborskii* (Hawkins *et al.*, 1985, 1997), *Umezakia natans* (Harada *et al.*, 1994) and *Aphanizomenon ovalisporum* (Banker *et al.*, 1997). In pure form, cylindrospermopsin mainly affects the liver, although crude extracts of *C. raciborskii* injected or given orally to mice also induce pathological symptoms in the kidneys, spleen, thymus and heart (see Chapter 4 for more details). Pure cylindrospermopsin has an LD_{50} in mice (i.p.) of 2.1 mg kg l^{-1} bw at 24 h and 0.2 mg kg l^{-1} bw at 5-6 days (Ohtani *et al.*, 1992). Recently, new structural variants of cylindrospermopsin have been isolated from an Australian strain of *C. raciborskii,* with one being identified as demethoxy-cylindrospermopsin (Chiswell *et al.*, 1999).

Dermatotoxic Alkaloids-Aplysiatoxins and Lyngbyatoxin

Benthic marine cyanobacteria such as *Lyngbya, Oscillatoria* and *Schizothrix* may produce toxins causing severe dermatitis among swimmers in contact with the filaments. The inflammatory activity of *Lyngbya* is caused by aplysiatoxins and debromoaplysiatoxin (Figure 6.3) which are potent tumour promoters and protein kinase C activators (Mynderse *et al.*, 1977; Fujiki *et al.*, 1990). Another strain of *Lyngbya majuscula* has caused dermatitis and severe oral and gastrointestinal inflammation. It was found to contain lyngbyatoxin-a (Figure 6.3) (Cardellina *et al.*, 1979). Debromoaplysiatoxin along with other toxic compounds has also been isolated from other Oscillatoriaceae, such as *Schizothrix calcicola* and *Oscillatoria nigroviridis.*

Irritant Toxins-Lipopolysaccharides

Weise *et al.* (1970) were the first to isolate LPS from the cyanobacterium *Anacystis nidulans* and numerous reports of endotoxins in cyanobacteria have followed. Lipopolysaccarides are generally found in the outer membrane of the cell wall of Gram negative bacteria, including cyanobacteria, where they form complexes with proteins and phospholipids. They are pyrogenic and toxic (Weckesser and Drews, 1979). Lipopolysaccarides, as the name implies, are condensed products of a sugar, usually a hexose, and a lipid, normally a hydroxy C_{14}-C_{18} fatty acid. The many structural variants of LPS are generally phylogenetically conserved, *i.e.* particular orders, genera and occasionally species, have identical or similar fatty acid and sugar components contained in their cell wall LPS. It is generally the fatty acid component of the LPS molecule that elicits an irritant of allergenic response in humans and mammals.

Debromoaplysiatoxin

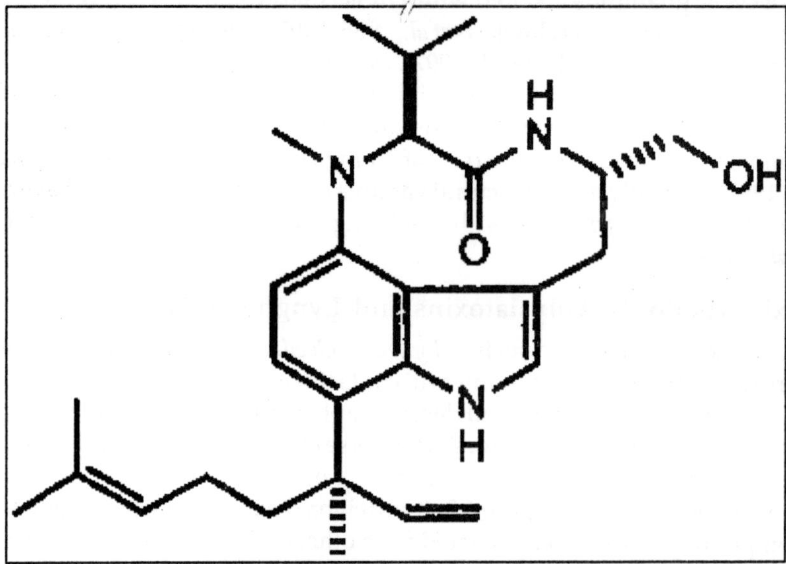

Lyngbyatoxin A

Figure 6.3: The Chemical Structures of Debromoaplysiatoxin and Lyngbiatoxin-a

Lipopolysaccharides are an integral component of the cell wall of all Gram negative bacteria, including cyanobacteria, and can elicit irritant and allergenic responses in human and animal tissues that come in contact with the compounds. There is considerable diversity of LPS composition among the cyanobacteria, but differences are largely related to phylogeny. Thus, different genera typically have distinct LPS compositions that are largely conserved within that genus (Kerr *et al.*, 1995). Cyanobacterial LPS are considerably less potent than LPS from pathogenic gram-negative bacteria such as, for example, *Salmonella*. The chemical stability of cyanobacterial LPS in surface waters is unknown.

Structurally, LPS is a complex polymer composed of four regions. Region I, the O-antigen region, consists of repeating oligosaccharide units that may vary in structure, with numerous combinations of different sugar residues and associated glycosidic linkages. As suggested by its name, the O-antigen also exhibits several antigenic determinants that constitute the receptor sites for a number of lysogenic bacteriophages. Regions II and III are the outer core and backbone of a core polysaccharide. There is generally only minor variation in core structure between species. The backbone of the polysaccharide is connected to a glycolipid, lipid A (Region IV), via a short link normally composed of 3-deoxy-D-mannoocmiosonic acid (KDO). Lipid A is a disaccharide of glucosamines highly substituted with phosphate, fatty acids and KDO, although the proportion of KDO is low or absent in cyanobacteria compared with other bacterial LPS. The lipid A component is also acetylated with amide and ester-linked hydroxy fatty acids.

Recent studies of the fatty acid composition of Australian species of cyanobacteria (Kerr *et al.*, 1995) show a range of β-OH fatty acids ranging in size from C_{10} to C_{22}. Normal, saturated and branched chain acids have been detected. There was a stark predominance of straight chain 14:0 and 18:0 β-OH acids in *Microcystis* strains that was quite distinct from *Anabaena* and *Nodularia* strains where 16:0 β-OH predominated the LPS fatty acid fraction.

Although comparatively poorly studied, cell wall components, particularly LPS endotoxins from cyanobacteria may contribute to human health problems associated with exposure to mass occurrences of cyanobacteria. The few results available indicate that cyanobacterial LPS is less toxic than the LPS of other bacteria, such as *Salmonella* (Keleti and Sykora, 1982; Raziuddin *et al.*, 1983). More studies are needed to evaluate the chemical structures and health risks of cyanobacterial LPS.

Other Bioactive Compounds

Cyanobacteria are known to produce several other bioactive compounds, some of which are of medical interest, as well as compounds toxic to other cyanobacteria, bacteria, algae and zooplankton. Severe intoxication of fish embryos by crude extracts of *Planktothrix agardhii* has been reported by Oberemm *et al.* (1997). Skulberg *et al.* (1994) reported the presence of an unidentified "protracted toxic effect" in cyanobacterial samples that caused death within 4-24 hours in mice. Whether this effect was due to a specific cyanotoxin is unclear.

Cyanobacteria have been found to be a rich source of biomedically interesting compounds and therefore screening programmes for new bioactivities are underway. Cyanobacteria are known to produce antitumour, antiviral, antibiotic and antifungal compounds. Of the cyanobacterial extracts screened by a Hawaiian research group, 0.8 per cent showed solid tumour selective cytotoxicity (Moore *et al.*, 1996). Depsipeptides (peptides with an ester linkage) called cryptophycins isolated from a cyanobacterium, *Nostoc* sp. strain GSV 224, are promising candidates for an anticancer drug (Trimurtulu *et al.*, 1995). Recently, several new cyclic or linear peptides and depsipeptides from cyanobacteria have been characterised. Some are protease inhibitors, but the biological activity of the others remains to be characterised (Namikoshi and Rinehart, 1996). Many of the cyanobacterial bioactive compounds possess structural similarities to natural products from marine invertebrates.

Occurrence of Cyanotoxins

Mass Occurrences of Toxic Cyanobacteria

The toxicity of cyanobacterial mass occurrences (blooms) was originally brought to the attention of scientists through reports of animal poisonings by farmers and veterinarians, with the first well documented case being reported from Australia in 1878 (Francis, 1878). In most, if not all, reported cases since that time, afflicted animals consumed water from water bodies where there was an obvious presence of a cyanobacterial scum on the water surface (see Ressom *et al.* (1994) and Yoo *et al.* (1995) for a list of reported animal poisonings). More recent measurements of cyanobacterial toxins using sensitive modern analytical methods have often revealed high frequencies of toxic blooms even when animal poisonings have not been reported (Table 6.4).

Table 6.4: Frequencies of Mass Occurrences of Toxic Cyanobacteria in Freshwaters

Country	*No. of Tested Samples*	*% of Toxic Samples*	*Type of Toxicity*	*Reference*
Australia	231	42	Hepatotoxic Neurotoxic	Baker and Humpage, 1994
Australia	31	84[1]	Neurotoxic	Negri *et al.*, 1997
Brazil	16	75	Hepatotoxic	Costa and Azevedo, 1994
Canada, Alberta	24	66	Hepatotoxic Neurotoxic	Gorham, 1962
Canada, Alberta	39	95	Hepatotoxic	Kotak *et al.*, 1993
Canada, Alberta (3 lakes)	226	74[1]	Hepatotoxic	Kotak *et al.*, 1995
Canada, Saskatchewan	50	10	Hepatotoxic Neurotoxic	Hammer, 1968
China	26	73	Hepatotoxic	Carmichael *et al.*, 1988b
Czech and Slovak Rep.	63	82	Hepatotoxic	Maršálek *et al.*, 1996
Denmark	296	82	Hepatotoxic SDF Neurotoxic	Henriksen *et al.*, 1996b
Former German Dem. Rep.	10	70	Hepatotoxic SDF	Henning and Kohl, 1981
Germany	533	72[1]	Hepatotoxic	Fastner, 1998
Germany	393	22	Neurotoxic	Bumke-Vogt, 1998
Greece	18	?	Hepatotoxic	Lanaras *et al.*, 1989
Finland	215	44	Hepatotoxic Neurotoxic	Sivonen, 1990a
France, Brittany	22	73[1]	Hepatotoxic	Vezie *et al.*, 1997
Hungary	50	66	Hepatotoxic	Törökné, 1991
Japan	23	39	Hepatotoxic	Watanabe and Oishi, 1980
Netherlands	10	90	Hepatotoxic	Leeuwangh *et al.*, 1983
Norway	64	92	Hepatotoxic Neurotoxic SDF	Skulberg *et al.*, 1994
Portugal	30	60	Hepatotoxic	Vasconcelos, 1994
Scandinavia	81	60	Hepatotoxic	Berg *et al.*, 1986
Sweden	331	47	Hepatotoxic Neurotoxic	Willén and Mattsson, 1997

Contd...

Table 6.4–Contd...

Country	No. of Tested Samples	% of Toxic Samples	Type of Toxicity	Reference
UK	50	48 28[1]	Hepatotoxic	Codd and Bell, 1996
USA, Minnesota	92	53	Unspecified Neurotoxic	Olson, 1960
USA, Wisconsin	102	25	Hepatotoxic Neurotoxic	Repavich *et al.*, 1990
Mean		59		
India			Hepatotoxic	Parkar *et al.*, 1997

1: HPLC was used to detect the toxin content of the samples.

Throughout the world, it appears that liver-toxic (hepatotoxic, microcystin-containing) freshwater blooms of cyanobacteria are more commonly found than neurotoxic blooms. Liver-toxic blooms have been reported from all continents and almost every part of the world where samples have been collected for analysis. Nevertheless, mass occurrences of neurotoxic cyanobacteria are common in some countries and these have been reported from North America, Europe and Australia, where they have caused several animal poisonings. Blooms which have caused both liver and kidney damage due to the toxin cylindrospermopsin (and possibly related cyanotoxins) have been reported in Australia, Japan, Israel and Hungary.

In recent years, surveys have been carried out in a number of countries in South America, Africa, Australia, Asia and Europe. The conclusion that can be drawn from these surveys is that toxic cyanobacteria are internationally ubiquitous, and that as further surveys are carried out more toxic cyanobacterial blooms and new toxic species will be discovered. This is particularly true of tropical and subtropical regions that are currently under-represented in the literature. It seems likely that every country in the world will have water bodies which support blooms of toxic cyanobacteria at some time or another. It is also important to note that mass occurrences of toxic cyanobacteria are not always associated with human activities causing pollution or "cultural eutrophication". For example, massive blooms of toxic cyanobacteria have been reported in Australian reservoirs with pristine or near-pristine catchments (watersheds), and toxic benthic cyanobacteria have killed cattle drinking from oligotrophic, high-alpine waters in Switzerland.

Species Composition and Variation Among Toxic Blooms

Cyanobacterial populations may be dominated by a single species or be composed of a variety of species, some of which may not be toxic. Even within a single-species bloom there may be a mixture of toxic and non-toxic strains. A strain is a specific genetic subgroup within a particular species, and each species may encompass tens or hundreds of strains, each with slightly different traits. Some strains are much more toxic than others, sometimes by more than three orders of magnitude. This can mean that one highly toxic strain, even when occurring in minor amounts amongst larger numbers of non-toxic strains, may render a bloom sample toxic (Sivonen *et al.*, 1989a,b; Bolch *et al.*, 1997; Vezie *et al.*, 1998).

Some of the studies shown in the table have been conducted over several years while others lasted only one season. The relative share of cyanobacteria in the samples varied; low frequency of cyanobacteria led to low percentages of toxic samples in some studies. In most of the studies the method used to detect toxicity is mouse bioassay, normally with a 4-hour time limit (or longer when slow death factors (SDF) have been included). SDF may indicate low hepatotoxicity of samples or other unknown toxicity.

Toxic and non-toxic strains from the same cyanobacterial species cannot be separated by microscopic identification. The use of molecular genetic methods, in particular the use of molecular probes and primers that target specific toxin production genes, will lead to the development of more precise identification methods for toxic cyanobacteria in the future. To confirm that a particular cyanobacterial strain is a toxin-producer, it is important to isolate a pure culture of that strain, preferably free of other bacteria; then to detect and quantify toxin concentrations in the pure culture (either by bioassay or chemical analysis); and, where possible, to purify and characterise fully the toxins (for such examples see Tables 6.2 and 6.3). It is likely that the list of confirmed toxic species will increase in the future due to the isolation of new species and strains, and because of the use of improved isolation, culturing and analytical methods.

Microcystis sp., commonly *Microcystis aeruginosa*, are linked most frequently to hepatotoxic blooms world-wide (see Tables 6.2 and 6.5 for details and references for all toxic species). *Microcystis viridis* and *Microcystis botrys* strains also have been shown to produce microcystins. As noted previously, *Microcystis* is a non-nitrogen-fixing genus which is often dominant under nutrient-rich conditions (especially where there is a significant supply of ammonia), although it also forms blooms in less polluted waters. Microcystin-producing *Anabaena* sp. have been reported from Canada, Denmark, Finland, France and Norway. A recent study from Egypt revealed that 25 per cent of 75 *Anabaena* and *Nostoc* strains isolated from soil, rice fields and water bodies contained microcystins. *Planktothrix agardhii* and *Planktothrix rubescens* (previously called *Oscillatoria agardhii* and *O. rubescens*) are common microcystin producers in the Northern Hemisphere; toxic strains of these have been isolated from blooms in Denmark, Finland and Norway. In addition, these species were frequently shown to be dominant in microcystin containing blooms in China, in Germany and in Sweden. In Swiss alpine lakes, *Oscillatoria limosa*, which is benthic (*i.e.* it grows attached to sediments and rocks), is a microcystin producer. In spite of the widespread occurrence of cyanobacterial blooms in Australia, *Planktothrix* blooms are rare there. This may be due to the higher temperature and tendency for elevated clay-derived turbidity in Australian water bodies.

The toxicity of the species listed in the table is in most cases verified by laboratory studies with isolated strains. A few bloom samples are also included from the new areas of occurrence where toxicity of the species is not verified by strain isolation but the toxins are determined in the bloom samples. The authors have suggested the listed species as the probable toxin producer (based on their dominance) but these reports should be treated as tentative until pure strains are studied.

Nostoc rivulare blooms in Texas, USA have caused poisoning of domestic and wild animals (Davidson, 1959) and, more recently, two unidentified *Nostoc* strains were shown to produce microcystins (Table 6.5).

The hepatotoxin, cylindrospermopsin, has been found in *Cylindrospermopsis raciborskii* in Australia and Hungary, in *Umezakia natans* in Japan, and in *Aphanizomenon ovalisporum* in Israel (Table 6.5). In spite of their occurrence in Europe, it appears that cylindrospermopsin-producing genera most commonly form toxic blooms in subtropical, tropical or arid zone water bodies. However, there have been reports of increasing occurrences of *Cylindrospermopsis raciborskii in* Europe and the USA (Padisák, 1997).

Table 6.5: Toxic Cyanobacteria Species and their Geographical Distribution

Toxic Species	*Cyanotoxin*	*Location*	*Reference(s)*
Anabaena flos-aquae	Microcystins	Canada	Krishnamurthy *et al.*, 1989; Harada *et al.*, 1991
Anabaena	Microcystins	Denmark	Henriksen *et al.*, 1996b
Anabaena spp.	Microcystins	Egypt	Yanni and Carmichael, 1997
Anabaena spp. (*flos-aquae, lemmermannii, circinalis*)	Microcystins	Finland	Sivonen *et al.*, 1990b; 1992a
Anabaena circinalis	Microcystins	France	Vezie *et al.*, 1998
Anabaena flos-aquae	Microcystins	Norway	Sivonen *et al.*, 1992a
Microcystis aeruginosa	Microcystins	Worldwide	Several; see Rinehart *et al.*, 1994 for a summary
M. viridis	Microcystins	Japan	Kusumi *et al.*, 1987; Watanabe *et al.*, 1986
M. botrys	Microcystins	Denmark	Henriksen *et al.*, 1996b
Planktothrix agardhii	Microcystins	China	Ueno *et al.*, 1996a
P. agardhii	Microcystins	Denmark	Henriksen *et al.*, 1996b
P. mougeotii	Microcystins	Denmark	Henriksen *et al.*, 1996b
P. agardhii	Microcystins	Finland	Sivonen, 1990b; Luukkainen *et al.*, 1993
P. agardhii	Microcystins	Norway	Krishnamurthy *et al.*, 1989; Mcriluoto *ot al.*, 1989
Oscillatoria limosa	Microcystins	Switzerland	Mez *et al.*, 1996
Nostoc sp.	Microcystins	Finland	Sivonen *et al.*, 1990a, 1992b
Nostoc sp.	Microcystins	England	Beattie *et al.*, 1998
Anabaenopsis millerii	Microcystins	Greece	Lanaras and Cook, 1994
Haphalosiphon hibernicus (soil isolate)	Microcystins	USA	Prinsep *et al.*, 1992
Nodularia spumigena	Nodularins	Australia	Baker and Humpage, 1994; Jones *et al.*, 1994
N. spumigena	Nodularins	Baltic Sea	Sivonen *et al.*, 1989b
N. spumigena	Nodularins	New Zealand	Carmichael *et al.*, 1988a; Rinehart *et al.*, 1988
Aphanizomenon ovalisporum	Cylindrospermopsin	Israel	Banker *et al.*, 1997
Cylindrospermopsis raciborskii	Cylindrospermopsin	Australia	Hawkins *et al.*, 1985; 1997
C. raciborskii	Cylindrospermopsin	Hungary	Törökné, 1997
Umezakia natans	Cylindrospermopsin	Japan	Harada *et al.*, 1994
Anabaena flos-aquae	Anatoxin-a	Canada	Carmichael *et al.*, 1975; Devlin *et al.*, 1977

Contd...

Table 6.5–Contd...

Toxic Species	*Cyanotoxin*	*Location*	*Reference(s)*
Anabaena spp.	Anatoxin-a	Finland	Sivonen *et al.*, 1989a
Anabaena blooms	Anatoxin-a	Germany	Bumke-Vogt, 1998
Anabaena sp.	Anatoxin-a	Ireland	James *et al.*, 1997
Anabaena sp.	Anatoxin-a (minor amounts)	Japan	Park *et al.*, 1993a
Anabaena planctonica bloom	Anatoxin-a	Italy	Bruno *et al.*, 1994
Aphanizomenon sp.	Anatoxin-a	Finland	Sivonen *et al.*, 1989a
Aphanizomenon blooms	Anatoxin-a	Germany	Bumke-Vogt, 1998
Cylindrospermum sp.	Anatoxin-a	Finland	Sivonen *et al.*, 1989a
Microcystis sp.	Anatoxin-a (minor amounts)	Japan	Park *et al.*, 1993a
Oscillatoria sp. benthic	Anatoxin-a	Scotland	Edwards *et al.*, 1992
Oscillatoria sp.	Anatoxin-a	Ireland	James *et al.*, 1997
Planktothrix sp.	Anatoxin-a	Finland	Sivonen *et al.*, 1989a
Planktothrix formosa	Homoanatoxin-a	Norway	Skulberg *et al.*, 1992
Anabaena flos-aquae	Anatoxin-a(S)	Canada	Matsunaga *et al.*, 1989; Mahmood and Carmichael, 1987
A. lemmermannii	Anatoxin-a(S)	Denmark	Henriksen *et al.*, 1997; Onodera *et al.*, 1997a
Anabaena circinalis	Saxitoxins	Australia	Humpage *et al.*, 1994; Negri *et al.*, 1995; 1997
Aphanizomenon flos-aquae	Saxitoxins	USA	Jackim and Gentile, 1968; Ikawa *et al.*, 1982; Mahmood and Carmichael, 1986
Cylindrospermopsis raciborskii	Saxitoxins	Brazil	Lagos *et al.*, 1997
Lyngbya wollei	Saxitoxins	USA	Carmichael *et al.*, 1997; Onodera *et al.*, 1997b
Microcystis		India	Parkar *et al.*, 1997

The neurotoxin, anatoxin-a, was first shown to be produced by *Anabaena flos-aquae* strains originating from Canada, and later by Finnish strains of unidentified *Anabaena* species, and in individual species of *Oscillatoria, Aphanizomenon,* and *Cylindrospermum,* by benthic *Oscillatoria* from Scotland, and by *Anabaena* and *Oscillatoria* in Ireland. It also was present in *Anabaena planctonica* blooms in Sardinia, Italy, in *Anabaena* and *Aphanizomenon* blooms in Germany, and in minor amounts in some Japanese bloom samples, as well as in *Anabaena* strains. Homoanatoxin-a has been characterised from an *Oscillatoria formosum* (*Phormidium formosum*) strain from Norway (Table 6.5). To date, anatoxin-a(S) has been found only from *Anabaena* species: *A. flos-aquae* in the USA and Scotland, and *A. lemmermannii* in Denmark.

Aphanizomenon flos-aquae blooms and strains were found to contain saxitoxins in the USA and this species was for a long time the only known saxitoxin producer amongst the cyanobacteria. More recently, saxitoxins have been shown to be common in Australian rivers and reservoirs and to be produced by *Anabaena circinalis.* In North America, a benthic freshwater *Lyngbya wollei* was found to produce saxitoxins, as was a strain of *Cylindrospermopsis raciborskii* in Brazil (Table 6.5).

Cyanotoxin Patterns in Strains and Species of Cyanobacteria

Cyanobacteria may produce several toxins simultaneously. In general, more than one microcystin has been characterised from the strains listed in Table 6.2. Among neurotoxic strains, several PSPs are found in the same strain, although there are considerable variations between species (Table 6.3). Furthermore, simultaneous neurotoxin and hepatotoxin production has been noted; the best example studied being the *Anabaena flos-aquae* strain NRC 525-17 which produces anatoxin-a(S) (Matsunaga *et al.*, 1989) and several microcystins (Harada *et al.*, 1991a).

Microcystin

Although many strains produce several microcystins simultaneously, usually only one or two of them are dominant in any single strain. Qualitative variation in the microcystins present is most frequently found among strains of *Anabaena* but also in *Microcystis* (Sivonen *et al.*, 1995). Some taxa have a number of microcystins in common, such as planktonic *Anabaena, Microcystis* and *Planktothrix* (*Oscillatoria*). However, there is evidence of microcystin variants that are typical for certain cyanobacterial taxa.

Planktothrix and some strains of *Anabaena* produce only demethylmicrocystins (Table 6.2). *Planktothrix* (*Oscillatoria*) isolates from Finland (13 strains studied and toxins fully characterised) seem to produce one of two types of microcystin (D-Asp^3-RR or Dha^7-RR) (Sivonen *et al.*, 1995).

German field samples dominated by *Planktothrix* have also shown these microcystins, with dominance of one major demethylated microcystin in populations of *P. rubescens*, and two or three of these variants in populations of *P. agardhii* (Fastner *et al.*, 1998).

Microcystis strains from Japan appear to contain chiefly microcystin-LR, -RR and -YR, with some cultures showing all three variants, and some strains being dominated by one of them. These three microcystins are the only variants reported in several studies on *M. aeruginosa* and *M. viridis* (*e.g.* Watanabe, 1996). Many of the microcystins listed in Table 6.2 have been found only in minor amounts or, to date, have been found to be produced only by individual isolates.

In natural samples which usually contain many strains, or more than one toxin-producing species, different combinations of microcystins can be found. For example, in a *Microcystis* bloom from Homer Lake, USA, 19 different microcystins were characterised (Namikoshi *et al.*, 1992a, 1995) and in one Australian bloom of *Microcystis aeruginosa,* 23 microcystins were detected by high pressure liquid chromatography (HPLC), none of which were microcystin-LR (Jones *et al.*, 1995).

Microcystin-LR is often mentioned as the most frequently occurring microcystin, although such observations may be biased by the fact that a chemical standard for the analysis of microcystin-LR was the earliest to be commercially available. It has been reported to be the major toxin in bloom and strain samples from Portugal (Vasconcelos *et al.*, 1995. 1996), France (Vezie *et al.*, 1997), Canada (Kotak *et al.*, 1993) and frequently co-occurring with microcystin-RR and -YR in Japan (Watanabe *et al.*, 1988, 1989).

Geographical patterns are indicated by some survey results. Wide variation among the L-amino acids of microcystins has been reported for South Africa (Scott, 1991), frequent presence of demethylmicrocystins (RR and LR) has been seen in Finnish strains (Sivonen *et al.*, 1995) and microcystins in Danish samples show wide variation (Henriksen, 1996a). In part, these patterns probably reflect regional differences in dominance of cyanobacterial species or strains. Water bodies with regular dominance of specific taxa are likely to exhibit characteristic patterns of microcystin variants.

Nodularin

The cyanotoxin, nodularin, is found in waters where *Nodularia spumigena* is present; the most prominent areas being the Baltic Sea and brackish water estuaries and coastal lakes of Australia and New Zealand. However, the best known *Nodularia spumigena* bloom location, Lake Alexandrina, Australia, has salinities which are only slightly elevated above normal river water and at levels still suitable for drinking water. The presence of variants of nodularin in environmental samples is usually rather insignificant. In the Baltic Sea, the collection of samples for several years has shown nodularin to be the major compound present. The same is true for the almost 90 hepatotoxic *Nodularia* strains isolated from the same source (Sivonen *et al.*, 1989b; Lehtimäki *et al.*, 1997). Analyses of several strains isolated from blooms across Australia have revealed similar results, with nodularin variants being found rarely, and then only at low relative abundance (Jones *et al.*, 1994; Blackburn *et al.*, 1997).

Saxitoxins

There is much diversity of saxitoxin distribution in cyanobacteria from around the world (Table 6.3). In addition, the lack of analytical standards for many saxitoxins has probably restricted findings in some countries. Saxitoxin-producing *Anabaena circinalis* blooms are widespread in Australian rivers and reservoirs, and the relative abundance of individual toxins is remarkably constant in toxin-producing strains, which is quite opposite to the microcystin-producing cyanobacteria. In all healthy *Anabaena circinalis* cultures examined in Australia, the relative composition of individual saxitoxins is very similar and dominated by C-toxins (Blackburn *et al.*, 1997). As blooms and cultures age, the proportion of decarbamoyl-gonyautoxins breakdown products increases at the expense of the C-toxins. In North American *Aphanizomenon flos-aquae* and in Brazilian *Cylindrospermopsis raciborskii* samples, mostly neosaxitoxin and smaller amounts of saxitoxin have been detected. In the case of the *Aphanizomenon flos-aquae* from North America, only bloom samples and strains from New Hampshire, USA have been found to contain saxitoxins. Mat-forming *Lyngbya wollei* from Alabama, USA was found to produce decarbamoyl saxitoxin (dcSTX), decarbamoylgonyautoxin-2 and -3 (dcGTX2 and dcGTX3) and six new saxitoxins.

Concentrations of Cyanotoxins in Surface Waters

Information on the concentrations of cyanotoxins in surface waters has been appearing only recently in the international literature. In early studies (pre-1990s), the toxicity of bloom samples was determined by mouse bioassays, but this method is unsuitable for measuring the low concentrations of cyanotoxins that usually prevail in cyanobacterial populations when they do not accumulate in scums. The development of better analytical methods, in the first instance HPLC and more recently enzyme linked immunosorbent assay (ELISA), (and for microcystins and nodularins also the protein phosphatase assay) has made the quantification of total and individual toxins possible.

The quantitative determination of toxin concentrations is mostly performed from lyophilised (freeze-dried) cultures, bloom samples or seston (particulate material suspended in water, which contains not only cyanobacterial cells but usually other algae, some zooplankton, and possibly inorganic material such as soil and sediment particles). Results are usually expressed as milligrams or micrograms of toxin per gram dry weight (dw). Whereas in cultures and bloom samples, the dry weight originates from cyanobacteria, it will encompass further particles (seston) in plankton samples taken outside of scum areas. The highest published concentrations of cyanotoxins from cyanobacterial bloom samples, measured by HPLC, are (Table 6.6):

- ☆ Microcystin–7,300 $\mu g\ g^{-1}$ dw from China and Portugal,
- ☆ Nodularin–18,000 $\mu g\ g^{-1}$ dw from the Baltic Sea,

☆ Cylindrospermopsin–5,500 μg g^{-1} dw from Australia,
☆ Anatoxin-a–4,400 μg g^{-1} dw from Finland,
☆ Saxitoxins–3,400 μg g^{-1} dw from Australia,
☆ Anatoxin-a(S)–3,300 μg g^{-1} dw from the USA.

Table 6.6: Toxin Concentrations Reported in Cyanobacterial Bloom or Water Samples

Location	*Period of Study*	*No. of Toxic Samples (Total no. of samples)*	*Toxins Identified*	*Range of Total Concentrations (μg g^{-1} dw, unless otherwise indicated)*	*Analysis Method*	*Reference*
			Microcystins			
Australia	1991	4	Microcystins, 24 unidentified	2,100-4,100[2]	HPLC	Jones *et al.*, 1995
Canada, Alberta	1990	37(50)	Microcystin-LR	4-610	HPLC	Kotak *et al.*, 1993
Canada, Alberta (3 lakes)	1990-93	168(226)	Microcystin-LR	1-1,550	HPLC	Kotak *et al.*, 1995
China	1988	5(10)	Microcystin-RR, -LR	200-7,300	HPLC	Zhang *et al.*, 1991
Czech and Slovak Rep.	1995-96	(63)	Microcystin-LR	4-6,835	HPLC	Maršálek *et al.*, 1996
Denmark	1992-94		Microcystin-RR, -LR	3-2,800	HPLC	Christoffersen, 1996
Denmark	1993-95	198(296)	Microcystins	5-1,900	HPLC	Henriksen *et al.*, 1996b
Finland	1994-95	17(20)	Microcystin-LR	> 10-800	HPLC	Lahti *et al.*, 1997
France	1994	16(22)	Microcystins	70-3,970	HPLC	Vezie *et al.*, 1997
France, L. Grand-Lieu	1994	19(30)	Microcystins	30-230	HPLC	Vezie *et al.*, 1998
Germany	1992	8(15)	Microcystin-LR	36-360	HPLC	Fastner, 1994
Germany	1993	17(18)	Microcystins	0.15-36[1,2]	ELISA	Ueno *et al.*, 1996b
Germany	1995-96	385(533)	Microcystins	1-5,000	HPLC	Fastner, 1998
Germany	1997	34	Microcystins, several	1-25,000[1]	HPLC	Chorus *et al.*, 1998
Japan	1990	12(14)	Microcystin-RR, -YR, -LR	160-950	HPLC	Watanabe *et al.*, 1992
Japan	1988-92	11(19)	Microcystin-RR, -YR, -LR, [Dha[7]] -LR	70-1,610	HPLC	Park *et al.*, 1993a
Japan, Lake Suwa	1980-91	13	Microcystin-RR, -YR, -LR	30-2,100	HPLC	Park *et al.*, 1993b
Japan	1986-88	4(4)	Microcystin-RR, -YR, -LR	100-860	HPLC	Shirai *et al.*, 1991
Japan	1992-95	18(22)	Microcystin-RR, -YR, -LR	0.04-480[1]	HPLC	Tsuji *et al.*, 1996
Japan	1993-95	46(57)	Microcystins	0.05-1,300[1,2]	ELISA	Ueno *et al.*, 1996b
Japan	1993-94	12(17)	Microcystins	0.06-94[1,2]	ELISA	Nagata *et al.*, 1997
Japan	1989-94	10(10)	Microcystins	300-15,600[1,2] 330-19,500[1,2]	ELISA HPLC	Nagata *et al.*, 1997

Contd...

Table 6.6–Contd...

Location	Period of Study	No. of Toxic Samples (Total no. of samples)	Toxins Identified	Range of Total Concentrations (μg g^{-1} dw, unless otherwise indicated)	Analysis Method	Reference
Portugal	1989-92	12(12)	Microcystin-LR plus six known and three unidentified microcystins	1,000-7,100	HPLC	Vasconcelos *et al.*, 1996
Portugal	1994-95	28(29)	Microcystins	0.1-37[1,2]	ELISA	Ueno *et al.*, 1996b
South Africa	1985-86		Microcystin-FR, -LR, -YR, -LA, -YA, -LAba	5-420	HPLC	Wicks and Thiel, 1990
South Africa	1988-89	9(9)	Microcystin-YR, -LR, -FR, -YA, -LA, -LAba	40-630	HPLC	Scott, 1991
UK	1992	3(3)	Microcystins, 3	17-131[1,2]	HPLC	Codd *et al.*, 1995
USA, Wisconsin	1993	9	Microcystins	1,900-12,800[2]	ELISA	McDermott *et al.*, 1995
			Nodularins			
Baltic Sea	1985-87	17(23)	Nodularin	< 100-2,400	HPLC	Sivonen *et al.*, 1989b
Baltic Sea	1990-91	6(16)	Nodularin	300-18,000	HPLC	Kononen *et al.*, 1993
Tasmania, Orielton Lagoon	1992-93	7(9)	Nodularin	2,000-3,500	HPLC	Jones *et al.*, 1994
			Anatoxins			
Denmark	1993-95	9(10)	Anatoxin-a(S)	4-3,300[3]	ChE inhibition assay	Henriksen *et al.*, 1997
Finland	1985-87	13(30)	Anatoxin-a	10-4,400	GC/MS	Sivonen *et al.*, 1989a
Finland and Japan		3(3)	Anatoxin-a	0.4-2,600	LC/MS	Harada *et al.*, 1993
Germany	1995-96	10(45)	Anatoxin-a	0.02-0.36[1]	GC-ECD	Bumke-Vogt, 1998
Ireland	1995	2(2)	Anatoxin-a	10-100	HPLC (fluorimetric)	James *et al.*, 1997
Japan	1988-92	9(14)	Anatoxin-a	0.3-16	TSP-LC/MS	Park *et al.*, 1993a
			Saxitoxins			
Australia	1990-92	11(11)	Saxitoxins	85-2,040	HPLC and FAB-MS	Humpage *et al.*, 1994
Australia	1992-94	24(31)	Saxitoxins	50-3,400	HPLC	Negri *et al.*, 1997
USA	1994	7(8)	Saxitoxins	5-60[4]	HPLC/AOAC	Carmichael *et al.*, 1997

Dw: Dry weight; HPLC: High pressure liquid chromatography; ELISA: Enzyme linked immunosorbent assay; GC/MS: Gas chromatography/mass spectrometry; LC/MS: Liquid chromatography/mass spectrometry; GC-ECD: Gas chromatography-electron capture detection; TSP-LC/MS: Thermospray-liquid chromatography/mass spectrometry; FAB-MS: Fast atom bombardment-mass spectrometry; AOAC: Mouse bioassay done according to the Association of Official Analytical Chemists.

1: Given as μg l^{-1}; 2: Microcystin-LR used as standard; 3: Measured by enzyme inhibition;
4: Micrograms of STX equivalents.

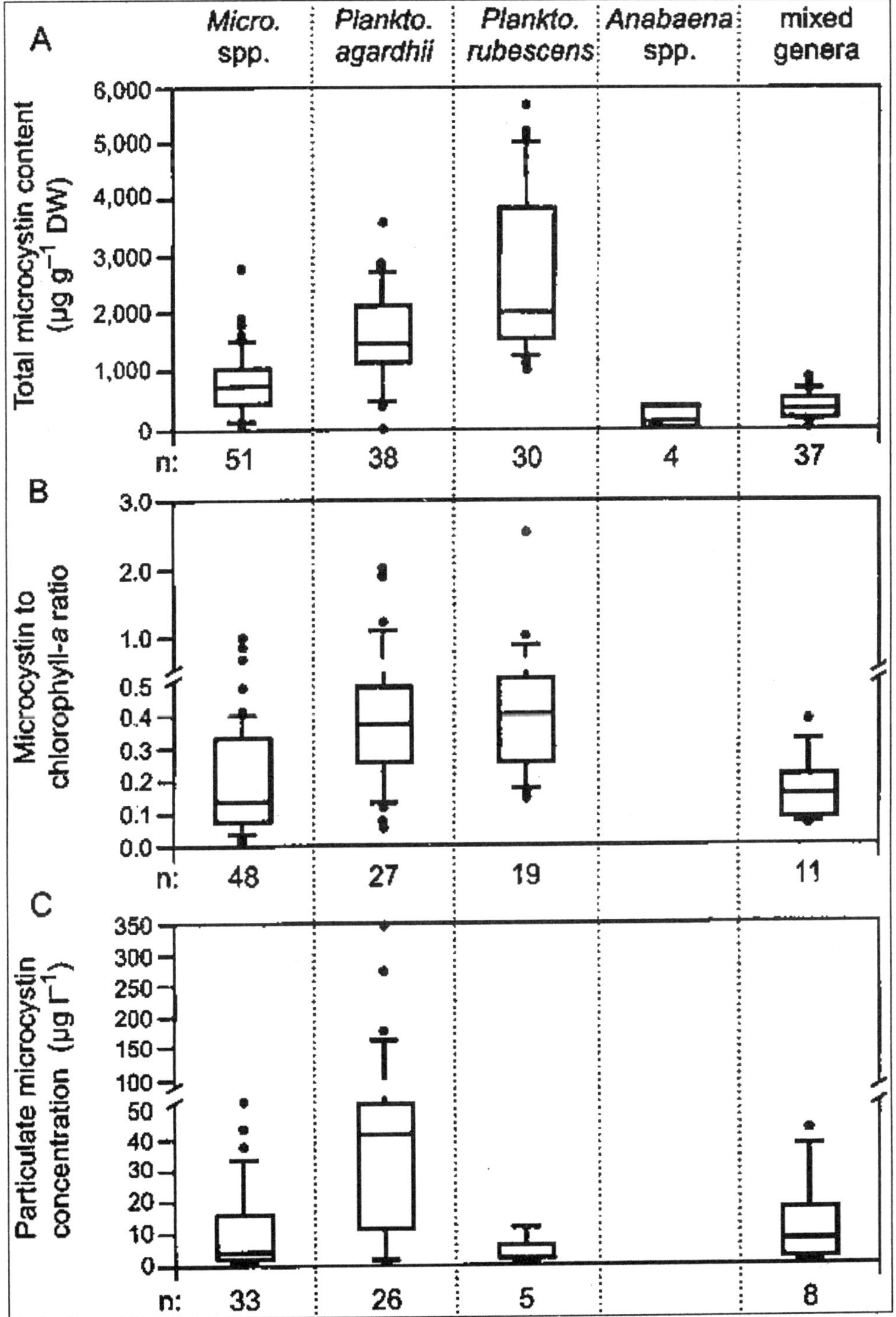
A
Micro. spp.
Plankto. agardhii
Plankto. rubescens
Anabaena spp.
mixed genera
Total microcystin content (µg g⁻¹ DW)
6,000
5,000
4,000
3,000
2,000
1,000
0
n: 51 38 30 4 37
B
Microcystin to chlorophyll-a ratio
3.0
2.0
1.0
0.5
0.4
0.3
0.2
0.1
0.0
n: 48 27 19 11
C
Particulate microcystin concentration (µg l⁻¹)
350
300
250
200
150
100
50
40
30
20
10
0
n: 33 26 5 8

Figure 6.4

Table 6.7: Dissolved (Extracellular) Toxin Concentrations Measured in Water Samples

Location	Period of Study	No. of Toxic Samples (Total no. of samples)	Toxin Identified	Concentration (μg l^{-1})	Analysis Method	Reference
Australia		24	Microcystins	3-1.800[1]	HPLC	Jones and Orr, 1994
China	1993-94	130(835)	Microcystins	0.05-1.6	ELISA	Ueno *et al.*, 1996a
Finland	1993-94	38(38)	Microcystin-LR	0.06-0,21	HPLC and ELISA	Lahti *et al.*, 1997
Germany	1993-94	11(19)	Microcystins	0.07-0.76	ELISA	Ueno *et al.*, 1996b
Japan	1992-95	9(22)	Microcystin-RR, -YR, -LR	0.02-3.8	HPLC	Tsuji *et al.*, 1996
Japan	1993-95	26(38)	Microcystins	trace-5.6	ELISA	Ueno *et al.*, 1996b
Japan	1993-94	4(13)	Microcystins	0.08-0.8	ELISA	Nagata *et al.*, 1997
Thailand	1994	7(10)	Microcystins	0.08-0.35	ELISA	Ueno *et al.*, 1996b
USA, Wisconsin	1993	27(27)	Microcystins	0.07-200	ELISA	McDermott *et al.*, 1995

HPLC: High pressure liquid chromatography; ELISA: Enzyme linked immunosorbent assay.

1 High range concentrations following treatment of a large bloom with algicide, which released intracellular microcystins.

Table 6.8: Laboratory Studies on Cellular Toxin Concentrations in Cyanobacteria

Parameter	Organism	Toxin(s)/ Analysis Method	Changes in Toxin Concentrations (dw)	Highest/ Lowest Toxin Production	Reference(s)
			Temperature (°C)		
12.5-30	*Anabaena* spp. (2 strains), batch cultures	Microcystins HPLC	3.5-30 fold[1]	Highest at 25, lowest at 30; different toxins at different temperatures	Rapala *et al.*, 1997
10-28	*Anabaena* spp. (2 strains), continuous cultures	Microcystins HPLC	3-10 fold	Lowest at 10, highest at 25	Rapala and Sivonen, 1998
15-30	*Anabaena* spp. (2 strains), batch cultures	Anatoxin-a HPLC	3 fold	Lowest at 30, highest at 20	Rapala *et al.*, 1993
10-28	*Anabaena* spp. (2 strains), continuous cultures	Anatoxin-a HPLC	4-7 fold	Highest at 19-21, lowest at 10 and 28	Rapala and Sivonen, 1998
15-30	*Aphanizomenon* sp. (1 strain), batch cultures	Anatoxin-a HPLC	3 fold	Lowest at 30, highest at 20	Rapala *et al.*, 1993
10,25,34	*Microcystis aeruginosa* (1 strain), batch cultures	Microcystins mouse bioassay	5 fold	Highest toxicity at 25, lowest at 10	Codd and Poon, 1988

Contd...

Table 6.8–Contd...

Parameter	Organism	Toxin(s)/ Analysis Method	Changes in Toxin Concentrations (dw)	Highest/ Lowest Toxin Production	Reference(s)
15-35	*Microcystis aeruginosa* (1 strain) batch cultures	Microcystins HPLC mouse bioassay	4 fold	Highest toxicity at 20; different toxins at different temperatures	van der Westhuizen and Eloff, 1985; van der Westhuizen *et al.*, 1986
18,25,35	*Microcystis aeruginosa* (1 strain), batch cultures	Microcystins mouse bioassay	1.4 fold	Highest toxicity at 18, lowest at 32	Watanabe and Oishi, 1985
10-30	*Nodularia spumigena* (2 strains), batch cultures	Nodularin HPLC	3-4 fold	Highest at 20, lowest at 10 or 30	Lehtimäki *et al.*, 1994
7-28	*Nodularia spumigena* (1 strain), batch cultures	Nodularin HPLC	3 fold	Highest at 19	Lehtimäki *et al.*, 1997
15-30	*Oscillatoria agardhii* (2 strains), batch cultures	Microcystins HPLC	7 fold	Strain dependent; lowest at 30	Sivonen, 1990b
		Light ($\mu mol\ m^{-2}\ s^{-1}$)			
2-100 continuous	*Anabaena* spp. (2 strains), batch cultures	Microcystins HPLC	3 fold	Highest at 25	Rapala *et al.*, 1997
7, 19, 42 continuous	*Anabaena* spp. (2 strains), continuous cultures	Microcystins HPLC	2.5-15	Lowest at 10, highest at 25	Rapala and Sivonen, 1998
2-128 continuous	*Anabaena* spp. (2 strains), batch cultures	Anatoxin-a HPLC	3 fold	Highest at 26-44, lowest at 2	Rapala *et al.*, 1993
7, 19, 42 continuous	*Anabaena* spp. (2 strains), continuous cultures	Anatoxin-a HPLC	No effect	Highest at 19, lowest at 7	Rapala and Sivonen, 1998
2-128 continuous	*Aphanizomenon* sp. (1 strain), batch cultures	Anatoxin-a HPLC	4 fold	Highest at 128, lowest at 2	Rapala *et al.*, 1993
5-50 continuous	*Microcystis aeruginosa* (1 strain), batch cultures	Microcystins mouse bioassay	2.4 fold	Highest toxicity at 20	Codd and Poon, 1988
20-75 continuous	*Microcystis aeruginosa* (1 strain), continuous cultures	Microcystins HPLC	2.5 fold	Highest at 40	Utkilen and Gjølme, 1992
21-205 continuous	*Microcystis aeruginosa* (1 strain), batch cultures	Microcystins mouse bioassay	1.2 fold	Highest toxicity at 142, lowest at 21	van der Westhuizen and Eloff, 1985
7.5, 30, 75 continuous	*Microcystis aeruginosa* (1 strain), batch cultures	Microcystins mouse bioassay	3.8 fold	Highest toxicity at 30, lowest at 7.5	Watanabe and Oishi, 1985
25, 50, 80 continuous	*Nodularia spumigena* (2 strains), batch cultures	Nodularin HPLC	No difference		Lehtimäki *et al.*, 1994

Contd...

Table 6.8–Contd...

Parameter	Organism	Toxin(s)/ Analysis Method	Changes in Toxin Concentrations (dw)	Highest/ Lowest Toxin Production	Reference(s)
2-155 continuous	*Nodularia spumigena* (1 strain), batch cultures	Nodularin HPLC	50 fold[1]	Higher at high irradiances, minimal at 2	Lehtimäki *et al.*, 1997
12-95 continuous	*Oscillatoria agardhii* (2 strains), batch cultures	Microcystins HPLC	2.5 fold	Highest at 12-44	Sivonen, 1990b
		***Phosphorus* (mg P l^{-1})**			
0.05-5.5	*Anabaena* spp. (2 strains), batch cultures	Microcystins HPLC	5 fold	Highest at 5.5, lowest at 0.05	Rapala *et al.*, 1997
0.05-5.5	*Anabaena* spp. (2 strains), batch cultures	Anatoxin-a HPLC	No difference	No statistically significant differences	Rapala *et al.*, 1993
0.05-5.5	*Aphanizomenon* sp. (2 strains), batch cultures	Anatoxin-a HPLC	2 fold	Lowest at 0.05-0.1, highest at 0.5-5.5	Rapala *et al.*, 1993
BG-11 and medium without P	*Microcystis aeruginosa* (1 strain), batch cultures	Microcystins mouse bioassay	1.7 fold	Higher toxicity without P	Codd and Poon, 1988
0.0025, 0.025	*Microcystis aeruginosa* (1 strain), continuous cultures	Microcystins HPLC	2.3 fold	More toxin at 0.025	Utkilen and Gjølme, 1995
MA medium 1/1; dilutions 1/10, 1/20	*Microcystis aeruginosa* (1 strain), batch cultures	Microcystins mouse bioassay	Less than 1	Highest toxicity with the original medium	Watanabe and Oishi, 1985
0.1-5.5	*Oscillatoria agardhii* (2 strains), batch cultures	Microcystins HPLC	1.8-2.5 fold	Lowest toxin at 0.1	Sivonen, 1990b
0.3, 0.6, 1.0	*Nodularia spumigena* (2 strains), batch cultures	Nodularin HPLC	Less than 1 fold	Lowest at 0.3	Lehtimäki *et al.*, 1994
0-5.5	*Nodularia spumigena* (1 strain), batch cultures	Nodularin HPLC	4 fold	Lowest at 0-0.02, highest at 0.2-5.5	Lehtimäki *et al.*, 1997
		***Nitrogen* (mg N l^{-1})**			
BG-11 medium, medium without N	*Microcystis aeruginosa* (1 strain), batch cultures	Microcystins mouse bioassay	5 fold	Higher toxicity with the medium containing N	Codd and Poon, 1988
0.05-1	*Microcystis aeruginosa* (1 strain), continuous cultures	Microcystins HPLC	3 fold	Higher at high N	Utkilen and Gjølme, 1995
MA medium 1/1; dilutions 1/10, 1/20	*Microcystis aeruginosa* (1 strain), batch cultures	Microcystins mouse bioassay	2.5 fold	Highest toxicity with the original medium	Watanabe and Oishi, 1985
0.42-84	*Oscillatoria agardhii* (2 strains), batch cultures	Microcystins HPLC	5 fold	Higher at high N, lowest at low N	Sivonen, 1990b

Contd...

Table 6.8–Contd...

Parameter	*Organism*	*Toxin(s)/ Analysis Method*	*Changes in Toxin Concentrations (dw)*	*Highest/ Lowest Toxin Production*	*Reference(s)*
			Micronutrients		
Al, Cd, Cr, Cu, Fe, Mn, Ni, Sn, Zn; various concentrations	*Microcystis aeruginosa* (1 strain), batch cultures	Microcystins HPLC	1.7 fold	Less toxins at low Fe concentrations	Lukac and Aegerter, 1993
0.1-3.4 μg Fe l^{-1}	*Microcystis aeruginosa* (1 strain), continuous cultures	Microcystins HPLC	1.5 fold	More toxin at high Fe concentrations	Utkilen and Gjølme, 1995
0.03-1.2 μg Fe l^{-1}	*Microcystis aeruginosa* (1 strain), continuous cultures	Microcystins HPLC	0-3 fold	Less toxin at low Fe concentrations	Lyck *et al.*, 1966
			Salinity (‰)		
3, 5, 8, 11	*Nodularia spumigena* (2 strains), batch cultures	Nodularin HPLC	No difference	No statistical difference	Lehtimäki *et al.*, 1994
0-30	*Nodularia spumigena* (1 strain), batch cultures	Nodularin HPLC	8 fold	Highest at 15, lowest at 0 and 30	Lehtimäki *et al.*, 1997
0-35	*Nodularia spumigena* (6 strains), batch cultures	Nodularin HPLC	5 fold	Highest at 12, lowest at 35	Blackburn *et al.*, 1996
			CO_2		
BG-11 medium, medium without CO_2	*Microcystis aeruginosa* (1 strain), batch culture	Microcystins mouse bioassay	6 fold	Higher toxicity with the medium containing CO_2	Codd and Poon, 1988
			pH		
1-14	*Microcystis aeruginosa* (1 strain), batch cultures	Microcystins mouse bioassay	1.8 fold	Toxicity highest at low and high pH	van der Westhuizen and Eloff, 1983

Dw: Dry weight; HPLC: High performance liquid chromatography.

1: When the growth of the strains was poor the amount of toxins was also very low (less than 0.1 mg g^{-1} dw of cells); when these cases were compared to maximal toxin production more than ten-fold differences could be seen

Biosynthesis

To understand how cyanotoxins are produced, it is necessary to study the biochemical and genetic basis of toxin production. Knowledge of the biosynthetic pathways of cyanotoxins is in its early stage and no complete biochemical pathways are known. Biosynthesis of several cyanotoxins has been studied by feeding labelled precursors to a cyanobacterial culture and following their incorporation into the carbon skeleton of the toxins. Shimizu *et al.* (1984) used an *Aphanizomenon flos-aquae* strain to study biosynthesis of saxitoxin analogues. They proposed a new pathway for neosaxitoxin biosynthesis, the key steps of which are the condensation of an acetate unit, or its derivative, to the amino group bearing an a-carbon of arginine or an equivalent, and a subsequent loss of the carboxyl carbon and imidazole ring formation on the adjacent carbonyl carbon. They established the origin of all the carbons in the toxin alkaloid ring system. The side-chain carbon was derived from methionine (Shimizu, 1986).

Anatoxin-a is related structurally to the tropane class of alkaloids found in higher plants. Based mainly on ^{14}C-labelled precursors and enzymatic studies, Gallon *et al.* (1990) and Gallon *et al.* (1994) suggested the biosynthesis of anatoxin-a to be analogous to that of tropanes. Anatoxin-a was proposed to be formed from ornithine/arginine via putrescine, which is oxidised to pyrroline, a precursor of anatoxin-a. Labelling experiments using ^{13}C NMR (nuclear magnetic resonance spectrometry) indicated that the carbon skeleton of anatoxin-a is derived from acetate and glutamate. The studies showed that C-1 of glutamic acid is retained during the transformation of anatoxin-a and not lost by decarboxylation, a finding incompatible with the tropane alkaloid theory (Hemscheidt *et al.*, 1995b). All of the carbons of anatoxin-a(S) are derived from amino acids. Three methyl carbons arise from L-methionine or other donors to the tetrahydrofolate C1 pool. L-arginine accounts for C-2, C-4, C-5 and C-6 carbons of the toxin (Moore *et al.*, 1992, 1993). The intermediate in the biosynthesis of anatoxin-a(S) from L arginine is (2*S*,4*S*)-4 hydroxyarginine (Hemscheidt *et al.*, 1995a). The structure of the cylindrospermopsin suggests a polyketide origin for the toxin (Moore *et al.*, 1993).

The origin of carbons in microcystin (Moore *et al.*, 1991) and in nodularin (Choi *et al.*, 1993; Rinehart *et al.*, 1994) have been studied by following the incorporation of labelled precursors into the toxins by NMR. Carbons C1-C8 of Adda in nodularin are acetate derived and the remaining carbons presumably originate from phenylalanine. Methyl groups in carbons 2, 4, 6, 8, and the O-methyl group in the Adda unit, originated from methionine. The D-Glu and L-Arg carbons C4-C5 were acetate derived, with C1-C2 being from glutamate. Methyldehydrobutyrine was possibly formed from threonine, its methyl group coming from methionine. The β-methylaspartic acid was found to originate from condensation of pyruvic acid (C3-C4) and acetyl-CoA (C1-C2) (Rinehart *et al.*, 1994). The studies on the carbon skeleton of nodularin, with some minor differences, agree with work on microcystin-LR by Moore *et al.* (1991). In their study, L-Leu and D-Ala units in microcystin had acetate incorporation. The dehydroamino acid in microcystin has been proposed to be formed from serine rather than from threonine (Rinehart *et al.*, 1994). Rinehart's group found linear nodularin, which was shown by culture experiments to be a precursor of cyclic nodularin. Three additional linear peptides were isolated from a bloom sample, one of them was possibly a precursor of cyclic microcystin-LR and the others possibly degradation products (Rinehart *et al.*, 1994).

Genetic Regulation of Cyanotoxin Production

The genes and enzymes involved in cyanotoxin production are still mostly unknown. The first molecular biological studies on toxic cyanobacteria investigated the possible involvement of plasmids in toxin production. Four toxic strains of *Microcystis aeruginosa* contained plasmids, and no plasmid could be shown in one toxic and in several non-toxic strains (Schwabe *et al.*, 1988). More recently, a similar study in Australia found no evidence for plasmid involvement in microcystin synthesis (Bolch *et al.*, 1997). Gallon *et al.* (1994) studied an anatoxin-a producing *Anabaena* strain NCR 44-1, which spontaneously became non-toxic. They found that the size of a plasmid was reduced in that non-toxic clone, but this work has not been repeated or confirmed.

Multi-enzyme complexes and peptide synthetase genes are involved in hepatotoxin production. Several cyclic and linear peptides, often with D-amino acids, are known to be produced, non-ribosomally, by multi-domain peptide synthetases via the so-called thiotemplate mechanism in bacteria and lower eukaryotes. The best characterised are the synthesis of gramicidin S and tyrocidin by *Bacillus*. Peptide synthetase genes have been detected and sequenced (partly) in *Microcystis aeruginosa*

(Meissner *et al.*, 1996) and in *Anabaena* (Rouhiainen *et al.*, 1994). Analogous polymerase chain reaction (PCR) products to the peptide synthetase genes have been shown by using DNA from *Microcystis* (Jacobs *et al.*, 1995; Arment and Carmichael, 1996) and *Nodularia* as a template. Dittman *et al.* (1997) showed, in knockout experiments, that peptide synthetase genes are responsible for microcystin production.

At least some strains which produce hepatotoxins also produce other small cyclic peptides (Namikoshi and Rinehart, 1996; Weckesser *et al.*, 1996) which are likely to be produced by nonribosomal peptide synthesis.

Fate in the Environment

Partitioning Between Cells and Water

It appears likely that cyanotoxins are produced and contained within the actively growing cyanobacterial cells (*i.e.* they are intracellular or particulate). Release to the surrounding water, to form dissolved toxin, appears to occur mostly, if not exclusively, during cell senescence, death and lysis, rather than by continuous excretion.

In laboratory studies, where both intracellular and dissolved toxins (microcystins/nodularin and saxitoxins) have been measured, it is generally the case that in healthy log phase cultures, less than 10-20 per cent of the total toxin pool is extracellular (Sivonen, 1990b; Lehtimäki *et al.*, 1997; Negri *et al.*, 1997; Rapala *et al.*, 1997). As cells enter stationary phase the increased rate of cell death may lead to an increase in the extracellular dissolved fraction. Even during log-phase cell growth in culture, a small percentage of cells in the population may be dying and lysing (and releasing intracellular toxins), even though there is an overall positive population growth. There are some indications that anatoxin-a may leak out of cells during growth especially in low light conditions. High concentrations of anatoxin-a, sometimes exceeding the intracellular pool of toxins, have been found in media in a batch culture study (Bumke-Vogt *et al.*, 1996).

In the field, healthy bloom populations produce little extracellular toxin. The range of measured concentrations for dissolved cyanotoxins, in all cases except those where a major bloom is obviously breaking down, is 0.1-10 $\mu g\ l^{-1}$ (Lindholm and Meriluoto, 1991; Jones and Orr, 1994; Tsuji *et al.*, 1996; Ueno *et al.*, 1996b; Lahti *et al.*, 1997b) Cell-bound concentrations are several orders of magnitude higher (Tables 6.6 and 6.7). In lakes or rivers, toxins liberated from cells are rapidly diluted by the large mass of water, especially if mixing of water by wind action or currents is vigorous (Jones and Orr, 1994). However, the concentration of dissolved toxins may be much higher in ageing or declining blooms. This is an important consideration for water treatment plant operators, because it means that removal of healthy cyanobacterial cells intact from the raw water supply may obviate or substantially reduce the need for additional adsorptive (activated carbon) or oxidative (ozone or chlorine) toxin removal processes.

The release of toxins from cells is enhanced by chemical treatments for the eradication of cyanobacteria, especially the use of algicides (either copper-based or organic herbicides). Treatment of a bloom with copper sulphate, for example, may lead to complete lysis of the bloom population within three days and release of all the toxins into the surrounding water (Berg *et al.*, 1987; Kenefick *et al.*, 1992; Jones and Orr, 1994). The efficacy of copper sulphate treatment is, however, very much dependent on water chemistry, especially alkalinity, pH and dissolved organic content.

Chemical Breakdown

The four main groups of cyanotoxins: microcystins, anatoxins, PSPs and cylindrospermopsins, exhibit quite different chemical stabilities and biological activities in water.

Microcystins

Microcystins, being cyclic peptides, are extremely stable and resistant to chemical hydrolysis or oxidation at near neutral pH. Microcystins and nodularin remain potent even after boiling. In natural waters and in the dark, microcystins may persist for months or years. At high temperatures (40 °C) and at elevated or low pH, slow hydrolysis has been observed, with the times to achieve greater than 90 per cent breakdown being approximately 10 weeks at pH 1 and greater than 12 weeks at pH 9 (Harada *et al.*, 1996). Rapid chemical hydrolysis occurs only under conditions that are unlikely to be attained outside the laboratory, *e.g.* 6M HCl at high temperature.

Microcystins can be oxidised by ozone and other strong oxidising agents, and degraded by intense ultra violet (UV) light. These processes have relevance for water treatment, although they are unlikely to contribute to degradation occurring in the natural environment.

In full sunlight, microcystins undergo slow photochemical breakdown and isomerisation, with the reaction rate being enhanced by the presence of water-soluble cell pigments, presumably phycobiliproteins (Tsuji *et al.*, 1993). In the presence of pigments the photochemical breakdown of microcystin in full sunlight can take as little as two weeks for greater than 90 per cent breakdown, or longer than six weeks, depending on the concentration of pigment (and presumably toxin, although this has not been tested). A more rapid breakdown under sunlight has been reported in the presence of humic substances (which can act as photosensitisers) in field concentrations ranging from 2-16 mg l^{-1} dissolved organic carbon (DOC). Approximately 40 per cent of the microcystins was degraded per day under summer conditions of insolation (Welker and Steinberg, 1998). In deeper or muddy waters, the rate of breakdown is likely to be considerably slower.

Anatoxins

Anatoxin-a is relatively stable in the dark, but in pure solution in the absence of pigments it undergoes rapid photochemical degradation in sunlight. Breakdown is further accelerated by alkaline conditions (Stevens and Krieger, 1991). The half-life for photochemical breakdown is 1-2 hours. Under normal day and night light conditions at pH 8 or pH 10, and at low initial concentrations (10 µg l^{-1}), the half-life for anatoxin-a breakdown was found to be approximately 14 days (Smith and Sutton, 1993). Anatoxin-a(S) decomposes rapidly in basic solutions but is relatively stable under neutral and acidic conditions (Matsunaga *et al.*, 1989).

Saxitoxins

In the dark at room temperature, saxitoxins undergo a series of slow chemical hydrolysis reactions. The C-toxins lose the N-sulphocarbamoyl group to form decarbamoyl gonyautoxins (dc-GTXs); while the dc-GTXs, GTXs and STXs slowly degrade to, as yet unidentified, non-toxic products. The half-lives for the breakdown reactions are in the order of 1-10 weeks, with more than three months often being required for greater than 90 per cent breakdown (Jones and Negri, 1997). Because dc-GTXs are much more toxic than C-toxins (by a factor of 10-100), a solution or water body containing a natural mixture of C-toxins and GTXs, for example from the lysis of an Australian bloom of *Anabaena circinalis*, will actually increase in toxicity over a period of up to three weeks, before toxicity begins to abate during the succeeding 2-3 months. Boiling an extract of *Anabaena* with predominant C-toxins may also substantially increase toxicity. Similar transformation reactions occur in living cells as they age in culture or in a natural bloom (Negri *et al.*, 1997). No detailed studies have been carried out on saxitoxin breakdown in sunlight, either with or without pigments.

Cylindrospermopsins

Cylindrospermopsin is relatively stable in the dark, with slow breakdown occurring at elevated temperature (50 °C) (Chiswell *et al.*, 1999). In sunlight and in the presence of cell pigments, breakdown occurs quite rapidly being more than 90 per cent complete within 2-3 days (Chiswell *et al.*, 1999). Pure cylindrospermopsin is relatively stable in sunlight.

Removal on Natural Sediments and Soils

Microcystins appear to be retained only weakly on natural suspended solids in rivers and reservoirs; usually no more than 20 per cent of the total microcystin concentration is adsorbed. In a laboratory experiment, some of the dissolved anatoxin-a and microcystins were reported by Rapala *et al.* (1993) to be adsorbed on lake sediments. Percolation through clay soils may provide some cyanotoxin removal, but this will depend greatly on the type of clay, surface charge, cation concentration of the water, etc. Cyanobacterial cells and microcystins were retained in soil columns, but less efficiently in sediment columns, in laboratory experiments simulating the fate of cyanobacterial toxins in artificial recharge of groundwater and bank filtration (Lahti *el al.*, 1996). No data are available for other cyanobacterial toxins, but some removal may be expected, again depending on the chemical conditions of soil and water.

Sedimentation of living cells without lysis, for example through grazing by zooplankton and sinking of faecal pellets, may lead to accumulation and persistence of toxin material in sediments, although this process has received little scientific attention. As discussed in more detail below, microcystins retained in intact cells may persist for several months. Cells deposited in sediments may be subject to fairly rapid breakdown by sediment bacteria and protozoa, with the resultant release of toxins.

Biodegradation

Microcystins

In spite of their chemical stability and resistance to eucaryotic and many bacterial peptidases, microcystins are susceptible to breakdown by aquatic bacteria found naturally in rivers and reservoirs. These bacteria appear to be reasonably common and widespread. Degradative bacteria have been found in sewage effluent (Lam *et al.*, 1995), lake water (Jones *et al.*, 1994; Cousins *et al.*, 1996; Lahti *et al.*, 1997a), lake sediment (Rapala *et al.*, 1994; Lahti *et al.*, 1997a) and river water (Jones *et al.*, 1994). Nonetheless, one Finnish study showed a complete lack of degradation of microcystin over a three-month period by an inoculum taken in winter from the Vantaanjoki river (Kiviranta *et al.*, 1991). There is usually an initial lag phase with little loss of microcystin and this period can be as short as two days or more than three weeks, depending on the water body, climatic conditions, the concentration of dissolved microcystin and in some cases, although not all, the previous bloom history of a lake (Jones *et al.*, 1994; Rapala *et al.*, 1994; Lahti *et al.*, 1997b). Once the biodegradation process commences, removal of microcystin can be more than 90 per cent complete within 2-10 days. This may vary depending on the water body, initial microcystin concentration and water temperature (Jones *et al.*, 1994; Lahti *et al.*, 1997b).

Jones *et al.* (1994) isolated a species of aquatic *Sphingomonas* that initiated ring-opening of microcystin-LR to produce linear (acyclo-)microcystin-LR as a transient intermediate (Bourne *et al.*, 1996). This compound was nearly 200 times less toxic than the parent toxin. The products of complete bacterial degradation were non-toxic to mice at doses up to 500 μg kg^{-1} (compared with an LD_{50} for microcystin-LR of about 60 μg kg^{-1}). The same bacterium, however, did not degrade the closely related cyclic pentapeptide nodularin. In a strain of *Pseudomonas aeruginosa* from a Japanese lake, microcystin degradation appeared to proceed by attack on the Adda side chain of microcystin (Takenaka and Watanabe, 1997). Several bacteria were isolated from lake water and sediment in Finland capable of degradation of microcystins and some strains also degraded nodularin. One strain was identified as a *Sphingomonas* sp. and two of the strains belonged to the beta-subgroup of *Proteobacteria*, although the genera remains to be determined (Lahti *et al.*, 1997a).

Other Cyanobacterial Toxins

Little work has been undertaken on the biodegradation of anatoxins, saxitoxins or cylindrospermopsin. Anatoxin-a may be readily degraded by bacteria associated with cyanobacterial filaments. Laboratory studies using non-axenic strains of cyanobacteria found low concentrations of dissolved anatoxin-a in the culture medium (Kiviranta *et al.*, 1991; Rapala *et al.*, 1993) whereas high concentrations of anatoxin-a were found in the medium of a continuous culture using an axenic strain (free of contaminating bacteria) of the same species (Rapala and Sivonen, 1998). A *Pseudomonas* sp. strain able to degrade anatoxin-a at a rate of 6-10 μg ml^{-1} per three days was isolated by Kiviranta *et al.* (1991). In the presence of lake sediment and natural bacteria, the half-life for breakdown of anatoxin-a in the laboratory was about five days (Smith and Sutton, 1993). In a recent study by Jones and Negri (1997) no bacterially-mediated degradation of saxitoxins from *Anabaena circinalis* was observed in a range of surface water samples.

Bioaccumulation

Microcystins bioaccumulate in common aquatic vertebrates and invertebrates, including fish (Carbis *et al.*, 1997; Beattie *et al.*, 1998), mussels (Eriksson *et al.*, 1989; Falconer *et al.*, 1992; Prepas *et al.*, 1997; Watanabe *et al.*, 1997) and zooplankton (Watanabe *et al.*, 1992). In mussels, the highest microcystin concentrations are found in the hepatopancreas, and in vertebrates they are found in the liver. Williams *et al.* (1997) have shown covalent binding and accumulation of microcystin-LR in salmon liver and crab larvae. Whether the levels of microcystin accumulation are sufficient to pose a risk to humans is uncertain, and will depend on levels of consumption and the severity of toxic blooms in the area where fish or shellfish are caught or collected. Common advice given by water authorities is that the viscera of the fish should not be eaten, but caution should be taken in all cases where major toxic blooms occur.

Saxitoxins from marine "red tide" dinoflagellates are well known for their propensity to bioaccumulate in marine vertebrates and invertebrates, often with disastrous consequences for animals and humans that consume them. Similarly, saxitoxins from the freshwater cyanobacterium *Anabaena circinalis* may bioaccumulate in an Australian species of freshwater mussel to concentrations exceeding international guidelines (Shumway *et al.*, 1995) during as little as seven days exposure to a cell density of 100,000 cells per ml of a toxigenic strain (Negri and Jones, 1995). This cell density is commonly encountered in natural blooms of this species.

Persistence and Stability in Cells

Culture studies indicate that microcystins and nodularin degrade only very slowly (time scale of weeks), if at all, whilst contained within living cells (Sivonen, 1990b; Lehtimäki *et al.*, 1994, 1997; Rapala *et al.*, 1997; Orr and Jones, 1998). Similarly, scums of *Microcystis aeruginosa* that dry on the shores of lakes may contain high concentrations of microcystin for several months (Jones *et al.*, 1995).

These toxins are released back into the water body when re-immersed. Thus there is the potential for significant localised concentrations of dissolved microcystin even in the absence of living cells or a recently collapsed bloom.

In a lake study carried out over two summer–autumn periods, Lahti *et al.* (1997b) found that dissolved microcystin was more persistent than particulate toxin, with 30 and 15 days respectively required for 90 per cent degradation to occur.

Impact on Aquatic Biota

Direct cyanobacterial poisoning of animals can occur by two routes: through consumption of cyanobacterial cells from the water, or indirectly through consumption of other animals that have themselves fed on cyanobacteria and accumulated cyanotoxins. Cyanotoxins are known to bioaccumulate in common aquatic vertebrates and invertebrates, including fish, mussels and zooplankton. Consequently, there is considerable potential for toxic effects to be magnified in aquatic food chains. Such toxicity biomagnification is well known for anthropogenic pollutants such as heavy metals and pesticides. There is no reason to suspect that the situation would be any different with natural cyanotoxins.

It is difficult to ascribe the deaths of natural populations of aquatic animals, especially fish, unequivocally to cyanotoxin poisoning. One of the main reasons for this is because the collapse of a large cyanobacterial bloom can lead to very low concentrations of oxygen in the water column as a consequence of bacterial metabolism; consequent fish deaths may be due to the anoxia. The best evidence for the potential for toxic effects on aquatic organisms comes from controlled laboratory trials with exposure of animals to toxic cyanobacteria or cell-free solutions of cyanotoxins.

Effects on Aquatic Bacteria

The influence of cyanobacterial toxins on bacteria is not fully understood and the scientific literature gives a number of contradictory statements. According to some authors neither an extract of *Microcystis aeruginosa* nor pure microcystin-LR have a biocidal effect on *Bacillus subtilis, Staphylococcus aureus, Escherichia coli* or *Pseudomonas hydrophila* (Foxall and Sasner, 1988). However, these limited tests should not be seen as general indicators of the potential impacts of cyanotoxins on aquatic bacteria. The majority of aquatic bacteria are yet to be cultured, and studies with common mammalian pathogens or "laboratory" bacteria should not be taken as all encompassing. It is quite possible that cyanotoxins impact on some species of aquatic bacteria and not others. Certainly, microcystins are not toxic to all bacteria because several species are known to degrade quite high concentrations of these toxins. It is even possible that the slow release of cyanotoxins from the cell surface or from senescent cells may stimulate associations of particular bacterial types which may even act as symbionts.

Attempts have been made to use bacterial toxicity tests (based on inhibition of bacterial phosphorescence) to screen for the presence of cyanotoxins, especially microcystins. However it appears that the inhibition of bacterial phosphorescence is not related to the commonly known cyanotoxins. It has been suggested that the negative effect may be related to the presence of unidentified LPS endotoxins in the cell wall of the cyanobacterial cells.

Effects on Zooplankton

Evidence of the potential effects of cyanotoxins on zooplankton from numerous studies, mostly in laboratory situations, is complex and inconsistent. The vast majority of published studies has been based on mouse bioassay data describing cyanobacterial toxicity, with only a few more recent studies having used analytical methods such as HPLC to quantify individual toxins. Overall, it appears that cyanobacteria may exhibit a deleterious effect on zooplankton, but the effect is highly variable between genera and species, and even between clones of individual zooplankton species. One of the main questions yet to be resolved is whether the observed inhibitory effects are due to the putative poor nutritional value of cyanobacteria, to the known cyanotoxins, or to other unidentified compounds. There is evidence in the literature to support all three effects as being significant, at least with particular species under experimental growth conditions. A major difference in study design is whether organisms are exposed to cyanotoxins dissolved in water, or fed with toxic cyanobacteria. The latter is likely to lead to a substantially higher dose. Furthermore, Jungmann and Benndorf (1994) reported that exposure of *Daphnia* to dissolved microcystins showed effects only at concentrations several orders of magnitude above those found in field samples. They did, however, observe toxicity to *Daphnia* by unidentified metabolites other than microcystins from *Microcystis.*

There is dramatic variation among zooplankton species in their response to toxic (and even non-toxic) cyanobacteria. For example, DeMott *et al.* (1991) showed that the four species of zooplankton differed in their sensitivity to hepatotoxins by almost two orders of magnitude, but toxicity was observed only at very high concentrations that are scarcely encountered in natural water bodies (48 h LC_{50} ranging from 450 to 21,400 µg of microcystin per litre). Snell (1980) found that there was a genotype-dependent response of the rotifer *Asplanchna girodi* to toxic *Anabaena flos-aquae* and *Lyngbya* sp. Hietala *et al.* (1997) observed a variation in susceptibility of more than three orders of magnitude in the acute toxicity of *Microcystis aeruginosa* to 10 clones of *Daphnia pulex.* Both DeMott *et al.* (1991) and Laurén-Määttä *et al.* (1997) suggested that clone and species differences between zooplankton susceptibilities to toxic cyanobacteria may lead to selection pressures in favour of resistant strains or species in water bodies where toxic cyanobacteria occur frequently.

Benndorf and Henning (1989) found that the toxicity of a field population of *Microcystis* was increased by the feeding activity of *Daphnia galeata* over a period of a few months. A possible explanation for this phenomenon is offered by DeMott *et al.* (1991) who demonstrated that a number of zooplankton species will avoid grazing on toxic cyanobacteria, but continue to graze on non-toxic species. Similar results have also been shown for grazing by the phytoplanktivorous fish *Tilapia* and silver carp. Thus, grazing pressure from zooplankton and some fish may lead to the selective enrichment of toxic cyanobacterial strains over time.

It is likely that under natural conditions in water bodies, certain species and strains of zooplankton may be affected by cyanotoxins, whereas others will be unaffected. As such, cyanotoxins may influence the zooplankton community structure, especially during times when cyanobacteria are dominant within the phytoplankton.

Effects on Fish

If fish are dosed with cyanotoxins by i.p. injections or by force-feeding, they develop similar symptoms of intoxication as laboratory mammals. The question relevant for field exposure is whether cyanotoxins enter healthy fish. For example, Tencalla *et al.* (1994) showed that gastrointestinal uptake by gavage (force-feeding) caused massive hepatic necrosis followed by fish deaths, whereas immersion of adults and juveniles in contaminated water did not cause toxic effects. Other reported evidence suggests that immersion in toxic cyanobacteria or cyanotoxins may be harmful to fish. Differences in sensitivity may be pronounced between species: goldfish were found to be nearly 30 times less susceptible to i.p. microcystin than mice (Sugaya *et al.*, 1990). Release of toxic compounds from mass developments of cyanobacteria was considered to be the cause of fish kills by Penaloza *et al.* (1990).

Histopathological investigations of fish deaths during cyanobacterial blooms in the UK, indicated that the cause of death was mostly due to damage of the gills, digestive tract and liver (Rodger *et al.*, 1994). The gill damage was probably caused by the high pH induced by cyanobacterial photosynthesis activity prior to the bloom collapse, together with the higher level of ammonia arising from the decomposition of the cyanobacteria. However, gill damage may have enhanced microcystin uptake and thus led to liver necrosis. Damage to gills by dissolved microcystin-LR has been shown experimentally in *Tilapia* and trout (Garcia, 1989; Gaete *et al.*, 1994; Bury *et al.*, 1996).

Other pathological symptoms ascribed to toxic cyanobacterial blooms include damage to the liver, heart, kidney, gills, skin and spleen (Garcia, 1989; Råbergh *et al.*, 1991). Garcia (1989) and Rodger *et al.* (1994) carried out experiments on trout, while Råbergh *et al.* (1991) experimented on carp. The latter study highlighted degenerative changes in kidney tubules and glomeruli. The effect of microcystins on European carp, *Cyprinus carpio,* under natural field conditions in Australia has been described by Carbis *et al.* (1997) as atrophy of hepatocytes, gills with pinpoint necrosis, epithelial ballooning, folded lamellar tips, exfoliation of the lamellar epithelium, elevated asparate aminotransferase activity and serum bilirubin concentrations. Laboratory studies indicate that dissolved microcystins may affect fish embryos (Oberemm *et al.*, 1997) and behaviour of fish (Baganz *et al.*, 1998). Recently Gupta and Gupta (2006) reported Microcystin toxicity in freshwater fish *Heteropneustes fossilis* (Bloch).

The most definitive effect of microcystin on fish concerns Atlantic Salmon reared in net pens in coastal waters of British Columbia and Washington State, USA. As yet unidentified microcystin-producing organisms produce a progressive degeneration of the liver in salmon smolts placed into open-water net pens (Anderson *et al.*, 1993). The disease, referred to as Net Pen Liver Disease (NPLD), has resulted in significant economic losses for the mariculture industry.

Effect on Fungi

The toxic cyanobacterium *Microcystis aeruginosa* was studied earlier for its antibacterial and antialgal properties. From the present study we deduce that though *Mycrocystis* extract is not only detrimental to fungal weeds but also kill *Pleurotus* mushrooms (Singh *et al.*, 2002), yet it should not be used either for irrigating of mushroom beds or controlling agents against fungal weeds occurred during the *Pleurotus* mushroom cultivation. Because, its toxin might spoil medicinal properties of the mushrooms, thus instead of getting good health people may suffer health hazards. Vyas (2007) reported deterimental effect of *Microcystis aeuroginosa* cell extract on *Phytopthora parasitica* and some species of AM fungi.

Table 6.9: Percent Growth Inhibition *in vitro* of Test Three *Pleurotus* spp. and Two Fungal Weeds by the Extract of Cyanobacterium *Microcystis eruginosa*

Extract Conc. (ppm)	*Percent Inhibition*				
	P.sajor-caju	*P.florida*	*P.ostreatus*	*A.niger*	*Penicillium sp.*
5	20	20.1	20.4	23.1	29.4
10	25.5	25.3	25.4	29.2	38.2
25	45.1	45.5	45.2	48.2	54.1
50	78.3	78.2	78.1	82.1	92.4
75	100	100	100	100	100

Table 6.10: Sporophore Initiation and Biological Efficiency of Three Test *Pleurotus* spp. Treated with Extract of Cyanobacterium *Microcystis aeruginosa* Under *in vivo* Condition

Extract Conc. (ppm)	*P.sajor-caju*		*P.florida*		*P.ostreatus*	
	Sporophore Initiation	*BE (%)*	*Sporophore Initiation*	*BE (%)*	*Sporophore Initiation*	*BE (%)*
Control	19	82.1	21	74.2	18	71.4
5	30	50.2	33	48.1	34	46.2
10	32	40.1	36	38.1	36	35.3
25	40	25.3	42	22.2	42	20.1
50	ND	ND	ND	ND	ND	ND
75	ND	ND	ND	ND	ND	ND

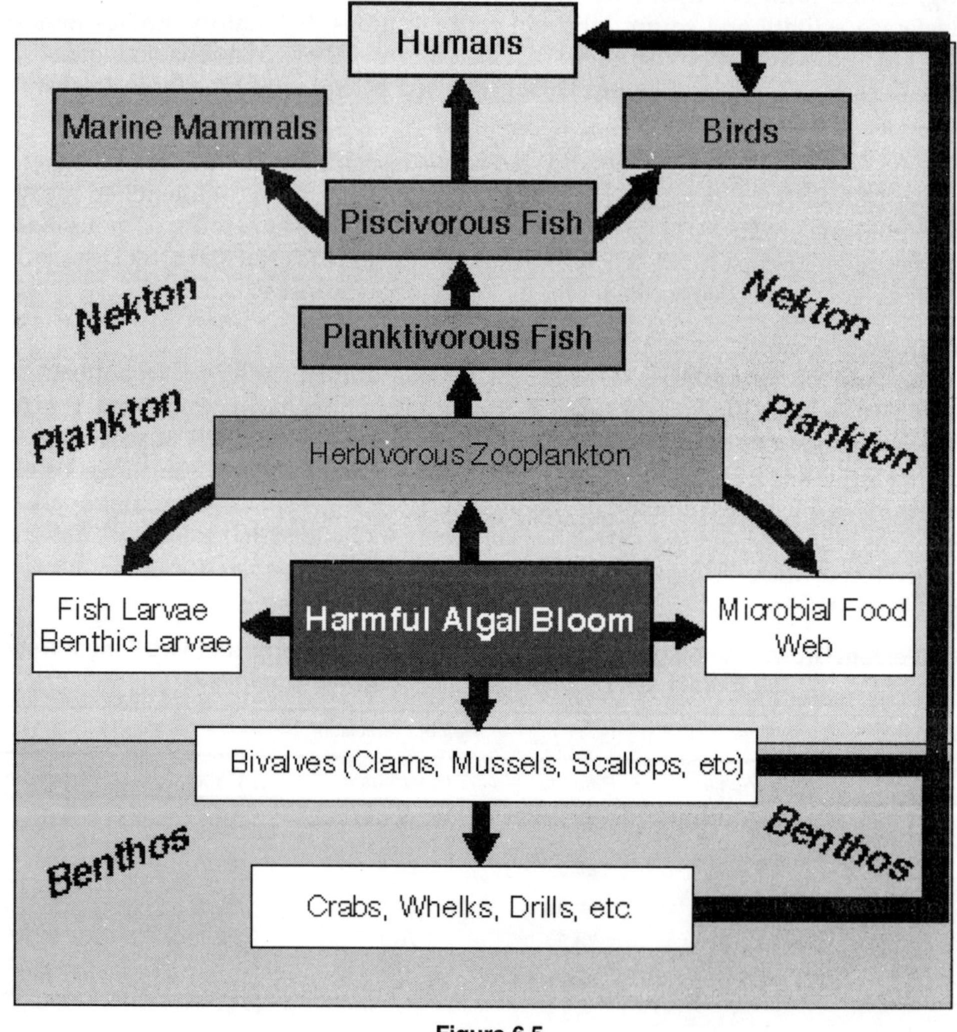

Figure 6.5

Table 6.11: Clinical Symptoms Produced by Cyanobacterial Toxins and their Median Lethal Doses (LD_{50}) (after Carmichael, 1994; Harada *et al.*, 1994)

Toxin Producing Cyanobacteria	*Types of Toxins*	*Symptoms*	*LD_{50}* (µg/Kg body wt.)*	*Test Organisms(s)*
		Neurotoxins		
Anabaena flosaquae	Anatoxin-a	Muscular fasciculation, decreased movement, collapse, cyanosis, convulsions, death	200	Mice, rat
Anabaena flosaquae	Anatoxin-a(s)	Hypersalvation, mucoid nasal, tremors, diarrhoea, cyanosis, death	20	Mice, pig, rat, duck
Aphanizomenon flosaquae, Anabaena circinalis	Saxitoxin and Neosaxitoxin	Irregular breathing, spasm, gasping, loss of coordination, tremors, death	10	Mice, rat
		Hepatotoxins		
Microcystis aenigiliosa M. viridis, M. wesenbergii, Nostoc sp., *Oscillatoria* sp., *Anabaena* sp.	Microcystins	Slow movement, increase in liver weight, hypovolemic shock, intrahepatic haemmorrage, death	50-100	Mice, rat
Nodularia spumigena	Nodu!arin	Slow movement, increase in liver weight, hypovolemic shock, intrahepatic haemmorrage, death	ND	Mice
Cylindrospermopsis raciborskii, Umezakia natans	Cylindros-permopsin	Liver swelling, hepatic necrosis, congestion in kidney and heart death	ND	Mice

Table 6.12: Species of Cyanophyceans with Recognized Toxin-producing Strains. The list presents species of cyanophyceans that have been confirmed lo have toxin-producing strains. The publication referred to represent selected key papers. The early publications cited cover primarily investigations of field cases of intoxications

Species	*References*
Unicellular	
Coeloshaerium kutzingianum Nag.	Fitch *et al.* (1934)
Gomphosphaeria lacustris Chod.	Gorham and Carmichael (1988)
Gumphosphaeria nageliana (Unger) Lemm.	Berg *et al.* (1986)
Microcystis areuginosa Kutz.	Hughes *et al.* (1958)
Microcystis cf. *botrys* Teil.	Berg *et al.* (1986)
Microcystis viridis (A. Br.) Lemm.	Watanabe *et al.* (1986)
Microcystis wesenbergii Kom.	Gorham and Carmichael (1988)
Synechococcus nageli sp. (strain Miami BCII 6S)	Mitsui *et al.* (1987)
Synechococcus nageli sp. (strain ATCC 18800)	Amann (1977)
Synechococcus sauvageau sp.	Lincoln and Carmichael (1981)

Contd...

Table 6.12–Contd...

Species	References
Multicellular	
Anabaena circinalis Rabcnh.	May and McBarron (1973)
Anabaena flos-aquae (Lyngb.) Breb.	Porter (1887)
Anabaena hassallii (Kutz.) Witttr.	Andrijuk *et al.* (1975)
Anabaena lemmermannii P. Richt.	Fitch *et al.* (1934)
Anabaena spiroides var. contracta Kleb.	Beasley *et al.* (1983)
Anabaena variabilis Kutz.	Andrijuk *et al.* (1975)
Anabaenopsis milleri Woron.	Lanaras *et al.* (1989)
Aphanizomenon flos-aquae (L.) Ralfs	Jackim and Gentile (1968)
Cylindrospermum Kutzing sp.	Sivonen *et al.* (1989)
Cylindrospermopsis raciborskii (Wolos.) Seenaya and Subba Raju	Hawkins *et al.* (1985)
Fischerella epiphytica Ghose	Ransom *et al.* (1978)
Gloeotrichia echinulata (J.E. Smith) P. Richter	Ingram and Prescott (1954)
Hapalosiphon fontinalis (Ag.) Born.	Moore *et al.* (1984)
Hormothamnion entromorphoides Grun.	Gerwick *et al.* (1986)
Lyngbya majuscula Harvey	Grauer and Arnold (1961)
Nodularia spumigena Mertens	Francis (1878)
Nostoc linckia (Roth) Born. et Flah.	Ransom *et al.* (1978)
Nostoc paludosum Kutz.	Andrijuk *et al.* (1975)
Nostoc rivulare Kutz.	Davidson (1959)
Nostoc zetterstedtii Areschoug	Mills and Wyatt (1974)
Oscillatoria acutissima Kuff.	Barchi *et al.* (1984)
Oscillatoria agardhii Gom.	Ostensvik *et al.* (1981)
Oscillatoria agardhii/rubescens group	Skulberg and Skulberg (1985)
Oscillatoria nigro-viridis Thwaites	Mynderse *et al.* (1977)
Oscillatoria vaucher sp.	Sivonen *et al.* (1989)
Oscillatoria formosa Bory (*Phormidium formosum* (Bory) Anagn. and Kom.)	Skulberg *et al.* (1992)
Pseudanabaena catenata Lauterb.	Gorham *et al.* (1982)
Schizothrix calcicola (Ag.) Gom.	Mynderse *et al.* (1977)
Scytonema pseudohofmnni Bharadw.	Moore *et al.* (1986)
Tolypothrix byssoidea (Hass.) Kirchn.	Barchi *et al.* (1983)
Trichodesmium erythraeum Ehrb.	Feldmann (1932)

Acknowledgements

D.V. gratefully acknowledge U.G.C. for awarding research award and financially support.

References

Anderson, D.M. (1994). Red tides. *Scientific American*, August, 52-58.

Anderson, R.J., Luu, H.A., Chen, D.Z.X., Holmes, C.F.B., Kent, M., LeBlanc, M., Taylor, F.J.R. and Williams, D.E. (1993). Chemical and biological evidence links microcystins to salmon "Netpen liver Disease". *Toxicon*, 31, 1315-1323.

Annila, A., Lehtimäki, J., Manila, K., Eriksson, J.E., Sivonen, K., Rantala, T.T. and Drakenberg, T. (1996). Solution structure of nodularin an inhibitor of serine/threonine specific protein phosphatases. *J. Bio. Chem.*, 271(28), 16695-16702.

Arment, A.R. and Carmichael, W.W. (1996). Evidence that microcystin is a thio-template product. *J. Phycol.*, 32, 591-597.

Azavedo, S.M.F.O., Evans, W.R., Carmichael, W.W. and Namikoshi, M. (1994). First report of microcystins from a Brazilian isolate of the cyanobacterium *Microcystis aeruginosa*. *J. App. Phycol.*, 6, 261-265.

Baganz, D., Staaks, G., Steinberg, C. (1998). Impact of the cyanobacteria toxin, microcystin-LR, on the behavior of zebrafish, *Danio rerio*. *Wat. Res.*, 32, 948-952.

Baker, P.D. and Humpage, A.R. (1994). Toxicity associated with commonly occurring cyanobacteria in surface waters of the Murray-Darling basin, Australia. *Aust. J. Mar. Freshwat. Res.*, 45, 773-786.

Banker, P.D., Carmeli, S., Hadas, O., Teltsch, B., Porat, R. and Sukenik, A. (1997). Identification of cylindrospermopsin in *Aphanizomenon ovalisporum* (*Cyanophyceae*) isolated from Lake Kinneret, Israel. *J. Phycol.*, 33, 613-616.

Barford, D. and Keller, J. (1994). Co-crystallization of the catalytic subunit of the serine/threonine specific protein phosphatase 1 from human in complex with microcystin-LR. *J Molecular Biol.*, 235, 763-766.

Bateman, K. P., Thibault, P., Douglas, D. J. and White, R. L. (1995). Mass spectral analyses of microcystins from toxic cyanobacteria using on-line chromatographic and electrophoretic separations. *J. Chromatog. A*, 712, 253-268.

Beattie, K.A, Kaya, K., Sano, T. and Codd, G.A. (1998). Three dehydrobutyrine (Dhb)-containing microcystins from the cyanobacterium *Nostoc* sp. *Phytochemistry*, 47(7), 1289-1292.

Benndorf, J. and Henning, M. (1989). *Daphnia* and toxic blooms of *Microcystis aeruginosa* in Bautzen Reservoir. *Int. Rev. ges. Hydrobiol.*, 74, 233-248.

Berg, K. Skulberg, O.M. and Skulberg, R. (1987). Effects of decaying toxic blue-green algae on water quality–a laboratory study. *Arch. Hydrobiol.*, 108, 549-563.

Berg, K., Skulberg, O.M., Skulberg, R., Underdal, B. and Willén, T. (1986). Observations of toxic blue-green algae (Cyanobacteria) in some Scandinavian lakes. *Acta. Vet. Scand.*, 27, 440-452.

Blackburn, S.I., Bolch, C.J., Jones, G.J., Negri, A.P. and Orr, P.T. (1997). Cyanobacterial blooms: why are they toxic? In: J.R.D. Davis (Ed.) *Managing Algal Blooms: Outcomes from the CSIRO Blue-Green Algal Research Program*. J.R.D. Davis (Ed.) CSIRO Land and Water, Canberra, 67-77.

Blackburn, S., McCausland, M.A., Bolch, C.J.S., Newman, S.J. and Jones, G.J. (1996). Effect of salinity on growth and toxin production in cultures of the bloom-forming cyanobacterium *Nodularia spumigena* from Australian waters. *Phycologia*, 35, 511-522.

Boland, M.P., Smillie, M.A., Chen, D.Z.X. and Holmes, C.F.B. (1993). A unified bioscreen for the detection of diarrhetic shellfish toxins and microcystins in marine and freshwater environments. *Toxicon*, 31, 1393-1405.

Bolch, C.J.S., Blackburn, S.I., Jones, G.J., Orr, P.T. and Grewe, P.M. (1997). Plasmid content and distribution in the toxic cyanobacterial genus *Microcystis* Kutzing ex Lemmermann (Cyanobacteria: Chroococcales). *Phycologia*, 36, 6-11.

Botes, D.P., Tuinman, A.A., Wessels, P.L., Viljoen, C.C. and Kruger, H. (1984). The structure of cyanoginosin-LA, a cyclic heptapeptide toxin from the cyanobacterium *Microcystis aeruginosa. J. Chem. Soc., Perkin Transactions*, I, 2311-2318.

Botes, D.P., Wessels, P.L., Kruger, H., Runnegar, M.T.C., Santikarn, S., Smith, R.J., Barna, J.C.J. and Williams, D.H. (1985). Structural studies on cyanoginosins-LR, -YR, -YA, and -YM, peptide toxins from *Microcystis aeruginosa. J. Chem. Soc., Perkin Transactions*, I, 2747-2748.

Bourne, D., Jones, G.J. Blakeley, R.L., Jones, A., Negri, A.P. and Riddles, P. (1996). Enzymatic pathway for the bacterial degradation of the cyanobacterial cyclic peptide toxin microcystin -LR. *Appl. Env. Microbiol.*, 62, 4086-4094.

Bruno, M., Barbini, D.A., Pierdominici, E., Serse, A.P. and Ioppolo, A. (1994). Anatoxin-a and previously unknown toxin in *Anabaena planctonica* from blooms found in Lake Mulargia (Italy). *Toxicon*, 32, 369-373.

Bumke-Vogt, C. (1998). Anatoxin-a and neurotoxic cyanobacteria in German lakes and reservoirs. *Env. Toxicol. Water Qual.* (In Press).

Bumke-Vogt, C., Mailahn, W., Retard, W. and Chorus, I. (1996). A highly sensitive analytical method for the neurotoxin anatoxin-a, using GC-ECD, and first application to laboratory cultures. *Phycologia*, 35(6, Supplement), 51-56.

Bury, N.R., Flik, G., Eddy, F.B. and Codd, G.A. (1996). The effects of cyanobacteria and the cyanobacterial toxin microcystin-LR on Ca^{2+} transport and Na^+/K^+–ATPase in Tilapia gills. *J. Exp. Biol.*, 199, 1319-1326.

Canter, H., Heaney, S.I. and Lund, J.W.G. (1990). The ecological significance of grazing on planktonic populations of cyanobacteria by the ciliate *Nassula. New Phytol.*, 114, 247-263.

Carbis, C.R., Rawlin, G.T., Grant, P., Mitchell, G.F., Anderson, J.W. and McCauley, I. (1997). A study of feral carp *Cyprinus carpio* L., exposed to *Microcystis aeruginosa* at Lake Mokoan, Australia, and possible implication on fish health. *J. Fish Diseases*, 20, 81-91.

Carbis, C.R. Simons, J.A., Mitchell, G.F., Anderson, J.W. and McCauley, I. (1994). A biochemical profile for predicting the chronic exposure of sheep to *Microcystis aeruginosa*, an hepatotoxic species of blue-green alga. *Res. Vet. Sci*,. 57(3), 310-316.

Cardellina II, J.H., Marner, F.J and Moore, R.E. (1979). Seaweed dermatitis, structure of lyngbyatoxin A. *Science*, 204, 193-195.

Carmichael, W.W. (1986). Algal toxins. In: J.A. Callow (Ed.) *Advances in Botanical Research, No. 12.* Academic Press, London, 47-101.

Carmichael, W.W. (1992). *A Status Report on Planktonic Cyanobacteria (Blue Green Algae) and their Toxins.* EPA/600/R-92/079, Environmental Monitoring Systems Laboratory, Office of Research and Development, US Environmental Protection Agency, Cincinnati, Ohio.

Carmichael, W.W. (1997). The Cyanotoxins. *Adv. Bot. Res.*, 27, 211-256.

Carmichael, W.W., Beasley, V.R., Bunner, D.L., Eloff, J.N., Falconer, I., Gorham, P., Harada, K.I., Krishnamurthy, T., Yu, M.J., Moore, R.E., Rinehart, K., Runnegar, M., Skulberg, O.M. and Watanabe, M. (1988a). Naming of cyclic heptapeptide toxins of cyanobacteria (blue-green algae). *Toxicon*, 26, 971-973.

Carmichael, W.W., Biggs, D.F. and Gorham, P.R. (1975). Toxicology and pharmacological action of *Anabaena flos-aquae* toxin. *Science*, 187, 542-544.

Carmichael, W.W., Eschedor, J.T, Patterson, G.M.L. and Moore R.E. (1988b). Toxicity and partial structure of a hepatotoxic peptide produced by the cyanobacterium *Nodularia spumigena* Mertens. *Appl. Env. Microbiol.*, 54, 2257-2263.

Carmichael, W.W., Evans, W.R., Yin, Q.Q., Bell, P. and Mocauklowski, E. (1997). Evidence for paralytic shellfish poisons in the freshwater cyanobacterium *Lyngbya wollei* (Farlow ex Gomont) comb. nov. *Appl. Environ. Microbiol.*, 63, 3104-3110.

Carmichael, W.W. and Gorham, P.R. (1981). The mosaic nature of toxic blooms of cyanobacteria. In: W.W. Carmichael (Ed.) *The Water Environment: Algal Toxins and Health*, Plenum Press, New York, 161-172.

Carmichael, W.W., Mahmood, N.A. and Hyde, E.G. (1990). Natural toxins from cyanobacteria (blue-green algae). In: S. Hall and G. Strichartz (Eds) *Marine Toxins, Origin, Structure and Molecular Pharmacology*, Vol. 418, American Chemical Society, Washington D.C., 87-106.

Carmichael, W.W., Yu, M. J., He, Z.R, He, J.W. and Yu, J-L. (1988c). Occurrence of the toxic cyanobacterium (blue-green alga) *Microcystis aeruginosa* in Central China. *Arch. Hydrobiol.*, 114, 21-30.

Chiswell, R.K., Shaw, G.R., Eaglesham, G.K., Smith, M.J., Norris, R.L., Seawright, A.A. and Moore, M.R. (1999). Stability of cylindrospermopsin, the toxin from the cyanobacterium *Cylindrospermopsis raciborskii*. Effects of pH, temperature and sunlight on decomposition. *Environ. Toxicol. Water Qual.* (In Press).

Choi, B.W., Namikoshi, M., Sun, F., Rinehart, K.L., Carmichael, W.W., Kaup, A.M., Evans, W.R. and Beasley, V.R. (1993). Isolation of linear peptides related to the hepatotoxins nodularin and microcystins. *Tetrahedron Letters*, 34, 7881-7884.

Chorus, I. (1998). Die Blaualgen ("Cyanobakterien")–eine Berliner Besonderheit welcher Zusammenhang besteht zwischen dem Massenhaften Auftreten von Blaualgen und der Nutzung von Badegewässern? In: *Nachhaltigkeit im Wasserwesen in der Mitte Europas.* Symposium 17-19 June, 1998, Berlin (In Press).

Christoffersen, K. (1996). Ecological implications of cyanobacterial toxins in aquatic food webs. *Phycologia*, 35(6 Supplement), 42-50.

Codd, G.A. and Bell, S.G. (1996). *The Occurrence and Fate of Blue-green Algae in Fresh-waters.* National Rivers Authority Research and Development Report 29, Her Majesty's Stationery Office, London, 30 pp.

Codd, G.A. and Poon, G.K. (1988). Cyanobacterial toxins. In: J. G. Gallon, and L. J. Rogers (Eds) *Proc. Phytochem. Soc. Europe*, 28, Oxford University Press, Oxford, 283-296.

Codd, G.A., Edwards, C., Beattie, K.A., Lawton, L.A., Campell, D.L. and Bell, S.G. (1995). Toxins from blue-green algae. The Pringsheim Lecture. In: W. Wiessner, E. Schnepf and R. C. Starr (Eds) *Algae, Environment and Human Affairs.* Biopress, Bristol, 1-17.

Costa, M.S. and Azevedo, S.M.F.O. (1994). Implantacao de um banco de culturas de cianoficeas toxicas. *Iheringia*, 45, 69-74 (in Portuguese).

Cousins, I.T., Healing, D.J., James, H.A., Sutton, A. (1996). Biodegradation of microcystin-LR by indigenous mixed bacterial populations. *Wat. Res.*, 30, 481-485.

Craig, M., McCready, L., Luu, H.A., Smillie, M.A., Dubord, P. and Holmes, C.F.B. (1993). Identification and characterization of hydrophobic microcystins in Canadian freshwater cyanobacteria. *Toxicon*, 31, 1541-1549.

Cremer, J. and Henning, K. (1991). Application of reversed-phase medium-pressure liquid chromatography to the isolation, separation and amino acid analysis of two closely related peptide toxins of the cyanobacterium *Microcystis aeruginosa* strain PCC 7806. *J. Chromatog.*, 587, 71-80.

Davidson, F.F. (1959). Poisoning of wild and domestic animals by a toxic waterbloom of *Nostoc rivulare* Kuetz. *J. Am. Water Works Ass.*, 51, 1277-1287.

DeMott, W.R. Zhang, Q. Carmichael, W.W. (1991). Effects of toxic cyanobacteria and purified toxins on the survival and feeding of a copepod and three species of *Daphnia. Limnol. Oceanog.*, 36(7), 1346-1357.

de Silva, E.D., Williams, D.E., Andersen, R.J., Klix, H., Holmes, C.F.B. and Alien, T.M. (1992). Motuporin, a potent protein phosphatase inhibitor isolated from the Papua New Guinea sponge *Theonella swinhoei* Gray. *Tetrahedron Letters*, 33, 1561-1564.

Devlin, J.P., Edwards, O.E., Gorham, P.R., Hunter, M.R., Pike, R.K. and Stavric, B. (1977). Anatoxin-a, a toxic alkaloid from *Anabaena flos-aquae* NCR-44h. *Cana. J. of Chem.*, 55, 1367-1371.

Dittman, E., Neilan, B.A., Erhard, M., v. Döhren, H. and Börner, T. (1997). Insertional mutagenesis of a peptide synthetase gene which is responsible for hepatotoxin production in the cyanobacterium *Microcystis aeruginosa* PCC 7806. *Mol. Microbiol.*, 26, 779-787.

Edwards, C., Beattie, K.A., Scrimgeour, C.M. and Codd, G.A. (1992). Identification of anatoxin-a in benthic cyanobacteria (blue-green algae) and in associated dog poisonings at Loch Insh, Scotland. *Toxicon*, 30, 1165-1175.

Ekman-Ekebom, M., Kauppi, M., Sivonen, K., Niemi, M. and Lepistö, L. (1992). Toxic cyanobacteria in some Finnish lakes. *Environ. Toxicol. Water Qual.*, 7, 201-213.

Elleman, T.C., Falconer, I.R., Jackson, A.R.B., and Runnegar, M.T. 1978). Isolation, characterization and pathology of the toxin from a *Microcystis aeruginosa* (=*Anacystis cyanea*) bloom. *Aust. J. Biol. Sci.*, 31, 209-218.

Endean, R., Monks, S.A., Griffith, J.K. and Llewellyn, L.E. (1993). Apparent relationship between toxins elaborated by the cyanobacterium *Trichodesmium erythraeum* and those present in the flesh of the narrow-barred Spanish mackerel *Scomberomorus commersoni. Toxicon*, 31, 1155-1165.

Entzeroth, M., Blackman, A.J., Mynderse, J.S. and Moore, R.E. (1985). Structures and stereochemistries of oscillatoxin B, 31-noroscillatoxin B, oscillatoxin D, and 30-methyloscillatoxin D. *J. Organic Chem.*, 50, 1255-1259.

Eriksson, J.E., Meriluoto, J.A., Lindholm, T. (1989). Accumulation of peptide toxin from the cyanobacterium *Oscillatoria agardhii* in the freshwater mussel *Anadonta cygnea. Hydrobiologia*, 183, 211-216.

Falconer, I.R., Choice, A. and Hosja, W. (1992). Toxicity of the edible mussel (*Mytilus edulis*) growing naturally in an estuary during a water-bloom of the blue-green alga *Nodularia spumigena J. Environ. Toxicol. Water Qual.*, 7,119-123.

Fastner, J. (1994). First evidence on the occurrence of microcystin-LR in Berlin and Brandenburg lakes. In: G. A. Codd, T. M. Jefferies, C. W. Keevil and E. Potter (Eds) *Detection Methods for Cyanobacterial Toxins*. The Royal Society of Chemistry, Cambridge, 149-151.

Fastner, J. (1998). Microcystins in German fresh-water bodies. *Environ. Toxicol. Water Qual.* (In Press).

Fastner, J., Neumann, U. and Erhard, M. (1998). Patterns of different microcystins in field samples dominated by different species of cyanobacteria. In: I. Chorus, (Ed.) *Cyanotoxins–Occurrence, Effects, Controlling Factors*. Springer Verlag, (In Press).

Foxall, T.L. and Sasner J.J. (1988). Effect of a hepatic toxin from the cyanophyte *Microcystis aeruginosa*. In: W.W. Carmichael (Ed.) *The Water Environment. Algal Toxins and Health*. Plenum Press, New York.

Francis, G. (1878). Poisonous Australian lake. *Nature*, 18, 11-12.

Fujiki, H., Suganuma, M., Suguri, H., Yoshizawa, S., Takagi, K., Nakayasu, M., Ojika, M., Yamada, K., Yasumoto, T., Moore, R.E. and Sugimura, T. (1990). New tumor promoters from marine natural products. In: S. Hall and G. Strichartz (Eds) *Marine Toxins, Origin, Structure and Molecular Pharmacology*, Vol. 418, American Chemical Society, Washington D.C., 232-240.

Fulton, R.S. (1988). Resistence to blue-green algal toxin by *Bosmina longirostris. J. Plankton Res.*, 10(4), 771-778.

Gaete, V., Canelo, E., Lagos, N., and Zambrano, F. (1994). Inhibitory effects of *Microcystis aeruginosa* toxin on ion pumps of the gill of freshwater fish. *Toxicon.*, 82, 121-127.

Gallon, J.R., Chit, K.N. and Brown, E.G. (1990). Biosynthesis of the tropane-related cyanobacterial toxin anatoxin-a: role of ornithine decarboxylase. *Phytochemistry*, 29, 1107-1 111.

Gallon J.R., Kittakoop, O. and Brown, E.G. (1994). Biosynthesis of anatoxin-a by *Anabaena flos-aquae:* examination of primary enzymic steps. *Phytochemistry*, 35, 1195-1203.

Garcia, G.O. (1989). Toxicity of the cyanobacterium *Microcystis aeruginosa* strain 7820 to trout and tilapia: a clinical and histopathological study. MSc Thesis, University of Stirling, UK.

Gathercole, P.S. and Thiel, P.G. (1987). Liquid chromatographic determination of the cyanoginosins, toxins produced by the cyanobacterium *Microcystis aeruginosa. J. Chromatog.*, 408, 435-440.

Gentile, J.H. and Maloney, T.E. (1969). Toxicity and environmental requirements of a strain of *Aphanizomenon flos-aquae* (L.) Ralfs. *Can. J. Microbiol.*, 15,165-173.

Goldberg, J., Huang, H.B., Kwon, Y.G., Greengard, P., Nairn, A.C. and Kuriyan, J. (1995). Three-dimensional structure of the catalytic subunit of protein serine/threonine phosphatase-1. *Nature*, 376, 745-753.

Gorham, P.R. (1962). Laboratory studies on the toxins produced by waterblooms of blue-green algae. *Am. J. Public Health*, 52, 2100-2105.

Gupta, U.S. and Guha, S. (2006). Microcystin toxicitiy in a freshwater fish, *Heteropneustes fossilis* (Bloch). *Current Science*, 19: 1261–1271.

Hahn, S.T. and Capra, M.F. (1992). The cyanobacterium *Oscillatoria erythraea* a potential source of toxin in the ciguatera food-chain. *Food Additives and Contaminants*, 9, 351-355.

Hammer, U.T. (1968). Toxic blue-green algae in Saskatchewan. *Can. Vet. J.*, 9, 221-229.

Harada, K-I., Matsuura, K., Suzuki, M., Watanabe, M.F., Oishi, S., Dahlem, A.M., Beasley, V.R. and Carmichael, W.W. (1990b). Isolation and characterization of the minor components associated with microcystins-LR and -RR in the cyanobacterium (blue-green algae). *Toxicon*, 28, 55-64.

Harada, K.I., Nagai, H., Kimura, Y., Suzuki, M., Park, H.D., Watanabe, M.F., Luukkainen, R., Sivonen, K. and Carmichael, W.W. (1993). Liquid chromatography/mass spectrometric detection of anatoxin-a, a neurotoxin from cyanobacteria. *Tetrahedron*, 49, 9251-9260.

Harada, K.I., Ogawa, K., Kimura, Y., Murata, H., Suzuki, M., Thorn, P.M., Evans, W.R. and Carmichael, W.W. (199 la). Microcystins from *Anabaena flos-aquae* NRC 525-17. *Chem. Res. Toxicol.*, 4, 535-540.

Harada, K.I., Ogawa, K., Matsuura, K., Murata, H., Suzuki, M., Watanabe, M.F., Itezono, Y. and Nakayama, N. (1990a). Structural determination of geometrical isomers of microcystins-LR and -RR from cyanobacteria by two-dimensional NMR spectroscopic techniques. *Chemical Research in Toxicology*. 3, 473-481.

Harada, K.-I., Ogawa, K., Matsuura, K., Nagai, H., Murata, H., Suzuki, M., Itezono, Y., Nakayma, N., Shirai, M. and Nakano, M. (1991b). Isolation of two toxic heptapeptide microcystins from an axenic strain of *Microcystis aeruginosa*, K-139. *Toxicon*, 29, 479-489.

Harada, K.I., Ohtani, I., Iwamoto, K., Suzuki, M., Watanabe, M.F., Watanabe, M. and Terao, K. (1994). Isolation of cylindrospermopsin from a cyanobacterium *Umezakia natans* and its screening method. *Toxicon*, 32, 73-84.

Harada, K-I., Tsuji, K, Watanabe, M.F. (1996). Stability of microcystins from cyanobacteria–III. Effect of pH and temperature. *Phycologia*, 35(6 Supplement), 83-88.

Hashimoto, Y., Kamiya, H., Yamazato, K. and Nozawa, K. (1976). Occurrence of a toxic blue-green alga inducing skin dermatitis in Okinawa. In: A. Ohsaka, K. Hayashi and Y. Sawai (Eds) *Animal, Plant, and Microbial Toxins*. Vol. 1, Plenum Publishing, New York, 333-338.

Hawkins, P. and Lampert, W. (1989). The effect of *Daphnia* body size on filtering rate inhibition in the presence of a filamentous cyanobacterium. *Limnol. Oceanog.*, 34(6), 1084-1089.

Hawkins, P.R., Chandrasena, N.R., Jones, G.J., Humpage, A.R. and Falconer, I.R. (1997). Isolation and toxicity of *Cylindrospermopsis raciborskii* from an ornamental lake. *Toxicon*, 35(3), 341-346.

Hawkins, P.R., Runnegar, M.T.C., Jackson, A.R.B. and Falconer, I.R. (1985). Severe hepatotoxicity caused by the tropical cyanobacterium (blue-green alga) *Cylindrospermopsis raciborskii* (Woloszynska) Seenaya and Subba Raju isolated from a domestic water supply reservoir. *Appl. Environ. Microbiol.*, 50, 1292-1295.

Hawser, S.P., Codd, G.A., Carpenter, E.J. and Capone, D.G. (1991). A neurotoxic factor associated with the bloom-forming cyanobacterium *Trichodesmium*. *Toxicon*, 29, 277-278.

Hemscheidt, T., Burgoyne, D.L. and Moore, R.E. (1995a). Biosynthesis of anatoxin-. (2*S*,4*S*)-4-hydroxyarginine as an intermediate. *J. Chem. Soc., Chemical Communications*, 205-206.

Hemscheidt T., Rapala, J., Sivonen, K. and Skulberg, O.M. (1995b). Biosynthesis of anatoxin-a in *Anabaena flos-aquae* and homoanatoxin-a in *Oscillatoria formosa*. *J. Chem. Soc., Chemical Communications*, 1361-1362.

Henning, M. and Kohl, J.G. (1981). Toxic blue-green algae water blooms found in some lakes in the German Democratic Republic. *Int. Rev. ges. Hydrobiol.*, 66, 553-561.

Henriksen, P. (1996a). Microcystin profiles and contents in Danish populations of cyanobacteria/blue-green algae as determined by HPLC, *Phycologia, (Supplement)*, 35(6), 102-110.

Henriksen, P. (1996b). Toxic cyanobacteria/blue-green algae in Danish freshwaters. Thesis, Dept. of Phycology, University of Copenhagen.

Henriksen, P., Carmichael, W.W., An, J. and Moestrup, Ø. (1997). Detection of an anatoxin-a(s)-like anticholinesterase in natural blooms and cultures of cyanobacteria/blue-green algae from Danish lakes and in the stomach contents of poisoned birds. *Toxicon*, 35, 901-913.

Henriksen, P., Kaas, H., Damsø, L. and Moestrup, Ø. (1995). Toxic cyanobacteria (blue-green algae) in Danish freshwaters. Poster presented in 1st International Congress on Toxic Cyanobacteria (Blue-green Algae), August, Rnne, Denmark, 20-24.

Henriksen, P., Sivonen, K., Kaas, H. and Moestrup, Ø. (1998). Toxic cyanobacteria/blue-green algae in Danish freshwaters. *J. Phycol.* (In Press).

Hietala, J., Laurén-Määttä, C. and Walls, M. (1997). Sensitivity of *Daphnia* to toxic cyanobacteria: effects of genotype and temperature. *Freshwat. Biol.*, 37, 299-306.

Humpage, A.R., Rositano, J., Bretag, A.H., Brown, R., Baler, P.D., Nicholson, B.C. and Steffensen, D.A. (1994). Paralytic shellfish poisons from Australian cyanobacterial blooms. *Aust. J. Mar. Freshwater Res.*, 45(5), 761-771.

Ikawa, M., Wegener, K., Foxall, T.L. and Sasner, J.J. (1982). Comparison of the toxins of the blue-green alga *Aphanizomenon flos-aquae* with the *Gonyaulax* toxins. *Toxicon*. 20, 747-752.

Jackim, E. and Gentile, J. (1968). Toxins of a blue-green alga, similarity to saxitoxin. *Science*, 162, 915-916.

Jacobs, D., Bass, R.A. and Neilan, B.A. (1995). Isolation and characterization of candidate genes responsible for toxins biosynthesis in cyanobacteria. Abstract, Presented at the Vth Cyanobacterial Molecular Biology Workshop, July, 1995, Asilomar, CA, USA, 98, 21-25.

James, K.J., Sherlock, I.R. and Stack, M.A. (1997). Anatoxin-a in Irish freshwater and cyanobacteria, determined using a new fluorimetric liquid chromatographic method. *Toxicon*, 35(6), 963-971.

Jones, G.J. and Falconer, I.R. (1994). Factors affecting the production of toxins by cyanobacteria. Final Grant Report to the Land and Water Resources Research and Development Corporation, Canberra, Australia.

Jones, G.J. and Negri, A.P. (1997). Persistence and degradation of cyanobacterial paralytic shellfish poisons (PSPs) in freshwaters. *Wat. Res.*, 31, 525-533.

Jones, G.J. and Orr, P.T. (1994). Release and degradation of microcystin following algicide treatment of a *Microcystis aeruginosa* bloom in a recreational lake, as determined by HPLC and protein phosphatase inhibition assay. *Wat. Res.*, 28, 871-876.

Jones, G.J., Blackburn, S.I. and Parker, N.S. (1994). A toxic bloom of *Nodularia spumigena* Mertens in Orielton Lagoon, Tasmania. *Australian J. Mar. Freshwat. Res.*, 45, 787-800. 1783

Jones, G.J., Falconer, I.F. and Wilkins, R.M. (1995). Persistence of cyclic peptide toxins in dried cyanobacterial crusts from Lake Mokoan, Australia. *Environ. Toxicol. Water Qual.*, 10, 19-24.

Jungmann, D. (1992). Toxic compounds isolated from *Microcystis* PCC 7806 that are more active against *Daphnia* than two microcystins. *Limnol. Oceanog.*, 37, 1777-1783.

Jungmann, D. and Benndorf, J. (1994). Toxicity to *Daphnia* of a compound extracted from laboratory and natural *Microcystis* spp., and the role of microcystins. *Freshwat. Biol.*, 32, 13-20.

Kaya, K. and Watanabe, M.M. (1990). Microcystin composition of an axenic clonal strain of *Microcystis viridis* and *Microcystis viridis*–containing waterblooms in Japanese freshwaters. *J. App. Phycol.*, 2, 173-178.

Keleti, G. and Sykora, J.L. (1982). Production and properties of cyanobacterial endotoxins. *Appl. Environ. Microbiol.*, 43, 104–109.

Kenefick, S.L., Hrudey, S.E., Peterson, H.G. and Prepas, E.E. (1992). Toxin release from *Microcystis aeruginosa* after chemical treatment. *Wat. Sci. Tech.*, 27, 433-440.

Kerr, T., Jones, G.J. and Negri, A. (1995). Hydroxy fatty acid analysis of lipopolysaccharides in cyanobacteria. CSIRO Division of Water Resources, Australia, Summer Studentship report, 73 pp.

Kiviranta, J., Sivonen, K., Luukkainen, R., Lahti K. and Niemelä, S. I. (1991). Production and biodegradation of cyanobacterial toxins; a laboratory study, *Arch. Hydrobiol.*, 121, 281-294.

Kononen, K., Sivonen, K. and Lehtimäki, J. (1993). Toxicity of phytoplankton blooms in the Gulf of Finland and Gulf of Bothnia, Baltic Sea. In: T. J. Smayda and Y. Shimizu (Eds) *Toxic Phytoplankton Blooms in the Sea*, Elsevier Scientific Publications, Amsterdam, 269-274.

Kotak, B.G., Kenefick, S.L., Fritz, D.L., Rousseaux, C.G., Prepas, E.E. and Hrudey, S.E. (1993). Occurrence and toxicological evaluation of cyanobacterial toxins in Alberta lakes and farm dugouts. *Wat. Res.*, 27, 5-506.

Kotak, B.G., Lam, A.K.Y., Prepas, E.E., Kenefick, S.L. and Hrudey, S.E. (1995). Variability of the hepatotoxin microcystin-LR in hypereutrophic drinking water lakes. *J. Phycol.*, 31, 248-263.

Krishnamyrthy, T., Szafraniec, L., Hunt, D.F., Shabanowitz, J., Yates, J.R., Hauer, C.R., Carmichael, W.W., Skulberg, O., Codd, G.A. and Missler, S. (1989). Structural characterization of toxic cyclic peptides from blue-green algae by tandem mass spectrometry. *Proceedings of National Academy of Sciences USA.*, 86, 770-774.

Kusumi, T., Ooi, T., Watanabe, M.M., Takahashi, H. and Kakisawa, H. (1987). Cyanoviridin RR, a toxin from the cyanobacterium (blue-green alga) *Microcystis viridis. Tetrahedron Letters*, 28, 4695-4698.

Lagos, N., Liberona, J.L., Andrinolo, D., Zagatto, P.A., Soares, R.M. and Azevedo, S.M.F.Q. (1997). First evidence of paralytic shellfish toxins in the freshwater cyanobacterium *Cylindrospermopsis raciborskii* isolated from Brazil. Abstract, VIII International Conference on Harmful Algae, June 25-29, 1997, Vigo, Spain, 115.

Lahti, K., Kilponen, J., Kivimäki, A.L., Erkomaa, K. and Sivonen, K. (1996). Removal of cyanobacteria and their hepatotoxins from raw water in soil and sediment columns. In: A.L. Kivimäki and T. Suokko (Eds) *Artificial Recharge of Groundwater*. NHP Report No. 38, Helsinki, 187-195.

Lahti, K., Niemi, M. R., Rapala J. and Sivonen, K. (1997a). Biodegradation of cyanobacterial hepatotoxins–characterization of toxin degrading bacteria. Proceedings of the VII International Conference on Harmful Algae.

Lahti, K., Rapala, J., Färdig, M., Niemelä, M. and Sivonen, K. (1997b). Persistence of cyanobacterial hepatotoxin, microcystin-LR, in particulate material and dissolved in lake water. *Wat. Res.*, 31(5), 1005-1012.

Lam, A.K.-Y., Fedorak, P.M. and Prepas, E.E. (1995). Biotransformation of the cyanobacterial hepatotoxin microcystin-LR, as determined by HPLC and protein phosphatase bioassay. *Environ. Sci. Technol.*, 29(1), 242-246.

Lampert, W. (1981). Inhibitory and toxic effect of blue-green algae on *Daphnia. Rev. Ges. Hydrobiol.*, 66, 285-298.

Lanaras, T. and Cook, C.M. (1994). Toxin extraction from an *Anabaenopsis milleri*–dominated bloom. *Sci. Total Environ.*, 142, 163-169.

Lanaras, T., Tsitsamis, S., Chlichlia, C. and Cook, C.M. (1989). Toxic cyanobacteria in Greek freshwaters. *J. Applied Phycol.*, 1, 67-73.

Laurén-Määttä, C., Hietala, J. and Walls, M. (1997). Responses of *Daphnia pulex* populations to toxic cyanobacteria. *Freshwat. Biol.*, 37, 635-647.

Lawton, L.A., Beattie, K.A., Hawser, S.P., Campbell, D.L. and Codd, G.A. (1994). Evaluation of assay methods for the determination of cyanobacterial hepatotoxicity. In: G.A Codd, T.M. Jeffries, C.W. Keevil, E. Potter (Eds) *Detection Methods for Cyanobacterial Toxins*. Proceedings of the First International Symposium on Detection Methods for Cyanobacterial Toxins, September 1993 The Royal Society of Chemistry, Cambridge, 111-116.

Leeuwangh, P., Kappers, F.I., Dekker, M. and Koerselman, W. (1983). Toxicity of cyanobacteria in Dutch lakes and reservoirs. *Aquat. Toxicol.*, 4, 63-72.

Lehtimäki, J., Moisander, P., Sivonen, K. and Kononen, K. (1997). Growth, nitrogen fixation, and nodularin production by two Baltic Sea cyanobacteria. *Appl. Environ. Microbiol.*, 63, 1647-1656.

Lehtimäki, J., Sivonen, K., Luukkainen, R. and Niemelä, S.I. (1994). The effects of incubation time, temperature, light, salinity, and phosphorus on growth and hepatotoxin production by *Nodularia* strains. *Arch Hydrobiol.*, 130, 269-282.

Lindholm, T. and Meriluoto, J.A.O. (1991). Recurrent depth maxima of the hepatotoxic cyanobacterium *Oscillatoria agardhii. Can. J. Fish. Aquat. Sci.*, 48, 1629-1634.

Lukac, M. and Aegerter, R. (1993). Influence of trace metals on growth and toxin production of *Microcystis aeruginosa. Toxicon*, 31, 293-305.

Luukkainen, R., Namikoshi, M., Sivonen, K., Rinehart, K.L. and Niemelä, S.I. (1994). Isolation and identification of 12 microcystins from four strains and two bloom samples of *Microcystis* spp.: structure of a new hepatotoxin. *Toxicon.*, 32, 133-139.

Luukkainen R., Sivonen, K., Namikoshi, M., Färdig, M., Rinehart, K.L. and Niemelä, S.I. (1993). Isolation and identification of eight microcystins from 13 *Oscillatoria agardhii* strains: structure of a new microcystin. *Appl. Environ. Microbiol.*, 59, 2204-2209.

Lyck, S., Gjølme, N. and Utkilen, H. (1996). Irom-starvation increases toxicity of *Microcystis aeruginosa* CYA 22/1 (Chroococcales, Cyanophyceae). *Phycologia*, 35(6 Supplement), 120-124.

Mahmood, N.A. and Carmichael, W.W. (1986). Paralytic shellfish poisons produced by the freshwater cyanobacterium *Aphanizomenon flos-aquae* NH-5.*Toxicon*, 24, 175-186.

Mahmood, N.A. and Carmichael, W.W. (1987). Anatoxin-a(S), an anticholinesterase from the cyanobacterium *Anabaena flos-aquae* NCR-525-17.*Toxicon*, 25, 1221-1227.

Marš álek, B., LeDu, A., Turánek, J. and Machala, M. (1995). The selection of bioassays for cyanotoxin detection. In: Proceedings 1st International Congress on Toxic Cyanobacteria, 20-24 August 1995, Rønne, Denmark, 45.

Marš álek, B., Turánek J. and Hindák F. (1996). Toxic cyanobacteria in Czech and Slovak republic. In: Proceedings 1st. European Phycological Congress, Cologne, August 11-18, 1996, *Eur. J. Phycol. Suppl.*, 42.

Matsunaga, S., Moore, R.E., Niemczura, W.P. and Carmichael, W.W. (1989). Anatoxin-a(s), a potent anticholinesterase from *Anabaena flos-aquae. J. Amer. Chem. Soc.*, 111, 8021-8023.

Mattson, R. and Willén, T. (1986). *Toxinbildande blågröna alger i svenska insjöar 1985* (Toxin producing blue-green algae in Swedish lakes in 1985). Naturvårdsverket rapport 3096 (2)/1986. Laboratoriet för miljökontroll, Uppsala, ISSN 0282-7298.26. pp. (In Swedish, English summary).

Matveev, V., Matveeva, L., and Jones, G.J. (1994a). Study of the ability of *Daphnia carinata* King to control phytoplankton and resist cyanobacterial toxicity: implications for biomanipulation in Australia. *Aust. J. Mar. Freshwat. Res.*, 45, 889-904.

Matveev, V., Matveeva, L. and Jones, G.J. (1994b). Phytoplankton stimulation by mosquito fish in the presence of large *Daphnia. Ver. Verein. fur Theor. Ang. Limnol.*, 25, 2193-2197.

McDermott, C.M., Feola, R. and Plude, J. (1995). Detection of cyanobacterial toxins (microcystins) in waters of northeastern Wisconsin by a new immunoassay technique. *Toxicon.*, 33, 1433-1442.

Meissner, K., Dittman, E. and Börner, T. (1996). Toxic and non-toxic strains of the cyanobacterium *Microcystis aeruginosa* contain sequences homologous to peptide synthetase genes. *FEMS Microbiology Letters*, 135, 295-303.

Meriluoto, J.A.O., Sandström, A., Eriksson, J.E., Remaud, G., Grey Craig, A. and Chattopadhyaya, J. (1989). Structure and toxicity of a peptide hepatotoxin from the cyanobacterium *Oscillatoria agardhii. Toxicon*, 27, 1021-1034.

Mez, K., Hanselmann, K., Naegeli, H. and Preisig, H.R. (1996). Protein phosphatase-inhibiting activity in cyanobacteria from alpine lakes in Switzerland. *Phycologia*, 35(6 Supplement), 133-139.

Moikeha, S.N. and Chu, G.W. (1971). Dermatitis-producing alga *Lyngbya majuscula* Gomont in Hawaii. II. Biological properties of the toxic factor. *J. Phycol.*, 7, 8-13.

Moore B.S., Ohtani, I., de Koning, C.B., Moore, R.E. and Carmichael, W.W. (1992). Biosynthesis of Anatoxin-a(s). Origin of the carbons. *Tetrahedron Letters*. 33, 6595-6598.

Moore, R.E., Corbett, T., Patterson, G.M.L. and Valeriote, F.A. (1996). The search for new antitumor drugs from blue-green algae. *Current Pharm. Design*, 2, 317-330.

Moore, R.E., Lu Chen, J., Moore, B.S. and Patterson, G.M.L. (1991). Biosynthesis of microcystin-LR. Origin of the carbons in the Adda and Masp units. *J. Amer. Chem. Soc.*, 113, 5083-5084.

Moore, R.E., Ohtani, I., Moore, B.S., de Koning, C.B., Yoshida, W.Y., Runnegar, M.T. and Carmichael, W.W. (1993). Cyanobacterial toxins. *Gazzetta Chimica Italiana*, 123, 329-336.

Mynderse, J.S., Moore, R.E., Kashiwagi, M. and Norton, T.R. (1977). Antileukemia activity in the Oscillatoriaceae, isolation of debromoaplysiatoxin from *Lyngbya. Science*, 196, 538-540.

Nagata, S., Tsutsumi, T., Hasegawa, A., Yoshida, F., Ueno, Y. and Watanabe, M.F. (1997). Enzyme immunoassay for direct determination of microcystins in environmental water. *J. AOAC Int.*, 80, 408-417.

Namikoshi, M., and Rinehart, K.L. (1996). Bioactive compounds produced by cyanobacteria. *J. Ind. Microbiol.*, 17, 373-384.

Namikoshi, M., Choi, B.W., Sakai, R., Sun, F., Rinehart, K.L., Carmichael, W.W., Evans, W.R., Cruz, P., Munro, M.H.G. and Blunt, J.W. (1994). New nodularins, A general method for structure assignment. *J. Org. Chem.*, 59, 2349-2357.

Namikoshi, M., Rinehart, K.L., Sakai, R., Sivonen, K. and Carmichael, W.W. (1990). Structures of three new cyclic hepatotoxins produced by the cyanobacterium (blue-green alga) *Nostoc* sp. strain 152. *J. Org. Chem.*, 55, 6135-6139.

Namikoshi, M., Rinehart, K.L., Sakai, R., Stotts, R.R., Dahlem, A.M., Beasley, V.R., Carmichael, W.W. and Evans, W.R. (1992). Identification of 12 hepatotoxins from a Homer lake bloom of the cyanobacteria *Microcystis aeruginosa, Microcystis viridis, Microcystis wesenbergii;* nine new microcystins. *J. Org. Chem.*, 57, 866-872.

Namikoshi, M., Sivonen, K., Evans, W.R., Carmichael, W.W., Rouhiainen, L., Luukkainen, R. and Rinehart, K.L. (1992b). Structures of three new homotyrosine-containing microcystins and a new homophenylalanine variant from *Anabaena* sp. strain 66. *Chem. Res. Toxicol.*, 5, 661-666.

Namikoshi, M., Sivonen, K., Evans, W.R., Carmichael, W.W., Sun, F., Rouhiainen, L., Luukkainen, R. and Rinehart, K.L. (1992c). Two new L-serine variants of microcystins-LR and -RR from *Anabaena* sp. strain 202 A1 and 202 A2. *Toxicon*, 30, 1457-1464.

Namikoshi, M., Sivonen, K., Evans, W.R., Sun, F., Carmichael, W.W. and Rinehart, K.L. (1992d). Isolation and structures of microcystins from a cyanobacterial water bloom (Finland). *Toxicon*, 30, 1473-1479.

Namikoshi, M., Sun, F., Choi, B.W., Rinehart, K.L., Carmichael, W.W., Evans, W.R. and Beasley, V.R. (1995). Seven more microcystins from Homer lake cells: application of the general method for structure assignment of peptides containing,-dehydroamino acid unit(s). *J. Org. Chem.*, 60, 3671-3679.

Namikoshi, M., Yuan, M., Sivonen, K., Carmichael, W.W., Rinehart, K.L., Rouhiainen, L., Sun, F., Brittain, S. and Otsuki, A. (1998). Seven new microcystins possessing two L-glutamic acit units, isolated from *Anabaena* sp. strain 186. *Chem. Res. Toxicol.*, 11, 143-149.

Negri, A.P. and Jones, G.J. (1995). Bioaccumulation of paralytic shellfish poisoning (PSP) toxins from the cyanobacterium *Anabaena circinalis* by the freshwater mussel *Alathyria condola. Toxicon*, 33(5), 667-678.

Negri, A.P., Jones, G.J., Blackburn, S.I., Oshima, Y. and Onodera, H. (1997). Effect of culture and bloom development and of sample storage on paralytic shellfish poisons in the cyanobacterium *Anabaena circinalis. J. Phycol.*, 33, 26-35.

Negri, A.P., Jones, G.J. and Hindmarsh, M. (1995). Sheep mortality associated with Paralytic Shellfish poisoning toxins from the cyanobacterium *Anabaena circinalis. Toxicon*, 33, 1321-1329.

Oberemm, A., Fastner, J. and Steinberg, C. (1997). Effects of microcystin-LR and cyanobacterial crude extracts on embryo-larval development of zebrafish (*Danio rerio*). *Wat. Res.*, 31(11), 2918-2921.

Ohtani, I., Moore, R.E. and Runnegar, M.T.C. (1992). Cylindrospermopsin, a potent hepatotoxin from the blue-green alga *Cylindrospermopsis raciborskii. J. Amer. Chem. Soc.*, 114, 7941-7942.

Olson, T.A. (1960). Water poisoning–a study of poisonous algae blooms in Minnesota. *Amer. J. Public Health*, 50, 883-884.

Onodera, H., Oshima, Y., Henriksen, P. and Yasumoto, T. (1997a). Confirmation of anatoxin-a(s) in the cyanobacterium *Anabaena lemmermannii* as the cause of bird kills in Danish lakes. *Toxicon*, 35, 1645-1648.

Onodera, H., Satake, M., Oshima, Y., Yasumoto, T. and Carmichael, W.W. (1997b). New saxitoxin analogues from the freshwater filamentous cyanobacterium *Lyngbya wollei. Natural Toxins* (In Press).

Orr, P.T. and Jones, G.J. (1998). Relationship between microcystin production and cell division rates in nitrogen-limited *Microcystis aeruginosa* cultures. *Limnol. Oceanogr.*, 43(8), (In Press).

Padisák, J. (1997). *Cylindrospermopsis raciborskii* (Woloszynska) Seenayya et Subba Raju, an expanding, highly adaptive cyanobacterium: worldwide distribution and review of its ecology. *Arch. Hydrobiol., Suppl.*, 107, 563-593.

Painuly, P., Perez, R., Fukai, T. and Shimizu, Y. (1988). The structure of a cyclic peptide toxin, cyanogenosin-RR from *Microcystis aeruginosa. Tetrahedron Letters*, 29, 11-14.

Park, H.-D., Watanabe, M.F., Harada, K.-I., Nagai, H., Suzuki, M., Watanabe, M. and Hayashi, H. (1993a). Hepatotoxin (microcystin) and neurotoxin (anatoxin-a) contained in natural blooms and strains of cyanobacteria from Japanese freshwaters. *Natural Toxins*, 1, 353-360.

Park, H.-D., Watanabe, M.F., Harada, K.-I., Suzuki, M., Hayashi, H. and Okino, T. (1993b). Seasonal variations of *Microcystis* species and toxic heptapeptide microcystins in Lake Suwa. *Environ. Toxicol. Water Qual.*, 8, 425-435.

Parkar, D.L., Kumar, H.D., Rai, L.C. and Singh, J.B. (1997). Potassium salts inhibits growth of the cyanobacteria *Microcystis* spp. in pond water and defined media. Implication for control of Microcystin producing aquatic bloom. *Applied and Environmental Microbiology*, 2324-2329.

Penaloza, R., Rojas, M., Vila, I. and Zambrano, F. (1990). Toxicity of a soluble peptide from *Microcystis* sp. to zooplankton and fish. *Freshwat. Biol.*, 24(2), 223-240.

Prepas, E.E., Kotak, *E.G.*, Campbell, L.M., Evans, J.C., Hrudey, S.E. and Holmes, C.F.B. (1997). Accumulation and elimination of cyanobacterial hepatotoxins by the freshwater clam *Anodonta grandis simpsoniana. Can. J. Fish. Aquat. Sci.*, 54, 41-46.

Prinsep, M.R., Caplan, F.R., Moore, R.E., Patterson, G.M.L., Honkanen, R.E. and Boynton, A.L. (1992). Microcystin-LR from a blue-green alga belonging to the Stignonematales. *Phytochemistry*, 31, 1247-1248.

Råbergh, C.M.I., Bylund, G., Eriksson, J.E. (1991). Histopathological effect of microcystin LR a cyclic polypeptide from the cyanobacterium *Microcystis aeruginosa* on common carp (*Cyprinus carpio L.*). *Aquat. Tox.*, 20,131-146.

Rapala, J. and Sivonen, K. (1998). Assessment of environmental conditions that favour hepatotoxic and neurotoxic *Anabaena* spp. strains in cultured under light-limitation at different temperatures. *Microbial. Ecol.*, 36, 181-192.

Rapala, J., Lahti, K., Sivonen, K. and Niemelä, S. I. (1994). Biodegradability and adsorption on lake sediments of cyanobacterial hepatotoxins and anatoxin-a. *Letters in Applied Microbiol.*, 19, 423-428.

Rapala, J., Sivonen, K., Luukkainen, R. and Niemelä, S.I. (1993). Anatoxin-a concentration in *Anabaena* and *Aphanizomenon* at different environmental conditions and comparison of growth by toxic and non-toxic *Anabaena* strains, a laboratory study, *J. App. Phycol.*, 5, 581-591.

Rapala, J., Sivonen, K., Lyra, C. and Niemelä, S.I. (1997). Variation of microcystins, cyanobacterial hepatotoxins, in *Anabaena* spp. as a function of growth stimuli. *App. Environ. Microbiol.*, 64, 2206-2212.

Raziuddin, S., Siegelman, H.W. and Tornabene, T.G. (1983). Lipopolysaccharides of the cyanobacterium *Microcystis aeruginosa. Eur. J. Biochem.*, 137, 333-336.

Reinikainen, M., Kiviranta, J., Ulvi, V. and Niku-Paavola, M.L. (1995). Acute toxic effects of a novel cyanobacterial toxin on the crustaceans *Artemia salina* and *Daphnia pulex. Arch. Hydrobiol.*, 133, 61-69.

Repavich, W.M., Sonzogni, W.C., Standridge, J.H., Wedepohl, R.E. and Meisner L.F. (1990). Cyanobacteria (blue-green algae) in Wisconsin waters: acute and chronic toxicity. *Wat. Res.*, 24, 225-231.

Ressom, R., Soong, F.S., Fitzgerald, J., Turczynowicz, L., El Saadi, O., Roder, D., Maynard, T. and Falconer, I. (1994). *Health Effects of Toxic Cyanobacteria (Blue-green Algae)*. National Health and Medical Council, The Australian Government Publishing Service, Canberra, Australia, 108 pp.

Rinehart, K.L., Harada, K.-I., Namikoshi, M., Chen, C., Harvis, C.A., Munro, M.H.G., Blunt, J.W., Mulligan, P.E., Beasley, V.R., Dahlem, A.M. and Carmichael, W.W. (1988). Nodularin, microcystin, and the configuration of Adda. *J. Amer. Chem. Soc.*, 110, 8557-8558.

Rinehart, K.L., Namikoshi, M. and Choi, B.W. (1994). Structure and biosynthesis of toxins from blue-green algae (Cyanobacteria). *J. App. Phycol.*, 6, 159-176.

Rodger, H.D., Turnbull, T., Edwards, C. and Codd, G.A. (1994). Cyanobacterial bloom associated pathology in brown trout *Salmo trutta L.* in Loch Leven, Scotland. *J. Fish Dis.*, 17, 177-181.

Rouhiainen L., Buikema, W., Paulin, L., Fonstein, M., Sivonen, K. and Haselkorn, R. (1994). Peptide synthetase genes from hepatotoxin producing Cyanobacteria. Abstract In: VIII International Symposium on Phototrophic Prokaryotes, 10-15, September, Urbino, Italy, 26.

Rudolph-Böhner, S., Mierke, D.F. and Moroder, L. (1994). Molecular structure of cyanobacterial tumour-promoting microcystins. *FEBS Letters*, 349, 319-323.

Schwabe W., Weihe, A., Börner, T., Henning, M. and Kohl, J.G. (1988). Plasmids in toxic and nontoxic strains of the cyanobacterium *Microcystis aeruginosa. Current Microbiology*, 17, 133-137.

Scott, W.E. (1991). Occurrence and significance of toxic Cyanobacteria in Southern Africa. *Wat. Sci. Techno.*, 23, 175-180.

Shimizu, Y. (1986). Toxigenesis and biosynthesis of saxitoxin analogues. *Pure Appl. Chem.*, 58, 257-262.

Shimizu, Y., Norte, M., Hori, A., Genenah, A. and Kobayashi, M. (1984). Biosynthesis of saxitoxin analogues: the unexpected pathway. *J. Amer. Chem. Soc.*, 106, 6433-6434.

Shirai, M., Ohtake, A., Sano, T., Matsumoto, S., Sakamoto, T., Sato, A., Aida, T., Harada, K.I., Shimida, T., Suzuki, M. and Nakano, M. (1991). Toxicity and toxins of natural blooms and isolated strains of *Microcystis* spp. (Cyanobacteria) and improved procedure for purification of cultures. *App. Environ. Microbiol.*, 57, 1241-1245.

Shumway, S.E., van Egmond, H.P., Hurst, J.W. and Bean, L.L. (1995). Management of shellfish resources. In: G.M. Hallegraeff, D.M. Anderson, A.D. Cembella and H.O Enevoldsen [Eds] *Manual on Harmful Marine Microalgae.* UNESCO Intergovernmental Oceanographic Commission, Manuals and Guides 33, United Nations Educational, Scientific and Cultural Organization, 433-457.

Singh, N., Jain, A.K. and Vyas, D. (2002). Effect of cyanobacterial extract on oyster mushroom *Pleurotus* Sojor Caju. *J. Mushroom Res.*, 11: 85–87.

Sivonen, K. (1990a). *Toxic Cyanobacteria in Finnish Freshwaters and the Baltic Sea.* Reports from Department of Microbiology, 39, University of Helsinki, Hakapaino, Helsinki, 87 pp.

Sivonen, K. (1990b). Effects of light, temperature, nitrate, orthophosphate, and bacteria on growth of and hepatotoxin production by *Oscillatoria agardhii* strains. *App. Environ. Microbiol.*, 56, 2658-2666.

Sivonen, K. (1996). Cyanobacterial toxins and toxin production. *Phycologia,* 35(6 Supplement), 12-24.

Sivonen, K., Carmichael, W.W., Namikoshi, M., Rinehart, K.L., Dahlem, A.M. and Niemelä, S.I. (1990a). Isolation and characterization of hepatotoxic microcystin homologues from the filamentous freshwater cyanobacterium *Nostoc* sp. strain 152. *App. Env. Microbiol.*, 56, 2650-2657.

Sivonen, K., Himberg, K., Luukkainen, R., Niemelä, S.I., Poon, G.K. and Codd, G.A. (1989a). Preliminary characterization of neurotoxic blooms and strains from Finland. *Tax. Assess.*, 4, 339-352.

Sivonen, K., Kononen, K., Carmichael, W.W., Dahlem, A.M., Rinehart, K.L., Kiviranta, J. and Niemelä, S.I. (1989b). Occurrence of the hepatotoxic cyanobacterium *Nodularia spumigena* in the Baltic Sea and the structure of the toxin. *App. Env. Microbiol.*, 55, 1990-1995.

Sivonen, K., Namikoshi, M., Evans, W.R., Carmichael, W.W., Sun, F., Rouhiainen, L., Luukkainen, R. and K.L. Rinehart. (1992a). Isolation and characterization of a variety of microcystins from seven strains of the cyanobacterial genus *Anabaena. App. Env. Microbiol.*, 58, 2495-2500.

Sivonen, K., Namikoshi, M., Evans, W.R., Färdig, M., Carmichael, W.W. and Rinehart, K.L. (1992b). Three new microcystins, cyclic heptapeptide hepatotoxins, from *Nostoc* sp. strain 152. *Chem. Res. Toxicol.*, 5, 464-469.

Sivonen, K., Namikoshi, M., Evans, W.R., Gromov, B.V., Carmichael, W.W. and Rinehart, K.L. (1992c). Isolation and structures of five microcystins from a Russian *Microcystis aeruginosa* strain CALU 972. *Toxicon.*, 30,1481-1485.

Sivonen, K., Namikoshi, M., Luukkainen, R., Färdig, M., Rouhiainen, L., Evans, W.R., Carmichael, W.W., Rinehart, K.L. and Niemelä, S.I. (1995). Variation of cyanobacterial hepatotoxins in Finland. In: M. Munawar and M. Luotola (Eds) *The Contaminants in the Nordic Ecosystem, Dynamics, Processes and Fate.* Ecovision World Monograph Series, SPB Academic Publishing, Amsterdam, 163-169.

Sivonen, K., Niemelä, S.I., Niemi, R.M., Lepistö, L., Luoma, T.H. and Räsänen, L.A. (1990b). Toxic cyanobacteria (blue-green algae) in Finnish fresh and coastal waters. *Hydrobiologia,* 190, 267-275.

Sivonen, K., Skulberg, O.M., Namikoshi, M., Evans, W.R., Carmichael, W.W. and Rinehart, K.L. (1992d). Two methyl ester derivates of microcystins, cyclic heptapeptide hepatotoxins, isolated from *Anabaena flos-aquae* strain CYA 83/1. *Toxicon.*, 30, 1465-1471.

Skulberg, O.M., Carmichael, W.W., Anderson, R.A., Matsunaga, S., Moore, R.E. and Skulberg, R. (1992). Investigations of a neurotoxic Oscillatorialean strain (cyanophyceae) and its toxin. Isolation and characterization of homoanatoxin-a. *Env. Toxicol. Chem.*, 11, 321-329.

Skulberg, O.M., Underdal, B. and Utkilen, H. (1994). Toxic waterblooms with cyanophytes in Norway–current knowledge. *Algol. Stud.*, 75, 279-289.

Smith, C. and Sutton, A. (1993). The persistence of anatoxin-a in reservoir water. Foundation for Water Research, UK Report No. FR0427.

Snell, T.W. (1980). Blue-green algae and selection in rotifer populations. *Oecologia Berlin,* 46, 343-346.

Stevens, D.K. and Krieger, R.I. (1991). Stability studies on the cyanobacterial nicotinic alkaloid anatoxin-a. *Toxicon*, 29, 167-179.

Stoner, R.D., Adams, W.H., Slatkin, D.N. and Siegelman, H.W. (1989). The effects of single L-amino acid substitutions on the lethal potencies of the microcystins. *Toxicon.*, 27, 825-828.

Sugaya, Y., Yasuno, M. and Yani, T. (1990). Effects of toxic *Microcystis viridis* and isolated toxins on goldfish. *Jpn J. Limnol.*, 51(3), 149-153.

Sugiura, N. Nishimura, O. Inamori, Y. Ouchiyama, T. Sudo, R. (1997). Grazing characteristics of musty-odour-compound-producing *Phormidium tenue* by a microflagellate, *Monasguttula. Wat. Res.*, 31(11), 2792-2796.

Swoboda, U.K., Dow, C.S., Chaivimol, J., Smith, N. and Pound, B.P. (1994). Alternatives to the Mouse Bioassay for Cyanobacterial Toxicity Assessment. In: G.A. Codd, T.M. Jeffries, C.W. Keevil and E. Potter (Eds) *Detection Methods for Cyanobacterial Toxins.* Proceedings of the First International Symposium on Detection Methods for Cyanobacterial Toxins, September 1993, The Royal Society of Chemistry, 106-110.

Takenaka, S. and Watanabe, M.F. (1997). Microcystin-LR degradation by *Pseudomonas aeruginosa* alkaline phosphatase. *Chemosphere*, 34, 749-757.

Tencalla, F.G., Dietrich, D.R. and Schlatter, C. (1994). Toxicity of *Microcystis aeruginosa* peptide toxin to yearling rainbow trout (*Oncorhynchus mykiss*). *Aqua. Toxicol.*, 30(3), 215-224.

Todorova, A. and Jttner, F. (1996). Ecotoxicological analysis of nostocyclamide, a modified cyclic hexapeptide from *Nostoc. Phycologia*, 35(6 Supplement), 183-188.

Törökné, A.K. (1991). Toxin producing cyanobacteria in Hungarian freshwaters. Doctoral Dissertation, Budapest, Hungary.

Törökné, A.K. (1997). Interlaboratory trial using Thamnotox kit for detecting cyanobacterial toxins. In: *Proceedings of VIII International Conference on Harmful Algae*, Vigo, Spain, 114.

Trimurtulu, G., Ogino, J., Helzel, C.E., Husebo, T.L., Jensen, C.M., Larsen, L.K., Patterson, G.M.L., Moore, R.E., Mooberry, S.L., Corbett, T.H. and Valeriote, F.A. (1995). Structure determination, conformational analysis, chemical stability studies, and antitumor evaluation of the cryptophycins. Isolation of 18 new analogs from *Nostoc* sp. strain GSV 224. *J. Amer. Chem. Soc.*, 117, 12030-12049.

Tsuji, K., Naito, S., Kondo, F., Ishikawa, N., Watanabe, M.F., Suzuki, M., Harada, K-I. (1993). Stability of microcystins from cyanobacteria: Effect of light on decomposition and isomerization. *Environ. Sci. Technol.* 28, 173-177.

Tsuji, K., Setsuda, S., Watanuki, T., Kondo, F., Nakazawa, H., Suzuki, M. and Harada, K.I. (1996). Microcystin levels during 1992-95 for lakes Sagami and Tsukui Japan. *Natural Toxins*, 4, 189-194.

Utkilen, H. and Gjølme, N. (1992). Toxin production by *Microcystis aeruginosa* as a function of light in continuous cultures and its ecological significance. *App. Environ. Microbiol.*, 58, 1321-1325.

Utkilen, H. and Gjølme, N. (1995). Iron-stimulated toxin production in *Microcystis aeruginosa. App. Environ. Microbiol.*, 61, 797-800.

Ueno, Y., Nagata, S., Tsutsumi, T., Hasegawa, A., Watanabe, M.F., Park, H.D., Chen, G.C., Chen, G. and Yu, S.Z. (1996a). Detection of microcystins, a blue-green algal hepatotoxin, in drinking water sampled in Haimen and Fusui, endemic areas of primary liver cancer in China, by highly sensitive immunoassay. *Carcinogenesis*, 17, 1317-1321.

Ueno, Y., Nagata, S., Tsutsumi, T., Hasegawa, A., Yoshida, F., Suttajit, M., Putsch M. and Vasconcelos, V. (1996b). Survey of microcystins in environmental water by a highly sensitive immunoassay based on monoclonal antibody. *Natural Toxins*, 4, 271-276.

Van der Westhuizen, A.J. and Eloff, J.N. (1983). Effect of culture age and pH of culture medium on the growth and toxicity of the blue green alga *Microcystis aeruginosa. Zeit. Planzenphysiol.*, 110, 157-163.

Van der Westhuizen, A.J. and Eloff, J.N. (1985). Effect of temperature and light on the toxicity and growth of the blue-green alga *Microcystis aeruginosa* (UV-006). *Planta*, 163, 55-59.

Van der Westhuizen, A.J., Eloff, J.N. and Krüger, G.H.J. (1986). Effect of temperature and light (fluence rate) on the composition of the toxin of the cyanobacterium *Microcystis aeruginosa* (UV-006). *Arch. Hydrobiol.*, 108, 145-154.

Vasconcelos, V.M. (1994). Toxic cyanobacteria (blue-green algae) in Portuguese freshwaters. *Arch Hydrobiol.*, 130, 439-451.

Vasconcelos, V.M., Sivonen, K., Evans, W.R., Carmichael, W.W. and Namikoshi, M. (1995). Isolation and characterization of microcystins (heptapetide hepatotoxins) from Portuguese strains of *Microcystis aeruginosa* Kutz emend Elekin. *Arch. Hydrobiol.*, 134, 295-305.

Vasconcelos, V.M., Sivonen, K., Evans, W.R., Carmichael, W.W. and Namikoshi, M. (1996). Microcystin (heptapeptide hepatotoxins) diversity in cyanobacterial blooms collected in Portuguese freshwaters. *Wat. Res.*, 30, 2377-2384.

Vezie, C., Brient, L., Sivonen, K., Betru, G., Lefeuvre, J.C. and Salkinoja-Salonen, M. (1997). Occurrence of microcystins containing cyanobacterial blooms in freshwaters of Brittany (France). *Arch. Hydrobiol.*, 139, 401-413.

Vezie, C., Brient, L., Sivonen, K., Bertru, G., Lefeuvre, J.C. and Salkinoja-Salonen, M. (1998). Variation of microcystin content of cyanobacterial blooms and isolated strains in Grand-Lieu lake (France). *Microbiol. Ecol.*, 35, 126-135.

Von Elert, E. and Juttner, F. (1996). Factors influencing the allelopathic activity of the planktonic cyanobacterium *Trichormus doliolum. Phycologia*, 35(6 Supplement), 68-73.

Vyas, D. (2007). Fungicidal activity of cyanobacterium microcystis aeruginosa. Abstract in National Symposium on Plant Pathogens: Exploitation and Management and 59th Annual Meeting of Indian Phytopathology, pp. 66.

Watanabe, M. F. (1996). Production of Microcystins. In: M.F. Watanabe, H. Harada, W. W. Carmichael and H. Fujiki, (Eds) *Toxic Microcystis*. CRC Press, London, 262 pp.

Watanabe, M.F. and Oishi, S. (1980). Toxicities of *Microcystis aeruginosa* collected from some lakes, reservoirs, ponds and moat in Tokyo and adjacent regions. *J. Limnol.*, 41, 5-9.

Watanabe, M.F. and Oishi, S. (1985). Effects of environmental factors on toxicity of a cyanobacterium (*Microcystis aeruginosa*) under culture conditions. *App. Environ. Microbiol.*, 49, 1342-1344.

Watanabe, M.F., Harada, K.I., Matsuura, K., Oishi, S., Watanabe, Y. and Suzuki, M. (1989). Heptapeptide toxins contained in natural samples of *Microcystis* species. *Tox. Assess.*, 4, 487-497.

Watanabe M.F., Oishi, S., Harada, K-.I., Matsuura, K., Kawai, H. and Suzuki, M. (1988). Toxins contained in *Microcystis* species of cyanobacteria (blue-green algae). *Toxicon*, 26, 1017-1025.

Watanabe, M.F., Oishi, S., Watanabe, Y. and Watanabe, M. (1986). Strong probability of lethal toxicity in the blue-green alga *Microcystis viridis* Lemmermann. *J. Phycol.*, 22, 552-556.

Watanabe, M.F., Park, H-D., Kondo, F., Harada, K-I., Hayashi, H. and Okino, T. (1997). Identification and estimation of microcystins in freshwater mussels. *Nat. Toxins*, 5, 31-35.

Watanabe, M.M., Kaya, K. and Takamura, N. (1992). Fate of the toxic cyclic heptapeptides, the microcystins, from blooms of *Microcystis* (cyanobacteria) in a hypertrophic lake. *J. Phycol.*, 28, 761-767.

Watanabe, M.M., Zhang, X and Kaya, K. (1996). Fate of toxic cyclic heptapeptides, microcystins, in toxic cyanobacteria upon grazing by the mixotrophic flagellate *Poterioochromonas malhamensis* (Ochromonadales, Chrysophyceae). *Phycologia*, 35(6 Supplement), 203-206.

Weckesser, J. and Drews, G. (1979). Lipopolysaccharides of photosynthetic prokaryotes. *Ann. Rev. Microbiol.*, 33, 215-239.

Weckesser, J., Martin, C. and Jakobi, C. (1996). Cyanopeptolins, depsipeptides from cyanobacteria. *System. App. Microbiol.*, 19, 133-138.

Weise, G., Drews, G., Jann, B. and Jann, K. (1970). Identification and analysis of lipopolysaccharide in cell walls of the blue-green algae *Anacystis nidulans*. *Arch. Microbiol.*, 71, 89-98.

Welker, M. and Steinberg, C.E.W. (1998). Indirect photolysis of cyanotoxins: one possible mechanism of their low persistence. *Wat. Res.* (In Press).

Wicks, R.J. and Thiel, P.G. (1990). Environmental factors affecting the production of peptide toxins in floating scums of cyanobacterium *Microcystis aeruginosa* in a hypertrophic African reservoir. *Environ. Sci. Technol.*, 24, 1413-1418.

Wiedner, C. and Nixdorf, B. (1997). *Verbreitung und Steuerung der Entwicklung von toxischen und nicht-toxischen Cyanobakterien in ostbrandenburgischen Gewässern unterschiedlicher Trophie und Hydrographie im Zuge der reduzierten Belastung*. WaBoLu-Hefte 4/97, Berlin ISSN 0175-4211.

Willn, T. and Mattsson, R. (1997). Water-blooming and toxin-producing cyanobacteria in Swedish fresh and brackish waters, 1981-1995. *Hydrobiologia*, 353, 181-192.

Williams, D.E., Craig, M., Dawe, S.C., Kent, M.C., Holmes, C.F.B. and Anderson, R.J. (1997). Evidence for a covalently bound form of microcystin-LR in salmon larvae and dungeness crab larvae. *Chem. Res. Toxicol.*, 10, 463-469.

Yanni, Y.G. and Carmichael, W.W. (1997). Screening of cyanobacteria isolated from soil, rice fields and water resources of the Nile Delta for production of cyanotoxins. Abstract, In: VIII International Conference on Harmful Algae, 25-29 June, 1997 Vigo, Spain, 216.

Yoo, S., Carmichael, W.W., Hoehn, R.C. and Hrudey, S.E. (1995). *Cyanobacterial (Blue-green Algal) Toxins: A Resource Guide.* American Water Works Association Research Foundation, Denver, Colorado.

Zhang, Q.X., Carmichael, W.W., Yu, M.J. and Li, S.H. (1991). Cyclic peptide hepatotoxins from freshwater cyanobacterial (blue-green algae) waterblooms collected in central China. *Env. Toxicol. Chem.*, 10, 313-321.

Zhang, X. Watanabe, M.M., Inouye, I. (1996). Light and electron microscopy of grazing by flagellate *Poterioochromonas malhamensis* (Chrysophyceae) on a range of phytoplankton taxa. *J. Phycol.*, 32, 37-46.

Microbial Biotechnology and Ecology (2011) *Pages* **150–161**
Editors: **Deepak Vyas, G.S. Paliwal, P.K.Khare and R.K Gupta**
Published by: **DAYA PUBLISHING HOUSE, NEW DELHI**

Chapter 7

The Toxins of Cyanobacteria

☆ ***Mukesh Kumar***

Department of Botany, Sahu Jain P.G. College, Najibabad – 246 763, U.P.

ABSTRACT

Cyanobacteria is a group of extraordinarily diverse Gram-negative prokaryotes that originated 3.5 billion years ago on the earth. They are prokaryotes with oxygen evolving photosynthetic system and are found in a wide range of environmental conditions including extreme ones. They constitute a larger and fascinating group of photosynthetic and nitrogen fixing prokaryotes. They colonize most aquatic and terrestrial ecosystems and are considered to be one of the potential organisms which can be useful to mankind in various ways. The morphology of Cyanobacteria ranges from unicellular to branch filamentous with a maximum of three cell types: vegetative cells, akinetes and heterocysts. Massive growth of Cyanobacteria in ponds, lakes, reservoirs or other freshwater systems has become serious water quality problem which also threaten human and animal health. Blooms can discolour water, form surface scums, produce unpleasant taste and odor to water, and create problems to aquatic life. They may vary in colour from green to blue, red, brown, dark green or black. Some of the cyanobacterial species are harmless while other produces toxins affecting nervous system and the liver of the animals. Many cyanobacterial species produce toxins that affect animals and humans. Cyanobacterial toxins are the group of organic compounds with very diverse chemical structure. They are divided into two groups *i.e.* cyanotoxins and biotoxins. Cyanotoxins are not lethal for people and animals. They are enzymes, antibiotics and anticarcinogenic factors with very complicated chemical structure. Biotoxins are very toxic for people and can even cause lethal effect. Cyanobacterial toxins can be controlled by the use of chemicals, biological means or by the use of microorganisms.

Introduction

The Cyanobacteria

Cyanobacteria were among the pioneer organisms of the early earth. They probably evolved as a group of organisms about 2,000 million years before the eukaryotic micro algae (Bisby 1995). They have the distinction of being the oldest known fossils, more than 3.5 billion years old. It is a group of extraordinarily diverse gram-negative prokaryotes that originated 3.5 billion years ago. Their diversity ranges from unicellular to multicellular, coccoid to branched filaments, nearly colourless to intensely pigmented, autotrophic to heterotrophic, psychrophilic to thermophilic, acidophilic to alkylophilic, planktonic to barophilic, freshwater to marine including hypersaline (salt pans). They are found both free living and as endosymbionts. Adapted to a wide range of environmental factors including extreme ones, these colonize most aquatic and terrestrial ecosystems. They are considered to be one of the potential organisms which can be useful to mankind in various ways. Based on the International Code of Botanical Nomenclature the class cyanophyceae contains about 150 genera and 2000 species. The micro algae investigated by Phycologists under ICBN (Greuter *et al.*, 1994) included organisms of both eukaryotic and prokaryotic cell types. The blue-green algae, constituted the largest group of the later category. The prokaryotic nature of these organisms and their fairly close relationship with eubacteria made work under provisions of the International Code of Botanical Nomenclature (Sneath 1992, Rippka *et al.*, 1999, Waterbury 1992).

Cyanobacteria are prokaryotes with oxygen evolving photosynthetic system and are found in a wide range of environmental conditions. Cyanobacteria inhabit a wide range of environments and ecological habitats, constitute a larger and fascinating group of photosynthetic and nitrogen fixing prokaryotes. Their morphology ranges from unicellular to branch filamentous with a maximum of three cell types: vegetative cells, akinetes and heterocysts. They occur naturally in ponds and other water reservoirs. The most important factor, which favors their distribution widely through out the world is their ability to survive in the extreme conditions of the environment. Along with this some environmental factors also play an important role in the growth of cyanobacteria as light, temperature, pH etc. The recent trend among microbiologist is to call these organisms cyanobacteria in order to emphasize their close relationship with bacteria. In fact, they are best defined as microorganisms that contain a typically prokaryotic cell, a photosynthetic apparatus structurally and functionally similar to that located within chloroplast of the eukaryotic red algae. One general attribute of most cyanobacteria is that they are morphologically conservative but metabolically versatile. Conceptual advances in microbiology during the 20th century included the realization that a discontinuity exits between prokaryotic and eukaryotic cellular organisms within the organization of their cells.

Cyanobacterial Toxins

A toxin is a poisonous substance produced by living cells or organisms. Although technically man is a living organism, man-made substances created by artificial processes usually aren't considered toxins by this definition. A toxin is simply a poison that can affect the body by internal or external means. A toxin can be a chemical which occurs naturally or in synthetic form. They can be small molecules, peptides, or proteins that are capable of causing disease on contact with or absorption by body tissues interacting with biological macromolecules such as enzymes or cellular receptors. Toxins vary greatly in their severity, ranging from usually minor and acute (as in a bee sting) to almost immediately deadly (as in botulinum toxin). External toxins, either chemical or microbial, enter the body through food, water, air, or physical contact with the skin or mucous membranes. Internal toxins, as the free radicals, are produced inside the body through normal metabolic processes or through the decomposition of foods in the small and large intestines. Bacterial toxins and yeast overgrowth can also form in cases of chronic constipation.

More than 120,000 human-made chemicals have been introduced into the environment, in one form or another, and this number continues to grow each year at a phenomenal rate. At the same time, microbial toxins, being influenced by the vast numbers of chemicals, are mutating beyond belief. Each category of microbes produces species that generates toxins in host cells. Evidence is proving a definitive link between the accumulation of toxins in body tissues and the development of chronic diseases. Massive growth of cyanobacteria in ponds, lakes, reservoirs or other freshwater systems has become serious water quality problem which also threaten human and animal health. Blooms of *Microcystis* species are known as one of the most common worldwide problems of freshwater bodies. Blooms can discolour water, form surface scums, produce unpleasant taste and odor to water, and create problems to aquatic life. They may vary in colour from green to blu , red, brown, dark green or black. Species of cyanobacteria or blue-green algae may dominate and increase excessively in water bloom conditions.

Some of the cyanobacterial species are harmless while other produces toxins affecting nervous system and the liver of the animals. Many cyanobacterial species produce toxins that affect animals and humans. Consumption of contaminated water by people in any form may cause cyanobacterial toxicity. The most frequently adverse health affects are caused by drinking water containing the toxins or by recreational water contact. Cyanobacteria are particularly troublesome organisms because apart from producing large amount of biomass, they secrete very toxic substances to water that are known as cyanobacterial toxins. Any release of toxin into surrounding water can present a significant hazard to humans drinking the same water.

Cyanobacterial toxins are the group of organic compounds with very diverse chemical structure. They are divided into two groups *i.e.* cyanotoxins and biotoxins. Cyanotoxins are not lethal for people and animals. They are enzymes, antibiotics and anticarcinogenic factors with very complicated chemical structure. Biotoxins are very toxic for people and can even cause lethal effect. They are divided into neurotoxins (affecting nervous system), hepatotoxins (affecting liver) and dermotoxins (affecting skin).

High pH of water, scarcity of CO_2 dissolved in water and high amount of phosphorus is conductive to the production of the biomass of cyanobacteria (Carmichael 1994, Gajdek 2000). Cyanobacteria survive in the periods of unfavorable conditions in the form of spores and then, in favorable conditions quickly achieve quantitative mass development. In this time they give water distinct colour, referred to as bloom.

Production and Structure of Cyanobacterial

One of the groups of toxins produced and released by cyanobacteria is called microcystin named from the species *Microcystis aeruginosa*. The microcystins are a group of cyclic heptapeptide hepatotoxins produced by a number of cyanobacterial genera. The peptide ring is made up of two protein amino acids and five non-protein amino acids. It is the two protein amino acids that distinguish microcystin types from each other, while the other amino acids are relatively constant.

By using amino acid single letter code classification, each microcystin is designated a name depending on the variable amino acids which complete their structure. For instance, one of the most common toxins found in water supplies around the world, microcystin-LR contains the amino acids Leucine (L) and Arginine (R) in these variable positions.

The most common of the toxins, microcystins are also the ones most often responsible for poisoning animals and humans who come into contact with toxic blooms. They are extremely stable in water because of their chemical structure, surviving in both warm and cold water and can tolerate radical changes in water chemistry, including pH. To date, approximately 75 different kinds of microcystins have been discovered.

These hepatotoxins inhibit the protein phosphatases inside hepatocytes. They damage the liver by affecting the maintenance of the cytoskeleton by disrupting the balance of phosphate groups on cytoskeletal proteins. The hepatotoxins cause the cytoskeleton to collapse, causing the hepatocytes to collapse inwards. The hepatocytes and also the capillary cells then pull apart, spilling blood into the liver. The blood pools in the liver, causing death.

Another cyanobacterial toxin is *Nodularia spumigena*, characterized as Nodularin. In 1878, George Francis issued the first scientific report of the potent toxicity of Nodularin cyanobacterial blooms. The structure of nodularin is closely related to that of the potent cyclic heptapeptide hepatotoxins, the microcystins. The difference lies in that nodularin is composed of only five amino acids in the peptide ring. Not only are the structures of these two cyanobacterial toxins similar, but they also show the same hepatotoxic effects through the potent inhibition of protein phosphatases.

It is speculated that low-level exposure to these toxins may promote the development of cancer in the liver and other chronic disorders of the gastrointestinal tract. This is likely to occur because the protein phosphatases that are inhibited by hepatotoxins play an important role in regulating cell division. While not initiating the cancers, these toxins have been shown to hasten the development of cancer in animals. Carmichael suggests that "the extraordinarily high rates of liver cancer in parts of China may be tied to the cyanobacterial toxins in water."

Analytical testing confirms the amount of cyanobacteria toxin in water samples. In recent years, HPLC, ELISA, and the protein phosphatase assay have made the quantification of total and individual toxins possible. Lyophilized cultures and bloom samples are used to determine the quantitative concentration of toxin. Results are expressed as milligrams or micrograms of toxin per gram of dry weight.

Microcystin LR

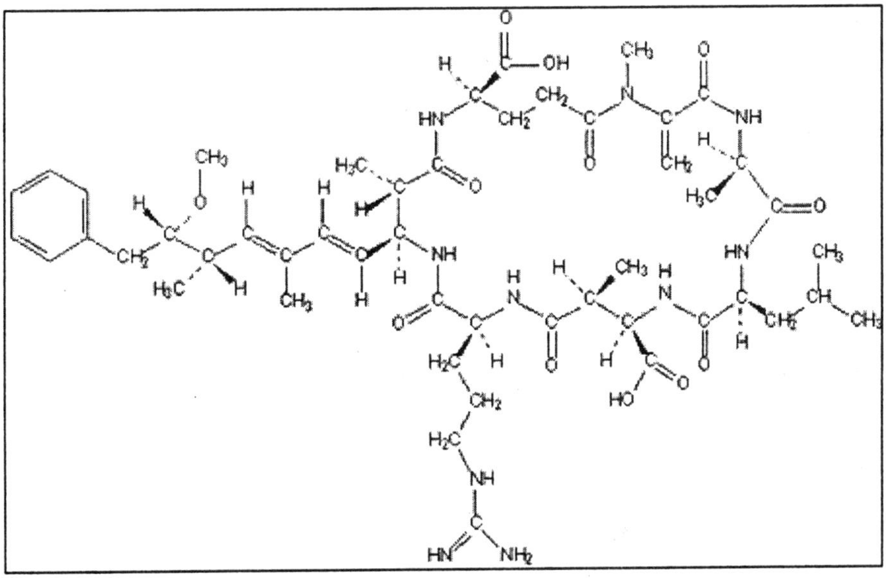

Microcystin LR

Potent inhibitor of protein phosphatase types 1 and 2A; has no effect on protein kinase.

Microcystin RR

Microcystin RR
Inhibitor of protein phosphatase type 2A with lower toxicity than microcystin LR.

Microcystin LA

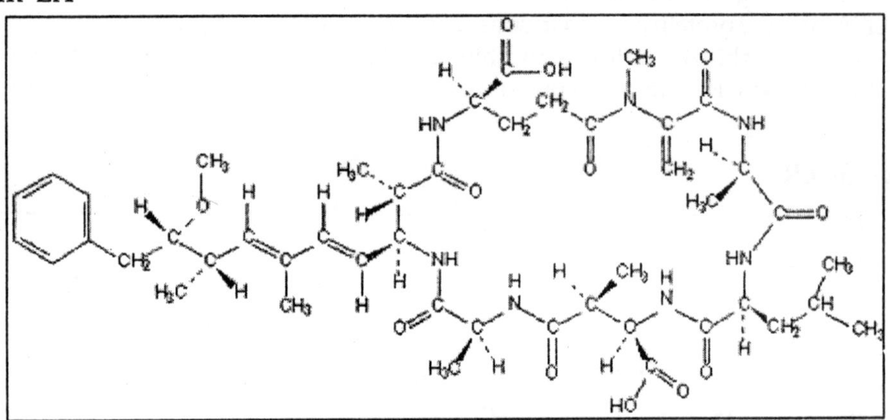

Microcystin LA
Inhibitor protein phosphatase type 2A and protein phosphatase type 3 more potently than protein phosphatase type 1 (order of potency PP2A > PP3 > PP1)

Cyanobacteria are capable of producing two kinds of toxin, the cyclic peptide hepatotoxin and the alkaloid neurotoxin. Serious illness such as hepatoenteritis, a symptomatic pneumonia and dermatitis may result from consumption of, or contact with water contaminated with toxin producing cyanobacteria (Hawkins *et al.*, 1985, Turner *et al.*, 1990). The neurotoxins include anatoxin-a, a depolarizing neuromuscular blocking agent; anatoxin-a [s], an anti–cholinesterase; and saxitoxin and neosaxitoxin that inhibit nerve conduction by blocking sodium channels (Carmicheal 1994).

Toxicity due to Cyanobacterial Toxins

Cyanobacterial toxins in drinking or recreational waters are also hazardous to human health. In India, the warm water temperature promotes dense *Microcystis* growth almost throughout the year.

Microcystin YR

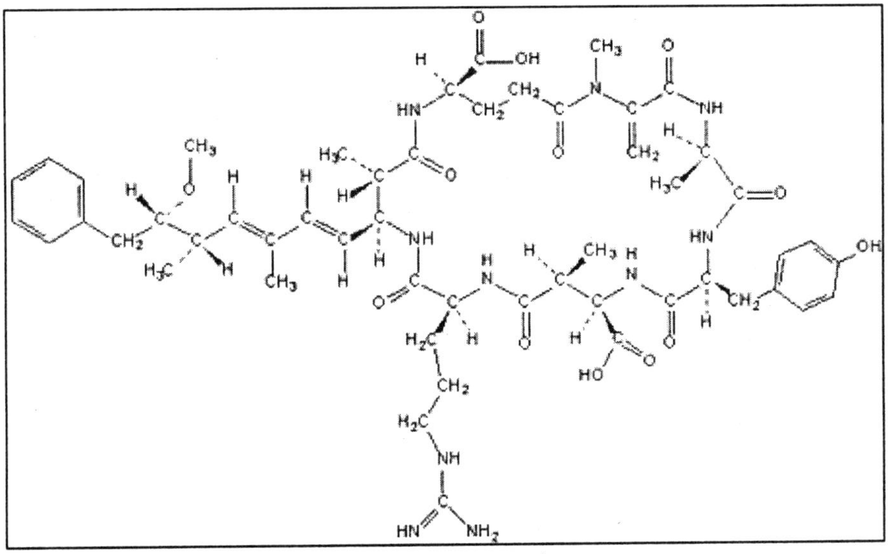

Microcystin YR
Inhibitor protein phosphatase type 2A and protein phosphatase type 1.

Cylindrospermopsin

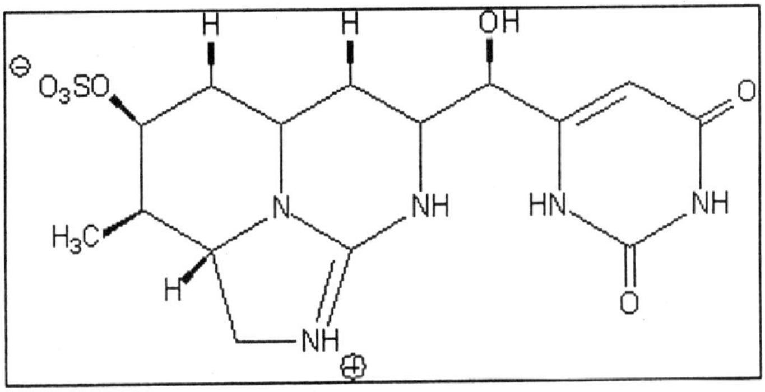

Cylindrospermopsin
Inhibition of protein synthesis. Target organ = liver

Although there is no evidence of human or animal lethality associated with these blooms, the occurrence of toxic blooms has been described in a few cases. In an epidemiologic study, it was found that patients with a history of bathing in *Microcystis*-infested ponds developed acute rhinosporidiosis, a disease caused by "pathogenic" strains of *Microcystis*. Several *Microcystis*-dominant phytoplankton materials collected from Central India have also been found to be toxic to the crustacean zooplankton *Moina macrocopa*. Accordingly, there have been many reports of the intoxication of birds, fish and other animals by cyanobacterial toxins (Vasconceles *et al.*, 2001, Alonso-Andicoberry *et al.*, 2002, Best *et al.*, 2002, Romanowska-Duda *et al.*, 2002, Krienitz *et al.*, 2003). As stated before, blooms of cyanobacteria

Nodularin

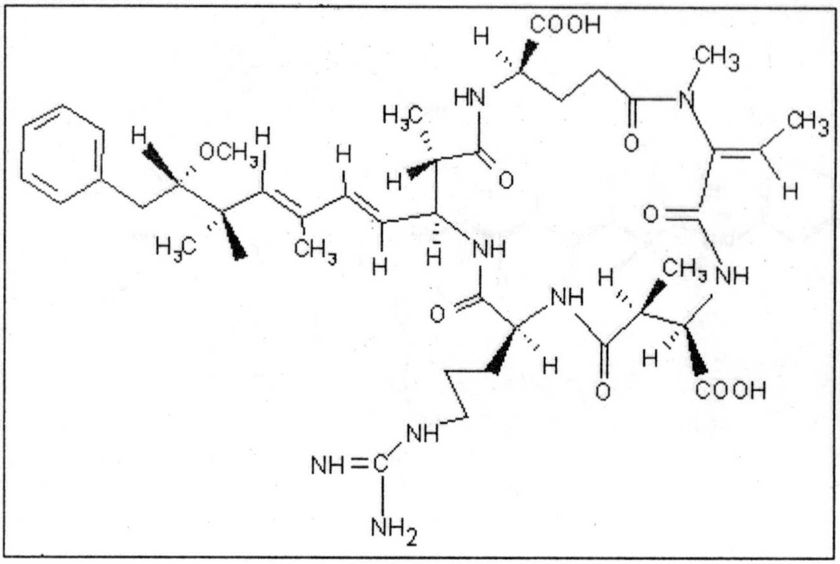

Nodularin
Potent inhibitor of protein phosphatases types 1 and 2A.

usually follow enrichment by nutrients such as phosphates and nitrates in the water. Most of these nutrients are derived from human wastes such as sewage and detergents, industrial pollution, run-off of fertilizers from agricultural land, and the input of animal or bird wastes from intensive farming (Bell and Codd 1994). Illnesses caused by cyanobacterial toxins to humans fall into three categories; gastroenteritis and related diseases, allergic and irritation reaction, and liver diseases. Microcystins have also been implicated as tumour-promoting substances (An and Carmichael 1994, Trogen *et al.*, 1996).

Impact of Toxins on Health of Man and his Pets

Microcystins are hepatotoxins (toxins that acts upon the liver) and known tumor promoters. If people drink water contaminated by microcystins, symptoms of exposure include nausea, vomiting and, in very rare but severe cases, acute liver failure. Reported health effects from cyanobacteria in humans are highly uncommon in the United States. Although the likelihood of people being affected by a *Microcystis* bloom is low, minor skin irritation can occur with contact, and gastrointestinal discomfort can also occur if water from a bloom is ingested.

Through the recreational use of contaminated water, cyanobacterial blooms of *Microcystis*, *Anabaena*, and others have been linked to incidence of human illness in many countries, but no fatalities have been reported (Lambert *et al.*, 1994b). In Canada, human illnesses have been reported in Saskatchewan, with symptoms including stomach cramps, vomiting, diarrhoea, fever, headache, pains in muscles and joints, and weakness (Dillenberg and Dehnel 1960). Similar symptoms as well as skin, eye, and throat irritation and allergic responses to cyanobacterial toxins in water have also been reported in other countries. The reported instances of illnesses are few, but, because they are difficult to diagnose, such illnesses may in fact be more common than has been reported (Carmichael and Falconer 1993).

Factors Affecting the Cyanobacterial Blooms

Physical Factors

Temperature

In general, cyanobacteria prefer warm conditions, and low temperatures are one of the major factors that end cyanobacterial blooms. Temperature alone may only partly determine bloom formation and it is accepted that a combination of factors are responsible for a bloom to develop. These are increasing temperatures, decreasing nutrients and increased water column stability. Van der Westhuizen and Eloff (1985) determined that temperature has the most pronounced effect on toxicity. At temperatures of 32°C and 36°C cell culture's toxicity was 1.6 and 4 times less than cells cultured at 28°C, suggesting that highest growth rate is not correlated with highest toxicity.

Light and Buoyancy

The effect of light intensity on the fine structure of *Microcystis aeruginosa* under laboratory conditions has been investigated. The optimal growth rate for *M. aeruginosa* cells was at 3,600-18,000 lux. At light levels in the excess of 18,000 lux the growth rate declined rapidly. Buoyancy is regulated by a number of mechanisms, such as the form of stored carbohydrates and turgor pressure regulation. Compositional changes in the protein: carbohydrate ratios during buoyancy reversals suggest a complex relationship between light and nutrients (N: P) (Villareal and Carpenter 2003). It however, seems that the regulation of gas vacuole synthesis is the most important. This almost unique feature of cyanobacteria gives these organisms a significant advantage over other phytoplanktons. In turbulent waters cyanobacteria loose this advantage and often this characteristic is used to control their blooms (Grobbelaar 2002).

Chemical Factors

Nitrogen and Phosphorus Ratios

It is becoming increasingly apparent that, notwithstanding the prevailing nitrogen and phosphorus ratio, the phytoplankton assemblage may be significantly altered through biomanipulation, and without any change whatsoever to the ambient availability of nitrogen and phosphorus (Harding and Wright 1999). Carmichael (1986) demonstrated that the omission of nitrogen causes approximately tenfold decrease in toxicity.

Iron and Zinc

Certain metal ions such as Zn^{2+} and Fe^{2+} significantly influence toxin yield. Zn^{2+} is involved in the hydrolysis of phosphate esters, the replication and transcription of nucleic acids, and the hydration and dehydration of CO_2 (Sunda 1991). All cyanobacteria require Fe^{2+} for important physiological functions such as photosynthesis, nitrogen assimilation, respiration and chlorophyll synthesis (Boyer *et al.*, 1987). It is not yet clear how Fe^{2+} deficiency modulates microcystin production, but it has been noted that as Cyanobacteria experience iron stress, they appear to compensate for some of the effects of iron loss by synthesizing new polypeptides (Lukac and Aegerter 1993).

Prevention and Control of Cyanobacterial Toxins

Chemical Control

Traditional methods for controlling algal blooms include use of copper sulfate and urea which have not only been found to be extremely expensive but cause adverse effects on aquatic biota when employed for the control of blooms in recreational water. Such treated water may also be unhealthy for further use. Few researchers were able to provide some basic information about the role of K^+ in controlling *Microcystis* growth. They conducted an extensive survey of over 21 Indian ponds and assayed the concentrations of various heavy metals (Cu, Cr, Ni, Zn, Pb, Mn), cations (Na^+, K^+, Ca^+) and nutrients (ammonium, phosphate, nitrate) commonly present in pond water of Varanasi, India. They came across very interesting results that Na^+ concentrations remain constant in almost all ponds surveyed but the K^+ concentration varied. Keeping in mind the above finding, these workers provided evidence that NaCl stimulates while KCl strongly inhibits the growth of *Microcystis* in both pond water and in defined media.

Biological Control

One alternative approach to the control of algal blooms involves the use of biological control (biocontrol) agents. Predatory bacteria that are indigenous to the lake environment have been isolated from algal blooms. Daft *et al.* (1985) proposed the following seven attributes that defined a good predatory bacterial agent:

1. Adaptability to variations in physical conditions
2. Ability to search for or trap prey
3. Capacity and ability to multiply
4. Prey consumption
5. Ability to survive low prey densities (switch or adapt to other food sources)
6. Wide host range, and
7. Ability to respond to changes in the host.

The practice of introduction of foreign microbial agents has raised some concern with regards to environmental safety due to the so-called host specificity paradigm involving host switching (HS) and host range expansion (HRE) (Secord 2003). Biocontrol of cyanobacteria, like other control measures for nuisance organisms, is often viewed with caution. This may be attributed to the experiences of plant pathologists who observed the destruction of important crops such as chestnut blight in the United States and potato blight in Ireland after the accidental release of pathogens (Atlas and Bartha 1998).

Viral pathogens would be ideal as biocontrol agents as they are target selective and specific for nuisance cyanobacteria. However, bacterial agents are considered more suitable than viruses as biocontrol agents because bacteria can survive on alternate food sources during non-bloom periods and the possibility of mutation within the host is not problematic, as bacterial predation is not reliant on unique attachment receptors (Rashidan and Bird 2001).

The Use of Microorganisms to Control Cyanobacterial Blooms

In the natural environment, there are predatory microorganisms that are antagonistic towards particular nuisance organisms (weeds, cyanobacteria) thus providing a natural means of controlling these nuisance organisms. Microbial agents antagonistic to algae (bacteria, fungi, virus and protozoa) have been isolated from harmful algal blooms (Burnham *et al.*, 1981, Ashton and Robarts, 1987, Yamamoto *et al.*, 1998, Sigee *et al.*, 1999, Walker and Higginbotham 2000, Rashidan and Bird 2001, Nakamura *et al.*, 2003a, Choi *et al.*, 2005). These microbial agents may play a major role in the prevention, regulation and termination of harmful algal blooms. Such microbial populations are called microbial herbicides (Atlas and Bartha 1998). The biological control of cyanobacteria provides a potential control measure to reduce the population of nuisance algal blooms to manageable levels. In many cases these bacterial agents are species- or genus-specific (Rashidan and Bird 2001), while others attack a variety of cyanobacteria (Daft *et al.*, 1985). The predatory bacteria are classified as members of the *Bacteroides-Cytophaga- Flavobacterium*, ranging from *Bacillus* spp. to *Flexibacter* spp., *Cytophaga* and *Myxobacteria.*

Choi *et al.* (2005) isolated the bacterium, *Streptomyces neyagawaensis*, which had a *Microcystis*-killing ability, from the sediment of a eutrophic lake in Korea. Under natural conditions, *Cytophaga* spp. was implicated in the demise of marine red tides caused by the flagellate *Chatonella* spp. in the Seto Inland Sea of Japan. *Bacillus cereus* N14 was isolated by Nakamura *et al.* (2003a) from a eutrophic lake in Japan and caused lysis of the *viridis.* Caiola and Pellegrini (1984) showed cells of *Microcystis aeruginosa* that were infected and lysed by *Bdellovibrio*-like bacteria in bloom containing water samples from Lake Varse Italy. Blakeman and Fokkerna (1982) observed that naturally occurring, resident microorganisms adapt to survive and grow in a specific habitat. If these organisms were effective antagonists against a pathogen, they would be preferred for biocontrol purposes. Organisms from other habitats, which may be equally antagonistic to the pathogen, would be less likely to survive, and consequently would have to be reapplied more frequently. The same would be true in other habitats, such as where antagonists are used to control cyanobacterial blooms.

However, there are disadvantages, which include the limited destruction of the target organism, limited survival of the microbial agent or its removal by other organisms, problems of large scale production, storage and application, as well as reluctance to apply microbial agents in a field environment.

References

Alonso-Andicoberry, C., Garcia-Villada, L., Lopez-Rodas, V. and Costas, E. (2002). Catastrophic mortality of flamingos in a Spanish National Park caused by cyanobacteria. *Veterinary Record* 151: 706-707.

An, J. and Carmichael, W.W. (1994). Use of a colorimetric protein phosphatase inhibition assay and enzyme linked immunosorbentassay for the study of microcystins and nodularins. *Toxicon* 32: 1495-1507.

Ashton, P.J. and Robarts, R.D. (1987). Apparent predation of *Microcystis aeruginosa* kutz emend elenkin by a Saprospira-like bacterium in a hypertrophic lake (Hartbeespoort dam, South Africa). *J Limnol Soc* S. Afr 13: 44-47.

Atlas, R.M. and Bartha, R. (1998). Microbial Ecology: Fundamentals and Applications. 4th edition. Benjamin/Cummings Science Publishers, 2725 Sand/Hill Road, Menlo Park, California 94025. p. 698.

Bell, S.G. and Codd, G.A. (1994). Cyanobacterial toxins and health hazards. Reviews in Medical Microbiology 5: 256-264.

Best, J.H., Pflugmacher, S., Wiegand, C., Eddy, F.B., Metcalf, J.S. and Codd, G.A. (2002). Effects on enteric bacterial and cyanobacterial lipopolysaccharides, and of microcystin-LR, on glutathione transferase activities in zebra fish (*Danio rerio*). *Aquatic Toxicol* 60: 223-231.

Bisby, F.A. (1995). Characterization of Biodiversity pp. 21-106 *In:* Global Biodiversity Assessment. (Eds.) Heywood V H and Waston R T. Cambridge University Press, Cambridge.

Blakeman, J.P. and Fokkerna, N.J. (1982). Potential for biological control of plant diseases on the phylloplane. *Ann Rev Phyopathol* 20: 167-192.

Boyer, G.L., Gillam, A.H. and Trick, C.G. (1987). Iron chelation and uptake. *In*: The Cyanobacteria. (Eds.) Van Baalen C and Fay P. Elsevier Science: New York, pp. 415-436.

Burnham, J.C., Collart, S.A. and Highison, B.W. (1981). Entrapment and lysis of the cyanobacterium *Phormidum luridum* by aqueous colonies of *Myxococcus xanthus* PCO2. *Arch Microbiol* 129: 285-294.

Caiola, M.G. and Pellegrini, S. (1984). Lysis of *Microcystis aeruginosa* (Kutz) by Bdellovibrio-like bacteria. *J Phycol* 20: 471-475

Choi, H.J., Kim, B.H., Kim, J.D. and Han, M.S. (2005). *Streptomyces neyagawaensis* as a control for the hazardous biomass of (cyanobacteria) in eutrophic freshwaters. *Biol Control* 33: 335-343.

Carmichael, W.W. (1994). The toxins of Cyanobacteria. Scientific American 270: 78-86.

Carmichael, W.W. and Falconer, I.R. (1993). Diseases related to freshwater blue-green algal toxins, and control measures. *In*: Falconer IR, (ed.) Algal Toxins in Seafood and Drinking Water. London, Academic Press, pp. 187-209.

Daft, M.J., Burnham, J.C. and Yamamato, Y. (1985). Algal blooms: conesquences and potential cures. J. Appl. Bacteriol Symp Suppl 175S-186S.

Daft, M.J., Mc Cord, S.B. and Stewart, W.D.P. (1975). Ecological studies on algal lysing bacteria in freshwaters. *Freshwater Biol* 5: 577-596.

Dillenberg, H.O. and Dehnel, M.K. (1960). Toxic water bloom in Saskatchewan. *Canadian Med Asso Journal* 83:1151-1154.

Gajdek, P. (2000). Mikrocystyny sinic W zbiornikach wodnych. Wiadomollci Chemiczne 54: 637-650.

Greuter, W., Barrie, F., Burdet, H.M., Chaloner, W.G., Demoulin, V., Hawksworth, D.L., Jorgensen, P.M., Nicholson, D.H., Silva, P.C., Trehane, P. and Mcneill, J. (1994). International Code of Botanical Nomenclature (Tokyo code), Koletz Scientific Books, Konigstein.

Grobbelaar, J.U. (2002). Dynamics of toxin production by Cyanobacteria. WRC Report: K5/1029/0/1.

Harding, W.R. and Wright, S. (1999). Initial findings regarding changes in phyto and zooplankton composition and abundance following the temporary drawdown and refilling of a shallow, hypertrophic South African costal lake. *J Lake Reservoir Manage* 15: 47-53.

Hawkins, P.R., Runnegar, M.T.C., Jackson, A.R.B. and Falconer, I.R. (1985). Severe hepatoxicity caused by the tropical cyanobacterium (Blue-Green alga) *Cylindrospermopsis reciborskii* (Wolonszynzka) Seenaya and Subba Raju isolated from a domestic water supply reservoir *Appl Environ Microbiol* 50: 1292-1295.

Krienitz, L., Ballot, A., Kotut, K., Wiegand, C., Putz, S., Metcalf, J.S., Codd, G.A. and Pflugmacher, S. (2003). Contribution of hot spring cyanobacteria to the mysterious deaths of Lesser flamingos at Lake Bogoria, Kenya. FEMS *Microbiol. Ecol* 43: 141-148.

Lambert, T.W., Holmes, C.F.B. and Hrudey, S.E. (1994). Microcystin class of toxins: health effects and safety of drinking water supplies. *Environmental review* 2:167-186.

Lukac, M. and Aegerter, R. (1993). Influence of trace metals on growth and toxin production of *Microcystis aeruginosa*. *Toxicon* 31: 293-305.

Nakamura, N., Nakano, K., Sungira, N. and Matsumura, M. (2003). A novel control process of cyanobacterial bloom using cyanobacteriolytic bacteria immobilized in floating biodegradable plastic carriers. *Environ. Technol* 24: 1569-1576.

Rashidan, K.K. and Bird, D.F. (2001). Role of predatory bacteria in the termination of a cyanobacterial bloom. *Microbial Ecol* 41: 97-105.

Rinehart, K.L. *et al.* (1988). Nodularin, microcystin and the configuration of Adda. *J. Am. Chem. Soc.,* 110(25): 8557-8558.

Rippka, R., Deruelles, J., Waterbury, J.B., Herdman, M. and Stanier, R.Y. (1979). Generic assignments strain histories and properties of pure cultures of cyanobacteria. *J Gen Microbiol* 111: 1–61.

Romanowska-Duda, Z., Mankiewicz, J., Tarczynska, M., Walter, Z. and Zalewski, M. (2002). The effect of toxic cyanobacteria (blue-green algae) on water plants and animal cells. *Polish J. Environ Studies* 11: 561- 566.

Secord, D. (2003). Biological control of marine invasive species: cautionary tales and land-based lesions. *Biol. Invasions* 5: 117-131.

Sigee, D.C., Glenn, R., Andrews, M.J., Bellinger, E.G., Butler, R.D., Epton, H.A.S. and Hendry, R.D. (1999). Biological control of cyanobacteria: principles and possibilities. *In*: The Ecological Bases for Lake and Reservoir Management, (Eds.) Harper DM, Brierley, Ferguson AJD, Philips G. Kluwer Academic Publishers, Netherlands 395 (396): 161- 172.

Sneath, P.H.A. (1992). International Code of Nomenclature of Bacteria, 1990 Revision. Amer Soc Microbiol Washington, D C.

Sunda, W.G. (1991). Trace metal interactions with marine phytoplankton. *Biol. Oceanogr* 6: 442-511.

Turner, P.C., Gammie, A.J., Hollinrake, K. and Codd, G.A. (1990). Pneumonia associated with contact with Cyanobacteria. *Brit Med J* 300: 1440- 1441.

Trogen, G.B., Annila, A., Eriksson, J., Kontteli, M., Meriluoto, J., Sethson, I., Zdunek, J. and Edlung, U. (1996). Conformational studies of microcystin-LR using NMR spectroscopy and molecular dynamics calculations. *Biochemistry* 35: 3197-3205.

Villareal, T.A. and Carpenter, E.J. (2003). Bouyancy regulation and the potential for vertical migration in the oceanic cyanobacterium *Trichodesmium. Microbial Ecol* 45: 1-10.

Van der, Westhuizen, A.J. and Eloff, J.N. (1985). Effects of temperature and light on toxicity and growth of the blue-green alga *Microcystis aeruginosa*[UV-006]. *Planta* 163: 55-59.

Vasconceles, V., Olivera, S. and Teles, F.O. (2001). Impact of a toxic and a non-toxic strain of *Microcystis aeruginosa* on the crayfish *Procambarus clarkii. Toxicon* 39: 1461-1470.

Waterbury, J.B. (1992). The Cyanobacteria isolation, purification and identification pp. 2058–2078. *In:* Balows H G, truper M, Dworkin M, Harder W and Schleifer K H (eds) *The Prokaryotes.* Second edition, Volume II. Springer Verlag, New York.

Yamamoto, Y., Kouchiwa, T., Hodoki, Y., Hotta, K., Uchida, H. and Harada, K. (1998). Distribution and identification of actinomycetes lysing cyanobacteria in a eutrophic lake. *J Appl Phycol* 10: 391-397.

Microbial Biotechnology and Ecology (2011) *Pages* **162–167**
Editors: **Deepak Vyas, G.S. Paliwal, P.K.Khare and R.K Gupta**
Published by: **DAYA PUBLISHING HOUSE, NEW DELHI**

Chapter 8

Antibacterial Potential of Diazotrophic Cyanobacteria: A Natural Strategy to Maintain Nitrogen Budget in Tropical Lowlands

☆ *Usha Pandey*

Faculty of Science and Technology, M.G. Kashividya Pith, Varanasi – 221 005, U.P.

ABSTRACT

Cyanobacteria are now considered as one of the most potential groups of organisms which can be useful to mankind in numerous ways. They are important component of soil microflora and contribute to nutrient enrichment in a variety of habitats including agricultural lands. For this reason, many species of cyanobacteria are used in the management of soil fertility. This study examined the antibacterial potential of four diazotrophic cyanobacteria namely *Oscillatoria limnetica*, *O. limosa*, *Nostoc calcicola*, and *N. piscinale* against the denitrifying bacterium *Pseudomonas denitrificans*. Addition of cell extracts (500 mg L^{-1}) of cyanobacteria in the growth medium resulted significantly lower growth and denitrification by *P. denitrificans*. *O. limnetica* showed superiority over rest of the species in this respect. Inhibition of growth of *P denitrificans* and its denitrification potential reduce N–losses in the ecosystem. This antagonistic potential of diazotrophic cyanobacteria can be exploited for management of soil fertility in tropical water–logged soils. On global scale, this natural strategy of cyanobacteria could help regulating N–cycle.

Introduction

Cyanobacteria, which constitute a versetille group of microorganisms, occur in divers habitats ranging from alkaline hot springs to permanent snow fields in poles. In addition to being primary producer, many cyanobacteria are capable of fixing molecular nitrogen. In tropics, where nitrogen often becomes a limiting factor for productivity in agriculture, diazotrophic cyanobacteria contribute significantly in maintaining nitrogen budget and fertility of agricultural lands. However, the process of denitrification, which converts nitrate into molecular nitrogen returning it back to the atmosphere, create an imbalance in soil nitrogen economy. The denitrification is especially rapid in tropical lowlands where elevated temperature coupled with low oxygen tension due to frequent water logging promotes the growth of denitrifying anaerobes. Spatial and temporal variations in field conditions and thus denitrifying activity are also caused by cycles of wetting and drying, which promote nitrification followed by denitrification (Knowles, 1982).

Denitrification is a process of dissimilatory reduction of NO_3^- and NO_2^- in which the major product is nitrous oxide (N_2O), which may further reduced to dinitrogen (N_2). In fact, N_2O is a free intermediate in the reduction of other nitrogen oxides to dinitrogen. When denitrification occurs under conditions favourable for this process, N_2O is produced only transiently. Denitrification is a major mechanism of loss of nitrogen in fertilizer use and release of N_2O to the atmosphere, where it involves in stratospheric reactions resulting in the depletion of ozone. Interestingly, however, denitrification is an essential mechanism to maintain global nitrogen budget (N–cycle). Nitrous oxide reductase (N_2O R) enzyme plays a significant role in reduction of nitrogen oxides. This is a membrane bound enzyme reported in *Pseudomonas perfectomarinus* (Payne *et al.*, 1971). The enzyme was present in the soluble fraction and, although extremely labile, has a half life of about 1h at room temperature. McCarthy *et al.* (1981) reported that electron transport to N_2O R generates a membrane potential only slightly smaller than that associated with O_2 utilization. It involves cytochromes of type b and c, which are membrane associated cytochromes in *Pseudomonas denitrificans*. Furthermore, continuous culture studies of energy yields in this organism growing on various nitrogen oxides suggest that energy conservation is associated with the use of N_2O as electron acceptor (Matsubara, 1975).

Certain cyanobacteria are known for their toxin production properties (McGregor and Fabbro, 2000; Pandey and Pandey, 2002). The capacity of some strains to release extracellular compounds that inhibit the growth of other microorganisms has now been considered as an important factor contributing to the formation and maintenance of cyanobacterial blooms (Bormans, 1999). Such mechanisms could be major determinants regulating nutrient balance, especially N–budgeting of a particular habitat. The antibacterial potential of cyanobacteria can affect the co–existing populations of microorganisms including denitrifying bacteria to minimize niche overlap and resource sharing and conservation. Such aspects of cyanobacteria are relatively less explored. In particular, no data so far is available on antagonistic potential of cyanobacteria against denitrifying anaerobes in Indian tropics. The present study is an effort in this direction with its possible relevance in maintaining nitrogen budget of tropical lowlands. In the present study, four strains of cyanobacteria namely, *Oscillatoria limnetica, Oscillatoria limosa, Nostoc calcicola*, and *Nostoc piscinale* were chosen for their antibacterial potential towards *Pseudomonas denitrificans*, an important denitrifying bacterium.

Materials and Methods

Cyanobacterial samples were collected from natural habitats and standard microbial techniques were employed for selection, isolation and clonal propagation of cyanobacteria. In brief, cyanobacterial mats collected from natural habitats were crushed with sterilized glass beads, diluted in sterilized double distilled water and spread on agar plates containing BG–11 medium and incubated until visible colonies appeared (Santra, 1993). Identification was made following Desikachary (1959). Colonies were picked up using sterilized micro-capillaries and transferred to culture tubes containing

10 ml liquid BG–11 medium. Growth was visible in tubes after 10 days of incubation. Such clonal cutures were washed thrice with sterilized double distilled water through repeated centrifugation and subsequently transferred to fresh BG–11 medium to obtain desirable population size. Cultures were incubated at 24 ± 1°C and illuminated for 10 days with cool day light fluorescent tubes (intensity 14.4 Wm^{-2}) on surface of the culture vessel with a 18/6 h night/dark cycle.

For the preparation of cyanobacterial cell extract, 10 g of 8 days old laboratory grown filaments of different strains were taken separately. Aqueous extracts of cyanobacteria, prepared as described in Pandey and Pandey (2002), were filtered separately through Whatman filter paper and filtrates were used for experiment.

The inhibitory effect of cell extracts of cyanobacteria on *Pseudomonas denitrificans* was studied following plate diffusion assay (Deora *et al.*, 2007). Actively growing bacterial culture was incorporated into presterilized cooled molten agar medium mixed thoroughly and dispersed into properly sterilized petri plates. After solidification, wells of 0.5 mm diameter were made using a sterilized cork borer and 10 ml of cyanobacterial extracts were carefully poured into wells. These plates were kept for 24h in bacteriological incubator at 28 °C. The inhibition zones formed due to allelopathic effect of cell extracts were measured. Bacterial growth was measured by Nephelo turbidity meter in the presence and absence of cyanobacterial cell extracts. Enzyme nitrous oxide reductase (N_2O R) was measured following the method of Kristjansson and Hollocher (1980). Percent reduction in denitrification was expressed in terms of loss of activity of nitrous oxide reductase in the presence of cyanobacterial cell extracts. Nitrous oxide reductase is the terminal enzyme that converts nitrous oxide to dinitrogen.

Data presented here represent the mean of three independent experiments. Variability is expressed in terms of standard error and paired t–test was used to represent significant differences from respective control.

Results and Discussion

Mean diameters of inhibition zone formed due to the antagonistic effects of cyanobacterial extracts are presented in Table 8.1. All the tested cyanobacteria inhibited the growth of *P. denitrificans* and the effect was maximum in case of *O. limnetica* followed by *O. limosa, N. piscinale* and minimum in *N. calcicola*. Suikkanen *et al.* (2006) have investigated the allelopathic effects of three cyanobacteria on phytoplankton and suggested it as a mechanism for the formation and maintenance of blooms by removing potential competitors. All the strains of cyanobacteria considered in this study are diazotrophs and commonly found in agricultural fields.

Cell extracts of all the four cyanobacteria were inhibitory to growth of *Pseudomonas denitrificans*. *Oscillatoria limnetica* cell extract was found to be the most effective in this respect (Table 8.2). At 500 ml L^{-1} concentration of *O. limnetica* cell extract the growth of the bacterium was almost negligible. For *O. limosa, N. calcicola* and *N. piscinale*, the effectiveness remained over 95 per cent at same concentration of cell extracts. These trends were consistent with those recorded for enzyme nitrous oxide reductase (N_2O R) activity (Figure 8.1). Denitrification measured in terms of

Table 8.1: Size of Inhibition Zones Formed in Cultures of *P. denitrificans* Resulting from Cyanobacterial Extracts. Values are mean ± 1SE.

Cyanobacteria	*Diameter of Inhibition Zone (mm)*
Oscillatoria limnetica	19.5 ± 1.35
Oscillatoria limosa	15.0 ± 1.26
Nostoc calcicola	9.5 ± 1.02
Nostoc piscinale	11.0 ± 1.04

nitrous oxide reductase activity was reduced by 78 per cent at 500 mg L^{-1} cell extract concentration of *O. limnetica*. For *O. limosa*, *N. calcicola* and *N. piscinale*, percent reductions in denitrification, in terms of N_2O R activity were 70, 61 and 68 respectively (Figure 8.1).

Table 8.2: Effect of Cyanobacterial Cell Extracts (500 mg L^{-1}) on Growth of *Pseudomonas denitrificans*

Time (h)	*Control*	*Growth of P. denitrificans (NTU)**			
		O. limnetica Cell Extract	*O. limosa Cell Extract*	*N. calcicola Cell Extract*	*N. piscinale Cell Extract*
0	0.03	0.03	0.03	0.03	0.03
24	3.5	0.04[a]	0.08[a]	0.09[a]	0.08[a]
48	7.5	0.04[a]	0.18[a]	0.23[a]	0.21[a]
72	7.9	0.04[a]	0.18[a]	0.23[a]	0.21[a]

*NTU: Nephelo Turbidity Unit.

a: Differences from respective controls are significant at $p < 0.01$ (analysis performed using paired t–test).

Denitrification is an essential process as for as N–cycle is concerned. However, from standpoint of agriculrure, denitrification is an undesirable process as it results in loss of nitrogen from the soil and hence a decline in nutrient available for plant growth. Because of the changing conditions and pulsed input associated with both natural and agricultural soils, denitrifying bacteria undergo flushes

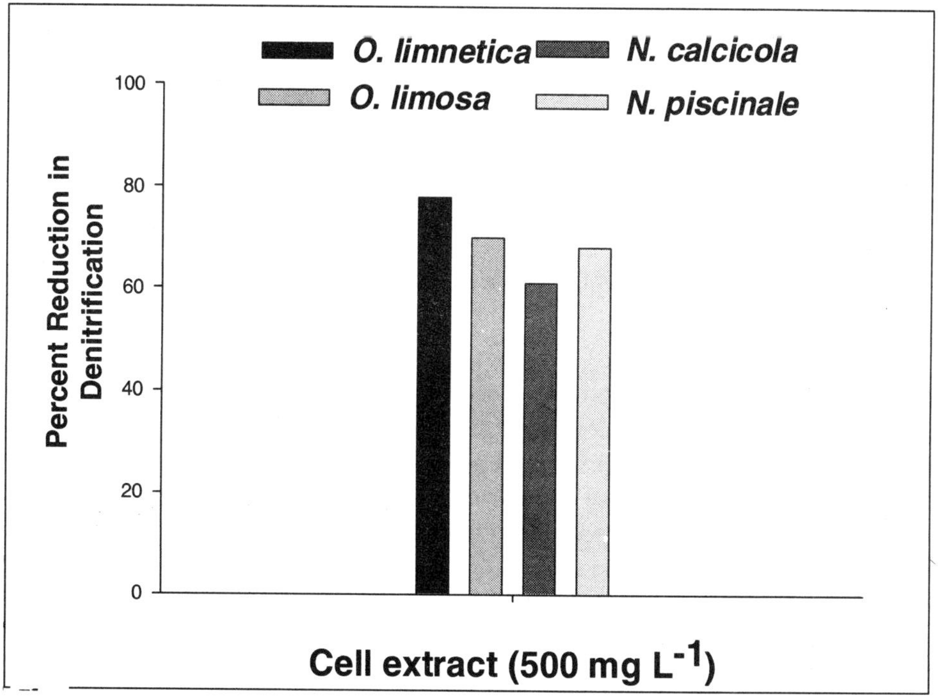

Figure 8.1: Percent Reduction in Denitrification (Measured in terms of N_2O R activity) in the Presence of Cyanobacterial Cell Extracts

of activity of short or long duration. Tropical lowland soils generally act as source of N_2O due to conditions favorable for denitrification. They can however act as N_2O sinks under complete anaerobic condition, readly availability of organic carbon and absence of NO_3^- (Knowles, 1982). The problem of denitrification is specially acute in tropical lowlands where elevated temperature, abundance of organic matter, neutral to alkaline pH and limited oxygen supply due to frequent water–logging, all together accelerate the process of denitrification. Data generated in this study suggest that continuous association of such cyanobacteria as *O. limnetica*, *O. limosa*, *N. calcicola* and *N. piscinale* with *P. denitrificans* may help maintaining nitrogen economy of lowland crop fields. As indicated in terms of growth and N_2O R activity, suppression of growth of *P. denitrificans* due to antagonistic activity of these diazotrophs suggests that these cyanobacteria have evolved strategy to maintain high nitrogen status of soil not only by fixing atmospheric N but also by conserving the fixed N in lowlands of tropics by reducing the growth of denitrifying anaerobes. In paddy fields, massive cyanobacterial mats could play significant role in inhibiting the growth of denitrifying anaerobes besides fixing atmospheric N_2.

Potential management of denitrification is essential for maintaining soil fertility stability especially in tropical water–logged soils. So far, the manipulation of soil conditions to inhibit denitrification is being used as the most general practice for management of denitrification in agriculture. Although more data may be required for field–scale verification, the present study clearly indicates that the antagonistic potential of diazotrophic cyanobacteria can be exploited as a management tool for N–addition as well as for minimizing denitrification–linked N–losses in agricultural fields. The study forms the first report of alleopathic effects of cyanobacteria towards denitrifying bacterium. This has relevance in budgeting the global nitrogen cycle as well as in generating genetically important strains of cyanobacteria to reduce N loss due to denitrification along with fixing dinitrogen.

References

Bormans, M. (1999). Controlling algal blooms in the Fitzroy River. *River for the Future* (10): 26–29.

Deora, G. S., Bhati, D. and Jain, N. S. (2007). Antibiotic effects of certain bryophytes on *Agrobacterium tumifacians*. *Journal of Pure and Applied Microbiology* (1): 215–219.

Desikachary, T. V. (1959). *Cyanobacteria*. Indian council of Agricultural Research, New Delhi. 1–686.

Knowles, R. (1982). Denitrification. *Microbiological Reviews* (46): 43–70.

Kristjansson, J. K. and T. C. Hollocher (1980). First practical assay for soluble nitrous oxide reductase of denitrifying bacteria and a partial kinetic characterization. *Journal of Biological Chemistry* (255): 704–707.

Matsubara, T. (1975). The participation of cytochromes in the reduction of N_2O to N_2 by denitrifying bacterium. *Journal of Biochemistry* (77): 627–632.

McCarthy, J. E. G., Ferguson, S. J. and Kell, D. B. (1981). Estimation with an iron selective electrode of the membrane potential in cells of *Paracoccus denitrificans* from the uptake of the butyltriphenyl–phosphorium cation during aerobic and anaerobic respiration. *Biochemistry Journal* (196): 311–321.

McGregor, G. B. and Fabbro, L. D. (2000). Dominance of *cylindrospermopsis raciborskii* (Nostocales, Cyanoprokaryota) in Queensland tropical and subtropical reservoirs : Implications for monitoring and management. *Lakes and Reservoirs : Research and Management* (5): 195–205.

Pandey, U. and Pandey, J. (2002). Antibacterial properties of cyanobacteria : A cost effective and ecofriendly approach to control bacterial leaf spot disease of chilli. *Current Science* (82): 262–264.

Payne, W. J. Riley, P. S. and Cox, C. D. (1971). Separate nitrite, nitric oxide and nitrogen oxide reducing fractions from *Pseudomonas perfectomarinus*. *Journal of Bacteriology* (106): 356–361.

Santra, S. C. (1993). *Biology of Rice Field Blue Green Algae*. Daya Publishing House. Delhi. 1- 84.

Suikkanen, S., Engström–Öst, J., Jokela, J., Sivonen, K. and Viitasalo, M. (2006). Allelopathy of Baltic Sea cyanobacteria: no evidence for the role of nodularin. *Journal of Plankton Research* (28): 543–550.

Microbial Biotechnology and Ecology (2011)
Editors: Deepak Vyas, G.S. Paliwal, P.K.Khare and R.K Gupta
Published by: DAYA PUBLISHING HOUSE, NEW DELHI

Pages 168–188

Chapter 9

Histochemical Studies on Some Petro-Plants Infected with AM Fungus (*Glomus fasciculatum*)

☆ *H.C. Lakshman*

Department of Botany, Microbiology Laboratory, Karnataka University, Dharwad – 580 003, Karnataka

Introduction

Imagine a day when you get up in the morning and read the newspaper headlines. 'The petroleum company has gone on strike' with this thought in your mind you start for your work. You are in your car driving towards your workplace and your car gives it up, you have to walk and further the entire day filled with hardship. Now multiply this intense feeling with the possibility of it lasting forever. In such a nightmare our so-called valuation lifestyle, rather our very existence shall be in a dilemma. We do not intent to exaggerate this worst-case scenario but to prove the grievousness of energy crisis.

The probability of such an extremity is evident in the future. This is because ever since the beginning of time Man has been depending extensively on fossil fuel for his every requirement and as time passed this requirement increased many folds and so did his dependency on this limited source of energy. As a result by the year 2020 the total fossil fuel supply will fall to a meager 10 per cent.

To meet this acute shortage, the technology aimed at the utilization of renewable energy that can serve to replace fossil fuel hydrocarbons needs to be expanded. The basic composition of these fossil fuels is hydrocarbons. In 1979 Dr. Calvin for the first time discovered hydrocarbons in latex of some plants, these hydrocarbons from plants have a great potential of replacing the fossil fuel hydrocarbon. Thus started the pioneering work towards the very obvious renewable source of petroleum, in the future–"The petrocrops"/petroplants. There are about 400 species of petrocrop plants in India itself, which are hoped to yield 40-45 barrels of fuel per acre.

A histochemical process is essential to study the structural organization of the vesicular-arbuscular mycorrhiza in cells and tissues. This technique is one of the useful tools in understanding basic biology of AM fungi and their interactions at the anatomical and physiological levels with host cells/tissues. Histochemical protocols have been integral components of investigation on AM fungi and their host plants. Gallaud (1905) for the first time explained, how fungal components could be stained by using cotton blue. AM inoculated strawberries gained the root sections by using Lactic acid and acid fuchsine with pioric acid O'Brien and McNaughton (1928). Daft and Nicolson (1966) used methylene blue. Such staining techniques were also proposed by other workers (Furlan *et al.*, 1973; Mossoe and Hopper, 1975; Davis and Menge, 1981). Philips and Hayman (1970) had given modified and improved staining procedure for rapid assessment of infection of root with vesicular arbuscular mycorrhizae. Kessler and Blank (1972) demonstrated the localization of phenolic substances and polyphosphates in *Eucalyptus* roots colonized by ecto and endo and ecto-endo mycorrhiza. Many workers are of the opinion that the localization of different chemical substances formed during physiological process are mainly due to AMF symbiosis (Mosse, 1973; Cox and Sanders, 1974; Kinden and Brown, 1975; Bonfante, Fosolo and Semerini, 1977). McDonald and Lewis (1978) reported the occurrence of some acid phosphates and sodium dehydrogenase activity in onion roots colonized with *Glomus mosseae*. Gianinazzi *et al.* (1979) have reported the acid phosphatase and alkaline phosphatase activity in onion roots colonized with *Glomus* species. Lakshman (1996); Senthlikumar and Krishnamurthy, (1999) have studied the peroxidase and acid phosphatase activities in some important timber trees species and ground orchid (*Spathoglottis*) with special reference to plant colonized with mycorrhizae. Solaiman *et al.* (1999) detected polyphosphates in intraradical and extraradical hyphae of *Gigaspora margarita*. Bago *et al.* (2002) have investigated the translocation of fungal storage lipids in mycorrhiza colonized roots of some important plants. Understanding mycorrhizal symbiosis is of great importance, as the fungal symbionts may play a key role in determining petroplants distribution and diversity. The relationship of petroplants with fungi is relatively unique in the plant kingdom. Petroplants such as *Jatropha curcas* L., *Jatropha gossypifolia* L., *Ricinus communis* L. and *Madhuca indica Gmel.* vary in their fungal specificity, both among the genera and over the course of their life cycle. AM mycorrhizal fungi are found intracellularly in cells of the cortex, and are confined to the roots (Hardley, 1992).

Histochemical preparations enable the identification and localization of certain classes of chemical substances. Morphologically the fungus penetrate the plant cell wall and develops an intimate contact with the plant protoplast in response to the infection, the fungus modifies its behavior to control and exploit its own advantage, Visualization of find structural details in cells interacting in mycorrhizal system is of major importance, structural-functional relationships can be understood when the structural organization is known. Conventional techniques could be used to complement other findings. Knowledge of the special distribution of macromolecular components in tissue and cells is another requisite for understanding of arbuscular mycorrhiza fungal interactions.

Materials and Methods

Seeds of four petro plants *viz.*, *Jatropha curcas* L., *Jatropha gossypifolia* L., *Ricinus communis* L. and *Madhuca indica Gmel.* were sown in earthen pots measuring 30×30 diameter. Each pot was filled with 4kg of sterilized garden soil containing 3 parts of soil and one part of pure sand in the ratio (3:1). When the seedlings were one week old, a 15g mixed inoculum of *Glomus fasciculatum* was inoculated to each pot in triplicate and were maintained in green house. Experiments were conducted after determining optimum VA-mycorrhizal colonization after 60, 120 and 180 days. Root bits were washed thoroughly in distilled water and were fixed in Corony's fluid (6 parts of ethyl alcohol +3 parts of chloroform +1 part of acetic acid) for fourty eight hrs and then washed with water before storing in 70 per cent alcohol. The fixed root bits were then dehydrated in a series of alcohol grades for two-hour interval between each grade (50 per cent alcohol, 70 per cent alcohol, 80 per cent alcohol). The fixed root bits were then dehydrated a series of alcohol grades for two-hour interval between each grade (50 per cent alcohol + butanol), 100 per cent alcohol + butanol (1:1), 100 per cent alcohol, 3:1 (alcohol + butanol), 100 per cent alcohol + butanol (1:3), pure butanol-2 changes. The dehydrated root bits were subjected to infiltration, and embedded in paraffin wax at 56°C to 58°C according to Johanson, (1940).

Infiltration, Embedding and Sectioning

The dehydrated root pieces were transferred to small vials containing pure butanol, then pieces of paraffin were added until the solvent (butanol) become saturated at room temperature then incubated by placing under table lamp (45 w) for 12 hrs. Then the vials containing material were transferred to oven and its temperature was at 58°C climate the traces of butanol. Subsequently, six to eight changes were given for all samples with an interval of 3 hrs was maintained for each molten paraffin change. Root bits were then embedded in paraffin. The paraffin blocks containing root bits were fixed to the wooden blocks. Serial microtome sections of 6 mm thickness were taken by using Lipstaw rotary microtome. The paraffin ribbons were affixed on to the slides flooded with gelatin adhesive. (Adhesive–1g of granular gelatin + 100ml of warm distilled water + pinch of potassium dichromate). The slides along with paraffin ribbons were kept on hot plate so that the sections were stretched to their original size. All the slides were labeled properly and kept in dust free boxes for drying for about 7 days. The slides were then subjected for staining. The following histochemical tests were conducted to understand the nature of cell wall and cellular components of the infected mycorrhizal roots.

Confirmation Test for Starch (Johanson, 1940)

In the present investigation this test is used to confirm the nature of Periodic Acid Schiff's (PAS) positive grains. It do not show that positive grains in the fungal hyphae and vesicles only a few small drops of Iodine is seen in arbuscules.

Test for Chitin

1000 ml of saturated potassium hydroxide solution was boiled. Hydrated sections were treated with warm KOH for 5-10 minutes and washed in 90 per cent alcohol. Chitin has been transformed into chitosan. It is tested later on with weak iodine solution. Red violet colouration indicates the presence of chitin.

Test for Total Proteins

This technique is excellent for the qualitative determination of proteins present in the cells and tissues.

Procedure

Deparaffinized sections were brought to water level and then immersed in mercuric bromophenol blue solution (prepared by adding 10g mercuric chloride and 100 mg of bromophenol blue in 100 ml of absolute alcohol) at room temperature for about 30 minutes. Stained sections were treated with 0.5 per cent acetic acid for about 5-10 min. which removes excess dye. On immersion in tap water, the stain in the sections became blue alkaline form. The sections were air dried, dehydrated in n-butanol, cleared in xylene and mounted with D.P.X.

Colour Indication

AMF fungus colonized root thin section sites of proteins stained blue.

Results

Blue colouration indicates the presence of total proteins in mycorrhizal roots. Blue colouration is not detected in non-mycorrhizal roots.

Test for Polysaccharides

PAS Method (Feder and O'Brien, 1968): Total inosoluble polysaccharides are localized by employing Periodic Acid Schiff's (PAS) method. In this method periodic acid ($IIIO_4$) will oxidize 1,2-glycol groups to produce aldehyde groups. Aldehyde groups thus formed react with leucobasic-fuchsin of Schiff's reagent to produce a visible purplish red (magenta) colour. Periodic Acid Schiff's reaction is highly recommended for the localization of total insoluble polysaccharides because of following characteristics.

1. Does not cause the breakage of polysaccharide chains.
2. Specific to polysaccharides.
3. Offers least interface and gives no false localization.
4. Forms intense and stable colour complex.

Preparations of Reagents

Periodic Acid 0.5 per cent

500 mg of periodic acid powder was dissolved in 100 ml of distilled water.

Schiff's Reagent (for Polysaccharides)

1g of basic fuchsin was dissolved in 100 ml of 0.15N HCl, agitated for three hours and then added with 1gm sodium metabisulphate and kept overnight. Treatment of this solution with activated charcoal produces straw colour Schiff's reagent.

Bleach (for Polysaccharides)

0.5 mg of sodium metabisulphate is dissolved in 95 ml of distilled water to which 5ml of 1N HCl is added.

Staining Procedure

1. Hydrated root sections were incubated in 0.5 per cent periodic acid for 15 minutes at room temperature.
2. Sections were washed in running water for about 5 minutes and incubated in Schiff's reagent for 30 minutes.
3. After incubation sections were rinsed with distilled water and were bleached with 2 per cent sodium meta bisulphate for a minute, dehydrated in alcohol series, cleared in xylene and mounted with DPX.

Results

The magenta red colouration of mycorrhizal roots indicates the presence of insoluble polysaccharides. Magenta red coloration was not detected in non-mycorrhizal roots.

Detection of DNA

Feulgen Method (Gomorol 1952): This method is based on Schiff's reaction for staining aldehydes, released from deoxyribose sugar, after the removal of purine at the level of purine-deoxyribose glucoside bonds of DNA by hydrolyzing in 1N HCl.

Staining Procedure

1. Hydrated sections were hydrolysed in 1N HCl at 60°C for 13 minutes.
2. Sections are rinsed in water and incubated with Schiff's reagent at room temperature for 30 minutes.
3. After rinsing in water sections are treated with bleach and again rinsed in water dehydrated, cleared in xylene and mounted in DPX colour indication.

Results

AMF colonized roots DNA appeared magenta–red and non-mycorrhizal roots do not colored with magenta–red.

Test for RNA: Toluidine Blue Method (O'Brien and McCully, 1981)

Preparation of Reagent

50 mg toluidine blue is dissolved in 100 ml of 0.05 M citrate phosphate buffer at pH 4.4.

Stock Solutions

1. 0.1 M solution of citric acid (19.21 gms in 1000 ml)
2. 0.2 M solution of disodium phosphate (53.65 gms of $Na_2HPO_{4,}7H_2O$ or $Na_2HPO_4 12H_2O$ in 1000 ml).
3. Citrate phosphate buffer 27.8 ml of B, diluted to a total of 100 ml with distilled water.

Staining Procedure

1. Deparaffinized and hydrated sections were immersed in 0.05 per cent toluidine blue for 5 minutes.
2. Sections were rinsed in distilled water, air dried, cleared in xylene and mounted in DPX.

Colour Indication

RNA appears purple and non-mycorrhizal root donot showed purple colour.

Test for Total Lipids

Free hand sections of fresh material were used. Root sections were treated with ethylene glycol for five minutes. Ethylene glycol was blotted out and treated with Sudan black B for ten minutes. Slides were washed 3-4 times in distilled water and sections were mounted on cleaned slides with glycerine jelly.

Control Test

Fresh freehand sections have been treated with heat cold alcohol in the reaction.

Preparation of Reagents

Sudan Black–B

0.7 g of Sudan black-B powder was dissolved in 100 ml of warm Ethylene glycol. Then the hot solution was filtered, cooled and stored in freezer. Free hand out sections of VAM colonized roots were used to prepare the histochemical slides for the localization of lipids and peroxidase.

Glycerine Jelly

10 g of Gelatin powder was dissolved in 60 ml of distilled water and followed by the addition of 70 ml of glycerol and 250mg phenol crystals.

Staining Procedure

VAM colonized fresh roots were selected and thoroughly washed with tap water and then with distilled water. The roots were macerated with 10 per cent KOH and washed with distilled water. The roots were treated with ethylene glycol for five minutes, excess ethylene glycol was blotted out and treated with Sudan black-B for 10 minutes, slides were washed 3-4 times in distilled water and sections were mounted on clean slides with glycerine jelly.

Results

The lipids appear blue to blue black colour in mycorrhizal roots. In non mycorrhizal roots blue to blue black colouration was not detected.

Test for Neutral Lipids

For this test freshly VAM colonized roots were used. Root sections were treated with ethylene glycol for five minutes. Ethylene glycol was blotted and later treated with III Sudan bland and IV Sudan black separately. The lipid bodies in hyphae, arbuscule and vesicles stained blue-black colouration indicates the presence of lipids.

Control Test

Sections are treated with cold pyridine for 30 minutes later they are transferred to hot pyridine for 30 minutes later they are transferred to hot pyridine at 60°C for 24 hrs then rinsed in water and stained in sudan black-B. The areas of lipids do not stain any colour *i.e.*, non-mycorrhizal root samples.

Toluidene Blue (for Polyphosphates)

0.05 per cent toluidene blue in citrate phosphate buffer of pH 4.4.

Results

Red coloured granular depositions indicate the presence of polyphosphates.

Test for Peroxidase Enzyme

Diaminobenzidinete trichloride (DAB) method (Graham and Karnovasky 1966): Root sections were incubated at room temperature for about 10-20 minutes in reactant solution and later they were washed thoroughly with distilled water and mounted in glycerine jelly.

Reactant solution was prepared by mixing 5 mg of 3.3 diaminobenzidinete trichloride (DAB) in 10 ml of 0.05M warm Tris-HCl buffer of 7.6pH and to this added 0.2ml of freshly diluted 1 per cent H_2O_2 then cooled, filtered and stored in brown bottle.

Results

Brown-black colour in mycorrhizal roots. Brown-black color was not detected in non-mycorrhizal roots.

Test for Polyphosphates

Fresh mycorrhizal infected root sections were used to localize polyphosphates. Sections were passed in to 0.1 per cent Toludine blue at pH-1-2 at room temperature. Sections rinsed in distilled water and mounted on clean glass slides with glycerine jelly. Red coloured granular deposition in hyphae arbuscules and vesicles gives the presence of polyphosphates.

Control Test

Fresh free hand sections have been treated with heat cold alcohol in the reaction.

Test for Cytochrome Oxidase Enzyme

Free hand sections of Fresh material were used. Sections were treated with stock solution A and B for one hour washed in distilled water and mounted on slides diluted glycerine jelly.

Stock solutions consists of (*a*) 315gms of Sodium phosphate dibasic dissolved and made it one litre and (b) 3.026 gms of Potassium phosphate monobasic dissolved and made it 1 liter. Mixed as shown below to get a particular pH?

Control Test

Fresh free hand sections have been treated with heat cold alcohol in the reaction.

Enzyme Esterase (Gomon 1950)

Esterases are enzymes which are capable of hydrolyzing esters, with in this group there are many different types of esters, acting upon a number of difficult substances. The method can be carried and employing the diazonium salt fast blue B as the coupling agent.

Reagent Required

1. Napthyl acetate, 2. Acetone, 3. 0.2 N phosphate buffer pH 7.4, 4. Diazonium salt fast blue B. Napthol acetate is dissolved in the acetone and the phosphate buffer was added, and the solution filtered and used immediately.

Procedure

Root sections were brought down to water placed incubating medium for 15-30 minutes at room temperature. Washed the sections on tap water for three minutes and counted in glycerine jelly. Reddish brown colour stained sections shows presence of enzyme esterase.

Test for Succinic Dehydrogenase

Freshly colonized mycorrhizal sections were flooded with incubating media 'a' and 'b' for 30 minutes each. After draining the media sections were mounted on clean slides with glycerin jelly.

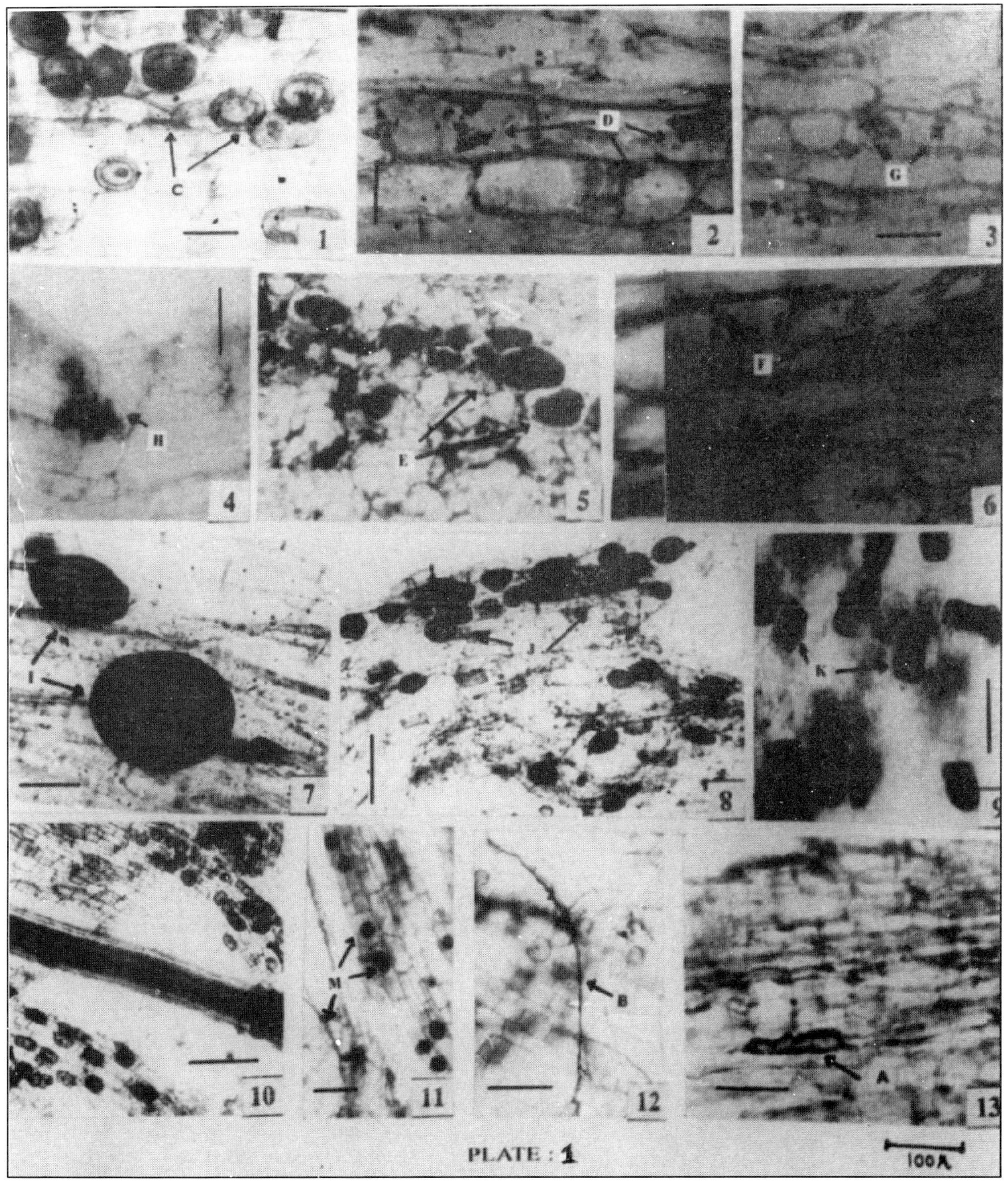

Plate 9.1

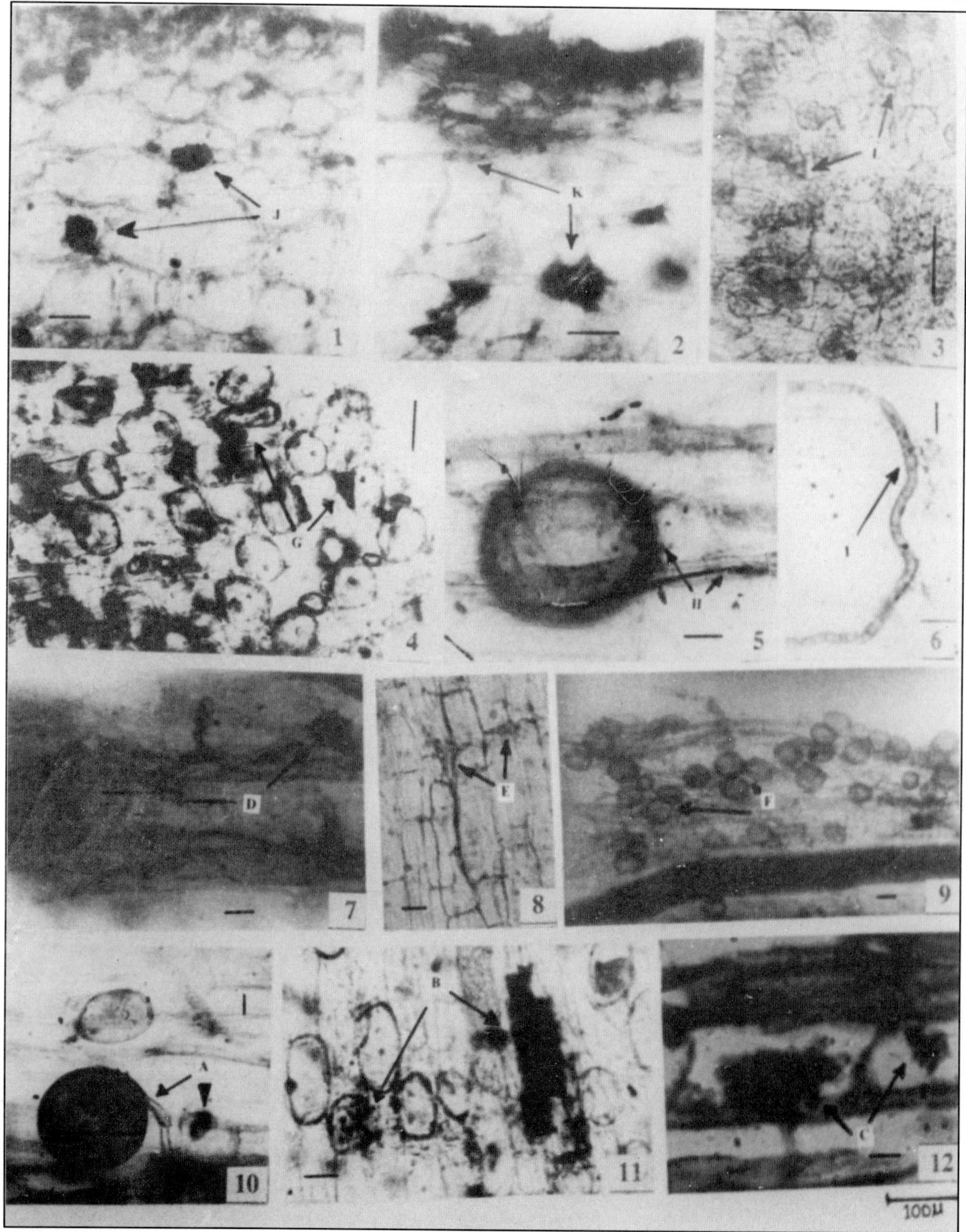

Plate 9.2

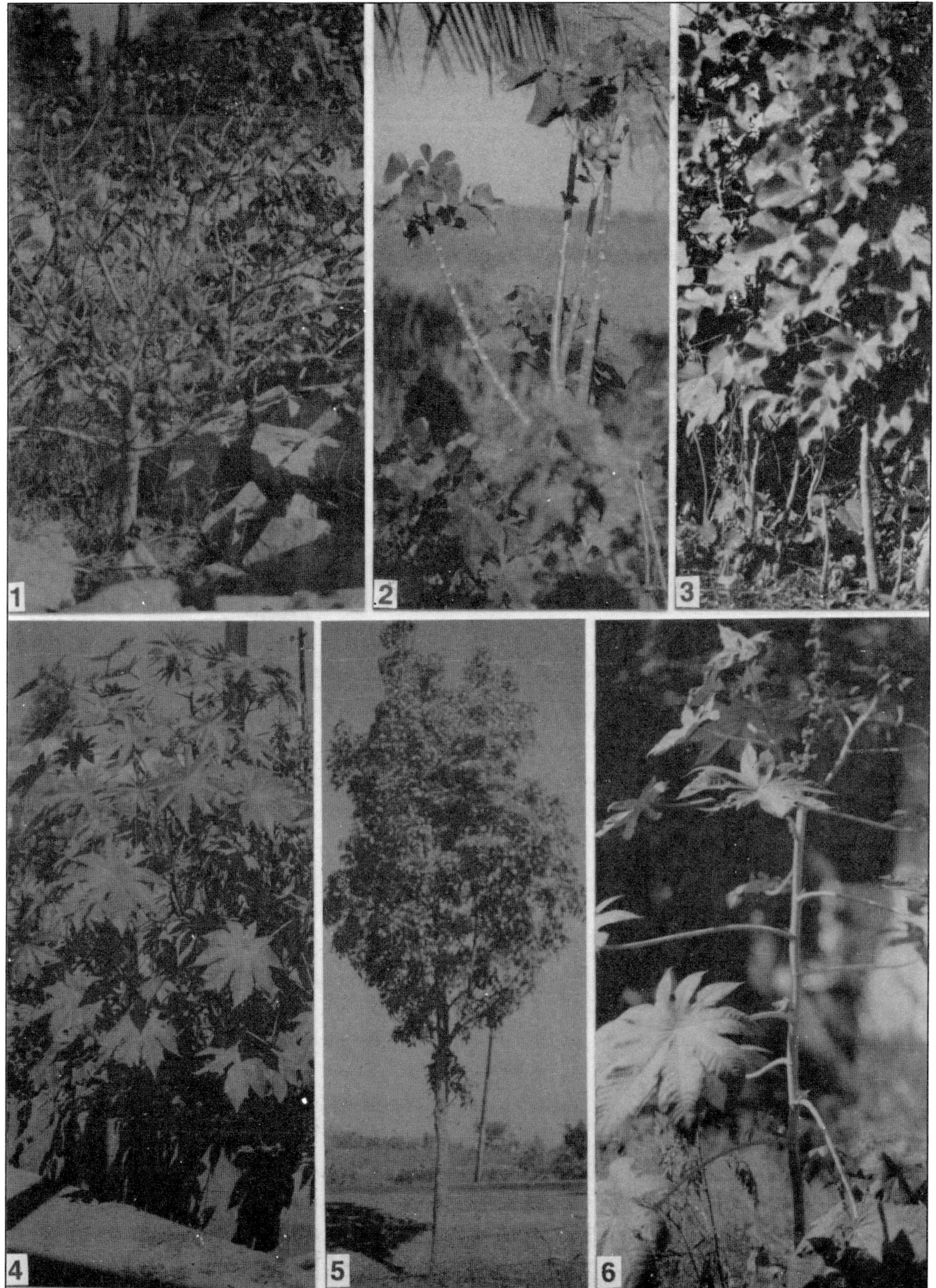

Plate 9.3

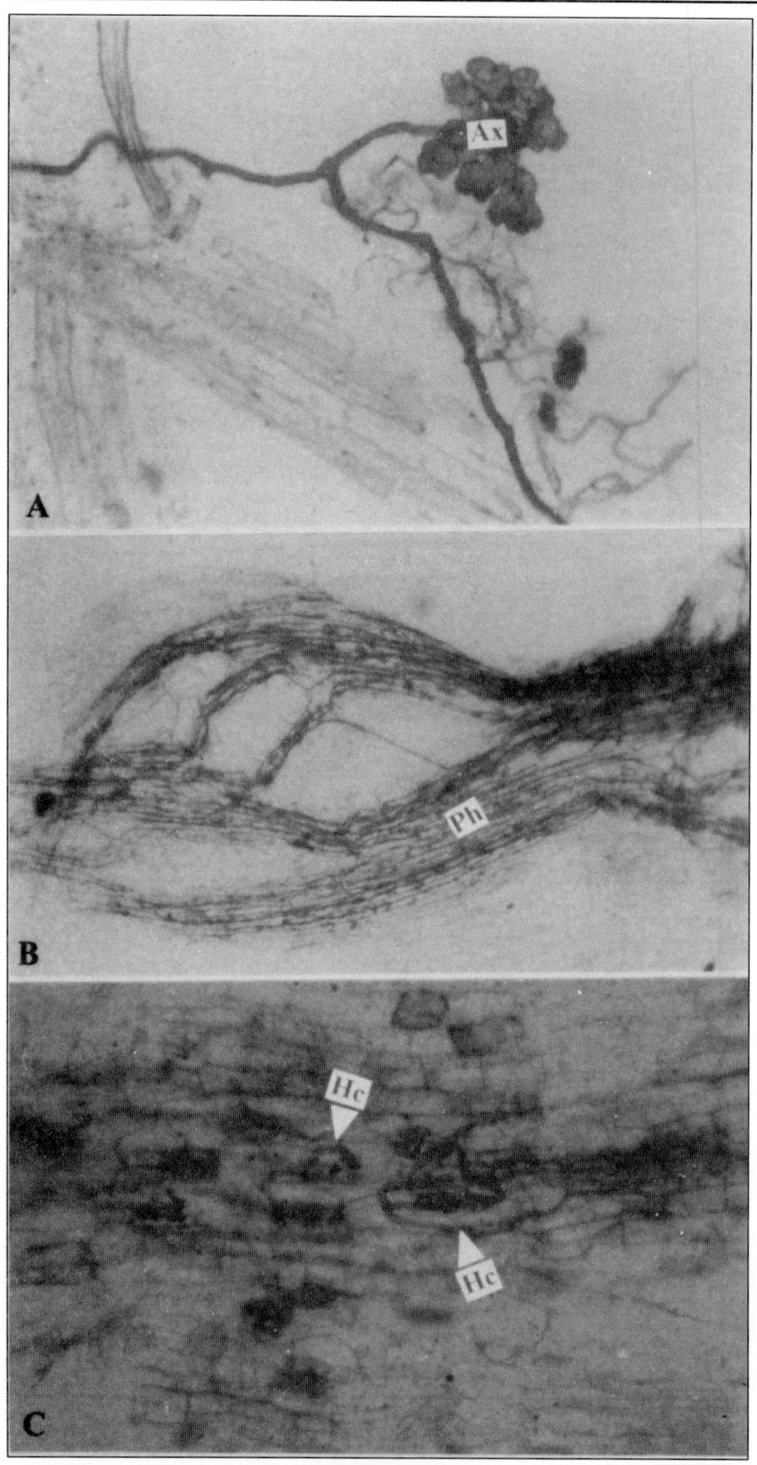

Plate 9.4

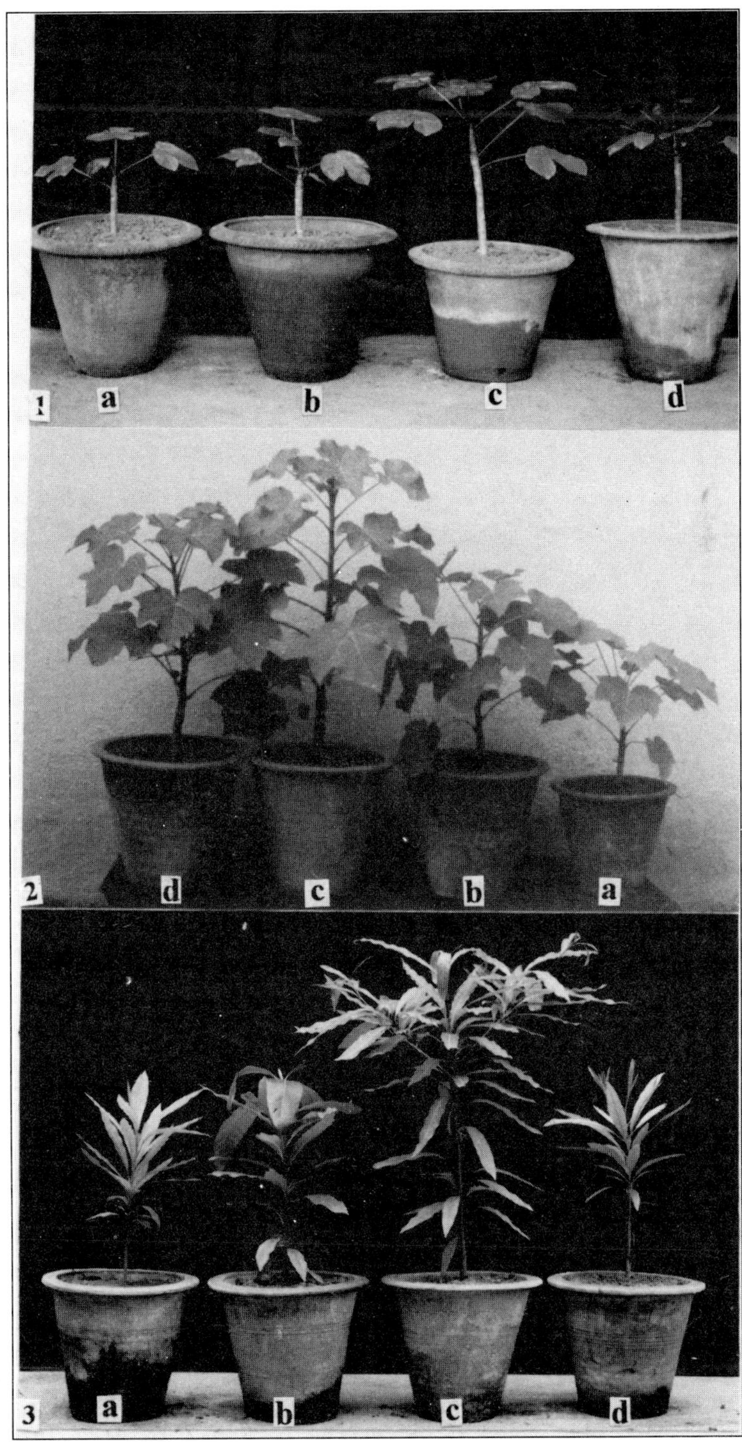

Plate 9.5

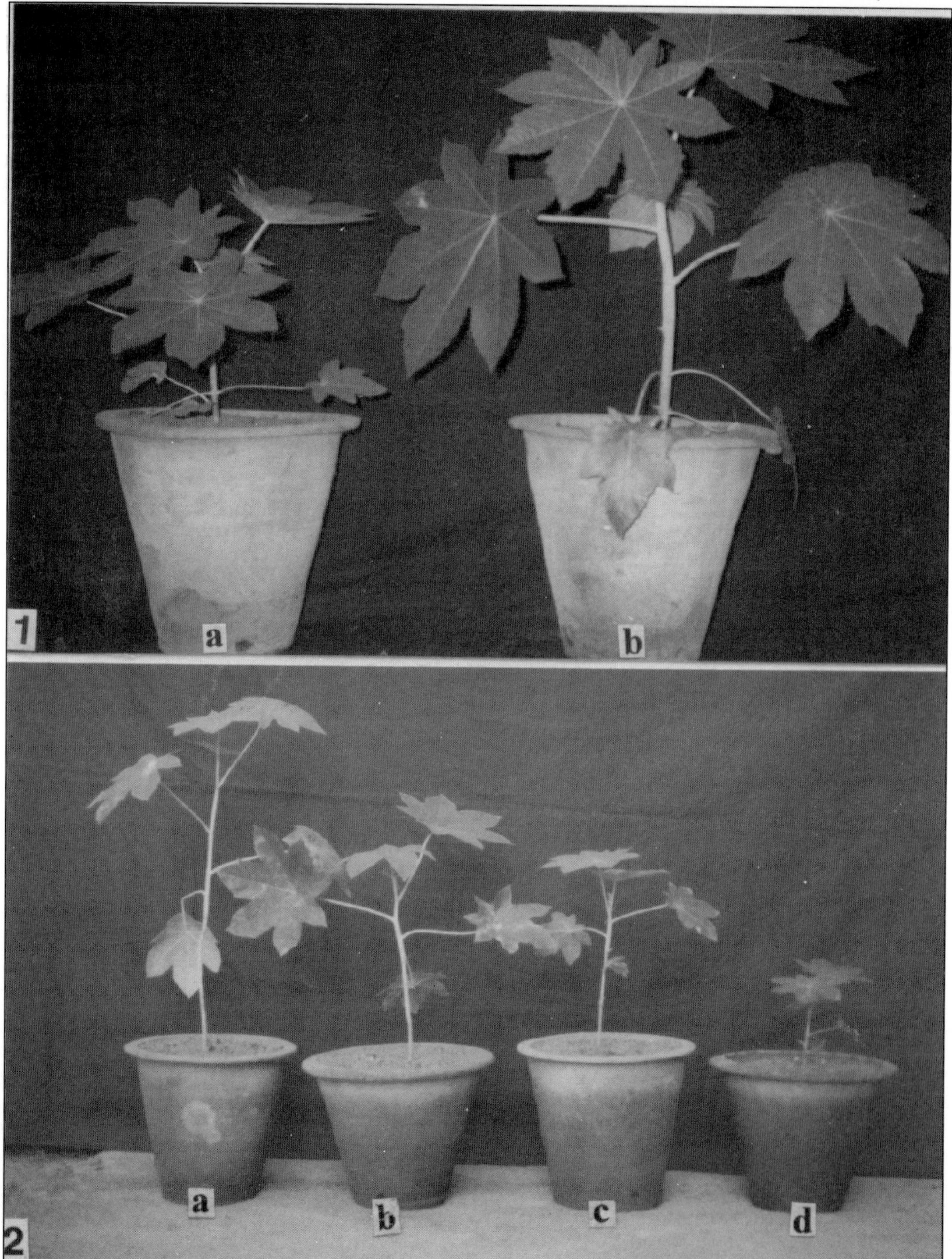

Plate 9.6

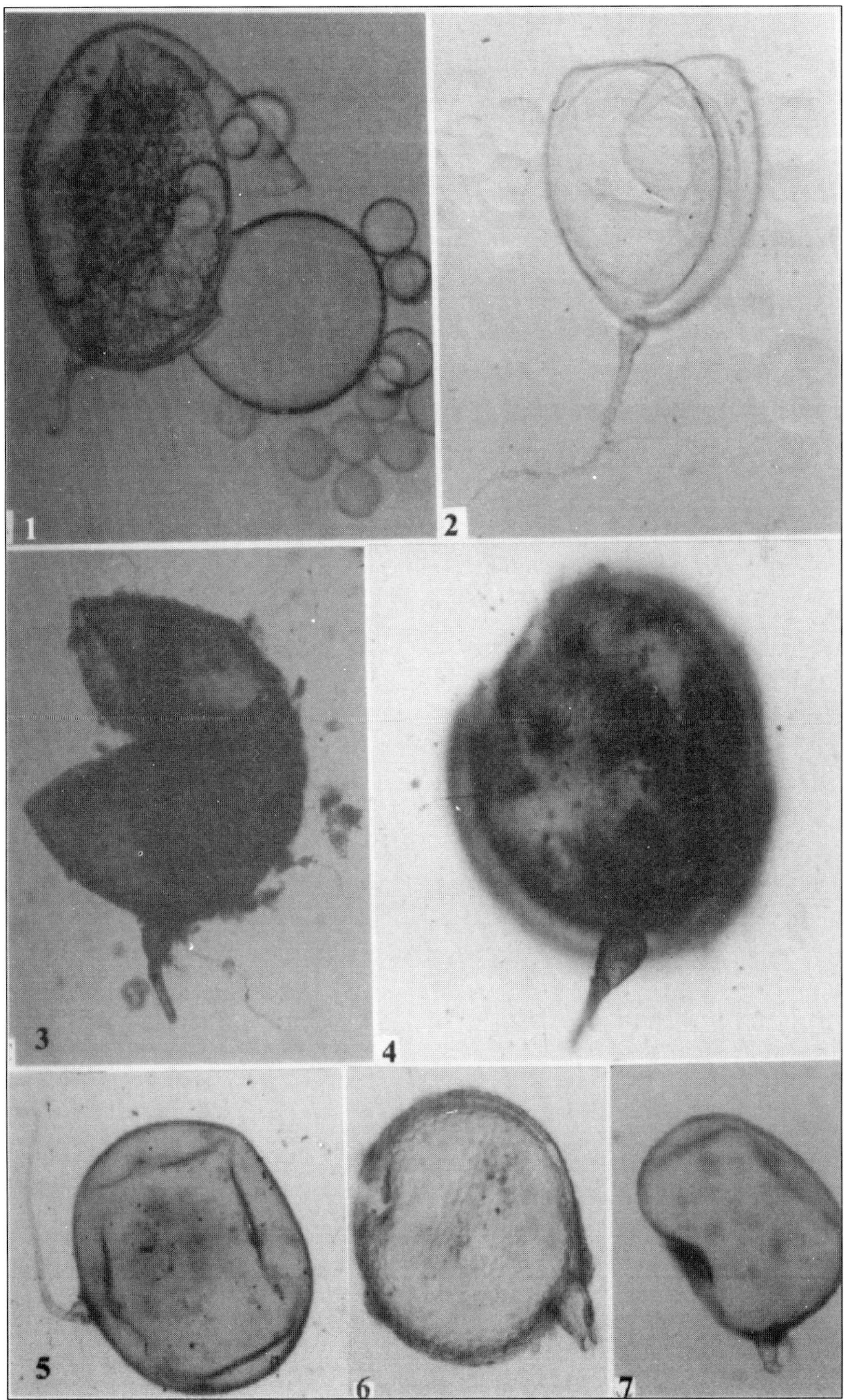

Plate 9.7

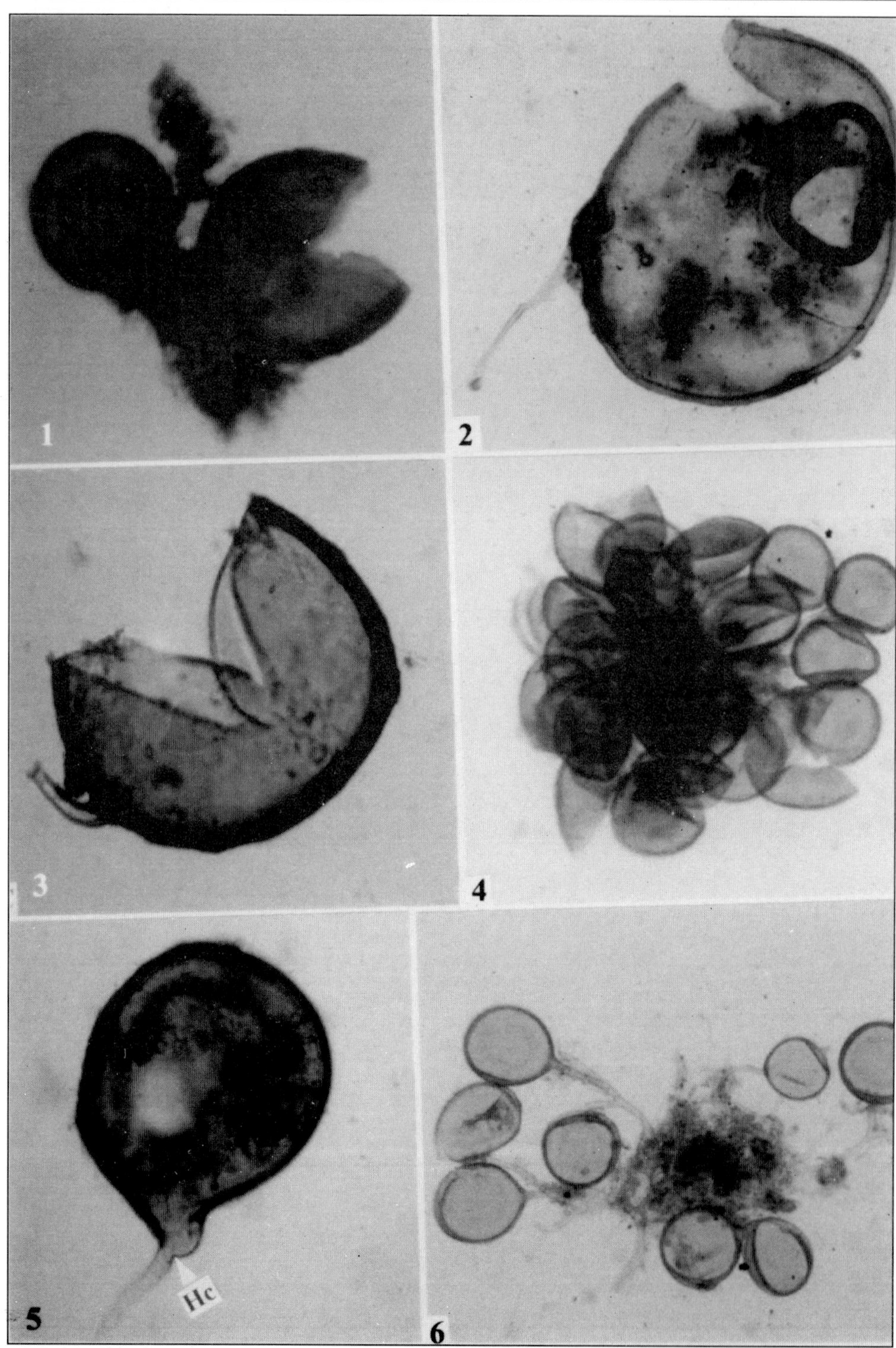

Plate 9.8

Media 'a'

6.75 g of sodium succinate was dissolved in 8 ml of water to which 0.05ml of 1N HCl was added. The pH was adjusted to 7.1 with 1N HCl.

Media 'b'

10 mg (powder) of NBT (4 mg/ml) was dissolved in 2.5 ml of distilled water with 0.2 M tris-buffer at pH 7.4 to this 1 ml of 0.05 ml of $MgCl_2$ was added followed by the addition of 3 ml distilled water Dark purple colouration of fungal components indicates the localization of succinic dehydragenase.

Test for Acid Phosphatase

Sections were incubated for 4-5 hrs in a substrate consisting of 0.1 M acetate buffer, plus 1mg ml^{-1} sodium 2 naphthyl acid phosphate, 1 mg ml^{-1} fast Garnet, 0.05 per cent $MgCl_2$ at pH 4 to 5 rinsed in distilled water. Extra pigmented root sections were bleached and washed in distilled water and mounted on clean slides with diluted glycerin jelly.

Test for Alkaline Phosphatase

Freshly colonized mycorrhizal sections were incubated overnight in a substrate. It consists of 0.05 tris-citric acid buffer at pH 8.5-9.2, plus 1mg ml^{-1} sodium 2-naphthyl acid (alkaline). 1 mg ml^{-1} fast blue, 0.05 per cent $MgCl_2$. Extra pigmented root sections were bleached and washed in distilled water and mounted on clean slide with diluted glycerin jelly.

Results and Discussion

Recent upsurge of interest and research on mycorrhiza associated plants exhibited various biochemical substances in their roots. It was noticed that translocation of materials takes place from host to fungus and vice versa. Specific observations such as localization of different chemical constituents in different components of VAM were made in the present study. Histochemical slides of freshly colonized roots clearly revealed the localization of RNA, polysaccharides (Plate 9.1: 1, 4, 6), polyphosphates (Plate 9.2: 5, 6 and 10) and protein, whereas lipids and peroxidase were localized by employing hand out section of fresh roots (Plate 9.1: 7 to 9). In the present study, mature arbuscules stained darkly for proteins test and remained negative in vesicles (Plate 9.1: 3) the inter/intracellular hyphae and mature arbuscules showed positive test for PAS, indicating high concentration of insoluble polysaccharide (Plate 9.1: 2 and 6 and Plate 9.2: 12). RNA was localized only in the arbuscules (Plate 9.1: 13). Accumulation of lipids in VAM localized roots imparts black colour, which had strong affinity for the general lipid stain called Sudan black-B. Accumulation of lipids in the form of very thick dark droplets was observed in hyphae and vesicles of mycorrhizal roots (Plate 9.1: 7, 10-11). Plate (2) shows the discontinuous localization of lipid droplets in hyphae which passes to the vesicles. Arbuscules shows the localization of lipid droplets in hyphae which passes to the vesicles. Arbuscules shows the localization of peroxidase (Plate 9.2: 1-3) and remain absent in vesicles. Cytochrome oxydase (Plate 2:4-5) Succinic dehydrogenase indiscontinuous arbuscule (Plate 9.2.2 and 4). Alkaline and acid phosphate are in (Plate 9.2: 7-8, 10-10). Plate 9.3 showing important petro plants selected by Lakshman (1996) these were 1) *Jatropha gossifolia* 2) *Jatropha curcas*, 3) enlarged *J. curcas*, 4) *Ricinis communis* var. 5) *Madhuca indica* 6) *Ricinis communis* var (Rosa). Plate 9.4 showing the macerated root sections and stained : A. axially cell with hyphae from *madhuca indica* soil sample B: numerous small vesicles hyphae from *Jatropha curcas* soil sample. C: Large vesicles with hyphae from *Ricinus communis*. (Plate 9.5) Inoculation of VAM with rock phosphate treatments 1:(A, B, C, D) showing the effect of *Glomus mosseae* with different levels of rock phosphate on *Jatropha gossifolia* 2: (A,B,C) showing the effect of

Glomus mosseae with different levels of rock phosphate on *Jatropha curcas*. 3: (A,B,C) showing the effect of *Glomus mosseae* with different levels of rock phosphate on *Madhuca indica*. (Plate 9.6) 1: (A,B) showing the growth response of *Ricinus communis* inoculated and non-inoculated plant. 2: (A,B,C,D) showing the effect of *Glomus mosseae* with different levels of rock phosphate on *Ricinus communis*. Some of the important AMF spores recovered from the rhizosphere soils of experimental plants. These were (Plate 9.7) 1: *Gigaspora margarita*, 2: *Gigaspora rosea*, 3: *Gigaspora decipiens*, 4: *Gigaspora gigentea*, 4: *Glomus fasiculatum*, 5: *Glomus mosseae*, 6: *Glomus lactum*. (Plate 9.8) 1: *Glomus citricola*, 2: *Glomus macrocarpum*, 3: *Scutellospora calospora*, 4: *Glomus aggregatum*, 5: *Glomus fulvum*, 6: *Glomus microcarpum*. showing the effect of Similar cytological changes were reported earlier. (Werner 1992; Senthilkumar and Krishnamurthy, 1999). The cytochemical study using coomassie brilliant blue (Fisher, 1968) showed positive staining of fungal hyphae, indicating high protein content (Plate No.1).

Striking increase of biochemicals, due to metabolic activities between host and fungus lead to biochemical reactions. This was detected and determined by staining procedure. The outcome of present work enabled us to understand the transformation of series of chemical substances due to host and symbiont interaction (Table 9.1), Lakshman (1996) who have demonstrated clearly that the various parameters in four Petrochemical plants. The results clearly demonstrated the translocation of materials from host to fungus and vice-versa. Basic proteins appeared to be most common type detected in immature arbuscules, vesicles and hyphal cytoplasm; these results are in conformity with that of Neneo, (1981). The periodic acid schiffs (PAS) reaction of polysaccharide with the arbuscular walls shows osmophilic and acidic properties and suggests that the wall is primarily made up of glycolipid in composition. The absence of starch grains in arbuscules and presence of starch grains in host cells lead to the conclusion that the carbohydrate materials has been taken by arbuscules, but not in the form of starch. Similar findings were also reported by the earlier workers in *Eucalyptsu* tree (Ling Lee *et al.*, 1977; Weete, 1974). The present study clearly demonstrates that the mycorrhizal roots were considerably large and cells were densely stained with PAS than non-mycorrhizal roots, this indicates that they are rich in polysaccharides (Junifer and Roberts, 1961; Harris and Northcote, 1971; Scannerini and Bonafonte-fasalo, 1979; Lakshman 1999, Inchal, 2002, Firoz, 2002). It has been pointed out that, VAM fungal hyphae and vesicles are rich in osmophillic substances (Bevente *et al.*, 1975; Cox *et al.*, 1975; Harley, 1975; Kinden and Brown, 1975; Holley Peterson, 1979). The accumulation of lipids in hyphae, vesicles and arbuscules has been observed in apple and Ericaceae members (Mosse, 1957). The present investigation supports the work of earlier workers that the vesicles and hyphae contain rich lipids probably of triglyceride. The vesicles acts as storage sink of lipids for the host plant (Cox *et al.*, 1975, Brannan and Losel, 1978). More accumulation of lipid in vesicles resulted in the transformation into triglycerides, monoglycerides, fats, sterols, etc. the potential role of polyphosphate uptake in hyphae is well documented by Callow *et al.* (1978). The VAM fungi synthesizes polyphosphates in granular form and transfer the same to arbusculus and ensure its availability to the host cell. Several workers demonstrated that the uptake and storage of phosphate might be a common phenomenon of all mutualistic mycorrhizal associations. Hence mycorrhizal plant utilizes more phosphate than non-mycorrhizal plants. Polyphosphate is a major 'P' reserve in VA-mycorrhizae. Root cortical cells of mycorrhizal plants contained arbuscules with high 'P' concentration. Whereas polyphosphate granules are commonly found in young proliferating arbuscules (Grey and Gerdmann, 1969; Bowen, 1968; Mosse 1973a). the peroxidiase activity was detected only in senescing arbuscules of all the experimental plants. It seems that mycorrhizal fungi colonize the host tissue by combination of mechanical interaction and enzymatic mechanism (Gianinazzi-Person *et al.*, 1996). Thus, VAM fungi can play an important role in developing the pathogen resistance host plant. The peroxidase

Table 9.1: Histochemistry Tests in Infected Roots of *Jatropha curcas* Plant Inoculated with *Glomus fasciculatum*

Sl.No.	Metabolic Localized	Test Reagent	Colour Indication	Localization in Fungal Structure			Reference
				Arbuscules	Hyphae	Vesicles	
1.	Polysaccharides	PAS	Magenta Red	+	–	–	Johnsen, 1992
2.	Starch	IKI solution	dissolved				Johnsen, 1940
3.	Chitin	KOH-IKI	Red Violet				Johnsen, 1940
4.	Nucleic acids (DNA)	Feulgen	Purple blue	+	+	+	
5.	RNA	Toluidine blue	Purple	+	–	–	O, Brein and McCully; 1981
6.	Protein (Total)	Mercuric bromophenol blue	Blue Blue blak	+	+	+	Pearse, 1960
7.	Lipids (Total)	Sudan black-B		+	+	+	Johnson, 1962
8.	Neutral Lipids	Sudan III or IV		+	+	+	Laxman, 1996
9.	Polyphosphates	Toluidine blue	Blue purple	+	+	+	Ashford *et al.*, 1975
10.	Cellulose	Calcoflour white	Fluorescence	–	–	–	Hughes and McCully, 1975
			Type of enzymes				
11.	Cytochrome oxidase	Nadireagent	Room temp. Bluish Purple	–	+	+	Chayen *etal.*, 1969.
12.	Peroxidase	Bensidine	blue turns brown	+	–	–	Jensen, 1962
13.	Succinic dehydrogense	Sodium succinate	Room temp. Bluish Purple	+	–	–	Bancroft, 1975
14.	Acid Phosphatase	Sodium B glycero phosphate	violet black	+	+	–	Pears, 1972
15.	Alkaline Phosphatase	Sodium B glycero phosphate	violet black	+	+	–	Pears, 1972

activity was detected only in senescing arbuscules in the present study and similar to the reports of Nemec (1981); Lakshman (1996) and Shanthikumar and Krishnamurthy (1999). It is concluded that the different chemical substances were accumulated in VAM fungi and and transferred to the host tissue. In finger millet, VAM colonized roots with arbuscules lead to be the path for the exchange of materials from fungus to host and vice versa.

References

Ashford, A. E, Ling lee, M and Chilvers G. A. (1975). Polyphosphate in mycorrhizas; A cytochemical demonstration. *New Phytol* 74: 447-453.

Bevege, D. I. (1968). A rapid technique for clearing tannins and staining intact roots for detection of mycorrhizas caused by *Endogone* spp., and some records of infection in Australian plants. *Trans. Bt. Mycol. Soc.* 51: 808-811.

Bevege, D. I. and Bowen, G. D. (1975). Endogone strain and host plant differences in development of vesicular-arbuscular mycorrhizas; 77-86 In. (Eds.) Sanders, F. E mosse, B and Tinker, P. B. *Endomycorrhizas*. Academic press, London. pp. 626.

Bonfanate-Fasolo, P. and Scannerient (1977). Cytological study of the VA-mycorrhiza in *orinthogallum umbellatum* L. *Allionia*. 22: 15-21.

Bonfante-Fasolo, P. and Scannerini, S. (1977). A cytochemical study of the vesicular-arbascular mycorrhiza clover. *Aust. J. Bot.*, 30: 485.

Callow, J. A. , Capaccio, L. C. M. , Parish, G. , and Tinker, P. B. (1978). Detection and estimation of polyphosphate in vesicular-arbuscular mycorrhizas. *New Phytol.* 80: 125-134.

Carling, D. E. , and white, J. A, and Brown, M. F. (1977). The influence of fixation procedure on the ultrastructure of the host endophyto interace of vascular-arbuscular mycorrhizae *Can. J. Bot.* 71: 48-51.

Chayen, J. L. Bitensky. R. G Butcher, and L. poulte. (1969). *A guide to practical histochemical*. Oliver and Boyd, Edinburgh, pp. 35.

Cox, G. , and Sanders, F. 1974. Ultrastructure of the host-fungus interface in vesicular-arbascular mycorrhiza. *New Phytol.* 73: 901-912.

Daft. M. J. , and Nicolson, T. H. (1966). Effect of Endogone mycorrhiza on plant growth. *New Phytol.* 65: 343-350.

Davis, R. M. , and Menge, J. A. (1981). Phytophthora parasitica inoculation intensity of vesicular-arbuscular mycorrhize in citrus. *New Phytol.* 87: 705-715.

Feder. N and O'Brien, T. (1968). Plant microtechnique some principals of new methods. *Am. J. Bot.* 55: 123.

Fisher, D. B. (1968). Protein staining of ribboned epon sections for light microscropy. *Histomchemie*. 16: 82-96.

Furlan, V. , and Fortin, J. Andre (1973). Formation of endomycorrhizae by Endogone calospora in Allium cepa under three temperature regimes. *Naturaliste Can.* 100: 467-477.

Gallaud, Etude. (1905). sur les mycorhizes endotrophes, *Rev. Gen. Bot.* , 17: 5-15.

Gianinazzi, S. , Gianiazzi-Pearson. , and Dexheimer, J. (1979). Enzymatic studies on the metabolism of vesicular-arbuscular mycorrhiza. III. Ultrastructural localization of acid and alkaline phosphatase in Onion roots fected by Glomus mosseae (Nicol. and Gerd). *New Phytol.* 82: 127-132.

Hardley, G. (1992). Orchid Mycorrhiza. In *Orchid Biology: Reviews and prospectives II*, pp. 83-113, edited by A. J. Corness, New York : University Press.

Harold, F. M. (1966). Inorganic polyphosphates in biology; structure, metabolism and function. *Bact. Rev.* 30: 772-976.

Holley, J. D., and Peterson, R. L. (1979). Development of a vesicular-arbascular mycorrhiza in bean roots. *Can. J. Bot.* 57: 1960-1978.

Jensen, W. A. (1962). *Botanical Histochemistry.* W. H. Freeman and Francisco. pp. 352.

Kessler, K. J, . and Blank, R. W. (1972). Endogone. Sporocarps associated with sugar maple. *Mycologia.* 64: 634-638.

Kinden, D. A. , and Brown, M. F. (1975). Electron microscope of vesicular-arbuscular mycorrhizae of yellow popular. III. Host-endophyte interaction during arbuscular development. *Can. J. Microbiol.* 21: 1930-1939.

Lakshman. H. C. (1996). Studies and histochemical on some tree species infected with Am-fungi in; *Ph.D. Thesis* Karnatak university Dharwad, India. pp. 249.

Lakshman. H. C. and Inchal. R. F. and Mulla. F. I. (2002). Histochemical studies on some medicinal plant infected with Am-fungi. *Eco. plan-Environment.* 91(4): 71-75.

Lev, R and Spicer S. S. (1964). Specific staining of sulphate group with alcian blue at low PH. *Histochem. Cytochem.* 12-309-312.

Lillie, R. D. (1965). *Histopathologic Technic and Practical Histochemistry.* Blakiston N. Y. 3rd edition.

Ling-Lee, Chilvers, G. A and Ashford. A. F. (1975a). A histochemical study of phenolic materials in mycorrhizal and infeeted roots of Eucalyptus fasitigiata deane and maden. *New Phytol.* 78-313-318.

Ling-lee, M. A. Ashford, and G. A. Chilvers. (1977). A histochemical study of saccharide distribution in eucalypt mycorrhizas. *New Phytol* 78-329-335.

Mosse, B. , and Hopper, C. (1975). Vesicular-arbuscular mycorrhizal infection in root organ cultures. *Physiol. Plant Pathol.* 5: 215-223.

Nemec, S. (1981). Histochemical characteristics of Glomus etunicatus infection of citrus *limon fibrous* root; *Can. J. Bot.* p. 609-617.

Pearse, A. G. E. (1968). *Histochemistry: Theoretical and Applied,* Vol. 1 Churchill. London. PP. 412.

Pearse, A. G. E. (1972). *Histochemistry: Theortical and Applied,* Vol. 2 Churcchill. Living stone Edinburgh, PP. 276.

Phillips, J. M. , and Hayman, D. S. (1970). Improved procedures for clearing roots and staining parasitic and vesicular-arbuscular mycorrhizal fungi for rapid assessment of infection. *Trans Bt. Mycol. Soc.* 55: 158-161.

Rao, J. (1973). Cytochemical localization of peroxidase in plant cell. *Physiol Plant.* 28: 132-133.

Scannerini, S. and Bonfante-Fasolo, P. (1979). Ultrastructural cytochemical demonstration. Of polysaccharides and proteins with in the host-arbuscul interfacical matrirx in an endomycorrhizae. *New Phytol.* 83: 87-94.

Scannerini, S. and P. Bonfante-Fasolo. (1977). Ultrastructural and cytochemical features of the matrix material in a vesicular-arbuscular. *Mycorrhiza caryologia*, 30(4): 499-500.

Senthlikumar and Krishnamurty. (1999). Peroxidase and acid Phosphatase activity in ground orchid Spathoglottis with reference to mycorrhiza. *Mycorrhiza News*, 10 (4): 11-13.

Werner, D. (1992). Orchid mycorrhiza. In: *Symbosis of Plants and Microbes*, pp. 367-380. Chapman and Hall, London.

Microbial Biotechnology and Ecology (2011) *Pages* 189–200
Editors: Deepak Vyas, G.S. Paliwal, P.K.Khare and R.K Gupta
Published by: DAYA PUBLISHING HOUSE, NEW DELHI

Chapter 10

Biodiversity of VAM Fungi Associated with Some Common Medicinal Plants of Bihar

☆ *A.K. Roy* and A.N. Singh*

Department of Botany, T.M. Bhagalpur University, Bhagalpur – 812 007

Introduction

Arbuscular mycorrhizal fungi are well distributed in both cultivated as well as barren areas. However, different types of soil show variation in the number and type of spores (Hayman, 1978). Distribution and diversity of AM fungi have been reported in diverse ecological conditions such as arctic (Kothari *et al.*, 1997), temperate (Smith and Bowen, 1979) and tropical regions (Singh *et al.*, 1994). Further these have been reported to occur in non-cultivated soil, cultivated soil, mining areas (Roy *et al.*, 2004), desert soils (Shanker *et al.*, 1990), scrub and grassland (Mukerji *et al.*, 1984). Moreover, these endophytes may also survive for years inside the living roots but the species composition of VAM population is found to vary with soil nature.

Thus, diversity is influenced by the several abiotic and biotic components including edaphic factors in an ecosystem which includes soil pH, soil moisture, soil temperature, soil depth, soil nutrients, soil disturbance, soil porosity, soil fertility and soil organic matter and climatic condition such as rainfall, atmospheric temperature, seasonal variation, humidity, light intensity, physical movement, and plant susceptibility. In general diversity of mycorrhizal fungi has also been observed in the same plant and also within the same plant species at different places (Allen and Booalis, 1983). Beside these, mycorrhizal activity like germination rate, growth of hyphal branching, recognition of the host,

* E-mail: botanyakr@yahoo.co.in.

penetration of the roots, growth of hyphae into the soil and sporulation have also been regulated by plant root exudates (Koske and Gemma, 1992).

The species of AM fungi are influenced by the soil temperature as *Gigaspora decipiens* produces highest number of spores at 21°C day temperature (Hari Kumar and Bagyaraj, 1988), where as, *Scutellospora calospora* prefers cooler northern zone (Koske, 1987). *Glomus* and *Gigaspora* were among the most commonly occurring genera in both tropical and temperate climate (Nicolson and Schenck, 1979). Trinick (1977) and Theodorou (1978) studied that the root colonization and spore number were less with higher level of moisture content. Similarly, more germination of spores in *Glomus epigeum* was observed at moisture levels above field capacity (Daniel and Trappe, 1980). The soil pH influences the VAM population in the forest soil (Abbott and Robson, 1991). Kruckelmann (1975) recorded that VAM spores were more influenced by soil pH than by any other factor.

The forest regions under study are found to have continuous pressure of human activities like implementation of developing projects, forest fire, over exploitation of medicinal plants and illegal felling of trees. The attempt to destroy forests and conversion of it in cultivable land results not only in the depletion of certain valuable taxa but also leads to substantial reduction in the density and extent of forest cover. During the course of unabated depletion of forest, there is possibility of drastic declination in the number of some valuable plants leading towards the category of rare or vulnerable. Medicinal plants growing under natural habitat also get victim of such natural and man made disasters which require regular surveillance along with strategy for their conservation and propagations. Growth promoting rhizosphere microbes or root symbionts associated with them may be exploited for the said purposes. Keeping this in view an attempt has been made here to study the present status of medicinal plants and diversity of root associated fungi *i.e.*,VAMF in the forest regions of eastern Bihar.

Methods Adopted

Extensive survey of forest areas of eastern Bihar (Bhagalpur, Banka and Jamui districts) was made at a regular interval of 3 months to get clear picture of diversification of medicinal plants in different seasons continuously for complete one year. The purpose of the survey was to collect detailed information *i.e.* distribution and population density, frequency, local name, useful parts of medicinal plants and their uses for health care. Collection of rhizosphere soil and root sample was also made during the survey for screening of AMF spore population and per cent root colonization. The frequency percentage and density of medicinal plants were also calculated with the help of $30 \times 30m^2$ quadrate by the following formula:

Frequency Percentage

$$\frac{\text{Total number of quadrates in which species occurred}}{\text{Total number of quadrates studied}} \times 100$$

Density

$$\frac{\text{Total number of quadrates studied}}{\text{Total number of individuals of the species}} \times 100$$

Documentation of Rare/Vulnerable Medicinal Plants

On the basis of frequency and density of individual plant species in the surveyed area, list of rare (taxon less in number or risk) and vulnerable (taxa of endangered category for a particular area) medicinal plant species was prepared.

Rhizosphere soil and feeder roots were collected separately in polythene bags at about 15 cm depth around the plant. Soil and root test samples were brought to the laboratory for assessment of mycorrhizal association and physico-chemical analysis of soil. Screening of soil was done by Wet Sieving and Decantation Method of Gerdemann and Nicolson (1963). 10g of soil samples were mixed in 50 ml luke warm tap water in 200 ml beaker, stirred the solution 1-2 min. properly and left it for 3 min. for setting of heavier particles. Suspension was allowed to pass through the sieves of various measurements (710 mm–45 mm) with course sieve on the top and fine at the bottom. This process was repeated twice or thrice, so that whole suspension decanted through mesh and majority of spores isolated from soil samples. Debris retained by the sieve was washed under a stream of water. The suspension was transferred into petriplates separately. The content was examined for the presence of spores or sporocarp under the dissecting or compound microscope. The spore population was determined either number of spores/gm. dried soil or/10 gm. dried soil.

Spores were isolated and identified on the basis of morphological features *i.e.*, spore colour, spore size, shape, thickness of the wall, lamination, number of the wall, attachment pattern of subtending hyphae and content of the spores as ascribed in the manual of Schenck and Perez (1988). Phillips and Hayman (1970) method was followed for determining per cent of AMF colonization. The root sample were washed carefully and cut into small pieces (1 cm), which were boiled in 10 per cent KOH solution for one hour, washed for 3 times and bleached in alkaline hydrogen peroxide (5 per cent NH_4OH, 0.5 per cent H_2O_2, H_2O v/v) for 12 hours. The root bits were again washed 2-3 times in tap water. The trypan blue (0.05 per cent) was used for staining and lactophenol for mounting. The treated root bits were tapped softly and examined AMF infection in terms of percentage root colonization (per cent RC) which was determined by the following formula.

$$\%\text{ Root colonization} = \frac{\text{Number of segments observed}}{\text{Number of positive segments}} \times 100$$

The garden soil was dried on room temperature, sieved and autoclaved at 15 lb./inch^2 pressure for 3 hours for 3 consecutive days. The soil was placed in oven for 3 days at 90°C. After proper sieving of sand treated with 10 per cent HCl left for 3 days and was then washed till whole HCl was removed.

Results and Discussion

Survey of Forest Regions and their Soil Profile

During the course of study, survey of forest areas of eastern Bihar (Bhagalpur, Banka and Jamui districts) was made at a regular interval of three months for a year. Field trips were arranged so as to cover most of the forest and hilly tracts of all the study sites.

The land surface as a whole is apparently a level tract sloping gently from south to north in Bhagalpur and Banka districts, where as Jamui district is full of hilly tracts covering major forest areas. On the basis of soil texture of the area understudy was classified into Clay, Loam, Sand or Sandy Loam. The area enjoys the monsoon climate with a hot summer and a pleasant winter season. The average annual rainfall of the area is 1131.26 mm with 82 per cent of the precipitation falling during the monsoon months of June to September.

Since the soil of this region is complex in origin, it possesses a very heterogeneous flora, which is essentially tropophilous but a tendency towards xerophilous structure in many of its species. The types of forest of the surveyed areas are categorized as follows: Bhagalpur and Banka Districts: Northern dry mixed deciduous forest, Jamui District: Moist deciduous Sal, *Boswellia* and Aegle forests. A large number of forest produce *viz.* Timber, Gum, Kendu leaf, Bamboo, Medicinal plants, fruits etc. has been reported from this region as the main source of income for local inhabitants but the present investigation is mainly concerned with the present status of medicinal plants.

A total number of 113 medicinal plants were recorded out of which 10 plants *viz.Achyranthes aspera, Andrographis paniculata, Asparagus racemosus, Catharanthus roseus, Costus specious, Euphorbia thymifolia, Rauvolfia serpentina, Rauvolfia tetraphylla, Woodfordia fruticosa* and *Withania somnifera* were found growing invariably in all the forest regions, which were selected for screening of their root symbionts *i.e.*,VAM fungi in different soil profile.

The soil types are almost same in all the surveyed sites *i.e.* alluvial, sandy loam and sandy silt. Macro- and micronutrients *viz.*, N, K, P, Na, Ca, organic carbon and organic matter of soil samples and their pH were determined and results are depicted in Table 10.1. The soil pH was found to range in alkaline side except the soil of Jamui district where it was 6.5 tending towards acidic side. The organic carbon of the soil was noticed to range between 3.0–4.1 per cent whereas organic matter ranged between 6.5–7.05. A comparative study of the data particularly related with N, K, P, Ca and Na contents of the soil samples reflects that the soil of Jamui and Bhagalpur have almost similar status whereas Banka soil is slightly poorer in nutrients. On the basis of quantity of macro and microelements *i.e.*, OC, OM, N, K, P, Ca and Na, soil samples of different sites may be categorised as good–best Banka > Bhagalpur > Jamui.

Table 10.1: Showing the Chemical Profile of Soil Samples Collected from Sites Under Study

Soil samples	*pH*	*OC (%)*	*OM (%)*	*P (%)*	*N (%)*	*K (%)*	*Ca (%)*	*Na (%)*
Bhagalpur	7.88	4.05	7.02	0.260	0.056	0.237	0.531	0.443
Banka	7.2	3.09	6.5	0.230	0.043	0.226	0.482	0.422
Jamui	6.5	4.10	7.05	0.265	0.055	0.250	0.602	0.472

OC: Organic carbon; OM: Organic matter; P: Phosphorus; N: Nitrogen; K: Potassium; Ca: Calcium; Na: Sodium.

Screening of Rhizosphere Soil Samples of Medicinal Plants Understudy

The rhizosphere soil sample and feeder roots of 10 commonly growing medicinal plants were collected to determine the root colonization, spore population and diversity of AM fungi. Results are presented in Tables 10.2–10.4. The study of root colonization is necessary to observe the degree of infectivity and to describe the morphology of specific mycorrhizal structure formed within the roots. It is also essential to evaluate the responses of various treatments such as the effectiveness of different inoculants on plant growth and the extent of host specificity in different host fungus combination. Furthermore, the anatomical features of some of the fungal structure inside the roots are diagnostic for certain species. It may be possible to differentiate AM fungi responsible for root colonization.

Root Colonization (RC)

The root samples of 10 medicinal plants were examined for percentage colonization. The results (Tables 10.2–10.4) show that in Bhagalpur region, the maximum RC was recorded in *A. racemosus i.e.*, 75 per cent, 83 per cent, 78 per cent and 70 per cent during 1st, 2nd, 3rd and 4th quarters respectively with yearly average of 76.5 per cent whereas it was found minimum in *E. thymifolia i.e.* 9 per cent, 15 per cent, 12 per cent and 10 per cent during 1st, 2nd, 3rd and 4th quarters respectively with yearly average of 11.5 per cent. In Banka region the maximum RC was recorded in *A. racemosus i.e.* yearly average of 75.25 per cent whereas *E. thymifolia* showed only 10 per cent root colonization. In Jamui forest region again *A. racemosus* plant showed maximum RC *i.e.*, 82 per cent while it was minimum *i.e.*, 14.5 per cent in case of *E.thymifolia*. The results also make it clear that the medicinal plants of Jamui region were found to have maximum fascination towards root infection followed by Bhagalpur and Banka sites. The reason behind this might be due to variation in soil texture.

Table 10.2: Showing Per cent Root Colonization and Spore Population of Medicinal Plants Understudy in Bhagalpur Region

Plant Species	*Jan-Mar (Q_1)*		*Apr-Jun (Q_2)*		*Jul-Sep (Q_3)*		*Oct-Dec (Q_4)*		*Yearly Average*	
	RC	*SP*	*RC*	*SP*	*RC*	*SP*	*RC*	*SP*	*RC*	*SP*
Achyranthes aspera	12	21	20	28	17	31	14	23	15.75	25.75
Andrographis paniculata	40	27	55	35	48	34	42	29	46.25	31.25
Asparagus racemosus	75	20	83	24	78	27	70	19	76.5	22.50
Catharanthus roseus	30	22	48	28	46	30	39	23	40.75	25.75
Costus specious	38	31	47	23	43	21	39	16	41.75	22.75
Euphorbia thymifolia	9	10	15	15	12	17	10	12	11.50	13.50
Rauvolfia serpentine	40	23	53	32	50	27	47	25	47.50	26.75
Rauvolfia tetraphylla	43	21	57	28	53	30	45	22	49.50	25.25
Woodfordia fruticosa	62	28	69	32	64	33	60	30	63.75	30.75
Withania somnifera	70	32	78	43	73	37	69	31	72.50	35.75

RC: Root Colonization; SP: Spore Population; Q: Quarter.

Table 10.3: Showing Per cent Root Colonization and Spore Population of Medicinal Plants Understudy in Banka Region

Plant Species	*Jan-Mar (Q_1)*		*Apr-Jun (Q_2)*		*Jul-Sep (Q_3)*		*Oct-Dec (Q_4)*		*Yearly Average*	
	RC	*SP*	*RC*	*SP*	*RC*	*SP*	*RC*	*SP*	*RC*	*SP*
Achyranthes aspera	10	19	17	28	15	26	12	21	13.50	23.50
Andrographis paniculata	37	26	49	35	40	33	38	28	41.00	30.50
Asparagus racemosus	70	18	82	24	77	20	72	20	75.25	20.50
Catharanthus roseus	29	20	37	28	33	24	30	19	32.25	22.75
Euphorbia thymifolia	7	8	13	15	11	14	9	12	10.00	12.25
Costus speciosus.	36	15	44	23	40	21	38	17	39.50	19.00
Rauvolfia serpentine	37	25	48	32	41	29	38	27	41.00	28.25
Rauvolfia tetraphylla	41	17	54	28	48	23	42	19	46.25	21.75
Woodfordia fruticosa	60	20	72	32	65	30	61	22	64.50	26.00
Withania somnifera	66	29	75	37	71	32	68	30	70.00	32.00

RC: Root Colonization; SP: Spore Population; Q: Quarter.

Table 10.4: Showing Per cent Root Colonization and Spore Population of Medicinal Plants Understudy in Jamui Region

Plant Species	Jan-Mar (Q_1)		Apr-Jun (Q_2)		Jul-Sep (Q_3)		Oct-Dec (Q_4)		Yearly Average	
	RC	SP	RC	SP	RC	SP	RC	SP	RC	SP
Achyranthes aspera	14	24	20	32	18	30	15	24	16.75	27.50
Andrographis paniculata	47	30	58	43	50	40	48	32	50.75	36.25
Asparagus racemosus	80	18	87	29	82	24	79	20	82.00	22.75
Catharanthus roseus	33	23	40	34	38	31	34	27	36.25	28.75
Euphorbia thymifolia	11	8	19	12	16	14	12	9	14.50	10.75
Costus speciosus	42	15	49	25	43	24	40	19	43.50	20.75
Rauvolfia serpentina	42	24	51	37	47	32	43	28	45.75	30.25
Rauvolfia tetraphylla	45	23	53	34	51	30	46	27	48.75	28.50
Woodfordia fruticosa	60	27	68	38	63	32	61	25	63.00	30.50
Withania somnifera	68	34	74	42	72	17	69	32	70.75	31.25

RC: Root Colonization; SP: Spore Population; Q: Quarter.

Spore Population (SP)

The rhizosphere soil samples of all the 10 medicinal plants were collected from survey sites at the interval of 3 months *i.e.*, January–March, April–June, July–September and October–December and were analyzed for AMF spore population for getting annual status of mycorrhizal population under the influence of variable survey site factors. Results are depicted in Tables 10.2–10.4. Spore population was noticed to vary with sites, plants, and period of study. In Bhagalpur region, *W. somnifera* showed presence of maximum number of spores/10 gm dry soil *i.e.* 32, 43, 37 and 31 during 1st, 2nd, 3rd and 4th quarters respectively with yearly average of 36 whereas the minimum SP was recorded in *E. thymifolia* with yearly average of 14. In Banka the maximum SP was recorded in *W. somnifera* with yearly average of 32, whereas it was found minimum in *E. thymifolia* with yearly average of 13. Similarly in Jamui samples it was highest (43) in case of *A. paniculata* and recorded minimum (8) in case of *E.thymifolia*. However, definite correlation could not be established between root colonization and spore population as *A. racemosus* showed maximum per cent of root colonization in all sites whereas spore population was highest in case of *W. somnifera* both in Bhagalpur and Banka soil samples and *A. paniculata* in Jamui.

Seasonal Variations

Investigation on seasonal variation of AM fungi has also been carried out by several earlier workers including Srinivas *et al.* (1988); Rachel *et al.* (1990); Mago and Mukerji (1994) and they confirmed variation in the incidence of AM fungi during different time periods of the year. Such seasonal variation in AMF population also affects the establishment of plants under field conditions (Boerner, 1986). There are reports on seasonal diversity in AM fungi associated with crops and other plant species (McGee, 1989; Lopez and Honrubia, 1992; Johnson–Green *et al.*, 1995 and Siguenza *et al.*, 1996); however, fragmentary report is available so far with regard to medicinal plants under natural habitat. In order to record it medicinal plants were screened from all the sites under study at a regular interval of 3 months representing different seasons such as Autumn (Jan-March), Summer (Apr- June), Rainy

(July- Sept) and Winter (Oct-Dec). The results are shown in Tables 10.2–10.4. The observation reveals that the degree of infectivity in terms of root colonization and spore population of AMF varied with seasons and also to some extent to the type of plants. The comparative study of results reflects that the summer season favours both the number of spores and root colonization in case of almost all plants. Of all *A. racemosus* showed maximum RC (83 per cent) during this period but spore population in rainy season. In general the spore population was found not always highest in the summer but in some cases it was also noticed maximum in rainy period. The winter season did not support comparatively better RC and SP than any other seasons in case of all plants. However, *Achyranthus aspera, Andrographis paniculata,* and *E. thymifolia* showed presence of minimum number of spores during autumn. The results clearly point out in general that the maximum RC and SP were noticed during summer followed by rainy, autumn and winter season. Mohan Kumar and Mahadevan (1984) have also recorded similar result that more number of spores were present in soil in summer whereas least number in rainy season. Maximum number of spores is encountered during July and October and further decreased in the subsequent months. To the contrary Verma (1999) observed that low temperature of winter season favoured the colonization of fine endophyte (*Glomus tenue*) in root cortex of *Eupatorium* species.

Taxonomy and Distribution of AMF

Morton and Benny (1990) proposed a revised classification of arbuscular mycorrhizal fungi with a new order Glomales, and two sub orders Glomineae and Gigasporineae and two new families Acaulosporaceae and Gigasporaceae. Gigasporaceae includes *Gigaspora* and *Scutellospora,* Glomaceae includes *Sclerocystis* and *Glomus* and Acaulosporaceae includes *Acaulospora* and *Entrophospora.* Morton (1998) has listed 126 species of AM fungi which includes 22 species of *Acaulospora,* 3 species of *Entrophospora,* 6 species of *Gigaspora,* 67 species of *Glomus,* 9 species of *Sclerocystis* and 19 species of *Scutellospora.* In India, important contributions on the taxonomy of AM fungi were made by Bakshi (1974) and Mukerji and Kapoor (1990). Since vesicles and arbuscules formation is not uniform in the genera of AM fungi. Berch (1986) proposed the use of term vesicular arbuscular mycorrhizae (VAM) for the genera *Glomus, Sclerocystis, Acaulospora* and *Entrophospora,* which produce both vesicles and arbuscules, whereas arbuscular mycorrhizae (AM) for the genera *Gigaspora* and *Scutellospora* which form arbuscules only.

A large number of species belonging to five genera of AMF *viz. Glomus aggregatum, Glomus australe, Glomus deserticola, Glomus fasciculatum, Glomus geosporum, Entrophosphora colombiana, Scutellospora calospora, Sclerocystis pakistanika, Gigaspora margarita, Glomus multicauli,* and *Glomus maculosum* were isolated from selected medicinal plants of forest areas of eastern Bihar.

The fungi were identified on the basis of morphology of Chlamydospore, Azygospore, Zygospore, subcellular structures, subtending hyphae and lamination/ornamentation of spore. One species each of *Sclerocystis, Entrophosphora, Gigaspora* and *Scutellospora* and seven species of *Glomus* were found to constitute all together 11 species of VAM fungal flora. Out of five genera, *Glomus* was found to present dominantly in all the surveyed forest areas. Several earlier workers (Kumaran and Santha Krishnan, 1995; Lekha *et al.,* 1995; Mehrotra, 1998; Trimurthulu and Johri, 1998) have also reported the dominance of *Glomus* in different plants. The identification of AM fungi is mainly based on the morphology of the resting spores. However, many investigators realized that they are insufficient to identify the genus or species. Spore wall structure and ornamentation characters are very frequently used to identify the species (Tiwari *et al.,* 1982). Some efforts have also been made to identify the AMF spore through serological tests (Aldwell *et al.,* 1983). Mosse (1990) stated that sequencing of DNA and RNA helps in determining the taxonomy of AM fungi. Allen (1991) investigated Restriction Fragment Length

Polymorphism (RFLP) technique is found highly specific and useful to differentiate AM fungi. Recently, Bonito *et al.* (1995) employed the PCR technology for the detection of an AM fungus in roots of different plant species.

Table 10.5: Distribution of AMF Species in Selected Medicinal Plants in Survey Sites

Plant Species	*Bhagalpur*	*Banka*	*Jamui*
Achyranthes aspera	*Glomus aggregatum, Glomus fasciculatum*	*Glomu smaculosum, Gigaspora margarita*	*Scutellospora calospora, Glomus deserticola*
Andrographis paniculata	*Glomus deserticola, Sclerocystis pakistanica*	*Glomus deserticola, G.multicauli*	*Glomus aggregatum, Glomus fasciculatum*
Asparagus racemosus	*Glomus maculosum, Gigaspora margarita*	*Scutellospora calospora, Glomus deserticola*	*Glomus deserticola, G.multicauli,*
Catharanthus roseus	*Glomus multicauli, Sclerocystis pakistanica*	*Glomus australe, Gigaspora margarita*	*Glomus multicauli, Sclerocystis pakistanica*
Euphobia thymifolia	*Scutellospora calospora, Glomus deserticola*	*Scutellospora calospora, Glomus deserticola*	*Glomus aggregatum, Glomus fasciculatum*
Costus specious	*Glomus australe, Gigaspora margarita*	*Entrophosphora colombiana, Glomus aggregatum*	*Glomus maculosum, Gigaspora margarita*
Rauvolfia serpentina	*Glomus multicauli, Sclerocystis pakistanica*	*Entrophosphora colombiana, Glomus aggregatum*	*Glomus australe Gigaspora margarita*
Rauvolfia tetraphylla.	*Glomus fasciculatum, Gigaspora margarita*	*Glomus multicauli, Sclerocystis pakistanica*	*Glomus geosporum, G.maculosum*
Woodfordia fruticosa	*Entrophosphora colombiana Glomus aggregatum*	*Glomus geosporum, G.maculosum*	*Entrophosphora colombiana, Glomus aggregatum*
Withania somnifera	*Glomus geosporum, G.maculosum*	*Glomus geosporum, G.maculosum*	*Entrophosphora colombiana, Glomus aggregatum*

Earlier scanty reports available so far confirms the AMF role in increasing the level of active components of the plants but in the last decade some workers reported the role of AMF on medicinal plants (Harley and Harley, 1987; Campurbi *et al.*, 1990; Sharma and Roy, 1991; Chaterjee, 1992; Harikumar, 2001; Babu and Manoharcharya, 2003;). Chaterjee (1992) studied the possibility to improve the quality of some important medicinal plants such as *Catharanthus roseus*, *Papaver* sp. and *Ageratum* sp. by the association of AMF. Babu and Manoharacharya (2003) also reported the presence of AM fungi in the roots of alkaloid rich medicinal plants (about 15 medicinal plant species of different families). Reports indicated the association of many AMF species with medicinal plants. In *Euphorbia rosea*, two *Glomus* species were reported *i.e. G. pubescence* and *G. monosporus*, *Croton sparsiflorus* showed the mycorrhizal association of *Glomus darus*, *Acalypha indica* showed the mycorrhizal association of *Glomus pubescence*. *Euphorbia heterophylla* was mycorrhizal for *Glomus citricolum* (Raghupathy, Mohan Kumar and Mahadevan, 1984). In *Phyllanthus fraturnus* invariable mycorrhizal colonization (75 per cent–80 per cent) with secondary root was noticed (Mulani *et al.*, 2002). *Acaulospora* sp., *Entrophospora* sp., *Glomus* sp., and *Sclerocystis* sp. were found to be colonizing in the root and root soil sample of *Abrus precatorious* and *Asparagus racemosus*. *Gigaspora* sp., *Acaulospora* sp., *Glomus* sp. and *Sclerocystis* sp. were isolated from the roots of *Withania somnifera* (Babu and Manoharacharya, 2003). Six species of AM fungi were found to colonize the roots of alkaloid bearing medicinal plants (Ratti and Janardhanan, 1995). *Convolvulus arvensis* (100 per cent) was found associated with VAM fungi (Rani and Bhaduria, 2001). During the present investigation different AMF spores were isolated from 10 selected medicinal plants. The results show that seven species of *Glomus* was found to be associated with most of the plants along with some other species. The results are depicted in the Table 10.5.

During the course of study it was noticed that most of the plants having association of minimum two AMF species, which clearly indicates the presence of mixed AMF in the rhizosphere soil of medicinal plants of survey sites. However, *Glomus* was recorded as the dominant AMF in all the three survey sites. Several earlier workers (Lekha *et al.*, 1995; Mehrotra, 1998; Trimurthulu and Johri. 1998) have also reported the dominance of *Glomus* in different plants.

Acknowledgements

Authors are thankful to Head, University Department of Botany, T.M. Bhagalpur University, Bhagalpur for providing laboratory facilities.

References

Abbott, L.K. and Robson, A.D. (1991). Field management of VAM fungi. In Keister D.L. and Cregan P.B. (eds.). *The Rhizosphere and Plant Growth*, Kluwer Academic publishers, Dordrecht, London, pp.355-362.

Abbott, L.K. and Robson, A.D. (1991). Field management of VAM fungi. In Keister D.L. and Cregan P.B. (eds.). *The Rhizosphere and Plant Growth*, Kluwer Academic publishers, Dordrecht, London, pp. 355-362.

Aldwell, F.E.B., Hall, I.R. and Smith (1983). The identification of VAM fungi using immuno-fluorescence. *Soil Biol. Biochem.*, 15:439-445.

Allen, M.F. (1991). *The Ecology of Mycorrhizae*. Cambridge University press, pp.184.

Babu, K.S. and Manoharachary, C. (2003). Occurrence of AM fungi in rhizosphere soils of some medicinal plants. *Indian Phytopath.*, 56(2): 223-227.

Bakshi, B.K. (1974). *Mycorrhiza and its role in forestry*, PL 480 Project report. Forest Research Institute, Dehradun, pp. 89.

Berch, S.M. (1986). Endogonaceae taxonomy, specificity, fossil record, phylogeny. *Front. Appl. Microbiol.*, 2: 161-188.

Boerner, R.E.J. (1986). Seasonal nutrient dynamics, nutrient re-absorption and mycorrhizal infection intensity of two perennial forest herbs. *Amer.J. Bot.*, 73: 1249-1257.

Bonito, R.D., Elliot, M.L. and Des Jardin, E.A. (1995). Detection of an AM fungus in roots of different plant species with the PCR. *Appl. Environ. Microbiol.* 61(7): 2809-2810.

Camprubi, A.; Estann, V.; Calvet.; Pera, J. (1990). Infectivity and affectivity of *Glomns mosseae* Mycorrhizal in four different species of medicinal plants, *Symbiosis (Rehorot)*, 9 (1-3): 305–307.

Chatterjee, T. (1992). In Abstract vol. of *Nat. sym. Management of Microbes*, Allahabad University.

Daniels, B.A. and Trappe, J.M. (1980). *Mycologia*, 72: 457-471.

Gerdemann, J.W. and Nicolsson, T. H. (1963). Spores of mycorrhizal *Endogone* species extracted from soil by wet sieving and decanting technique. *Transactions of British Mycological Society*, 46: 235-243.

Hari Kumar, K. M. and Bagyaraj, D. J. (1988). Effect of intercropping and organic Soil amendments on native VAM. Mycorrhizae for Green Asia. *Proceedings of the first Asian Conference on Mycorrhizae*, pp. 207-208.

Hari kumar, V.S. (2001). Arbuscular Mycorrhizal synthesis in some wetland plants in Kerala *Mycorrhizal News*. 12(4): 14–15.

Harly, J.L. and Harley, E.L. (1987). A checklist of mycorrhiza in the British flora. The phytologist. *Can. J. Bot.*, 73(9): 1318–1327.

Hayman, D. S. (1978). *Endomycorrhizal* pp. 401–442 in interaction between non-pathogenic sol microorganizeam and plants Edited by X. R. Dommergues and S. K. Kyup, Elsevier, Amsterdam (1978).

Johnson-Green, P.C., Kenkel, N.C. and Booth, T. (1995). The distribution and phenology of arbuscular mycorrhizae along an inland salinity gradient.*Can.J. Bot.* 73 (9): 1318-1327.

Koske R. E. and Gemma, J. N. (1992). In mycorrhizal functioning: A Integrative plant fungal process (eds., Allen M. F.), Chapman and Hall, New York, USA, pp. 3–36.

Koske, R. E. (1987). Distribution of VAM fungi along a latitudinal temperature gradient. *Mycologia*, 79: 55–68.

Kothari, I. L. Udhyaya Joseph and Patel, C. R. (1997). Mycorrhizal biodiversity of petro effluents irrigated fields. *J. Mycol. Plant Pathol.*, 27(3): 275–278.

Kruckalmann, H.W. (1975). Effect of fertilizer, soils tillage and plant species on the frequency of *Endogone* chlamydospores and mycorrhizal infection in arable soils, In: *Endomycorrhizas* (Eds., Samders F. E., Mosse, B. and Tinker P. B.) Academic Press, London, pp. 511–525.

Kumaran, K. and Santha Krishnan, P. (1995). Vesicular arbuscular mycorrhizal fungi in tea (*Camellia sinensis* L.O. Kuntz.) soil. In: *Mycorrhizae: Biofertilizer for the Future* (eds.) Alok Adholeya, Sujan Singh. *Proceedings of the Third National Conference on Mycorrhiza*, pp. 33-37.

Lekha K. S., prasad, Joseph P. and Vejayan M. (1995). *Glomus fasciculatum* a predominant VAM fungus associated with Black pepper in forest soil of Kerala. In: *Mycorrhizae: Biofertilizer for the Future. The Proceedings of Third National Congress on Mycorrhizal* (Eds. Adholeya, Alok and Singh, Sujan) TERI, pp. 81-85.

Lopez–Sanchez E. and Honrubia M. (1992). Seasonal variation of VAM in eroded soils from southern Spain, *Mycorrhiza*, 2: 33–39.

Mago, P. and Mukerji, K. G. (1994). VAM in Lamiaceae: I. Seasonal variation in some member. *Phytomorphology*, 44(102): 83–88.

Mc Gee, P. A. (1989). Variation in propagule members of VAM fungi in a semi–arid soil. *Mucol. Res.* 92: 28–33.

Mehrotra, V. S. (1998). Arbuscular mycorrhizal associations of plants colonizing coalmine spoil in India. *Science*, Cambridge, 130: 124.

Mohan Kumar, V. and Mahadevan, A. (1984). Do secondary substances inhibit mycorrhizal association. *Current Science*, 53: 377-378.

Morton, J. B. and Benny, G. L. (1990). Revised classification of AMF (Zygomycetes). A new order Glomales two new suborders Glomineae and Gigasporineae and two new families Acaulosporaceae and Gigasporaceae with identification of Glomaceae. *Mycotaxon*, 37: 471–494.

Morton, J.B. (1998). Taxonomy of VAM fungi: Classification, nomenclature and identification. *Mycotaxon*, 32(Jul-Sept). 267-324.

Mosse, B. (1990). Mycorrhizal symbiosis and plant growth. *Procedings of the 2nd National Congress on Mycorrhizal*. (Eds. D.J. Bagyaraj and A.Manjunath). Bangalore (Abstract).

Mukerji, K. G. and Kapoor, A. (1990). Taxonomy of VAM fungi with special reference to Indian taxa. In G. P. Agrawal (Ed) *Perspectives in Mycological Research*. Today and Tomorrow's Printers and Publishers, New Delhi, PP. 7-16.

Mukherjee, K.G., Sabharwal, A., Kochar, B. and Ardey, J. (1984). VAM. Concepts and Advances. In K.G.V.P. Agnihotri and R.P.Singh (Eds.) *Progress in Microbial Ecology*, pp. 489-525.

Mulani, R.M., Prabhu, R. Rajendra and Manjusha Dinkaran (2002). Occurrence of VAM in the roots of *Phyllanthus fraternus* Webster. *Mycorrhizal News*, 14(2): 11-14.

Nicolson, T.H. and Schenck, N. C. (1979). *Mycologia*, 71: 178-198.

Phillips, J. M., Hayman, D.S. (1970). Improved procedures for clearing roots and staining parasites and vesicular-arbuscular mycorrhizal fungi for rapid assessment of infection. *Transactions of the British Mycological Society* 55: 15-161.

Raghupathy, S.; Mohankumar, V. and Mahadevan, A. (1988). Distribution of VAM in Thanjavur district flora pp. 96–98. In: *Mycorrhizae for Green Asia*, edited by A. Mahadevan; N. Raman and K. Natarajan Madras; University of Madras (351pp.)

Rachel, E. K., Reddy, S. R. and Reddy.S. M. (1990). Seasonal variation in the colonization and spore population of VAM fungi in semi arid of A. P., *Nat. Acad. Sci. Letters.*, pp. 13–16.

Rani, V. and Bhaduria, S. (2001). VAM association with some medicinal plants growing on alkaline soils of Mainpuri district, Uttar Pradesh, *Mycorrhiza News*, 13(2): 12–14.

Ratti, Neelima and Janardhanan, K. K. (1995). VAM association in some alkaloid bearing plants. Mycorrhizae : biofertilizers for the future, *Third National Conference on mycorrhiza* (eds. Adholeya, Alok and Singh, Sujan) pp. 407–409.

Roy, A. K., Singh, A. N. and A. Arshi (2004). Dynamics of rhizosphere microflora in nutrient deficient OBD soil of ECL. *Proceedings of National Symposium on Current Perspective in Stress Biology*. 6–8 Feb. 2004, NBU, Siliguri.

Schenck, N. C. and Perez, Y. (1988). *Manual of the Identification of VA Mycorrhizal Fungi*, University of Florida, Gainesville, GL, 245pp.

Shanker, A., Mathew J. Neeraj Kaur, Mehrotra, R. S. and Verma, A. (1990). Mycorrhizal status of some desert plants and their physiological significance. In: *Trends in Mycorrhizal Research. Proceeding of the National Conference on Mycorrhizae*, HAU, Hissar, pp. 160–161.

Sharma, M. and Roy, A. K. (1991). VAM in hypoglycaemic plants. *Nat. Acad. Sci. Letters*, 14(12): 467–468.

Siguenza, C., Espejel, I. And Allen, E. B. (1996). Seasonality of mycorrhizae in coastal sand dunes of Baja California. *Mycorrhiza*, 6(2): 151–157.

Singh, C. S. Deepa Jha and Jha D. (1994). Mass inoculum production of VAM effect of various bacteriological media and fertilizer solutions. *Microbiol. Res.*, 149: 27–29.

Smith, S. E. and Bowen, G. D. (1979). Soil temperature, mycorrhizal infection and nodulation of *Medicago trumcalila* and *Trifolium subterraneum*. *Soil Biol and Biochemistry*. 11: 469–473.

Srinivas, K. Shanmugam, N. and Ramraj, B. (1988). Effect of VAM fungi on growth and nutrient uptake of forest tree seedlings. *Proc. 1st Asian conf. Mycorrhizae*, Madras. India. pp. 294–297.

Tiwari, J. P., Skorpod, W. P., Mukherji, K. G. and Mishra, S. (1982). *Trans. Br. Mycol. Soc.* 76: 207–304.

Trinick, M. J. (1977). *New Phytologist*, 78: 207–304.

Trimurthulu, N. and Johri, B. N. (1998). Prevalence and distribution of VAM spore population in different tarai soils of Uttar Pradesh. *J. Mycol. Pl. Pathol.* Vol. 28 No. 3, 236–239.

Verma, A. (1999). In Verma, A., Hock, B. (eds.) *Mycorrhiza*. Springer-Verlag, pp. 521–556.

Microbial Biotechnology and Ecology (2011)
Editors: Deepak Vyas, G.S. Paliwal, P.K.Khare and R.K Gupta
Published by: DAYA PUBLISHING HOUSE, NEW DELHI

Pages 201–208

Chapter 11

Association of Vesicular Arbuscular Mycorrhizal Fungi with Ornamental Plants

☆ ***Bhaskar Chaurasia and P.K. Khare***

Department of Botany, Dr. H.S. Gour Vishwavidyalaya, Sagar – 470 003, M.P.

ABSTRACT

The present chapter deals with the analysis of root and rhizosphere soil samples for composition of VAM population in ten selected ornamental plants. The VAM colonization in the root samples ranged from 63 to 100 per cent with maximum colonization in *Narcissus poeticus*. The maximum and minimum spore population in the rhizosphere soil were found in *Narcissus poeticus* (126 spores 25^{-1} g soil) and *Rosa* sp. (77 spore 25^{-1} g soil), respectively. Further, maximum number of vesicles (47 vesicles cm^{-1} root bit) were also observed in *Narcissus poeticus* and the lowest (21 vesicles cm^{-1} root bit) in *Rosa* sp.

A total number of 23 VAM species were identified belonging to five genera *i.e. Acaulospora, Gigaspora, Glomus, Sclerocystis* and *Scutellispora*. Genus *Glomus* was found dominant in the rhizosphere soil samples of all the ornamental plant species. *Glomus* species constituted 66 per cent of total VAM species composition followed by *Sclerocystis* (13 per cent), *Acaulospora* (13 per cent), *Gigaspora* (4 per cent) and *Scutellispora* (4 per cent). Alongwith three species of *Glomus i.e. G. aggregatum, G. ambisporum, G. fasciculatum, Acaulospora scrobiculata* and *Sclerocystis pakistanika* were found most frequent and abundant VAM species in the rhizosphere soil of all ornamental plants studied.

Observation of the present investigation indicates that VAM population attributes *i.e.* no. of spores and vesicles, species diversity and colonization, were more in herbaceous plants as compared to woody species.

Introduction

Vesicular Arbuscular Mycorrhizal (VAM) fungi have extremely wide host range due to their non specificity. Vascular plants of all life forms association with VAM fungi and its importance for plant growth have been fully appreciated. The VAM fungi exhibit a perfect symbiosis and this interaction in turn increase plant growth, enhance accumulation of plant nutrients through greater soil exploration (Abbot and Robson, 1989) and improve soil health (Hodge *et al.*, 2001). The primary benefit for the plant is the increase in phosphorus and nutrient uptake from soil, although protection against certain pathogens, production of plant growth hormones and the increased solubility of soil minerals are also regarded as important benefits (Ahmadjian, 1986). Further, due to their wide ecological amplitude, they are found in diverse habitats ranging from arctic to tropics (Dalpe and Aiken, 1998; Chaurasia, 2001), arid to aquatic (Ba *et al.*, 1996) and climax to highly disturbed communities (Chaurasia *et al.*, 2007; Sastry and Johri, 1999). In view of the above importance and needs of VAM associations and also the paucity of work done there is a need to screen each and every habitat for VAM population and their distribution. The present work was carried out to study the isolation, and identification of indigenous VAM species associated with the rhizosphere soil of ornamental plants.

Materials and Methods

Study Site

The Botanic Garden of Dr. H.S. Gour Vishwavidyalaya is recognized by Botanic Garden Conservation International. This site was selected with a view that it consists of plants from different climatic region *i.e.*, Himalayan, Southern, Sea shore, desert and vegetation of Central India. Since it is actively managed for soil and fertility, the soil is clay loam. A number of forest, ornamental and rare plants are maintained and propagated here. Plants from all facets of groups *i.e.*, angiosperms, gymnosperms, pteridophytes, bryophytes are growing here luxuriantly. Further, plants from different habitats *i.e.*, forest, grassland, desert, aquatic, high altitude regions, are maintained.

Collection of Soil and Root

The soil and root samples were randomly collected from rhizosphere of selected plants. Soil samples were taken by digging out a small amount of soil close to a plant to a depth of 10-15 cm after removing the top soil. The samples were taken in three replicates. All the samples were brought to the laboratory in labelled polyethylene bags.

Roots were excavated carefully with the help of hoe and care was taken to prevent damage to the fine roots. Fine feeder roots were separated and lightly shaked. Root samples were collected in three replicates from each plant species and kept in labelled polyethylene bags.

Processing and Assessment of Colonization of Root Samples

Freshly collected root samples were rinsed with tap water several times to wash the roots thoroughly. Roots were cut into small bits of about 1 cm pieces and modified procedure (Kormanik *et al.*, 1980) was used for clearing and staining. Alternatively presence or absence of colonization was recorded in each of the 10 pieces. Minimum 100 root segments were used for this method.

Extraction, Estimation and Identification of VAM Spores

Gerdemann and Nicolson's (1963) wet- sieving and decanting procedure was adopted for isolation of VAM spores. For estimation of VAM spores, a modified method of Smith and Skipper (1979) by Gour and Adholeya (1994) was followed. VAM fungal identification was done following different identification keys (Hall, 1984; Morton, 1988; Schenck and Perez, 1990; Mehrotra and Baijal, 1994).

Analysis of Data

VAM colonization (per cent): The per cent VAM colonization was calculated by using following formula:

$$\text{Per cent VAM colonization} = \frac{\text{Total no. of infected root pieces}}{\text{Total no. of root pieces studied}} \times 100$$

Relative density: Relative density of VAM species with each host species was calculated following the under mentioned formula.

$$\text{Relative Density} = \frac{\text{No. of VAM species associated with the host species}}{\text{Total no. of VAM species associated with the entire host considered}} \times 100$$

Results and Discussion

As evident from the results that there existed consistency in almost all ornamental plant species in having higher VAM colonization, number of vesicles and spore population (Table 11.1).

Narcissus poeticus showed 100 per cent VAM colonization and maximum number of vesicles (47 cm^{-1} root bit) in their roots and highest VAM spore population (126 spores $25g^{-1}$ soil) occurred in its rhizosphere soil. *Rosa* sp. comes out to be the poorest host for VAM fungi as the colonization, number of spores, vesicles (Figure 11.1) and number of VAM species associated with it were minimum (Table 11.1). All ornamental plants selected for study are herbaceous in nature except *Rosa* species. Several workers reported that herbaceous plants are extensively colonized by VAM fungi (Jain *et al.*, 1997, Chaurasia and Khare, 1999).

Table 11.1: Different Attributes of VAM Fungi Associated with Some Ornamental Plants

Sl.No.	Name of Species	Colonization (per cent)	Average Number of Vesicles (cm^{-1} root bit.)	Spore Population ($25g^{-1}$ soil)	Total Number VAM Fungal Species	Dominant VAM Species
1.	*Calendula officinalis*	75	37	105	12	ASCB, LAGR, LMCC
2.	*Chrysanthemum morifolium*	85	39	80	16	LFSC, ASCB, LAGR, SPKS
3.	*Dahelia pinnata*	95	24	105	10	ASCB, LABS, LFSC, SPKS
4.	*Dianthus caryophyllatus*	84	42	91	9	LAGR, LFSC, LABS, SPKS
5.	*Gerbera gamsoni*	87	41	110	15	LAGR, LFSC, ASCB, LMSS, SSNS
6.	*Narcissus poeticus*	100	47	126	20	ASCB, LMCC, LAGR, LFSC, SSNS
7.	*Phlox* sp.	94	40	95	9	ASCB, LAGR, LFSC, SPKS
8.	*Polianthes tuberosa*	66	37	87	7	LAGR, LABS, LFSC, SSNS
9.	*Rosa* sp.	63	21	77	6	LFSC, SPKS, LAGR, LABS
10.	*Tagates erectus*	74	28	102	12	ASCB, LHTS, LFSC, SPKS

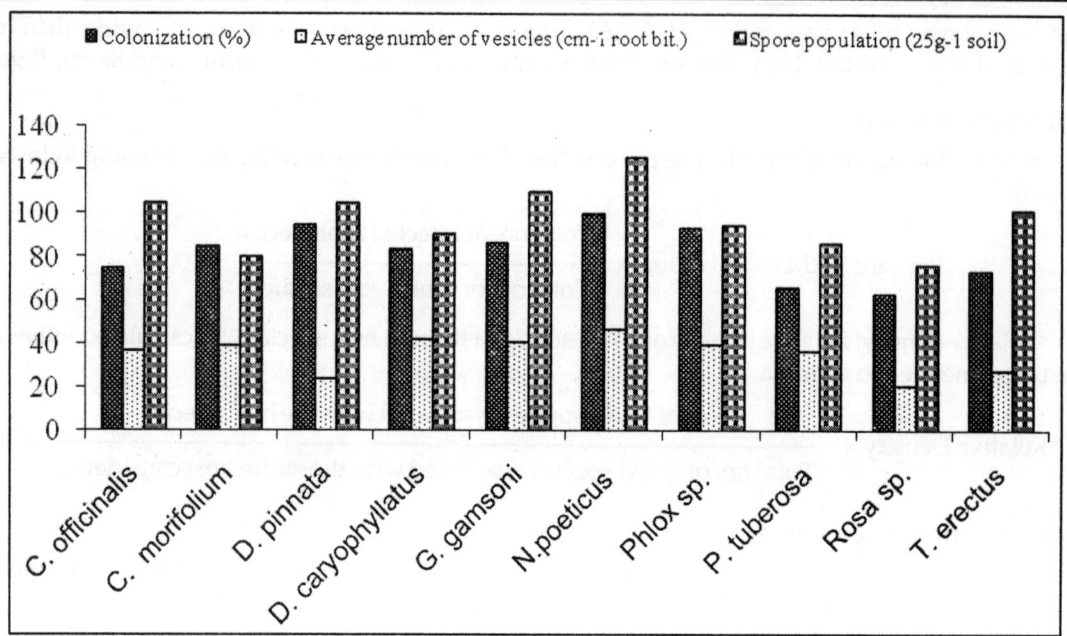

Figure 11.1: Different Attributes of VAM Fungi in the Rhizosphere Soil of Different Ornamental Plants at Botanical Garden

23 VAM species were recovered from rhizosphere soil of different ornamental plants at Botanical Garden. About 66 per cent of total VAM isolates of VAM fungi included *Glomus* species followed by *Acaulospora* (3 species), *Sclerocystis* (3 species), *Gigaspora* and *Scutellispora* (each with one species) (Table 11.2 and Figure 11.2).

Several workers reported predominance of *Glomus* species in different habitats (Bhadauria and Yadav, 1999; Lingon *et al.*, 1999, Chaurasia 2001, Chaurasia *et al.*, 2005 a and b; 2007). Predominance of *Glomus* at the present study sites as well as the reports given by a number of workers cannot be assertively interpreted due to paucity of data pertaining to the physiology and adaptiveness of this species.

Five other species *e.g. Calendula officinalis, Dahelia pinnata, Gerbera gamsoni, Narsissus poeticus* and *Tagatus erectus* possessed higher VAM spore population (>100 spore $25g^{-1}$ soil). It is evident from results that *A. scrobiculata, G. aggregatum, G. ambisporum, G. fasciculatum* and *S. pakistanica* were the dominant VAM species (Tables 11.2 and 11.3). Except for *Glomus* species other VAM species showed a poor frequency distribution. Similar to present findings, several workers reported predominance of *Glomus* species *viz. G. aggregatum* and *G. fasciculatum* species in different rhizosphere soil (Kunwar *et al.*, 1999; Lingon *et al.*, 1999, Chaurasia *et al.*, 2005 a and b; 2007). Besides these two *Glomus* species some other *Glomus* species were frequently distributed in the rhizosphere soils. Wide occurrence and distrubution of *Glomus* species in the rhizosphere soil may be attributed to its early evolution and can be considered one of the few plant fungus associations with a fossil record (Pirozynski and Dalpe, 1989; Taylor *et al.*, 1995; Phipps and Taylor, 1996; Helgason *et al.*, 1998). Allen (1991) reported that uneven distribution of VAM fungi in rhizosphere of different species may be dependent on the nature of host, host growth pattern and age of plant.

Table 11.2: Distribution of Different VAM Fungi in Rhizosphere Soil of some Important Ornamental Plant Species at Botany Garden

Sl.No.	VAM Sp. Code	Plant Species										Frequency %
		Calendula officinalis	*Chrysanthemum morifolium*	*Dahelia pinnata*	*Dianthus caryophyllatus*	*Gerbera gamsoni*	*Naricissus poeticus*	*Phlox* sp.	*Polianthes tuberosa*	*Rosa* sp.	*Tagates erectus*	
1.	ASCB	+	+	+	+	+	+	+	+	+	+	100.00
2.	ASPN	–	–	–	–	–	–	+	–	–	–	10.00
3.	AUDL	+	+	–	–	–	+	–	–	–	–	30.00
4.	GRSA	+	+	–	–	–	+	–	–	–	+	40.00
5.	LAGR	+	+	+	+	+	+	+	+	+	+	100.00
6.	LABS	+	+	+	+	+	+	+	+	+	+	100.00
7.	LCST	+	+	–	+	+	+	–	–	–	–	50.00
8.	LETC	–	+	–	–	+	+	+	–	–	–	40.00
9.	LFSC	+	+	+	+	+	+	+	+	+	+	100.00
10.	LGSP.	+	+	–	–	–	+	+	–	–	+	40.00
11.	LHTS	–	+	+	+	–	+	–	–	–	+	50.00
12.	LINR	–	+	+	–	+	+	–	–	–	+	50.00
13.	LMCC	+	+	–	–	+	+	–	–	–	–	40.00
14.	LMAG	–	–	–	–	+	+	+	–	–	–	30.00
15.	LMSS	–	+	+	–	+	+	–	–	–	+	50.00
16.	LOCT	–	–	+	+	–	+	–	–	–	–	30.00
17.	LTNB	–	+	–	–	–	+	–	–	–	+	30.00
18.	G.sp.B.	+	–	–	+	+	–	–	–	–	–	30.00
19.	G.sp.C.	–	–	–	–	–	–	–	+	+	–	20.00
20.	SMRC	–	–	–	–	+	+	–	–	–	+	30.00
21.	SPKS	+	+	+	+	+	+	+	+	+	+	100.00
22.	SSNS	+	+	–	–	+	+	–	+	–	–	50.00
23.	CARN	–	–	+	–	+	+	–	–	–	–	30.00

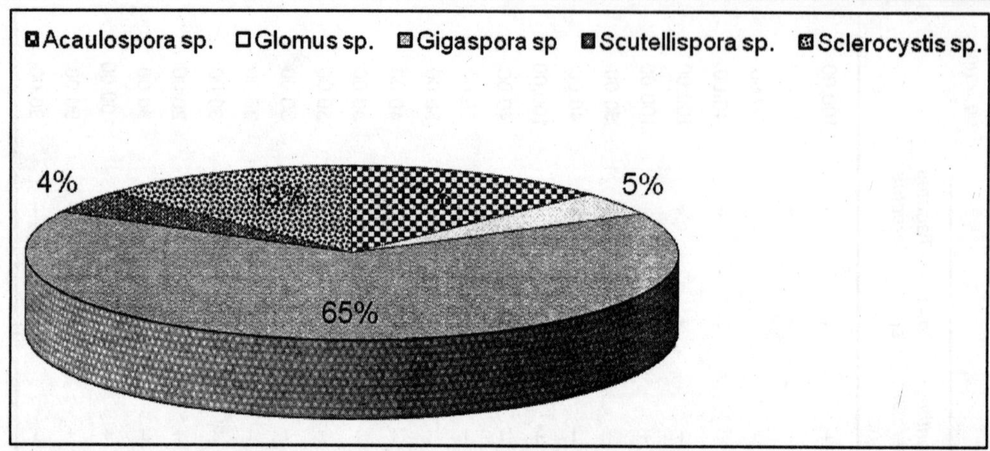

Figure 11.2: VAM Species Composition in the Rhizosphere Soil in the Ornamental Plants

Table 11.3: Association of VAM Species and their Relative Densities with Different Ornamental Plants

Sl.No.	Name of Plants Species	No. of VAM Species Associated	Relative Density
1.	*Calendula officinalis*	12	10.34
2.	*Chrysanthemum morifolium*	16	13.79
3.	*Dahelia pinnata*	10	8.62
4.	*Dianthus caryophyllatus*	9	7.75
5.	*Gerbera gamsoni*	15	12.93
6.	*Narcissus poeticus*	20	17.24
7.	*Phlox* sp.	9	7.75
8.	*Polianthes tuberosa*	7	6.03
9.	*Rosa* sp.	6	5.17
10.	*Tagates erectus*	12	10.34

In conclusion the important observation of the present investigations are (1) there is no correlation among per cent colonization, spore population, species diversity and (2) herbaceous species having higher VAM attributes in comparison to woody ornamental plants. This report gives a preliminary account of VAM fungi associated with ornamental plant species. Ornamental plants are economically important and role of VAM fungi in their productivity still needs considerable attention.

References

Abbott, L.K. and Robson, A.D. (1984). The effect of mycorrhizae on plant growth, 113-130. In: *VA mycorrhiza*, (eds) CL, Powell, D. J. Bagyaraj. CRC Press, Boca Raton, Florida USA..

Ahmadjian, V. (1986). *Symbiosis*. University Press of New England, Hanover, New Hampshire, pp. 212.

Allen, M. F. (1991). *The ecology of mycorrhizae*. Cambridge University Press England.

Ba A.M., Dalpe Y., Guissou T. (1996). Glomales of Acacia holosericea and Acacia mangium. *Bios For Trop*. 25: 5-18.

Bhadauria, S. and Yadav, R. (1999). Vesicular-arbuscular mycorrhizal associations in fuel wood trees growing in alkaline soil, *Mycorrhiza News*, 10 (4): 14-15.

Chaurasia B. (2001). Ecological study of tropical forests with special reference to vesicular Arbuscular mycorrhizal (VAM) association. *Ph. D. Theis*, Dr. H.S. Gour V.V. Sagar, M.P.

Chaurasia B. and Khare P. K. (1999). VAM fungi associations in a protected grassland. *Mycorrhiza News*, 11 (1): 13-14.

Chaurasia B, Pandey A. and Palni L.M.S. (2007). Arbuscular mycorrhizal species diversity in Kumaun region of Indian Central Hiamlaya. In: *The Mycorrhizae: Diversity, Ecology and Application* (eds) Tiwari M. and Sati S. C., Daya Publishing House, New Delhi-110 035. 286-294.

Chaurasia B, Pandey A. and Palni L.M.S. (2005a). Occurrence of arbuscular mycorrhizae in the rhizosphere of Himalalayan Yew (*Taxus baccata* L. subsp. Wallichiana (Zucc.) Pilger)- a case study. In: *Basic Research and Applications of Mycorrhizae*. (eds) Podila G.K. and Verma A.K., IK International Publication, New Delhi, pp. 26-35.

Chaurasia B, Pandey A. and Palni L.M.S. (2005b). Distribution, colonization and diversity of arbuscular mycorrhizal fungi in Rododendrons of Central Himalayan region of India. *Forest Ecology and Management* 207: 315-324.

Dalpe Y. and Aiken S.G. (1998). Arbuscualr mycorrhizal fungi associated with *Festuca* species in the Canadian High Arctic. *Canadian Journal of Botany* 76: 1930-1938.

Gerdemann, J.W. and Nicolson, T.H. (1963). Spores of mycorrhizal Endogone species extracted from soil by wet sieving and decanting. *Trans Br. Mycol. Soc.* 46: 235-244.

Gour, A., Adholeya, A., Mukerji, K. G. (1998). A comparison of AM fungi inoculants using *Capsicum* and *Polianthes* in marginal soil amended with organic matter. *Mycorrhiza*, 7 (6): 307-312.

Hall, I.R. (1984). Taxonomy of VA mycorrhizal fungi, pp.57-94. In: *VA mycorrhiza*, ed. by C.L.Powell and D.J. Bagyaraj. CRC Press, Boca Raton, FL.

Helgason, T., Daniell, T. J., Husband, R., Fitter, A. H. and Young, J. P. W. (1998). Ploughing up the wood wide web ?. *Nature*. 394 (30): 431.

Hodge A., Campbell C.D., and Fitter A.H. (2001). An arbuscular mycorrhizal funbgus accelerates decomposition and acquires nitrogen directly from organic material. *Nature* 413: 297-299.

Jain, R.K., Hasan, N., Singh,R.K., and Pandey, S.N. (1997). Vesicular-arbuscular mycorrhizal (VAM) associations in some weeds of forage legumes, *Mycorrhiza News*, 9(1): 10-12.

Kormanik, P.P., Bryan, W.C. and Schultz, R.C. (1980). Procedure and equipment for staining large number of plant roots for endomycorrhizal assay. *Can. J. Microbiol.* 26: 536-538.

Kunwar, J.K., Reddy, J.P.M. and Manoharachary, C. (1999). Occurrance and distribution of AMF associated with garlic rhizosphere soil. *Mycorrhiza New*. 11(2): 4-6.

Lingan, V.K., Tholkappian, D., and Sundaram, M.D. (1999). VA mycorrhizal fungi occurring in the mangrove vegetation of Pichavaram forest. *Mycorrhiza News*. Vol.1 (2): 6-7.

Mehrotra, V.S. and Baijal, U. (1994). Advances in the taxonomy of vesicular-arbuscular mycorrhizal fungi. *Biotechnology in India*. pp. 227-286.

Morton, J.B. (1988). Taxonomy of VA mycorrhizal fungi: Classification nomenclature, and indetification. *Mycotaxon*. 32: 267-324.

Phipps, C.J. and Taylor, T.N. (1996). Mixed arbuscular mycorrhizae from the triassic of Antartica. *Mycologia*. 88(5): 707-714.

Pirozynski, K.A. and Dalpe, Y. (1989). Geological history of the Glomaceae with particular reference to mycorrizal symbiosis. *Symbiosis*, 7: 1-36.

Sastry M.S.R. and Johri B.N. (1999) Arbuscular mycorrhizal fungal diversity of stressed soils of Bailadila iron ore sites in Bastar region of Madhya Pradesh. Current Science 77: 1095-1100.

Schenck, N.C. and Perez, Y. (1990). A manual for identification of vesicular-arbuscular mycorrhizal fungi. INVAM University of Florida. Gainesville, FL. 286 pp.

Smith, G.W. and Skipper, H.D. (1979). Comparison of methods to extract spores of vesicular-arbuscular-mycorrhizal fungi. *Soil. Sci. Soc. J.* 43: 722-725.

Taylor, T.N., Remy, W., Hass, H. and Kerp., H. (1995). Fossil arbuscular mycorrhizae from the early Devonian. *Mycologia*. 87: 560-573.

Microbial Biotechnology and Ecology (2011) *Pages* 209–224
Editors: Deepak Vyas, G.S. Paliwal, P.K.Khare and R.K Gupta
Published by: DAYA PUBLISHING HOUSE, NEW DELHI

Chapter 12

Perspective of AM Fungi in Agroforestry Systems

☆ *Ashok Shukla*[1]*, *A. Kumar*[1], *D. Vyas*[2], *A. Jha*[1], *M. Kamalvanshi*[1] *and N. Chakravarty*[1]

[1]*National Research Centre for Agroforestry, Jhansi – 284 003, U.P.*
[2]*Dr. H.S. Gour University, Sagar – 470 003, M.P.*

ABSTRACT

Arbuscular mycorrhizal (AM) fungi form symbiotic association with most economically important plants. These fungi improve plant growth under low fertility conditions, increase tolerance against plant pathogens, improve water balance of the plants, contribute to the formation of soil structure and help plants to establish in new areas. In agroforestry systems trees are deliberately planted on the same unit of land with agricultural crops for rehabilitation of the degraded areas. The potential benefit of AM fungi in rehabilitation of degraded lands by use of agroforestry system is more apparent than ever before. The need to increase food, fiber and fuel wood production to keep pace with the fast growing population is crucial. The low biomass production of agroforestry tree species in degraded areas can, therefore, be circumvented by the use of AM fungi. The role of AM fungi in enhancing plant growth and yield, resistance to drought and salinity and tolerance to pathogens is well documented, but little is known about their interactions with agroforestry systems. The present chapter enlighten the potential benefit of AM fungi in rehabilitation of degraded lands by use of agroforestry systems.

Introduction

In 1885 A. B. Frank was the first to describe the symbiosis between a fungus and the roots of trees and he coined the term *Mycorrhiza.* The term originates from the Greek *mycos*, meaning 'fungus' and

* E-mail: ashokshukla06@gmail.com.

rhiza, meaning 'root'. Mycorrhiza is a symbiotic mutualistic relationship between special soil fungi and fine plant roots; it is neither the fungus nor the root, but rather the structure formed from these two partners. Since the association is mutualistic, both organisms benefit from the association. The fungus receives carbohydrates (sugars) and growth factors from the plant, which in turn receives many benefits, including increased nutrient absorption. In this association, the fungus takes over the role of the plant's root hairs and acts as an extension of the root system.

Mycorrhizal fungi are an important group of soil-borne microorganisms that contribute substantially to the establishment, productivity, and longevity of natural or man-made ecosystems (Harley and Smith, 1983). These fungi form symbiotic association with most terrestrial plant families (Trappe, 1977). In natural ecosystems mycorrhizal fungi can colonize much of the root system. Colonization is restricted to the root cortex and does not enter the vascular cylinder. The symbiosis is so well balanced that, although many of the host cells are invaded by the fungal endophyte, there is no visible tissue damage and under certain conditions it enhances the growth and vigour of the host plant. Because most economically important plants form mycorrhizae, the subject is currently attracting much attention in agricultural, horticultural, and forestry research. There are different types of mycorrhizae. The present chapter is concerned with AM fungi, information available in literature on its benefits, occurrence, taxonomy, ecology, culturing techniques and their role in agroforestry are being reviewed and being presented here, in short.

Arbuscular mycorrhizal fungi (AMF) are by far the most abundant of all mycorrhizas. They are characterized by the formation of an extraradical mycelium and branched haustorial structures within the cortical cells termed arbuscules. The latter are the main sites of exchange between the two symbiotic partners (Hock and Varma, 1995). In contrast to ectomycorrhizal fungi, AMF are considered to be obligate biotrophic microorganisms and cannot be cultured axenically. The general differentiation between symbiosis and pathogenicity is not easy and this is particularly true for mycorrhizas. Depending on environmental conditions, root colonization with AM fungi can either stimulate or inhibit plant growth (Sanders, 1993) and during the formation of the AM symbiosis several defence responses have been observed in the plant (Gianinazzi-Pearson *et al.*, 1996; García-Garrido and Ocampo, 2002).

Beneficial Effects of Mycorrhizae

The most prominent effect of AM fungi is that it plays an important role in enhancing the plant growth and yield due to an increase supply of phosphorus to the host plant. Mycorrhizal plants can absorb and accumulate several times more phosphate from the soil or solution than non–mycorrhizal plants. However uptake of nitrogen, zinc, copper and minor nutrients are enhanced as well. Improved plant nutrition is due to (i) increased root surface through extraradical hyphae, (ii) degradation of organic material and (iii) alteration of the microbial composition in the rhizosphere (Marschner, 1998; Hodge and Campbell, 2001). In exchange for the nutrients, the fungus is supplied with photosynthates (about 20 per cent of the plant assimilation capacity) and these assimilates are either respired or released into the soil. As a result of higher carbon drain, microbial rhizosphere composition is altered and therefore the term "mycorrhizosphere" was coined (Rambelli, 1973). As the majority of all plants are mycorrhizal, mycorrhizosphere versus rhizosphere might be the rule rather than the exception (Linderman, 1988). In addition, mycorrhizas increase drought resistance (Augé and Stodola, 1990) and heavy metal tolerance (Brundrett, 1991), improve soil aggregation (Andrade *et al.*, 1998) and promote overall plant health (Linderman, 1992).

Mycorrhiza increase root surface area for water and nutrients uptake. The use of mycorrhizal bio-fertilizer helps to improve higher branching of plant roots, and the mycorrhizal hyphae grow from the root to soil enabling the plant roots to contact with wider area of soil surface, hence, increasing the absorbing area for water and nutrients absorption of the plant root system. Therefore, plants with mycorrhizal association will have higher efficiency for nutrients absorption, such as nitrogen, phosphorus, potassium, calcium, magnesium, zinc and copper and also increase plant resistance to drought. Benefits of mycorrhizal bio-fertilizer are as follows:

- ✰ Allow plants to take up nutrients in unavailable forms or nutrients that are fixed to the soil, especially phosphorus which are immobile in the soil. In addition, mycorrhiza help to absorb other organic substances that are not fully soluble for plants to use, and also help to absorb and dissolve other nutrients for plants.
- ✰ Enhance plant growth, improve crop yield and increase income for the farmers.
- ✰ Reduce the use of chemical fertilizer.
- ✰ Improve plant resistance to root rot and collar rot diseases. Mycorrhizal association in plant roots will help plant to resist root rot and collar rot diseases caused by other fungi.
- ✰ Enhance water transport in plants, decrease transplant injury and promote establishment of plants in wasteland. Mycorrhizal plants recover better following moisture stress, more efficient in water use and frequently have higher root-shoot ratio than non-mycorrhizal plants.
- ✰ Increase plant growth by 20-30 per cent in terms of bio-mass.
- ✰ Enable the plants to grow and survive better under various stress conditions, like those in coal spoils, sand dunes, saline-alkaline soils, eroded- degraded sites and lands polluted by industrial wastes.

Table 12.1: Different Types of Mycorrhizae and their Hosts

Types of Mycorrhizae	*Host Plant/Families*
Ecto	Pinaceae, Fagaceae, Betulaceae, Leguminaceae, mostly Caesalpinoid legumes, Salicaceae, Tiliaceae, Rosaceae, Juglandaceae, etc.
Arbuscular	Majority of the plants including those important in agriculture, horticulture, pasture and tropical forests
Ericoid	Ericaceae and Epacridaceae
Orchidaceous	Orchidaceae
Arbutoid	Arbutus and Monotropha

Occurrence

VAM fungi have the widest host range and distribution of all the mycorrhizal associations. It is estimated that about 90 per cent of vascular plants normally establish mutualistic relationship with VAM fungi. VAM fungi have been observed in 1000 genera of plants representing some 200 families. There are at least 300,000 receptive hosts in the world flora (Kendrick and Berch, 1985) and there are about 120 species of VAM fungi (Schenck and Perez, 1987). If the hosts are divided up evenly among the fungi with no overlap in host range, each fungus would have more than 2500 potential partners. We know that host ranges overlap extensively, suggesting that some individual VAM fungi may well have access to thousands of hosts (Kendrick and Berch, 1985).

According to Gerdemann (1975), it is easier to list most plant families that do not form VAM than to list those that do. Families not forming vesicular arbuscular mycorrhizal fungi include Pinaceae, Betulaceae, Orchidaceae, Fumariaceae, Commelinaceae, Urticaceae, and Ericaceae (Table 12.2). Families that rarely form vesicular-arbuscular mycorrhiza include the Brassicaceae, Chenopodiaceae, Polygonaceae, and Cyperaceae. Families that form both ectomycorrhizae and vesicular arbuscular mycorrhizal fungi include Juglandiaceae, Tilliaceae, Myrtaceae, Salicaceae, Fagaceae, and Caesalpiniaceae (Gerdemann, 1975). Important crops with VAM fungi include wheat, maize, all millets, potatoes, beans, soybeans, tomatoes, apples, oranges, grapes, banana, castor, tobacco, tea, coffee, cocoa, sugarcane, mango, asparagus, rubber, cardamom, pepper, etc. Most of the tropical rain forest trees are arbuscular mycorrhizal (Janos, 1983). Harley (1969) has listed the gymnosperms in which VAM fungi have been observed. They are found in Pteridophytes (Cooper, 1976) and Bryophytes (Parke and Linderman, 1980). Recently, arbuscular mycorrhizal colonization has been reported in floating (Bagyaraj *et al.*, 1979) and submerged aquatic plants (Clayton and Bagyaraj, 1984). Usually arbuscular mycorrhizae are confined to the roots; they have been reported in diverse structures such as the modified leaves of water fern *Salvinia cucullata* (Bagyaraj *et al.*, 1979), fruiting peg of peanut (Graw and Rehm, 1977) and modified scale like leaves and rhizomes of ginger and canna (Selvaraj *et al.*, 1986).

Table 12.2: Important Plant Families and Tree Genera Known to Form Mycorrhizal Associations

Family	*Genus*	*ECM*	*VAM*
Betulaceae	*Alnus* (alder)	√	√
	Betula (birch)	√	√
Caesalpinoideae	*Cassia*	√	
	Non N-fixing trees	√	√
Casuarinaceae	*Casuarina*	√	√
Dipterocarpaceae	*Shorea*	√	√
Ebenaceae	*Diospyros*		√
Fagaceae	*Fagus* (beech)	√	
	Quercus (oak)	√	
Juglandaceae	*Carya* (hickory, pecan)	√	
Meliaceae	*Cedrela*		√
	Khaya (African mahogany)		√
	Swietenia (mahogany)		√
Mimosoldeae	*Acacia*		√
	Albizia		√
Myrtaccae	*Eucalyptus*	√	√
Paplionoideae	*Dalbergia* (rosewood)		√
	Pterocarpus		
Rosaceae	*Malus* (apple)		√
Rutaceae	*Citrus* (orange, lemon)		√
Sallcaceae	*Salix* (willow)	√	√
Commercial crops	*Caria* (papaya)		√
	Coffee (coffee)		√
	Hevea (rubber)		√
	Most palms		√

VAM fungi, in addition to their widespread distribution throughout the plant kingdom, are also geographically ubiquitous and occur in plants growing in arctic, temperate, and tropical regions (Mosse *et al.*, 1981). In general, VAM population is more in cultivated soil compared to virgin soil (Mosse and Bowen, 1968). They are mostly seen in the top 15-30 cm of soil, and their numbers decrease markedly below the top 15 cm (Redhead, 1977). They are normally not found in depths beyond the normal root range of plants (Mosse *et al.*, 1981). The distribution of species of VAM fungi varies with climatic and edaphic environment as well as with land use. For example, *Acaulospora laevis* is common in Western Australia (Abbott and Robson, 1977) and New Zealand (Mosse and Bowen, 1968) but occurs less frequently in soils of Eastern Australia (Mosse and Bowen, 1968). *Glomus* species appear to have widest distribution. *Gigaspora* and *Sclerocystis* species are more common in tropical soils. *Acaulospora* seems to be better adapted to soils with pH <5.0. In fact, certain VAM fungi have been linked to particular kinds of soil: *Glomus mosseae* with fine textured, fertile, high pH soils; *Acaulospora leavis* with coarse-textured, acid soils, and *Gigaspora* species with sand dune soils (Kendrick and Berch, 1985).

Classification of VA Mycorrhizal Fungi

VAM fungi, being obligate biotrophs, do not grow on synthetic media and hence are classified according to morphological characteristics of the spores formed in the soil. One hundred and twenty species have been described by Schenck and Perez (1987), and they are all grouped in a single family, the Endogonaceae. The family is considered to be in an order of its own, the Endogonales tentatively placed in the class Zygomycetes in the subdivision Zygomycotina (Benjamin, 1979). The seven genera, *Endogone, Glomus, Sclerocystis, Entrophospora, Acaulospora, Scutellospora and Gigaspora,* presently constitute the Endogonaceae. Of these, only *Endogone* forms zygospores characteristic of Zygomycetes, while others probably lack sexual reproduction, species of *Endogone* do not form VAM fungal association. The other six genera form vesicular-arbuscular mycorrhizal associations.

The main features of VAM fungi are summarized by Trappe and Schenck (1982) and Hall (1984). Hall and Abbott (1983) compiled photographic transparencies illustrating diagnostic features of the Endogonaceae. Walker (1983) has suggested a standardized terminology for use in description of endogonaceous spore walls involving a stylized graphic representation of the wall structure ("murograph"). This concept is recommended for future descriptions of new species. Recently, Schenck and Perez (1987) published a manual for the identification of VAM fungi.

Glomus, the most common genus of VAM fungi, has over 50 species, which form globose, ellipsoid or rather irregularly shaped spores that range from 20-400 µm. These spores are thick-walled (up to 30 µm) and hyaline, yellow, red-brown, brown or black. Spores are attached to a single subtending hypha (or to two, three, or more in exceptional species) and produced in the soil near plant roots, at the soil surface, or occasionally in roots, and they may form singly, in groups of a few to many, or in large aggregates called sporocarps. Sporocarps are most commonly found in undisturbed forest communities with perennial plants and accumulated organic material. Sporocarpic species, when grown on plants in pot culture, usually produce spores singly or in small aggregates. Some *Glomus* species (*e.g. Glomus lacteum*) are not known to form spores in sporocarps, while others form spores outside the plant root only infrequently (*e.g. Glomus intraradices*). The spores of most species germinate by emergence of a germ tube directly through the subtending hypha.

Sclerocystis species produce chlamydospores that are very similar to those of *Glomus*, except that they tend to be clavate rather than globose. All *sclerocystis* species form spores only in sporocarps up to 700 µm in diameter. The spores, which can be up to 125 µm long, develop in a single layer, radially arranged around a central plexus of sterile and sporogenous hyphae. The sporocarps may group together in masses up to several cm in diameter on the soil surface, on leaves, twigs, and mosses. There is no published information on the germination of *Sclerocystis* spores.

Spores of the genus *Acaulospora* appear to form laterally on the neck of a small thin-walled saccule, called variously a mother spore, a vesicle, a hyphal terminus, a soporiferous saccule, or a sporogenous saccule (Walker, 1987). When mature, the spore does not display a subtending hypha because the vesicular structure that gives rise to it loses its cytoplasm and collapses during development of the spore. The spores are globose or ellipsoid, from <100 to >400 μm in diameter, and hyaline, yellow, or reddish-brown. The surface of the sporewall may be ornamented with pits, projections of various shapes, folds, spines, or reticulations, and the wall is up to 12 μm thick. One species of *Acaulospora* is now known to produce sporocarps, but in other species, spores are normally found in the soil of the rhizosphere, *Entrophospora* is more or less similar to *Acaulospora* except that the spore is formed inside the parent hypha just below the vesicle.

Scutellospora spores can be greater than 600 μm in diameter, and the smallest ones are just under 200 μm in diameter. Spores develop terminally on a bulbous hyphal suspensor, which remains attached at maturity and may bear short lateral projections. Spores are usually globose but can be ovoid, obovoid, pyriform or irregular. Spores are hyaline, white, yellow, pinkish, grey-green, or brown. Spore wall structure is composed of at least two wall groups, with one or more flexible membranous or coriaceous walls in the inner group or groups. The genus is characterized in particular by its mode of spore germination. Germination is by means of one or more germ tubes produced near the spore base from a germination shield formed within or upon a flexible inner wall. Thin walled, knobby, or broadly papillate auxiliary cells (vesicles) are borne in soil on straight or coiled hyphae, formed singly or in clusters. *Gigaspora* produces spores which are superficially similar to those of *Scutellospora* spores. The striking difference is the germination of spores, which is by direct growth of one or more germ tubes through the spore wall. It is possible that this genus evolved from *Scutellospora* (Walker, 1987).

Another fungus, or group of fungi, that forms endomycorrhizae has been referred to in the literature as "the fine endophyte," since its hyphae are <4 μm wide, compared to 10-20 μm for typical VAM fungi. This anomalous endophyte has been described as *Glomus tenue*, though it does not resemble the other species of *Glomus*. Its spores are 10-15 μm in diameter, and when young are hyaline and indistinguishable from the vesicles that form in the roots; when mature, however, they are pigmented. Because of their small size as compared to those of other VAM fungi, the spores of *Glomus tenue* are not often recorded in nature, though mycorrhizae of this type are common, particularly in dry regions.

Morphology and Histology

Arbuscular mycorrhizal roots are surrounded by an extensive loose hyphal network that may extend into the soil for as much as 1 cm. Hyphae also grow along root surface tightly appressed to the epidermis. However, they are never abundant enough to form a fungal mantle comparable to that of ectotrophic mycorrhizae. Vesicles and large thick walled spores are borne on hyphae in the soil. During mycorrhiza formation, the AM fungus undergoes several developmental stages. In the asymbiotic stage, spores germinate and AM fungi show limited hyphal development in the absence of a host plant. However, in the presence of root exudates, they switch to the presymbiotic stage which is characterized by extensive hyphal branching (Figure 1; Buee *et al.*, 2000). Subsequent to hyphal branching, the fungus contacts the root surface via appressorium formation before hyphal penetration of the root epidermis. This is followed by symbiotic colonization of the root cortex tissue, which involves formation of intracellular arbuscules (tree-like heavily branched structures) or hyphal coils and concomitantly, the production of a sporulative extraradical mycelium (Smith and Read, 1997).

Histology of mycorrhizal roots can easily be observed by examining whole mounts under relatively low power of a compound microscope. The hyphae penetrate the epidermal cells of young roots behind the meristematic region. The fungus grows throughout the cortex, but it does not invade the endodermis, stele or root meristem. Cells containing chloroplast are not infected. Shortly after infection, the fungus forms arbuscules within cortical cells. Vesicles are inter or intracellular, depending on the host species. Some species of the endophyte produce vesicles that remain relatively thin walled. In others the vesicles become thick walled, and do not differ in any important respect from chlamydospores produced in the soil. Vesicles function as food-storage organs, or if they develop into thick-walled chlamydospores, they may function as reproductive structures.

Production of VAM Inoculum

Identification of efficient indigenous strains of VAM fungi along with suitable host and substrate is a pre-requisite for mass production of VAM inocula. Plant growth period of 2-3 months gives a large crop of mycorrhizal spores to produce sizable amount of inoculum. VAM inoculum can also be produced under sterile environment by using hydroponic cultures and transferred organ culture techniques. Although, these techniques have not reached commercialization due to certain limitations.

Inoculation Methods

For successful mycorrhizal infection, the inoculum is placed in the root zone of actively growing plants, which are not heavily fertilized. The quantity of infection by the introduced endophytes depends on placement, inoculum potential, inoculum density, type of inoculum and environmental factors. Various methods proposed for placement of the inoculum are as follows:

Layering or Pads

Inoculum is placed in layers or pads beneath seeds such that the roots penetrating the inoculum will get infected. Presently, it is one of the most effective methods of inoculating plants with VAM fungi. Layering on small and large scale can be done by using manual planters and tractor drawn seeders, respectively.

Banding or Side Dressing

In this method, VAM inoculum is placed to sides of seedling or seeds in the zone of root proliferation. Banding mycorrhizal inoculum 5 cm deep and 5 cm away from 2 month old citrus seedling was found to be as effective as placing the inoculum directly on the roots at transplanting and more effective than seed pelleting.

Mixing Soil with Inoculum

Mixing mycorrhizal inoculum with soil is the most natural method for inoculating plants. However, it requires large amount of inoculum to obtain rapid infection. Generally, this method is used for inoculating plants in nursery.

Seed Pelleting

In this method, inoculum is extracted from a pot culture by wet sieving and decantation, root retained on 1 mm sieve are fragmented and added to the inoculum. Five ml aqueous solutions (1 per cent w/v) of methyl cellulose and calcium carbonate are mixed with 35 ml of mycorrhizal sievings. This material is poured over seeds (amount depending upon the crop species), mixed thoroughly and seeds are dried.

Pre-inoculation of Transplanted Seedlings

In this method, inoculum is placed in the seedbeds and seedlings are transplanted when these get adequately infected. The method is useful with crops like onion and tomato.

Ecology

Factors Affecting VAM Symbiosis in Field

Initial studies have shown that temperature, moisture, pH, amendments and some management practices like fallowing, cropping pattern, fertilizers and pesticides may all affect the conduciveness of soil to mycorrhizal symbiosis. In general, long fallowing, excessive secondary tillage, high inputs of fertilizers and pesticides especially broad-spectrum fumigants, substituted aromatic hydrocarbons and benzimidazoles leads to a decline in the inoculum and VAM colonization. Further, maintaining a plant cover on soil help in building up the inoculum of VAM in soil. Since, crop species differ in association with VAM fungi, selection of appropriate crop/cultures in the cropping sequences can be expected to help raise the population of VAM in soil.

Biological Interactions with VAM Fungi

In 1904, Hiltner coined the term *rhizosphere* to denote the region of the soil subjected to the influence of plant roots and characterized by intense microbial activity. Many workers have subsequently shown that the microflora of the rhizosphere differs both quantitatively and qualitatively from that in the soil beyond the influence of the root (Parkinson, 1967; Bowen, 1976; Bagyaraj *et al.*, 1972). The rhizosphere effect was greatest with bacteria followed by actinomycetes and fungi. The increased microbial activity in the rhizosphere has been attributed to the extra nutrients available in the region. The extra nutrient supply comes from the root exudates, sloughed-off parts of the root cap, mucigel, root hair residues and abraded epidermal cells (Rovira, 1979 and Tinker, 1980). The microflora of the rhizosphere could influence plant growth in many ways as all plant nutrients pass through this region (Rovira, 1967 and Nye, 1977).

Of the various microorganisms colonizing the rhizosphere, VAM fungi occupy a unique ecological position as they are partly inside and partly outside the host. The internal phase of a mycorrhizal fungus does not encounter competition and antagonism from other soil microorganisms and has an ensured source of nutrients from the host. This advantage enables them to achieve a large and more functional biomass in more intimate contact with the root and thus increases their chances of exerting a greater effect on plants than other microbial species restricted only to the rhizosphere.

Certain generalizations and conclusions about the interactions of VAM fungi with other soil organisms can be drawn. VAM markedly improve nodulation and nitrogen fixation by legume bacteria mainly by providing high phosphorus required for the fixation process. Mycorrhizal plants also allow introduced populations of beneficial soil organisms like *Azotobacter* and phosphate solubilising bacteria to maintain higher numbers than around non-mycorrhizal plants and to exert synergistic effects on plant growth. In general, VAM fungi decrease the severity of root diseases. Summary of some important interactions between VAM fungi and beneficial soil organisms are presented in Table 12.3.

Table 12.3: Summary of Important Interactions Between VAM Fungi and Beneficial Soil Microorganisms

Groups	*Species*	*Interactions*
N-fixation bacteria	*Rhizobium* sp.	Increased VAM infection level, nodulation, N-fixation and plant growth
Free living N-fixation bacteria	*Azotobacter* sp. *Beijerinkia* sp. *Clostridium* sp. *Azospirillum* sp.	Increased VAM infection level, AM spore production and bacterial population
Phosphate solubilizing bacteria	*Pseudomonas* sp. *Agrobacterium* sp.	Good bacterial population in rhizosphere of mycorrhizal plants
Phosphate solubilizing fungi	*Aspergillus niger* *Penicillum funiculosum*	Availability of P increased by P-solubilizing fungi and uptake increased by VAM

Research Work Carried Out by Authors at NRCAF, Jhansi

The role of VAM fungi in enhancing plant growth and yield, resistance to drought and salinity and tolerance to pathogens is well documented, but little is known about their interactions with agroforestry systems. Studies are being carried out in this regard at National Research Centre for Agroforestry, Jhansi. The results obtained so far showed the presence of VAM fungi in roots of 19 forestry trees, 7 horticultural trees, 10 field crops and 8 fodder crops. The colonization index varied from 20.4 to 95.9 per cent (Kumar, 1992). Local soils were found to be rich in VAM spore populations. *Glomus* was predominant genus, apart from this *Acaulospora, Gigaspora* and *Sclerocystis* were also present (Kumar *et al.*, 2006; Jha *et al.*, 2008 and Kamalvanshi *et al.*, 2008). Cultures of 11 *Glomus* and 2 *Acaulospora* species were purified from tree rhizosphere. Inoculation of tree seedlings (*Acacia nilotica, Pongamia pinnata, Jatropha curcas, Eucalyptus tererticornis, Albizia procera, Dalbergia sissoo, Leucaena leucocephala, Emblica officinalis, Zizyphus mauritiana, Buchanania lanzan* and *Cordia dichotoma*) and intercrops (*Phaseolus mungo, P. vigna, Zea mays, Triticum aestivum, Cicer arietinum* and *Pisum sativum*) with suitable VAM species recorded substantial increase in plant growth and phosphorus (P) uptake (Kumar *et al.*, 2007). This resulted in a benefit comparable to high input levels of P in *P. mungo, T. aestivum, E. tererticornis* and *A. procera* at much lower P concentrations (Shukla *et al.*, 2008).

In agroforestry systems, trees acted as VAM inoculum reservoir for intercrops (Kumar *et al.*, 2007). Cross inoculation test performed by using VAM fungi isolated from trees showed that these could colonize the roots of important rainy season (*P. mungo, P. vigna* and *Z. mays*) and winter (*C. arietinum, P. sativum* and *T. aestivum*) intercrops (Kumar *et al.*, 2007). VAM fungi also cross infected the plant species under agroforestry situations. Intercropping increased VAM activity in rhizosphere of trees (Kumar *et al.*, 2007). Tree shade reduced the rate of mycorrhization of intercrops, especially during winter months. VAM inoculations enhanced the growth and phosphorus uptake of intercrops in shade and the tree canopy management increased this advantage. Use of excessive shading (25 per cent of full sun or more) in nurseries reduced mycorrhization of tree seedlings (Shukla *et al.*, 2008). VAM activity in terms of spore population and mycorrhizal diversity was more in light soils as compared to heavy soils. Pruning/canopy management of trees reduced their VAM colonization (Shukla, 2009). Excessive stagnation of water during rainy season in plantations (*E. officinalis* and

Table 12.4: List of Efficient Vesicular Arbuscular Mycorrhizal Fungi for Different Plant Species

Plant Species	*Efficient Mycorrhizal Fungus/Fungi*	*Mycorrhizal Fungi Tested*	*Parameters Evaluated*	*References*
		Agriculture crops		
Allium cepa (Onion)	*Gigaspora margarita*	*G. margarita*, *G. calospora*, and a known VAM fungus	Leaf number, dry matter, P-uptake, bulb yield	Ramana and Babu (1999)
	G. calospora	*G. margarita*, *G. calospora*, and a known VAM fungus	Root colonization	Ramana and Babu (1999)
Amorphophallus paeonufolius	*Glomus mosseae* + *G. aggregatum*	*G. mosseae*, *G. aggregatum*, *Gigaspora albida*, *Pisolithus tinctorius*	Tuber yield/plant	Ganesan and Mahadevan (1994)
Ananas comosus	*Glomus fasciculatum*	*G. fasciculatum*, *Glomus* sp., *Acaulospora* sp., *Scutellospora* sp.	Plant growth, nutrition	Jaizme-Vega and Azcon (1995)
Acacia nilotica	*Glomous mosseae* + *Gigaspora gilmorei*	*G. mosseae*, *G. constrictum*, *Gigaspora gilmorei*, and their combinations	Collar diameter, root–shoot dry weight and length	Mandal and Kaushik (1994)
Acacia auriculaeformis	*Glomus etunicatum*, *G. macrocarpum*	*G. etunicatum*, *G. macrocarpum*, *G. fasciculatum*, *G. mosseae*	Height, diameter, biomass, P-uptake	Aggangan, Lorilla, and Cruz (1990)
Acer saccharum (Sugar maple)	*Glomus macrocarpum*	*G. macrocarpum*, *G. clarum*, *G. epigaeum*, *G. mosseae*	Leaf number, mean lateral root number	Reid, Parker, Mitchell *et al.* (1988)
Azadirachta indica (neem)	*Glomus mosseae*	*Glomus mosseae*, *G. fasciculatum*, and seven other VAM fungi	Plant height, stem girth, biomass, P-content, zinc concentration, root colonizations	Sumana and Bagyaraj (1999)
Cajanus cajan	*Glomus clarum*	*G. fasciculatum* and seven other VAM fungi	Plant growth	Diederichs (1992)
	Glomus etunicatum	*G. etunicatum*, *Gigaspora margarita*	Shoot dry matter, nutrient uptake	Ahiabor and Hirata (1994)
Capsicum	*Glomus intraradices*	*G. intraradices*, indigenous mixed culture, commercial inoculum (Mycorise and C)	Fruit yield	Gaur, Adholeya, and Mukerji (1998)
Carica papaya	*Glomus fasciculatum*	*G. fasciculatum*, *Glomus* sp., *Acaulospora* sp., *Scutellospora* sp.	Plant growth, nutrition	Jaizme-vega and Azcon (1995)
Cacocasia esculenta	*Glomus mosseae* + *G. aggregatum*	*G. mosseae*, *G. aggregatum*, *Gigaspora albida*, Pisolithus tinctorius	Tuber yield/plant	Ganesan and Mahadevan (1994)
Cucumis sativus	*Glomus caledonium*	*G. caledonium*, *Glomus* sp.	P-uptake	Joner and Jokobsen (1994)

Contd...

Table 12.4–Contd...

Plant Species	Efficient Mycorrhizal Fungus/Fungi	Mycorrhizal Fungi Tested	Parameters Evaluated	References
Eleusine coracana	*Glomus caledonicum*	*G. caledonicum, G. mosseae, G. fasciculatum, G. epigaeum* (*G. versiforme*), *Gigaspora calospora, G. margarita*	Mycorrhizal efficacy, root colonization	Tewari, Johri, and Tandon (1993)
Fragaria xananassa (micropropagated)	*Glomus versiforme* 36-366	*G. versiforme* (2 isolates), *G. mosseae, G. etunicatum*	Yield, production of runners	Taube-Baab and Baltruschat (1996)
Glycine max	*Acaulsopora scrobiculata*	*A. scrobiculata, Glomus intraradices,* and four other AM fungi	Plant growth, crop yield	Vasuvat, Nopamornbodi, and Thamsurakul (1987)
Lycopersicum esculentum	*Glomus etunicatum*	*Glomus etunicatum, G. mosseae*	Shoot dry weight, plant height	McGraw and Schenck (1981)
cv. *Manapal*	*G. mosseae*	*Glomus etunicatum, G. mosseae*	Root colonization	McGraw and Schenck (1981)
cv. *Walter*	*G. mosseae*	*Glomus etunicatum, G. mosseae*	Shoot weight, plant height	McGraw and Schenck (1981)
Manihot esculenta (cassava)	*G. fasciculatum*	*G. fasciculatum,* G. *mosseae, G. constrictum, Glomus etunicatum, Acaulsopora morrowea*	Root colonization, plant weight, shoot and root dry weight	Sivaprasad, Sulochana and Nair (1990)
Manihot esculenta (cassava)	*G. mosseae + G.aggregatum*	*G. mosseae, G aggregatum, Gigaspora albida, Pisolithus tinctorius*	Tuber yield/plant	Ganesan and Mahadevan (1994)
Medicago sativa	*Glomus intraradices*	*G. intraradices, G. mosseae, Gigaspora margarita*	Root colonization, fungal sporulation	Douds, Galvez, Becard *et al.* (1998)
Musa acuminata	*Glomus fasciculatum*	*G. fasciculatum, Glomus* sp., *Acaulospora* sp., *Scutellospora* sp.	Plant growth, nutrition	Jaisme-Vega and Azcon (1995)
Oryza sativa cv. Prakash	*Glomus intraradices*	*G. intraradices, G. fasciculatum*	Grain yield	Secilia and Bagyaraj (1994)
Orzya sativa (upland rice)	*Acaulospora spinosa*	*Acaulospora spinosa, A. scrobiculata*	Plant biomass, grain yield, root colonization	Ammani and Rao (1996)
Persea Americana	*Glomus fasciculatum*	*G. fasciculatum, Glomus* sp., *Acaulospora* sp., *Scutellospora* sp.	Plant growth, nutrition	Jaizme-vega and Azcon (1995)
Polianthes tuberosa (rajnigandha)	*Glomus intraradices*	*G. intraradices*, indigenous mixed cultures, commercial inoculum (Mycorise)	Fruit yield, spike length	Gaur, Adholeya, and Mukerji (1998)

Contd...

Table 12.4–Contd...

Plant Species	*Efficient Mycorrhizal Fungus/Fungi*	*Mycorrhizal Fungi Tested*	*Parameters Evaluated*	*References*
Trifolium (Clover)	*Acaulospora trappei*	*A. trappei, A. laevis, Acaulospora* sp.,	Root colonization	Gazey, Abbott, and Robson (1992)
Triticum aestivum wheat (var. Swift)	*Glomus intraradices*	*G. intraradices, Gigaspora margarita*	Plant yield, number of grains/spike	Asif Khan, Khan *et al.* (1995)
Vigna mungo (black gram)	*Glomus epigaeum* (*G. versiforme*)	*G. epigaeum, Acaulospora spinosa, A. morrowae*	Root colonization, shoot dry weight, N and P concentrations	Rao and Rao (1996)
Vigna radiata (green gram)	*Glomus epigaeum* (*G. versiforme*)	*G. epigaeum, Acaulospora spinosa, A. morrowae*	Root colonization, shoot dry weight, N and P concentrations	Rao and Rao (1996)
Vigna unguiculata	*G. etunicatum*	*G. etunicatum, Gigaspora margarita*	Shoot dry matter, nutrient uptake	Ahiabor and Hirata (1994)
Vigna unguiculata cv. Katumanu K80	*G. etunicatum*	*Glomus etunicatum, G. claroideum, Glomus* sp.	Top dry weight	Obura, Skipper, and Wagner (1987)
Vigna unguiculata *cv.* California No. 5 black eye	*G. claroideum*	*Glomus etunicatum, G. claroideum, Glomus* sp.	Top dry weight	Obura, Skipper, and Wanger (1987)
Zea mays (pioneer 3905)	*Glomus etunicatum*	*G. etunicatum, G. mosseae, G. aggregatum, G. versiforme*	Leaf mass, protein concentrations	Boucher, Dalpe and Charest (1999)
Nephrolepis exaltata var. whitmanii (fern) micropropagated plants	*Glomus intraradices, G. clarum*	*G. intraradices, G. clarum, G. versiculiferum, G. versiforme*	Root infection	Ponton, Piche, Parent *et al.* (1990)
		Tree Crops		
Malus domestica (apple)	*Glomus mosseae*	*G. mosseae, G. macrocarpum*	Root colonization, plant height, plant growth	Miller, Bodmer, and Schuepp (1989)
Hevea brasiliensis	*Glomus clarum, Glomus* sp.	*G. clarum, Glomus* sp., *A. spinosa, Gigaspora margarita, Entrophospora colombiana, Glomus* sp., and three other species	Dry weight	Ikram, Mahmud, and Othman (1993)
Tectona grandis	*Glomus leptotichus*	Not mentioned	Seedling growth parameters	Rajan, Reddy, and Bagyaraj (2000)
Zizyphus mauritiana	*Glomus fasciculatum*	*G. fasciculatum, G. mosseae, Scutellospora calospora*	Growth, root colonization, nutrient uptake	Mathur and Vyas (1996)
Citrus jambhiri (rough lemon)	*Glomus fasciculatum*	*G. fasciculatum, G. mosseae, G. etunicatum*	Plant height, top weight, root weight, chlamydospores in soil	Nemec (1979)
Persea American (avocado)	*Glomus fasciculatum*	*Glomus fasciculatum, Acaulospora* sp., *Scutellospora* sp.	Plantlet growth and nutrition	Jaizme-vega and Azcon (1995)

Hardwikia binata) was found to be harmful for colonization of plants. *Glomus* was more adapted to such conditions in *E. officinalis* plantations (Kumar *et al.*, 2009). Inoculation of intercrops (*P. mungo* and *T. aestivum*) and tree seedlings (*E. tererticornis* and *A. procera*) with a suitable VAM consortium was found more beneficial than individual VAM fungi in *P. mungo, T. aestivum, E. tererticornis* and *A. procera*.

Conclusions

Mycorrhizal symbiosis has lately created a keen interest among biological scientists of the country involving mycologists, soil scientists, agronomist, plant physiologists, plant geneticists, environmentalist, foresters and microbiologists alike. Major efforts are now being concentrated towards the production of bulk inoculum of mycorrhizal bio-fertilizers for use in forestry, horticulture, floriculture, agriculture, etc. While many ectomycorrhizal fungi have been brought in pure cultures, VAM fungi till now, defied all attempts to bring them in pure culture on synthetic media. Many efforts are being made all over the world to decode the genetic barrier to grow these fungi on synthetic media. In India, though fundamental studies on molecular and biochemical level are scarce, much headway has been achieved in selecting suitable VAM fungi for different crops and for different site conditions (Table 12.4). Special attempts are being made to determine the role of VAM fungi in ameliorating soils polluted with industrial wastes. Subjects on which more information is needed are as follows:

- ✰ Distribution of mycorrhizal fungi under varying edapho-climatic conditions.
- ✰ Plant growth responses and mycorrhizal dependency.
- ✰ Role of mycorrhiza on difficult/disturbed sites.
- ✰ Tripartite biological interactions involving rhizosphere flora, mycorrhizal fungi and plant roots.
- ✰ Physiology and biochemistry.
- ✰ Management of pests, mycorrhizae and biocides for increased plant productivity.
- ✰ Soil/water pollution and mycorrhizae.

References

Abbott, L.K. and Robson, A.D. (1977). Growth stimulation of subterranean clover with vesicular arbuscular mycorrhizas. *Ausraliant Journal of Agricultural Research* 28: 639-649.

Bagyaraj, D.J. and Rangaswami, G. (1972). Studies on the rhizosphere microflora of *Eleusine coracana* under the influence of foliar chemicals sprays. I. Quantitative incidence of microorganisms. *Madras Agricultural Journal* 59: 517.

Bagyaraj, D.J., Manjunath, A. and Patil, R.B. (1979). Occurrence of vesicular-arbuscular mycorrhizas in some tropical aquatic plants. *Transactions of British Mycological Society* 72: 164-167.

Benjamin, R.K. (1979). Zygomycetes and their spores. in B Kendricks (ed). The Whole Fungus. National Museums of Canada, Ottawa. pp. 573-616.

Bowen, G.D. and Rovira, A.D. (1976. Microbial colonization of plant roots. *Annual Review of Phytopathology* 14: 121-144.

Clayton, J.S. and Bagyaraj, D.J. (1984). Vesicular-arbuscular mycorrhizas in submerged aquatic plants of New Zealand. *Aquatic Botany* 19: 251-262.

Cooper, K.M. (1976). A field survey of mycorrhizas in New Zealand ferns. *New Zealand Journal of Botany* 14: 169-181.

Frank, A.B. (1985). Uber die auf Werzelsymbiose beruhende Ernahrung gewisser Baume durch unterirdische. Pilze. *Ber. Dtsch. Bot. Ges.* 3: 128-145.

Gerdemann, JW. (1975). Vesciular arbuscular mycorrhizae. in JG Torrey and Glarkson DT (eds) *The Development and Function of Roots*. Academic Press, London. pp. 576-591.

Graw, D. and Rehm, S. (1977). Vesicular-arbuscular Mycorrhiza in den Fruhttragern von *Arachis hypogea. L.Z. Acker Und Pflanzenbau* 144: 75-78.

Hall, I.R. and Abbott, L.K. (1983). Photographic slide collection illustrating features of Endogonaceae. *Bulletin of British Mycological Society* 17: 54-55.

Hall, I.R. (1984). Taxonomy of VA mycorrhizal fungi. in CL Powell and Bagyaraj DJ (eds) VA mycorrhiza. CRC Press, Boca Raton, FL. pp. 57-94.

Harley, J.L. (1969). *The Biology of Mycorrhiza*, 2nd ed. Leonard Hill, London.

Harley, J.L. and Smith, S.E. (1983). *Mycorrhizal Symbiosis*, 1st edn. Academic, London.

Hiltner, L. (1904). Uber neure Erfahrungen und Probleme auf dem Gebiet der Bodenbakteriologie und unter besonderer Beruksichtigung der Grundingung und Brache. *Arb Dtsch Landwirtsch Gesellschaftswiss* 98: 59-78.

Janos, DP. (1983). Tropical Mycorrhizas. In SL Sutton, TC Whitemore and AC Chadwick (eds) *Tropical Rain Forest: Ecology and Management*. Blackwell Scientific Publications, Oxford. pp. 327-345.

Jha, A, Kumar, A., Saxena, R. K., Kamalvanshi, M. and Shukla, A. (2008). Occurrence of Arbuscular Mycorrhizal Fungi in Selected Agroforestry Tree Species of Bundelkhand Region. National Symposium on Agroforestry Knowledge for Sustainability, Climate Moderation and Challenges Ahead. Dec.15-17. NRCAF, Jhansi. 60.

Kamalvanshi, M., Kumar, A., Jha, A. and Shukla, A. (2008). Occurrence of arbuscular mycorrhizal (AM) fungal species in *Pongamia pinnata, Jatropha curcas* and *J. gossypifolia*. National Symposium on Agroforestry Knowledge for Sustainability, Climate Moderation and Challenges Ahead. Dec.15-17. NRCAF, Jhansi 167.

Kendrick, B. and Berch, S. (1985). Mycorrhizae: Applications in Agriculture and Forestry. in CW Robinson (ed) *Comprehensive Biotechnology*, Vol. 4. Pergamon Press, Oxford. pp.109-150.

Kumar, A. (1992). Occurrence of VAM among some plant important in agroforestry under semiarid conditions. *Agroforestry Newsletter* 4(1): 7.

Kumar, A., Hashmi, S., Shukla, A. and Jha, A. (2006). Colonization of some important intercrops by Vesicular Arbuscular Mycorrhizae isolated from minor fruit crops. National Symposium on Agroforestry for Livelihood Security, Environment Protection and Bio fuel Production. Dec.16 - 18. NRCAF, Jhansi. 20.

Kumar, A., Hashmi, S. and Shukla, A. (2006). Occurrence of vesicular arbuscular mycorrhizae in *Buchanania lanzan* and *Cordia dichotoma*. *Range Management and Agroforestry* 27(1): 84-86.

Kumar, A., Shukla, A. Hashmi, S., Jha, A. and Kamalvanshi, M. (2007). Studies on arbuscular mycorrhizal fungi in agroforestry. *Agroforestry Newsletter* January- March, 2008, Vol. 20(1) pp. 5.

Kumar, A., Hashmi, S., Shukla, A. and Chaturvedi, O.P. (2007). Effect of intercropping on inoculum potential of arbuscular mycorrhizal fungi in agroforestry systems. *Annals of Arid Zone* 46(1): 31-36.

Kumar, A., Shukla, A., Hashmi, S. and Tewari, R.K. (2007). Effect of trees on colonization of intercrops by vesicular arbuscular mycorrhizae in agroforestry systems. *Indian Journal of Agricultural Sciences* 77(5): 291-298.

Mosse, B. and Bowen, G.D. (1968). The distribution of Endogone spores in some Australian and New Zeland soils and in the experimental field soil at Rothamsted. *Transactions of British Mycological Society* 51: 485-492.

Mosse, B., Stribley, D.P. and Le Tacon, F. (1981). Ecology of mycorrhizae and mycorrhizal fungi In M Alexander M (ed) *Advances in Microbial Ecology*. Plenum Press, New York. pp. 5: 137-209.

Nye, P.H. (1977). The rate limiting step in plant nutrient absorption from soil. *Soil Science*. 123: 292.

Parke, J.L. and Linderman, R.G. (1980). Association of vesicular-arbuscular mycorrhizal fungi with the moss *Funaria hygrometrica*. *Canadian Journal of Botany* 58: 1898-1904.

Parkinson, D. (1967). Soil microorganisms and plant roots in A Urges, F Raw (eds) *Soil Biology*. Academic Press, London, 449.

Redhead, J.F. (1977). Endotrophic mycorrhizas in Nigeria. Species of the Endogonaceae and Their distribution. *Transactions of British Mycological Society* 69: 275-280.

Rovira, A.D. and McDougall, B.M. (1967). Microbiological and biochemical aspects of the rhizosphere in: AD McLaren, GH Peterson (eds) *Soil Biochemistry*. Marcel Dekker, New York. pp.1: 417-493.

Rovira, A.D. (1979). Biology of soil-root interface in JL Warley, SR Russel (eds) *The Soil-Root Interface*. Academic Press, London 145-160.

Schenck, NC and Perez, Y. (1987). *Manual of the identification of VA Mycorrhizal Fungi*. University of Florida, Gainesville, Florida, USA. pp. 1-245.

Selvaraj, T., Kannan, K. and Lakshminarasimhan, C. (1986). Vesicular-arbuscular mycorrhizal fungi in roots and scale-like leaves of *Canna indica* L. (Cannaceae). *Current Science* 55: 728-730.

Singh, S. (2001). Mycorrhizal dependency, Part 1: Selection of efficient mycorrhizal fungi. *Mycorrhiza News* 13(1): 2-16.

Shukla, A., Kumar, A., Jha, A., Chaturvedi, O.P., Prasad, R. and Ajit (2008). Effect of shade on arbuscular mycorrhizal colonization and growth of crops and tree seedlings in Central India. *Agroforestry Systems* doi: 10.1007/s10457-008-9182-x.

Shukla, A., Kumar, A., Jha, A., Kamalvanshi, M. and Gupta, G. (2008). The effects of phosphorus application on growth and arbuscular mycorrhizal colonization of crops and tree seedlings. National Symposium on Agroforestry Knowledge for Sustainability, Climate Moderation and Challenges Ahead. Dec.15-17. NRCAF, Jhansi 41.

Shukla, A. (2009). Effect of tree introduction in agricultural fields on vesicular-arbuscular mycorrhizal status of component crops of agroforestry systems. *Ph.D Theis*, Bundelkhand University, Jhansi.

Tinker, P.B. (1980). Role of rhizosphere microorganism in phosphorus uptake by plants in FE Khasawneh, EC Sample and EJ Kamprath (eds) *The Role of Phosphorus in Agriculture*. American Society of Agronomy, Madison, wisc. pp. 617-647.

Trappe, J.M. (1977). "Biogeography of hypogeous fungi: Trees, mammals and continental drift" In HE Bigelow and EG Simmons (eds) *Abstr. 2nd Int. Mycol. Congr. Inc.* University of South Florida, Tampa. pp. 675.

Trappe, J.M. and Schenck, N.C. (1982). Taxonomy of the fungi forming endomycorrhizae. A. Vesicular-arbuscular mycorrhizal fungi (Endogonales) in NC Schenck (ed) Methods and Principles of Mycorrhizal Research. *American Phytopathological Society Publication*, St. Paul, MN. pp.1-10.

Walker, C. (1983). Taxonomic concepts in the Endogonaceae: Sproe wall characteristics in species description. *Mycotaxon* 18: 443-455.

Microbial Biotechnology and Ecology (2011) *Pages* 225–255
Editors: Deepak Vyas, G.S. Paliwal, P.K.Khare and R.K Gupta
Published by: DAYA PUBLISHING HOUSE, NEW DELHI

Chapter 13

Arbuscular Mycorrhizal Fungi: The Hidden Heroes of the Soil

☆ *Deepak Vyas[1]*, Meenakshi Mishra[1], Pradeep Singh[1], Ashok Shukla[1] and R.K. Gupta[2]*

[1]*Lab of Microbial Technology and Plant Pathology, Department of Botany Dr. H.S. Gour University Sagar – 470 003, M.P.*
[2]*Govt. P.G. College, Rishikesh, Uttarakhand*

ABSTRACT

Soil is not a pile of dirt but is a treasure house of earthy materials and home of many microorganisms as it was rightly said that "we think that we are standing on the earth but reality is that we are standing on the roof of another world". Rhizospheric region of the soil is one of the important room where plant, soil and microbes interact. However, these interactions are of many types but among these, mutualistic interactions are of great importance. Arbuscular mycorrhizal symbiosis is one of the mutualistic relationship among the plant, soil and other microbes.

In this review we have tried to summerize some of the multifacet roles performed by the AMF fungi in the soil for the benefit and better plant growth, soil remediation, disease control, dialogue among the co-organisms and their importance in the modern biology such as molecular biology, genetics, genomics, proteomics and fluxomics.

Introduction

AM symbioses are the most widespread mycorrhizal association, with a very long evolutionary history. Fossil survey and molecular data have demonstrated that the evolutionary history of AM fungi goes back at least to the Ordovician, about 460 million years ago (Redecker, 2002). The earliest

---

* E-mail: dvyas64@yahoo.co.in.

land plants show an association with fungi that formed vesicles and arbuscules that was very similar to today's AM fungi (Nicolson, 1975; Remy *et al.*, 1994). Recently Vyas *et al.* (2007-2008) reported occurrence of arbuscules and vesicles in bryophytes. This type of plant-fungal association is formed with 80 per cent of angiosperms (Harley and Harley, 1987). The fungi are obligate symbionts and they need a living plant root (or equivalent structure) in order to grow and reproduce. AM fungal development in roots of host plants starts when fungal hyphae grow from spores or from colonized roots toward the uncolonized roots. After contact of the hyphae with the root surface, the fungus is stimulated to change in morphology from an original simple branching pattern to irregularly septate pattern with reduced interhyphal spacing (Giovannetti *et al.*, 1993; Harrison, 1998). The fungus produces swollen appressoria on the root surface and spreads between and into the root cortical cells. There are two major morphological types of AM, *Arum* and *Paris* type, they are characterised by differences in fungal development within the roots (Gallaud, 1905; Smith and Smith, 1997). In general, internal hyphae branch and make four recognizable structures, intracellular hyphae that may be coiled, intercellular hyphae, arbuscules and spherical or ovoid vesicles (Smith and Smith, 1997). In *Arum-type* associations, intercellular hyphae penetrate between the root cortical cells and spread rapidly, then lateral branch-hyphae penetrate the root cortical cells and branch dichotomously and produce arbuscules. In *Paris-type* associations intracellular hyphae spread from cell to cell within the root cortex and form extensive intracellular hyphal coils and arbusculate coils (Gallaud, 1905). The types of internal structures that develop depend on the plant/fungal combination (Smith and Smith, 1997; Cavagnaro *et al.*, 2001).

About 83 per cent of dicotyledonous and 79 per cent of monocotyledonous plants is associated with mycorrhizal fungi (Wilcox, 1991). Mycorrhizal associations are found in a very wide range of habitats, including aquatic ecosystems, deserts, lowland tropical rain forests, high altitudes, high latitudes and in canopy epiphytes (Allen, 1991). Bi-directional movement of nutrients characterizes the fungus-plant symbioses, where carbon flows to the fungus and inorganic nutrients move to the plant, thereby providing a critical linkage between the plant root and soil. This association is a survival mechanism for both the fungi and plants, allowing each to survive in different environments (Gupta *et al.*, 2000). Mycorrhizal plants, in comparison with non mycorrhizal plants, have greater nutrient uptake because they possess a network of external hyphae (Sanders and Sheikh, 1983). The hyphae are the interface between soil and plant and have a large surface area that acts as an extension of the root absorbing area (Rhodes and Gerdemann, 1975; Owusu-Bennoah and Wild, 1979; Li *et al.*, 1991). This not only increases the volume of soil from which nutrients are absorbed, but also overcomes problem of depletion of nutrients (Nurlaeny *et al.*, 1996; Smith and Read, 1997) and water (Marulanda *et al.*, 2003) depletion close to actively absorbing roots, and plays a significant role in stabilizing soil structure. Mycorrhizal fungal associations have several advantages for their hosts, including increased growth and yield and reproductive success due to enhanced nutrient acquisition (Mosse *et al.*, 1973; Diederichs, 1990; Lewis and Koide, 1990; Stanley *et al.*, 1993). They may also increase disease and pest resistance, improve water relations (Allen and Allen, 1986; Davies *et al.*, 1993; Subramanian *et al.*, 1997), soil structure (Tisdall and Oades, 1979; Thomas *et al.*, 1986; Degens *et al.*, 1994; Beaden and Petersen, 2000) and tolerance of extreme pH (Sidhu and Behl, 1997; Douds *et al.*, 2000). This literature review will concentrate on structure and function of AM and their potential role in revegetating saline soils.

AMF in Carbon Sequestration

Arbuscular mycorrhizal fungi (AMF) comprising fungi in order Glomales (Zygomycota), ubiquitous symbionts of the majority of higher plants. AMF have been shown to have numerous effect on plant physiology and plant communities (Allen 1991; Smith and Read, 1997), which can lead to indirect effect on soil carbon storage. AMF are also very important in the process of soil aggregate stabilization (Tisdall and Oades, 1982). Relatively labile carbon can be protected inside soil aggregates which means AMF have yet another indirect influence on soil carbon storage (Miller and Jastrow, 1992).

Recently, a glycoprotein named glomalin was discovered using specialized protocols for soil that revealed amount up to several mg protein per gram of soil (Wright and Upadhyaya, 1996). Glomalin is produced by hyphae of all members of AM genera, but not by other groups of soil fungi so far tested. Although concentration of glomalin in soil seem to be responsive to global change factors such as elevated atmosphere CO_2 (Rillig *et al.*, 1999).

ERH (Extra Radical Hyphae) and Soil Aggregation

Indeed the influences of ERH on soil aggregation might be even more important to the carbon stock than the influence of the hyphal standing crop along (Miller *et al.*, 2000). Through their role in soil microaggregate stabilization, the ERH appear to contribute to the certain of an aggregate hierarchy. In doing so they help to create mechanism for increasing the residence time of organic debris within soil macroaggregates.

Mechanistically, the ERH contribution to soil aggregation can be viewed as 'Stioky string bag' mechanism, in which the hyphae help to etangle and enmesh soil particles to form macroaggregate structures (Miller *et al.*, 2000; Oades *et al.*, 1991). The physical dimensions of ERH allow them to grow and to remify through soil pores the size of those between macroaggregates. The contribution of AMF hyphae to carbon cycling lies not only with ERH but also, with exudates from hyphae. Arbuscular mycorrhizal fungi (AMF) take up photosynthetically fixed carbon from plant roots and translocate it to their external myceliumAMF are also responsible for directing the movement of huge quantities of photosynthate to the soil (for review, Douds *et al.*, 2000; Graham, 2000). Carbon in the root flows from plant to fungus in the form of sugars (Shachar-Hill *et al.*, 1995; Solaiman and Saito, 1997), and together with the transfer of mineral nutrients from fungus to root (Koide and Schreiner, 1992; George *et al.*, 1995; Jakobsen, 1995), this is the nutritional mainstay of what is arguably the world's most important mutualistic symbiosis. AM fungi obtain most or all of their carbon within the host root. Here, they acquire hexose and transform it into trehalose and glycogen, typical fungal carbohydrates (Shachar-Hill *et al.*, 1995). Triacylglyceride (TAG) is the main form of stored carbon in AM fungi (Beilby and Kidby, 1980; Jabaji-Hare, 1998), and this is mostly or exclusively made in the intraradical mycelium (IRM; Pfeffer *et al.*, 1999). Some of this stored lipid flows from the IRM to the extraradical mycelium (ERM; Pfeffer *et al.*, 1999), and in vivo microscopic observations indicate that the rate of export is sufficient to account for the high levels of *stored* lipid in the ERM (Bago *et al.*, 2002). The glyoxylate cycle is active in the ERM (Lammers *et al.*, 2001), and this pathway appears to be important in using exported TAG to make carbohydrate in the ERM.

The structure of glomalin has not been completely defined. The molecule appears to be a complex of a repeated monomeric structures bound together by hydrophobic interactions (Nichols, 2003) that, attaches to soil to help stabilize aggregates. The molecule contains tightly bound iron (0.04-8.8 per cent) (Rillig *et al.*, 2001; Nichols, 2003; Wright and Upadhyaya, 1998), and does not contain phenolic compounds such as tannins (Rillig *et al.*, 2001). Preliminary evidence (Wright and Upadhyaya, 1998; Nichols, 2003) suggests that cations are bound to glomalin in amounts that vary *for* different soils.

Rhizodeposition

The release of carbon compounds from living plant roots rhizodeposition into the surrounding soil is a ubiquitous phenomenon (Curl and Trueglove, 1986). The loss of C from root epidermal and cortical cells leads to a proliferation of microorganisms within endorhizosphere on the surface (rhizoplane) and outside the root (ectorhizosphere). C release also result in the rhizosphere having different chemical, physical and biological characteristics to the bulk soil (Barber, 1995).Theoretically, almost any soluble component present inside the root can be lost to the rhizosphere; however current evidence suggests that exudation is dominated by low molecular weight solutes such as sugars, amino acids and organic acids that are present in the cytoplasm at high concentrations (Farrar *et al.*, 2003). Influence of AM formation upon roots exudates following AM colonization root exudation patterns may be expected to alter because the AM fungus is a considerable C sink (Douds *et al.*, 2000; Graham, 2000). AM colonization alters the carbohydrate metabolism of the roots (Shachar-Hill *et al.*, 1995; Douds *et al.*, 2000; Bago *et al.*, 2003) and increases root respiration (Douds *et al.*, 2000; Shachar-Hill *et al.*, 1995). Hyphal exudation from the AMF will also occur.

AMF in Nutrient Sequestration

Enhanced uptake of P is generally regarded as the most important benefit that AMF provide to their host plant and plant P is often the main in plant fungal relationship (Thompson, 1987; Smith and Read, 1997; Graham, 2000). AMF can play a significant role in crop P nutrition, increasing total uptake and in some cases P use efficiency (Koide *et al.*, 2000). This may be associated with increased growth and yield (Vosatka, 1995, Ibibijen *et al.*, 1996; Koide *et al.*, 2000).

Where colonization by AMF is disrupted, uptake of P, growth and in some cases yield can be significantly reduced (Thompson, 1987, 1991 and 1994).

In many cases, this is due to a high concentration of (phyto) available soil P (Bethlenfalvay and Barea, 1994; Hetrick *et al.*, 1996; Thingstrup *et al.*, 1998; Soren Sen *et al.*, 2005). Under such conditions, the colonization of roots by AMF is often suppressed (Jensen and Jakobsen, 1980; Al-Karaki and Clark, 1999; Kahiluoto *et al.*, 2001). Where strong AMF colonization still occurs under condition of high soil P concentration it may reduce crop growth (Gavito and Varela, 1995; Kahiluoto *et al.*, 2001).

AMF play significant role in the uptake of other nutrients by the host plant, zinc (Zn) nutrition is most commonly reported as being influenced by the AM association, though uptake of copper (Cu), iron, N, K, Ca and Mg have been reported being as enhanced (Smith and Read, 1997; Clark and Zeto, 2000). AMF may also enhance plant uptake of N from organic sources (Hodge *et al.*, 2001). In many cases AMF cause a change in the absorption of soil nutrients by host simultaneously, though the effect on different nutrients is rarely the some (Lambert *et al.*, 1979, Kothari *et al.*, 1990; Wellings *et al.*, 1991; Thompson, 1987, 1991, 1994; Azaizeh *et al.*, 1995; Smith and Read, 1997; Srivastava *et al.*, 2002; Mohammad *et al.*, 2003).

The apparently contradictory evidence regarding the effect of AMF on plant nutrient absorption may be connected to the increasing realization that there is a degree of selectivity between host and the fungi and that different AMF have varying effects on different plant species, from strongly positive increases in nutrient uptake and or growth to strongly negative. (Monzon and Azcon, 1996; Bever *et al.*, 2001; Vander Heijden, 2002; O'Connor *et al.*, 2002.; Munkvold *et al.*, 2004). There is a good evidence for a substantial capacity of external hyphae to absorb NH_4-N and deliver it to the host plant. In the hyphosphere as in the rhizosphere, uptake of NH_4-N is associated with substrate acidification.

Increase of K/Na Ratio

Some previous studies on the effects of salinity on mycorrhizal plants have shown that AM roots had higher Na concentrations but also higher K concentrations and thus maintained a high K/Na compared to non-mycorrhizal plants. Scientists have found that mycorrhizal roots of salt grass plant

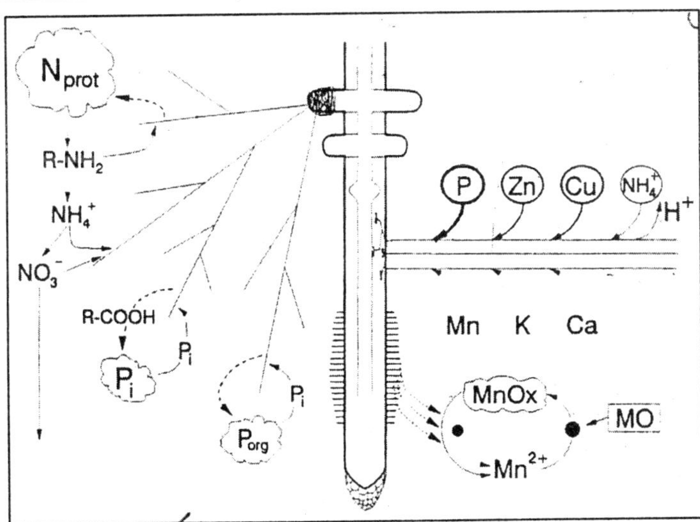

Figure 13.1: Schematic Presentation of some Established Components (Processes) of the Nutrient Dynamics in the 'Hyphosphere' of Ecto- and VA-mycorrhizal Roots. N_{prot}: Protein Nitrogen; MO: Microorganism. (H. Narchner, 1991)

(*Distichlis spicata*) had higher sodium, potassium and phosphorus concentrations than non-mycorrhizal roots. In contrast, the results of other studies have shown that Na uptake decreased in AM plants compared to controls. Sodium content of shoots of mycorrhizal halophytic *Aster tripolium* plants was lower than non-mycorrhizal plants under salinity stress (Rozema *et al.*, 1986). K/Na ratio increased in mycorrhizal barley (moderate salinity tolerant plant) at high levels of salinity by decreasing Na concentration, rather than by increasing K concentration (Mohammad *et al.*, 2003). Dwivedi 2003 and Soni 2006, reported potassium play an important role in mycorrhization in wheat, legumes and rice plants.

Increased Uptake of Other Mineral Nutrients

Concentrations of Ca, Mg and Zn in onion plants inoculated with *Glomus fasciculatum* increased in saline conditions and improved the nutritional status, which was at least partially responsible for increased plant growth (Ojala *et al.*, 1983). The improved growth and nutrient acquisition (P, K, Zn, Cu and Fe) in tomato demonstrate the potential of AM fungi for protecting plants against salt stress in arid and semiarid areas (Al-Karaki, 2000; Al-Karaki and Hammad, 2001). Although effects of AM fungi in increasing some toxic elements (*e.g.*, Na, CI and Mn) have been reported (Pfeiffer and Bloss, 1988; Cantrell and Linderman, 2001), a direct effect of AM fungi in rednenon of others has also been reported. Mycorrhizal fungi decreased sodium concentration in barley (*Hordeum vulgare*) when grow in saline conditions (Mohammad *et al.*, 2003), and Mn can be reduced in mycorrhizal plants when it occurs at toxic levels compared to non-mycorrhizal plants (Sanders and Fitter, 1992; Cardoso *et al.*, 2003).

AMF in Metal Sequestration

The use of living organism for the remediation of soils contaminated with heavy metals, radionuclide or polycyclic hydrocarbon is known as bioremediation (Kumar *et al.*, 1995; Brooks and

Robinson, 1998; Salt *et al.*, 1998, Baker *et al.*, 2000). AM fungi are involved in bioremediation through phytoremediation, the technique based on the use of plants for soil remediation (Leyval *et al.*, 1997; Turnau *et al.*, 2005). Depending on the type of pollutant different strategy for phytoremediation, such as phytostabilization, phytodegradation and phytoextraction has been used. For phytoremediation of soil polluted with heavy metals, the phytostabilization strategy involves the immobilization of heavy metals in the soil by establishing plants.

AMF can help phytoremediation activities, particularly in phytostabilization (Goncalves *et al.*, 1997; Leyval *et al.*, 1997, 2002; Orlowska *et al.*, 2002; Regvar *et al.*, 2003; Turnau *et al.*, 2005). Among possible mechanism by which AM fungi improve the resistance of plants to heavy metal is the ability of AM fungi to sequester heavy metals through the production of chelates or by absorption AM plants typically less translocate heavy metal to their shoots than the corresponding non AM control. Among the diverse type of mycorrhizosphere interactions known to benefit plant growth and health, those related to phytoremediation process. As rhizobacteria and AM fungi interact synergistically to the benefit of phytoremediation. A key point in phytoremediation is the use of heavy metal adapted microbes, soil microbial diversity and activity both negative affected by excessive concentratic of heavy metals. Indigenous bacterial population (Giller *et al.*, 1998) and AM fungi (Del Val *et al.*, 1999) must be adapted to metal toxicity and have evolved abilities to enable them to survive in polluted soil.

Various authors have reported isolating spores of arbuscular mycorrhizal fungal taxa such as *Glomus* and *Gigaspora* associated with most of the plants growing in heavy metal polluted habitats (Raman *et al.*, 1993; Chaudhry *et al.*, 1999). Identified *Glomus* and *Gigaspora* spp. in the mycorrhizospheres of fourteen plant species colonising a magnesite mine spoil in India. Whereas *Glomus mosseae* was isolated only and Duek *et al.* (1986) isolated *Glomus fasciculatum* alone from the heavy metal polluted soils. Pawlowska *et al.* (1996) surveyed a calamine spoil mound rich in Cd, Pb and Zn in Poland and recovered spores of *Glomus aggregatum, G. fasciculatum* and *Entrophospora* spp. from the mycorrhizospheres of the plants growing on spoil. Joner and Leyval (1997) reported that extra-radical hyphae of AM fungus G. *mosseae* can transport Cd from soil to subterranean clover plants growing in compartmented pots, but that transfer from fungus to plant is restricted due to fungal immobilization. It was also reported also reported no restriction of fungal hyphal growth into soil with high extractable Cd levels. It have been also showed very little, if any, translocation of Zn absorbed by mycorrhizal maize seedlings grown in contaminated soil, to the shoots. It was studied that localization of heavy metals within the fungal mycelium and mycorrhizal roots of *Euphorbia cyparissias* from Zn contaminated wastes and found higher concentrations of Zn as crystaloids deposited within the fungal mycelium and cortical cells of mycorrhizal roots. Studies by various researchers (Galli *et al.*, 1994; Hetrick *et al.*, 1994) have shown that mycorrhizal fungal ecotypes from heavy metal contaminated sites seem to be more tolerant to heavy metals (and have developed resistance) than reference strains from uncontaminated soils Galli *et al.* (1995) reported that although there was an increase in the contents of cystein, gamma EC and GSH in the mycorrhizal maize roots grown in quarto sand with added Cu, no differences in Cu uptake were detected between non-mycorrhizal and mycorrhizal plants. These results do not support the idea that AM fungi protects maize from Cu-toxicity. Mycorrhizae are also known to produce growth stimulating substances for plants, thus encouraging mineral nutrition and increased growth and biomass necessary for phytoremediation to become commercially viable strategy for decontamination of polluted soils. In addition to the damaging effects on plants, the effect of heavy metals on the soil microorganisms and soil microbial activity also need to be considered. Various soil factors such as the clay contents and mobility of heavy metals effect plants and soil biota. As metal uptake by plant roots depends on soil and their associated symbionts, it is important to monitor metal mobility and availability to plant and its symbionts when assessing the effect of soil contamination on plant uptake and related phytotoxic effects The prospect of symbionts existing in heavy metal contaminated soils has important implications for phytoremediation.. The potentials of phytoremediation of contaminated soil can be enhanced by inoculating hyper-accumulator plants with mycorrhizal fungi most appropriate for contaminated site. It is further suggested that the potential of phytoremediation of contaminated soil can be enhanced by inoculating hyper-accumulator plants with mycorrhiza.

AMF as Phytoprotector

The establishment of AM fungi in plant roots has been shown to reduce damage caused by soil borne plant pathogens with an enhancement of plant resistance/tolerance in mycorrhizal plants. The effectiveness of AM in biocontrol is dependent on the AM fungus involved as well as the substrate and the host plant (Azcon–Aguliar and Barea, 1996; Linderman, 1994, 2000, Elmer 2002).

Several AM fungal species have been found to control soil borne pathogens, for example under green house conditions.

Glomus faciculatum and *Gigaspora margarita* are shown to reduce root rot disease caused by *Fusarium oxysporum f.* sp. *asparagi* and *Helicobasidium mompa* in asparagus (*Asparagus officinalis L.*) (Matsubsara *et al.*, 2000; Matsubara *et al.*, 2001, Singh 2008).

Glomus clarum is shown to reduce root necrosis due to *Rhizcotonia solani* in cow pea (*Vigna unguiculata L.*) (Abdel-Fattah and Shabana, 2002).

In pasteurised soil AM fungi have been shown to decrease the root damage caused by root rot fungus *Cylindrocladium spathiphylli* in bananas, although the pathogen decreased the intensity of AM fungal root colonization (Declerck *et al.*, 2002). Since AM are formed in the roots of plants, maximum attention has been paid towards mycorrhizae disease incidence interactions in relation to soil and root borne pathogens (Table 13.1). AM fungi impart resistance to host plant against root pathogens. Root pathogens are major limiting factor for plant production. Most widespread root borne pathogens belong to genera, *Phytophthora, Fusarium, Pythium* and *Rhizoctonia*. They kill roots or reduce their ability to absorb water and nutrients by penetrating root tissues and producing toxins.

Different AM fungi are known to confer variable tolerance to *Phytophthora parasitica*. Davis and Menge (1980, 1981) used five different AM fungal species on three different plants. They observed that maximum resistance to the pathogens was due to two AM fungi namely *G. fasciculatum* and *G. constrictum* in *Citrus* sp. Arbuscular mycorrhizal peanut plants become resistant to root rot pathogen *Sclerotium rolfsii* (Krishna and Bagyaraj, 1983). Number of sclerotia produced by the pathogen were reduced on the mycorrhizal roots. Biomass production and phosphorus content were maximum in mycorrhizal plants and minimum in pathogen inoculated plants.

Take all disease of wheat, caused by *Guamannomyces graminis* var. tritici was reduced when mycorrhizal fungus was inoculated in plants. The disease is favoured by inadequate plant nutrition leading to mineral deficiency especially phosphorus (Graham and Menge, 1981).

AM fungi are able to increase nutritional status of the host plant thereby improving resistance against the pathogens. Recently Singh *et al.* (2008, 2009, 2010) reported inoculation of AM fungi before *Fusarium oxysporum* causing wilt disease protect the tomato plants. AM fungi and *Trichoderma* sp. produced more significant biocontrol effect (Singh, 2008). Vyas *et al.* (2010) reviewed mechanism phytoprotection by AM fungi in various plant diseases.

Table 13.1: Inhibitory Influence of VAM Fungi on Soil-Borne Fungal Pathogens

Host	*Disease*	*Pathogen*	*Reference*
Tobacco	Root rot	*Phytophthora cinnamomae*	Bartschi *et al.*, 1981
Onion	Wilt	*Pyrenochaeta terrestris*	Becker, 1976
Onion	Wilt	*Fusarium oxysporum f. sp. cepi*	Dehne, 1982
Tomato	Wilt	*Fusarium oxysporum f.sp. lycopersici*	Dehne and schonbeck, 1979
Wheat	Take-all disease	*Gaeumannomyces graminis var tritici*	Graham and Menge, 1982
Soybean	Root rot	*Macrophomia phaseolina, Rhizoctonia solani, Fusarium solani*	Zambolim and Schenck, 1983
Brassica	Root rot	*Olpidium brassicae*	Schonbeck, 1979
Casia tora	Wilt	*Fusarium oxysporum*	Chakrabarty and Mishra, 1986
Tomato	Root rot	*Fusarium oxysporum f.sp. redicis lycopersici*	Caron *et al.*, 1986
Brinjal	Wilt	*Verticillium albo-atrum*	Melo *et al.*, 1985

P Gossling, A Hodge, G Goodlaur and GD Bending, 2005.

Table 13.2: Inhibitory Effect of VAM Fungi on Nematodes

Host	*Disease*	*Nematode*	*Reference*
Phaseolus vulgaris	Root knot	*Meloidogyne javanica*	Oliveira and Zambolim, 1987
Barley	Root decline	*Aphalenchus avenae*	Hussey and Roncadori, 1981
Soybean	Root knot	*Meloidogyne spp.*	Kellam and Schenck, 1980
Tobacco	Root knot	*M. hapla*	Sikora
Tomato, Oat	Root knot	*M. incognita*	Schonbeck, 1975
Cotton	Root knot	*M. incognita*	Roncadori and Hussey, 1977
Tomato	Root knot	*M.incognita, M. Javanica*	Bagyaraj *et al.*, 1979
Soybean	Root knot	*M. incognita*	Kellam and Schenck, 1980
Cotton	Root knot	*M. incognita*	Salch and Sikora, 1984
Tomato	Root knot	*M. incognita*	Suresh and Bagyaraj, 1984
Cotton	Root knot	*M. incognita*	Smith *et al.*, 1986
Beans	Root knot	*M. javanica*	Olivera and Zambolim, 1987

KG Mukerji, BP Chamola and Mamta Sharma, 1997

Mycorrhiza-induced Resistance

Different mechanisms have been shown to play a role in plant protection by AMF, namely, improved plant nutrition, damage compensation, competition for colonization sites or photosynthates, changes in the root system, changes in rhizosphere microbial populations, and activation of plant defense mechanisms. Several mechanisms can be operative simultaneously, with contributions depending on environmental conditions, timing of the interaction and partners involved (Azcon Aguilar and Barea, 1996).

There is evidence for the accumulation of defensive plant compounds related to mycorrhization, although to a much lower extent than in plant-pathogen interactions. Accumulation of reactive oxygen species, activation of phenylpropanoid metabolism, and accumulation of specific isoforms of hydrolytic enzymes such as chitinases and glucanases has been reported in mycorrhizal roots. There reactions, however, are generally localized, suggesting. Concerning aboveground effects, accumulation of insect antifeedant compounds and transcriptional regulation of defense-related genes (Pozo *et al.*, unpublished data) have been described in the shoots of mycorrhizal plants. Furthermore, the volatile blends released by AM plants can be more attractive to aphid parasitoids than those from non-mycorrhizas. Nevertheless, accumulation of PR proteins, salicyclic acid, or expression of marker genes associated with systemic acquired resistance has not been reported in systemic tissues.

AMF as Communicators

The most important AM fungal structure for plant nutrition is represented by the extra radical mycelium spreading from mycorrhizal roots into the surrounding soil which is able to uptake nutrients N, P, S, Ca, K, Fe, Cu, Zn and to transfer them to root cells (Smith and Read, 1997; Cox *et al.*, 1980). Mycorrhizal mycelium has been investigated in different experimental studies, based on either destructive extraction from soil or root observation chambers or in vitro system which yielded only qualitative data on its structure and growth (Jakobson *et al.*, 1990; Jones *et al.*, 1998).

The first visualization of intact AM mycelium extending from mycorrhizal roots into the extraradical environment was obtained by means of a bidimensional model system which utilized two cellulose esters members "sandwiched" around the roots of individual plantlets. After only seven days growth, a fine network of extramatrical hyphae growing on the membrane was visible to the naked eye, and its length extended from 5169 to 7471 mm (hyphal length in *Thymus vulgaris* and *Allium porum*, respectively).

The experimental system divided to visualize the mycorrhizal mycelium also evidenced that the mechanism allowing the formation of the network was self recognition and hyphal anastomosis.

It is important to stress that the viability of mycorrhizal networks was 100 per cent and that all the anastomoses showed protoplasmic continuity and nuclear occurrence in hyphal bridges, confirming the occurrence of nuclear exchange also during fusion between extraradical symbiotic hyphae. AM fungi are known to infect a wide range of host species. They have a large geographical distribution (Malloch *et al.*, 1980), being found even in the Arctic tundras and the Antarctic region (DeMars and Boerner 1995b; Gardes and Dahlberg 1996). Unlike most ectomycorrhizal species, AM are not host specific. This enables them to form associations with a large number of plant species.

AM fungi regulate plant communities by affecting competition, composition and succession (Allen and Allen 1984; Kumar *et al.*, 1999). Limited resources and the struggle of the plants for a share of these is the primary selection pressure operating on plant species (St. John and Coleman, 1983). In competition between plants, mycorrhizae in the soil favour the growth of one species and are detrimental to other competing species. Fitter (1977) demonstrated this in competition between two grasses *Lolium perenne* and *Holcus lanatus*. Inoculation with mycorrhizae favoured the growth of *H. lanatus*. This was an indirect effect as infection with mycorrhizae reduced the root length of *L. perenne* by 40 per cent. AM may regulate competition between plants by making available to mycorrhizal plants, resources that are not available to non-mycorrhizal neighbours (Allen and Allen, 1984). AM symbiosis increases intraspecific competition (Facelli *et al.*, 1999). As a result, density of individuals of a single species would be reduced thereby allowing the co-existence of individuals of different species. This would lead to an increase in species diversity.

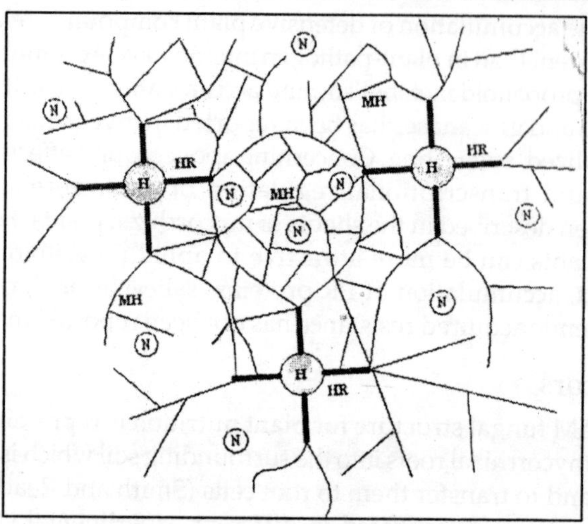

Figure 13.2: AM Hyphae Form a Network the Wood-Wide Web

Table 13.3: Extension and Interconnectedness of Extraradical Mycelial Networks Produced by AM Fungi Living

Plant Species/Fungal Species	*Hyphal Density (mm mm^{-2})*	*No. of Anastomoses per Hyphal Length*	*Anastomosis Frequence (per cent)*	*Reference*
Allium porum/Glomus mosseae	2.7	4.6	75.0	Giovannetti M *et al.*, 1999
Allium porum/Glomus mosseae	3.5	3.8	59.3	Giovannetti M *et al.*, 2004
*Daucus carota/Gigaspora margarita**	-	0.0075	9.8	De la Providencia IE *et al.*, 2005
*Daucus carota/Gigaspora rosea**	-	0.012	4.2	De la Providencia IE *et al.*, 2005
*Daucus carota/Glomus hoi**	-	0.057	100	De la Providencia IE *et al.*, 2005
*Daucus carota/intraradices**	-	0.076	100	Giovannetti M *et al.*, 2004
Daucus carota/Glomus mosseae	3.9	2.5	45.5	Giovannetti M *et al.*, 2004
*Daucus carota/Glomus proliferum**	-	0.066	100	De la Providencia IE *et al.*, 2005
*Daucus carota/Scutellospora reticulate**	-	0.0079	5.2	De la Providencia IE *et al.*, 2005
Gossypium hirsutum/Glomus mosseae	6.8	6.2	53.1	Giovannetti M *et al.*, 2004
Lactuca sativa/Glomus mosseae	2.9	3.0	63.8	Giovannetti M *et al.*, 2004
Petrosslinum cripsum/Glomus caledonium	3.8	1.5	18.6	Unpublished data
Petroselinum cripsum/Glomus intradices	2.3	5.5	56.9	Unpublished data
Petroselinum cripsum/Glomus mosseae	3.5	4.7	62.3	Unpublished data
Prunus cerasifera/Glomus mosseae	2.4	5.1	64.0	Giovannetti M *et al.*, 2001
Solanum melongena/Glomus mosseae	4.1	2.1	47.0	Giovannetti M *et al.*, 2004
Thymusvulgaris/Glomus mosseae	2.1	5.1	78.0	Giovannetti M *et al.*, 2001

*: Ri-TDNA transformed carrot root.

M Giovanetti, L Avio, P Fortuna, EP Sbrana, P Sterani, 2006.

Mycorrhizae govern species composition in communities by influencing plant fitness at the establishment phase. AM prevent non-mycorrhizal plants from growing in soils colonized by them. This has a selective advantage for the fungus. Maintaining a high proportion of compatible host species at the expense of non-compatible species provides the fungus with an undisturbed carbon supply (Francis and Read, 1994).

Succession is a chain of predictable processes whose course is influenced by nutrient availability. Mycorrhizae, owing to their role in nutrient uptake, may play an important part in determining the rate and direction of the process (Smith and Read, 1997a). They influence the outcome of succession by amending the composition of species or by affecting species diversity (Gange *et al.*, 1990).

AM fungi have been reported to be active in mediating nutrient transfer among plants (Chiariello *et al.*, 1982; Francis and Read, 1984; Grime *et al.*, 1987; Watkins *et al.*, 1996; Graves *et al.*, 1997; Lerat *et al.*, 2002) mainly through the extensive mycelial networks, which due to the lack host specificity may link the roots of contiguous plant species (Graves, *et al.*, 1997; Van der Heijden 1998). Recent studies showed a novel mechanism by which plants may become interconnected, that is hyphal fusion between extraradical hyphae originating from different individual plant root systems of different species, genera and families (Giovannetti, 2004).

AMF in Biotechnology

Introduction of AMF on micropropagate plantlets improves its establishment and growth in the field. Unfortunately not much work has been conduced in this line. But the few convincing reports decisively prove that successful hardening and *ex vitro* establishments of plantlets could be achieved by inoculation with AM fungi at the time of plants out.

One of the earliest report on the effect of growth and leaf mineral content of two apple clones propagated *in vitro* were increased substantially. Similarly enhanced effect on the growth of *in vitro* cultured strawberry plantlets could be achieved due to the association of AMF. The rooting of plantlets of garlic regenerated from called was significantly enhanced due to inoculation with *Glomus mosseae.* The transplant success and growth of *Robus idaeus* and *Pistacia integerrima* were achieved with mycorrhiza inoculation.

Effect of AMF on these culture flowers is also encouraging. In a different study at Vellayani, evaluated the effect of AMF in enhancing of survival, growth characteristic and uptake of nutrients by micropropagated Anthurium. AMF was incorporated into the rooting medium at the time of planting out through infected root bits. The study was conducted with *Glomus constrictum* and *G. etunicatum.* Micropropagated avocado plants generally exhibit low survival and very slow rate of growth during acclimatization. Inoculation of *G. fasciculatum* on micropropagated avocado planlets improved the formation of well developed root system, shoot growth, shoot root ratio and NPK content in plant tissue which helped plants to tolerate environmental stress transplanting. It was concluded that inoculation of AMF seems to be the key factor for subsequent growth and development of micropropagated plants of avocado.

AMF in Genetics

"Several constitutively expressed genes were shown to be expressed at the rhizodermis level, including root hairs and around the root tip. Moreover, a loss-of-function mutant defective in two *Phtl* transporters, normally expressed at the root periphery, in *Arabidopsis* exhibited a strong reduction of phosphate uptake by 75 per cent (Shin *et al.*, 2008), strongly indicating a role for *Phtl* transporters in the 'direct' uptake pathway. In the AM symbiosis, phosphate uptake by the fungus from soil is the first step in the process of phosphate transport to the root. Two AMF phosphate transporters (*GvPT* and *GiPT* from *Glomus versiforme* and *Glomus intraradices*, respectively (Harrison *et al.*, 1995; Maldonado-Mendoja *et al.*, 2001) form a common clade with transporters identified in fungal species from the Basidiomycota and Ascomycota. At least two members of this clade (pH084 and *GvPT*) exhibit high affinity towards phosphate, with *Km* values of 8 µM and 18 µM, respectively (Harrison *et al.*, 1995; Bun-Ya *et al.*, 1991). The *GvPT* and. *GiPT* genes are predominantly expressed in the extraradical fungal mycelium exposed to micromolar phosphate concentrations (Maldonado-Mendoja *et al.*, 2001). And so their encoded proteins are likely to participate in phosphate uptake at the fungus-soil interface.

AMF in Genomics and Proteomics

In recent years, outstanding molecular approaches have been used for the identification of genes and functions involved in plant-microbe endosymbioses. Following the first completion of genome sequencing projects, biological research has developed high throughout genetic programs with multiparallel analyses of gene transcripts, proteins and metabolites, that are now tentatively transposed to the world of mycorrhizal and rhizobial symbioses (Franken and Requena 2001; Colebatch *et al.*, 2002a, 2002b).

Table 13.4: Proteomic Studies in the Field of Plant-Microbe Symbioses

Biological Models	*Proteins Characterized by 2 DE*	*Identified Proteins*	*References*
	Endomycorrhizal symbioses		
Allium cepa/Glomus mosseae	15	0	Garcia-Garrido *et al.* (1993)
Nicotiana tabacum/G. mosseae/ Glomus instraradices	34	0	Dumans-Gaudot *et al.* (1994)
Lycopersicon esculentum/G. intraradices	5	0	Simoneau *et al.* (1994)
Pisum sativum/G. mosseae	42	0	Samra *et al.* (1997)
L. esculentum/G. mosseae	44	0	Benabdellah *et al.* (1998)
L. esculentum/G. mosseae	14	0	Dassi *et al.* (1999)
L. esculentum/G. mosseae	26	1	Benabdellah *et al.* (2000)
Triticum aestivum/G. mosseae	1	1	Fester *et al.* (2003)
Medicago truncatula/G. mosseae	55	8	Bestel-Corre *et al.* (2002)
P. sativum/G. mosseae	7	6	Repetto *et al.* (2003)
M. truncatula/G. mosseae	34	6	Bestel-Corre (2002)
Ri T-DNA Daucus carota/G. Intraradices	8	2	Bestel-Corre (2003)
G. intraradices	450	6	Dumas-Gaudot *et al.* (2003b)
Acaulospora laevis/Gigaspora rosea/ Scutellospora castanea/G. mosseae	12	0	Samra *et al.* (1996)

Franken and Requena, 2001

AM fungi bear large and highly repeated genomes, a feature that completely hinders the development of genomic analyses. Due to their obligate symbiotic status, the amount of accessible mRNA material is very limited; however, many limitations have been overcome with the help of polymerase chain reaction (PCR)-based methods (Franken and Requena, 2001) and *in vitro* monoxenic cultures (St-Arnaud *et al.*, 1996). Several EST libraries have thus been constructed using activated spores of *Gigaspora rosea* (Stommel *et al.*, 2001; Tamasloukht *et al.*, 2003), *Glomus mosseae* (Requena *et al.*, 2002), presymbiotic mycelium of *Gigaspora margarita* (Lanfranco *et al.*, 2000) and extra radical hyphae of *Glomus intradices* (Sawaki and Saito, 2001).

Concerning mycorrhizas, pioneering studies were achieved with ectomycorrhizas in the early 1990s (Hilbert *et al.*, 1991; Simoneau *et al.*, 1993; Burgess *et al.*, 1995; Burgess and Dell, 1996) allowing researchers to detect symbiosis-related (SR) polypeptides, up-regulated or newly induced in mycorrhizal roots, as well as down-regulated polypeptides, by comparison to control roots and mycelium extracts. Recently some SR proteins were identified by mass spectrometry and N-terminal sequencing (Tarka *et al.*, 2000), as well as mycelial proteins (Vallorani *et al.*, 2000). Arbuscular mycorrhizas, a similar progression was followed, from descriptive studies (Garcia-Garrido *et al.*, 1993; Dumas-Gaudot *et al.*, 1994; Simoneau *et al.*, 1994; Samra *et al.*, 1997; Benabdellah *et al.*, 1998; Dassi *et al.*, 1999) to the first identifications of a vacuolar H^+-ATPase and a Myk15 protein with an unknown function (Benabdellah *et al.*, 2000; Fester *et al.*, 2003). Additionally, protein profiles of both dormant and germinated spores of several fungi were compared (Samra *et al.*, 1996). Now, proteome analysis is used as a powerful tool to reveal more and more proteins involved in mycorrhiza development and functioning including proteins involved in defence response, root physiology and the respiratory pathway (Dumas-Gaudot *et al.*, 2001; Bestel-Corre *et al.*, 2002).

Fluxomics

The goal of fluxomics is to quantify all the metabolic fluxes in a cell, tissue or organism (Sauer *et al.*, 1999; Sauer, 2004). Investigation of the flow of matter through biochemical systems has always been central to the study of metabolism, and analysis of the rates of metabolic transformations–the study of enzyme kinetics–is likewise a long-established aspect of understanding any biological system in detail. However, the conceptual, experimental and computational tools for quantifying the integrated functioning of metabolic networks began to become available only in recent decades, and are still very much under development. Like many other omic approaches, fluxomics has yet to attain the goal of generating comprehensive system-wide data sets. However, progress in the last 10 year has been rapid and fluxomics has grown beyond is origins in bacterial systems and has begun to make significant contributions to the study of plant systems (Kruger *et al.*, 2003; Schwender *et al.*, 2004a; Ratcliffe and Shachar-Hill, 2006).

The analysis of multiple flows through a network involves both direct and indirect determination of metabolic and transport fluxes. Direct determination fluxes involves individually measuring the rates of substrate uptake, product secretion, and the accumulation of storage or structural compounds (lipids, carbohydrates and proteins) of known composition. Indirect determination of fluxes is performed in two ways. In the first method, fluxes measured directly are used to deduce other net fluxes; this is done by balancing the influxes and effluxes from individual metabolite pools using the known stoichiometries of biochemical reactions (flux balancing). The second method is based on interpreting the results of labeling experiments. Labeling measurements using radioactive isotypes are made by fractionation or chromatographic separation methods followed by scintillation counting of different intermediate and product metabolites. Measurements of stable isotopic labeling usually involve ^{13}C (or less commonly ^{15}N or ^{2}H) and are made by nuclear magnetic resonance (NMR) spectroscopy and mass spectrometry. The interpretation of labeling and flux measurement data in terms of multiple fluxes is nontrivial and almost always involves computer-aided modeling. Models are used to estimate fluxes by finding the values that result in a best fit of computed (simulated) to experimental results.

This reliance on fitting to a metabolic model means that a fluxomic investigation requires some prior knowledge of and assumptions about the metabolic architecture of the system. This knowledge is certainly much less complete in mycorrhizas than in many bacteria or model fungi and plants. However, progress in delineating metabolic and transport networks in mycorrhizal systems has been steady in recent years and has reached a point where models can be constructed for the quantitative interpretation of labeling data in the best-studied cases (Chalot and Brun, 1998; Bago *et al.*, 2000; Bucking and Shachar-Hill, 2005; Govindarajulu *et al.*, 2005). The outline of a working model of central metabolism and transport in the arbuscular mycorrhizal symbiosis that could serve as a starting point for flux analysis is shown in Figure 13.3. The advent of mycorrhizal plant and fungal genome sequences will be of enormous help in building and in filling in the molecular mechanisms of such models. When transcript and proteomic data sets for mycorrhizas become much more complete than they are at present–which can be expected to happen sooner rather than later–they too will be important in defining and validating model networks for use in flux analysis.

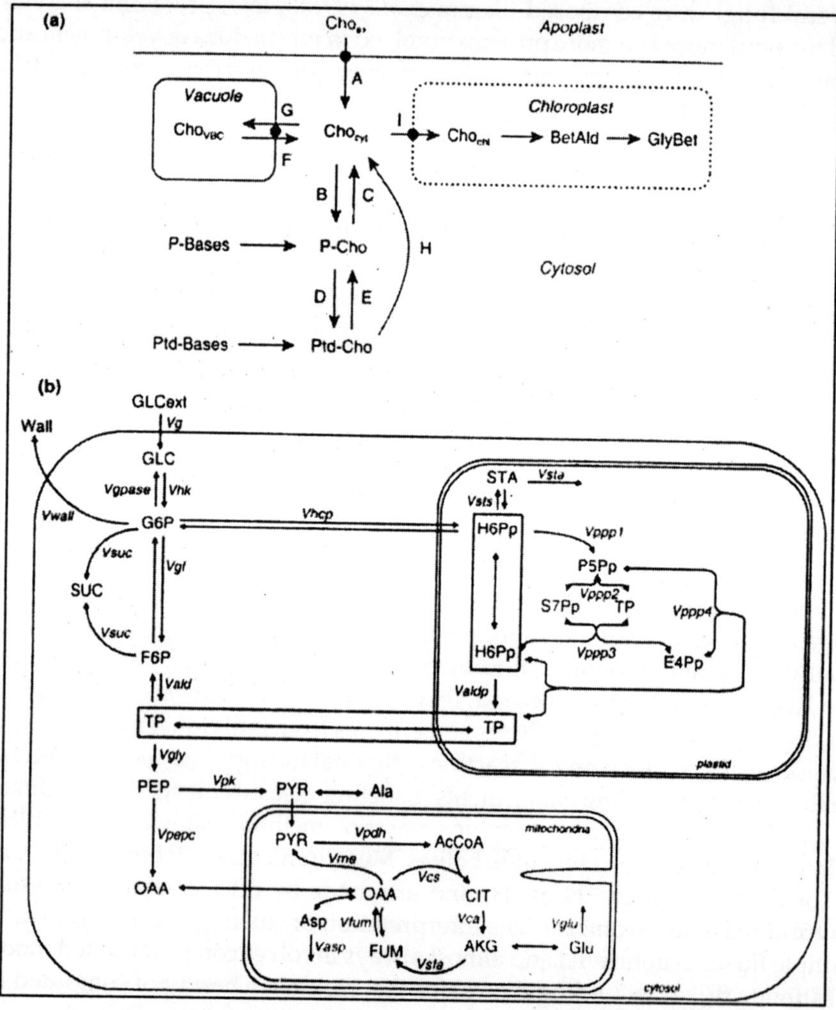

Figure 13.3: A Model Used in a Dynamic Laboring of the Glycine Betaine Synthesis in Transgenic Tobacco (*Nocotiana tabacum*) (Hill, 2000)

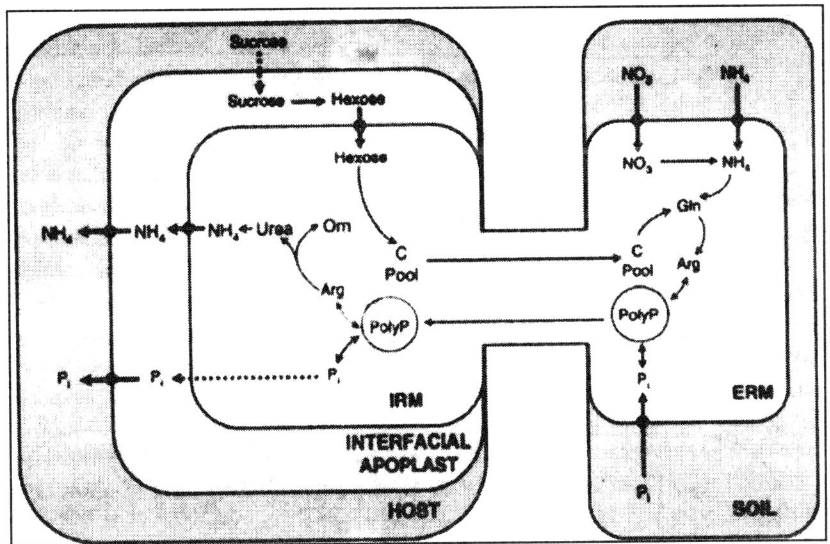

Figure 13.6: A Model of Nitrogen Flow in the Arbuscular Mycorrhizal Symbiosis, Suitable for Initiating a Fluxomics Analysis (Hill, 2000)

Conclusions

1. Soil is the major sink of carbon and AM fungi have shown that, they have also potential to sequester the carbon from the soil.
2. Deposition of heavy metal in the soil is troublesome affair which resulted into the toxicity, which is not only harmful for the plants but also unsafe for organism dependent on their food from plants. Here also AM fungi provide release from the heavy metal toxicity by sequestring heavy metals from the soil.
3. Control of plant disease was remain challenge for scientist and farmer both. Use of pesticide no longer remain the healthy affair, therefore, biological control was searched as an alternative, among the biocontrol agents, role of AMF have been recognized a fruitful one.
4. As it has been established that microbes and plants have very strong communication in the from of signal transduction, here also AMF provided evidences that they are best communicators in microbial world and have developed wood wide-web for their communication.
5. Biotechnology is the talk of hour and therefore role of AMF fungi have also been explored and recognised in the field of morden biology and have been tried to elucidate their relevance in biotechnology, molecular biology, genomics, proteomics and fluxomics.

Acknowledgements

Authors are thankful to Head, Department of Botany, Dr. H.S. Gour University, Sagar, RKG and AKS thankfully acknowledge UGC and DS Kothari for financial assistance respectively.

References

Al-Karaki GN and Clark RB. (1999). Varied rates of mycorrhizal inoculum on growth and nutrient acquisition by barley grown with drought stress. *J. Plant Nutrion* 22: 1775-1784.

Al-Karaki GN and Hammad R. (2001). Mycorrhizal influence on fruit yield and mineral content of tomato grown under salt stress. *Journal of Plant Nutrition* 24: 1311-1323.

Al-Karaki GN. (2000). Growth of mycorrhizal tomato and mineral acquisition under salt stress, *Mycorrhiza* 10: 51-54.

Allen EB and Allen MF. (1984). The competition between plants of different succession all stages: mycorrhizal as regulators. *Canadian J. of Botany* 62: 2625-2692.

Allen EB and Allen MF. (1986). Water relations of xeric grasses in the field: interaction of mycorrhizas and competition. *New Phytologist* 104: 559-571.

Allen EB and Cunningham GL. (1983). Effects of vesicular-arbuscular mycorrhizae on *Distichlis spicata* under three salinity levels. *New phytologist* 93: 227-236.

Allen R and Read DJ. (1994). The contribution of mycorrhizal fungi to the determination of plant community structure. *Plant and soil* 159 : 11-25.

Allen MF. (1991). *The Ecology of Mycorrhizae.* Cambridge: Cambridge University Press.

Azaizeh HA, Marschner H, Romheld V, Wittenmayer L. (1995). Effects of vesicular-arbuscular mycorrhizal fungus and other soil microorganisms on growth, mineral nutrient acquisition and root exudation of soil grown maize plants. *Mycorrhiza* 5: 321-327.

Azcon-Aguilar C and Barea JM. (1996). Arbuscular mycorrhizas and biological control of soil borne plant pathogens- an overview of the mechanisms involved. *Mycorrhiza* 6: 457-458.

Bago B, Azcon-Aguliar C, Goulet A, Piche Y. (1998). Branched absorbing structure (BAS): a feature of the extradical mycelium of symbiotic arbusculsar mycorrhizal fungi. *New Phytol* 139: 375-388.

Bago B, Pfeffer PE, Douds DD, Brouillette J, Becard G, Shachar-Hill Y. (1999). Carbon metabolism in spores of the arbuscular mycorrhizal fungus *Glomus intraradices* as revealed by nuclear magnetic resonance spectroscopy. *Plant Physiolz*121: 263-271.

Bago B, Pfeffer PE, Shachar-Hill Y. (2000). Carbon metabolism and transport in arbuscular mycorrhizas. *Plant Physiol* 128: 949-957.

Bago B, Zipfel W, Williams R, Jun J. Arreola R, Lammer P, Pfeffer PE, Shachar-Hill Y. (2002). Translocation and utilization of fungal lipid in the arbuscular mycorrhizal symbiosis. *Plant Physiol* 128: 108-124.

Bago B, Pfeffer PE, Abubaker J, Jun j, Allen JW, Brouillette, Douds DD, Lammers PJ and Sachar Hill. (1995). Carbon export from arbuscular mycorrhizal roots involves the translocation of carbohydrate as the translocation of carbohydrate as well as lipid. *Plant physiology*131: 1469-1507.

Bagyaraj DJ. (1984). Biological interactions with mycorrhizal fungi: I*n VA mycorrhiza* (eds). CLO Powell and DJ Bagyaraj (New York: CRC Press), 131-153.

Bagyaraj DJ, Manjunath A and Reddy DDR (1979). Interaction of vesicular arbuscular mycorrhizae with root knot nematode in tomato. *Plant soil.* 51: 397-403.

Baker AJM, MC Grath SP, Reeves RD, Smith JAC. (2000). Metal hyperaccumulator plants: a review of the ecology and physiology of a biological resource for phytoremediation of metal polluted soils. In: *Phytoremediation of contaminated soil and water*. (eds., Terry N, Banuelos G, Vangronsveld J,). Boca Ratton, Fl, USA: CRC Press, 85-107.

Barber S (1975). Soil nutrient bioavailability: A mechanistic approach. New York USA, John Wiley and Sons.

Bartschi H, Gianinazzi Pearson V and Vegh I. (1981). Vesicular arbuscular mycorrhizae formation and root disease (*Phytophthora cinnamomi*). development in *Chamaecyparis lawso. Phytopatho. Z.* 102: 213-218.

Beaden BN and Peterson L. (2000). Influence of arbuscular mycorrhizal fungi on soils structure and aggregate stability of vertisol. *Plant and Soil*. 218: 173-188.

Becker WN (1976). Quantification of onion vesicular-arbuscular mycorrhiza and their resistance to *Pyrenochaeta- terretris*. Ph.d. dissertation. Duke Uni, Durham.

Beilby JP, Kidby DK. (1980). Biochemistry of ungerminated and germinated spores of the vesicular-arbuscular mycorrhizal fungus, *Glomus caledonium*: changes in neutral and polar lipids. *J. Lipid Res*, 21: 739-750.

Benabdellah K, Azcon-Aguilar C, Ferrol N. (1998). Soluble and membrane symbiosis related polypeptides associated with the development of arbuscular-mycorrhizas in tomato (*Lycopersicon-esculentum*). *New phytol*.140: 15-143.

Benabdellah K, Azcon-Aguilar C, Ferrol N. (2000). Alterations in the plasma membrane polypeptide pattern of tomato roots (*Lycopersicon esculentum*). during the development of arbuscular mycorrhiza. *J Ex. Bot*. 51: 747-754.

Bestel Corre G, Dumas-Gaudot E, Gianinazzi S. (2004). Proteomics as at pool to monitor plant–microbe endosymbioses in the rhizosphere, 14: 1-10.

Bestel–corre G. (2002). La proteomique: un outil d' etude des interactions dans la rhizosphere. Identification de proteines reliees a la mycorrhization et a nodulation et evaluation de I' impact boues de I' impact de boues d' epuration sur les symbiosis. PhD Thesis. Universite de Bourgogne, Dijon.

Bethlenfalavy, GJ and Barea JM. (1994). Mycorrhizae in sustainable agricultural. J. Effects on seed yield and soil aggregation. *Am. J. Agric*.9: 157-161.

Bever JD, Schulatz PA, Pringle A, Morton JB. (2001). Arbuscular mycorrhizal fungi: more diverse than meets the eye, and the ecological tale of why. *Bioscience*, 51: 923-931.

Blilou I, Ocampo JA, Garcia-Garrido JM. (2000). Induction of Ltp (lipid transfer protein). and Pal (phenylalanine ammonia-lyase). gene expression in rise roots colonized by the arbuscular mycorrhizal fungus *Glomus mossease. J. Exp. Bot.*, 51: 1969-77.

Brooks RR and Robinson BH. (1998). The potential use of hyperaccumulators and other plants for phytomining. In: Brooks RR, ed., *Plants that hyperaccumulate heavy metals their role in phytoremediation, microbiology, archeology, mineral exploration, and phytomining*. Cambridge: CAB International, 327-356.

Bucking H, Sachar Hill Y. (2005). Phosphate uptake, transport and transfer by the arbuscular mycorrhizal fungus *Glomus* Abdel- Fattah GM and Shabana YM. (2002). Efficacy of the arbuscular mycorrhizal fungus *Glomus* in protection of cowpea plants against root rot pathogen *Rhictonia solani. Journal of Plant Disease Protection* 109: 207-215.

Bun-Ya M. (1991). The pho84 gene of *Saccharomyces cerevisiae* encodes an inorganic phosphate transporter.*Mol.Cell. Biol.*11: 3229-3238.

Burgess T, Laurent P, Dell B, Malajczuk N, Martin F. (1995). Effect of fungal isolate aggressivity on the biosynthesis of symbiosis related polypeptides in differentiating eucalypt mycorrhizas.*Can.J. Bot.*195: 408-417.

Burgess T and Dell B. (1996). Changes in protein biosynthesis during the differentiation of *Pisolithus-Eucalyptus grandios* ectomycorrhiza. *Planta* 74: 553-560.

Cantrell IC and Linderman RG. (2001). Preinoculation of lettuce and onion with VA mycorrhizal fungi reduces deleterious effects of soil salinity. *Plant and Soil* 223: 269-281.

Cantrell IC and Linderman RG. (2001). Preinoculation of lettuce and onion with VA mycorrhizal fungi reduces deleterious effects of soil salinity. *Journal of Environmental Quality* 30: 1822-1828.

Canvagnaro TR, Gao LL, Smith FA, Smith SE. (2001). Morphology of arbuscular mycorrhizas is influenced by fungal identity. *New Phytologist* 137: 373-388.

Cardoso E, Navarro RB, Nogueira MA. (2003). Charges in manganese uptake and translocation by mycorrhizal soyabean under increasing Mn doses. *Revista Brasileira De Ciencia Do Solo*, 27: 415-423.

Caron M, Fortin JA and Richard C. (1986). Effect of phosphorous concentration and *Glomus intraradices* on *Fusarium* crown and root rot of tomatoes. *Phytopathology* 76: 942-946.

Chakravarty P and Mishra RR. (1986). Influence of enditrophic mycorrhizae on the fusarial wilt of *Cassia tora L. J.phytopatho.*115: 130-133.

Chalot M, Blaudez D, Brun A. (2006). Ammonia: a candidate for nitrogen transfer at the mycorrhizal interface. *Trends in Plant Science*, 11: 263-266.

Chalot M and Brun A. (1998). Physiology of organic nitrogen acquisition by ectomycorrhizal fungi and ectomycorrhizas. *FEMS Microbiology Reviews* 22: 21-44.

Chaudhary TM, Hill, Khan AG, Duek C. (1999). Colonization of iron and zinc-contaminated dumped filter-cake waste by microbes, plants and association mycorrhizae. In: Remediation and management of Degraded Land. (eds Wong MH, Wong JWC Baker, AJM). CRC press, Boca, Chap, 27: 275-283.

Chiariello N, Hickman JC, Mooney HA. (1982). Endomycorrhizal role for interspecific transfer of phosphorous in a community of annual plants, *Science* 217: 941-943.

Clark RB and Zeto SK. (2000). Mineral acquisition by arbuscular mycorrhizal plants. *J. Plant Nutron.* 23: 867-902.

Colebatch G, Trevaskis B, Udvardi M. (2002a). Functional genomics: tool of the trade. *New phytol.* 153: 27-36.

Cox G, Moran KJ, Sanders F, Nockolads C, Tinker PB. (1980). Translocation and transfer of nutrients in vesicular-arbuscular nutrients in vesicular arbuscular mycorrhizas III Polyphosphate granules and phosphorous translocation. *New Phytologist*. 84: 649-659.

Curl EA and Trueglove B. (1986). The rhizosphere advanced series agricultural series in agriculture science 15. Berlin. Germany: Springer–Verlag.

Dassi B, Samara A, Dumas-Gaudat E, Gianinazzi S. (1999). Different polypepetide profiles from tomato polypeptide profiles from tomato roots following interaction with arbuscular mycorrhizal (*Glomus mosseae*). or pathogenic (*Phytophthora parasitica*). fungi.*Symbiosis*.26: 65-77.

Davies FT, Jr.Potter JR, Linderman RG. (1993). Drought resistance of mycorrhizal pepper plants independent of leaf p concentration–response in gas exchange and water relations. *Physiologia-Plantarum* 87: 45-53.

Davis RM and Menge JA. (1981). *Phytophthora parasitica* inoculation and intensity of vesicular–arbuscular mycorrhizae in citrus .*New Phytol*. 87: 705-715.

De la Providenica IE, de Souza FA, Fernandez F, Sejalon Delmas N, Declerck F, Sejalon Delmas N, Declerck S. (2005). Arbuscular mycorrhizal fungi reveal distnict patterns of anastomosis formation and hyphal healing mechanism between different pathogenic groups. *New phytol*. 165: 261-271.

De mars BG and Boerner REJ. (1995). Arbuscular mycorrhizal development in three crucifers. *Mycorrhiza*. 5: 405-408.

Declerck S, Risede JM and Rufyikiri G and Delvaux B. (2002). Effect of arbuscular mycorrhizal fungi on severity of root rot of bananas caused by *Cylindrocladium Spathiphylli*. *Plant Pathology* 51: 109-115.

Degans B, Sparling G, Abott LK. (1994). The contribution from hyphae,roots and organic carbon constituients to the aggregation of a sandy loam under long term clover based and grass pastures., *European Journal of Soil Science* 45: 459-490.

Dehne HW and Schonbeck F (1979). Untersuchungen zun Einfluss der Endotrophen Mycorrhiza auf pflanzen krankheiten.II phenolstaff-wechsel und Linifizierung (The influence of endtrophic mycorrhiza on plant diseases.II.phenol metabolism and lignifications. *Phytopathol.Z*.95: 210-216.

Dehne HW. (1982). Interaction between vesicular–arbuscular mycorrhizal fungi and plant pathogens. *Phytopathology*.72: 1115-1119.

Del Val C, Barea JM and Azcon-Aguilar C. (1999). Diversity of arbuscular mycorohizal fungus population in heavy metal contaminated soil. *Applied and Environmental Microbiology* 65: 718-723.

Dewivedi OP and Vyas D. (2002). Effect of potassium on the occurrence of AM fungi. *Basic and Appli. Mycol*. 1: 233-235.

Diedrich C. (1990). Improved growth of *Cajanus cajan* (L). Millsp. In an unsterile tropical soil by three mycorrhizal fungi.*Plant and soil* 123: 261-266.

Douds DD, Pfeffer PE, Shachar-Hill Y. (2000). Carbon partitioning, cost eds. Arbuscular mycorrhizae. In: Douds DD, Kapulnik Y, eds. *Arbuscular mycorrhizas physiology and function*. Dordrecht, The Netherlands: Kluwer Academic Publishers, 197-130.

Douds DD, Gadkar V, Adholeya A. (2000). Production of VAM fungus biofertilizer. In: Mukerji KG, Chamola BP, Singh J, Mycorrhizal Biology. New York Academic Publisher.

Duek TA, Viser P, Ernst WHO, Schat H. (1986). Vesicular-arbuscular-mycorrhizae decrease zinc toxicity to grasses growing in zinc-polluted soil. *Soil Biol. Biochem.* 18: 331-333.

Dumas–Gaudot E, Bestel Corre G, Valot B, Lenogue S, Amiour N, St-Arnaud M, Fontain B, Dieu M, Raes M, Gianiazzi S. (2003b). Use of in vitro grown *Glomus intraradices* to sensor the effect of agricultural amendment. In proceeding of the IVth international congress on mycorrhiza, Montreal.

Dumas Gaudot E, Guillaume P, Tahiri-Alaoui A, Gianinazzi–pearson V, Gianinazzi S. (1994). Changes in polypeptide patterns in tobacco root colonized by two *Glomus* species.*Mycorrhiza* 4: 215-221.

Dumas-Gaudat E, Bestel-Corre G, Gianinazzi S. (2001). Proteomics, a powerful approach towards under standing functional plant root interactions with arbuscular mycorrhizal fungi: In: Pandilai SG (ed). Recent research developments in plant biology. Research Signopost, Trivandrum, India, pp. 95-104.

Dwivedi OP. (2003). Studies in soil microorganisms with special reference to vesicular-arbuscular mycorrhizal (VAM) fungal association with wheat crop of Sagar region. Ph.D. Thesis. Dr. H.S. Gour University, Sagar (M.P.). 176.

Elmer WH. (2002). Influence of formononetin and NaCl on mycorrhizal colonization and *Fusarium* crown and root rot of asparagus. *Plant Disease* 86: 1318-1324.

Facelli E, Facelli JM, Smith SE, Mclaughlin MJ. (1999). Interaotive effects of arbuscular mycorrhizal symbiosis intraspecific competition and resource availability on Trifolium subterranean cv. Mt. Barker. *New Phytol.* 141(3): 535-547.

Farrar SC, Hawes M, Jones D, Lindo S. (2003). How roots control the flux of carbon to the rhizosphere. *Ecology* 84: 827-833.

Fester MK and Strack D. (2003). Amycorrhizae–responsive protein in wheat roots. *Mycorrhiza* 12: 219-222.

Francis R and Read DJ. (1994). The contributions of mycorrhizal fungi to the determination of plant community structure. *Plant and soil* 159 : 11-25.

Francis Rand Read DJ. (1984). Direct transfer of carbon between plants connected by vesicular-arbuscular mycorrhizal mycelium *Nature*; 307: 53-56.

Franken P and Requena N. (2001). Analysis of gene expression in arbuscular mycorrhizas: New approaches and challenges. New *phytol.* 150: 517-523.

Gallaud I (1905). Etudes surles mycorrhizes endotrophes.Revue Generale de Botanique.17: 5-48,66-83,123-135;223-239-313-325,425-433,479-500.

Galli U, Schuepp H, Brunold C. (1994). Heavy metal binding by mycorrhizal fungi. *Physiol. Plantarum* 92: 364-368.

Garcia- Garrido JM, Toro N, Ocampo JA. (1993). Presence of specific polypeptides in onion roots colonized by *Glomus mosseae*. *Mycorrhizae*. 2: 175-177.

Garcia-Garrido JM, Ocampo JA. (2002). Regulation of the plant defence response in arbuscular mycorrhizal symbiosis. *J. Exp. Bot.* 53: 1377-1386.

Gavito ME and Varela L. (1995). Response of criolla maize to single and mixed species inoculation of arbuscular mycorrhizal fungi. *Plant soil.* 176: 101-105.

George E, Marschner H, Jakobsen I. (1995). Role of arbuscular mycorrhizae fungi in uptake of phosphorus and nitrogen from soil. *Crit Rev. Biotechnol* 15: 257-270.

Gianinazzi-Pearson V. (1996). Plant cell to arbuscular mycorrhizal fungi: getting to the roots of the symbiosis. *Plant Cell.* 8: 1871-83.

Giller K. (1998). Toxicity of heavy metals to microorganisms and microbial processes in agricultural soils: reviews: *Soil Biology and Biochemistry* 30: 1389-1414.

Giovannetti, Sbrana C, Avio L, Citernesi AS, Logi C. (1993). Differential hyphal morphogenesis in arbuscular mycorrhizal fungi during pre–infection stages. *New Phytologist* 125: 587-593.

Giovannetti M, Sbrana C, Avio L. (2004). Patterns of below ground plant interconnection established by means of arbuscular mycorrhizal networks. *New Phytologist.* 164: 175-181.

Giovannetti M, Azolini D, Citer nesi AS. (1999). Anastomosis formation and nuclear and protoplasmic exchange in arbuscular mycorrhizal fungi. *Applied Eviron Microbiol.* 69: 616-624.

Giovannetti M, Fortuna P, Citernesi AS, Morini S, Nuti MP. (2001). The ocurrence of anastomosis formation and nuclear exchange in arbuscular mycorrhizal network. *New phytol.*151: 171-124.

Goncalves SC, Goncalves MT, Freitas H, Martin-S, Loucao MA. (1997). Mycorrhizae in a Portuguese serpentine community. In: *The ecology of ultarmafic and metalliferous areas,* (eds. Jaffre T, Reeves RD, Becquer T), Proceedings of the second International Conference on Serpentine Ecology in Noumea, 87-89.

Gonzalez-Chavez C, D'Haen J, Vangronsveld J, Dodd JC. (2001). Copper sorption and accumulation by the extraradical mycelium of different *Glomus* spp. (arbuscular mycorrhizal fungi) isolated from the same polluted soil. *Plant and soil,* 240: 287-297.

Govindarajulu M, Pfeffer P, Jin HR, Abubaker J, Douds DD, Allen JW, Bucking H, Lammers PJ, Shachar-Hill Y. (2005). Nitrogen transfer in the arbuscular mycorrhizal symbiosis. *Nature* 435: 819-823.

Graham JH and Menge JA. (1982). Influence of vesicular-arbuscular mycorrhizae and soil phosphorous on the take all disease of wheat. Phytopathplogy 72: 95-98.

Graham JH, Leonard RT and Menge JA. (1981). Membrance mediated decrease in root exudation responsible for phosphorous inhibition of vesicular-arbuscular mycorrhiza formation. *Plant Physiology.* 68: 548-552.

Graham JH. (1982). Effect of citrus root exudates on germination of chlamydospores of the vesicular-arbuscular mycorrhizal fungus *Glomus epigacum. Mycologia* 74: 831-835.

Graham JH.. (2000). Assessing costs of arbuscular mycorrhizal symbiosis in agroecosystems. In: Podila GK, Douds DD, eds. *Current advances in mycorrhizae research.* St. Paul, MN, USA: American Phytopathological Society Press, pp. 127-140.

Graves JD, Walkins NK, Fitter AH, Robinson D, Scrimgeour C. (1997). Interspecific transfer of carbon between plants linked by a common mycorrhizal network. *Plant Soil* 192: 153-159.

Grime JP, Mannkey JML, Hillersh, Read DJ. (1987). Floristic diversity in a model system using experimental microcosms, *Nature* 328: 420-422.

Gupta V, Satyanarayana T, Sandeep G. (2000). General aspects of mycorrhiza. In: Mukerji KG, Chamola BP, Singh J, Mycorrhizal *Biology*. New York: Kluwer.

Harley JL and Harley EL. (1987). A check list of mycorrhizae in British flora. *New Phytologist* 105: 1-102.

Harrison MJ. (1999). Molecular and cellular aspects of the arbuscular mycorrhizal symbiosis. *Ann. Rev. Plant Physiol. Plant Mol. Biol.* 50: 361-89.

Harrison MJ andVan Burren ML. (1995). A phosphate transporter from the mycorrhizal fungus *Glomus vesiforme*. *Nature* 378: 626-629.

Harrison MJ. (2005). Signaling in the arbuscular mycorrhizal symbiosis. *Annu. Rev. Microbiol.* 59: 19-42.

Harrison MJ. (1998). Development of the arbuscular mycorrhizal symbiosis. *Current opinion in plant Biology* 1: 360-365.

Hetrick BAD, Wilson GWT and Todd TC. (1996). Mycorrhiza response in wheat cultivars, relationship to phosphorous, *Can. J. Bot.* 74: 19-25.

Hetrick BAD, Wilson GWT, Figge DH. (1994). The influence of mycorrhizal symbiosis and fertilizer amendment on establishment of vegetation in heavy metal mine spoil. *Environ. Pollut.* 86: 171-179.

Hilbert JL, Cista G, Martin F. (1991). Ectomycorrhizin synthesis and polypeptide changes during the early stage of *Eucalyptus* mycorrhiza development. *Plant Physiology* 97: 977-984.

Hill. (2007). Quantifying flows through metabolic networks and the propects for fluxomic studies of mycorrhizas, *New phytologist* 175: 235-240.

Hodge A, Campbell CD, Fitter AH. (2000). An arbuscular mycorrhizal fungus accelerates decomposition and acquires nitrogen directly from organic material. *Nature*. 413: 297-299.

Hussey RS and Roncodori RW. (1981). Influence of Aphelenchus avenae on vesicular-arbuscular endomycorrhizal growth response in cotton. *J.Nematol.*13: 48-52.

Ibijbijen J, Urguiaga S, Ismaili M, Alves BJR and Boddey MR. (1996). Effect of arbuscular mycorrhizas an uptake of nitrogen by *Brachiaria arrecta* and Sorghum vulgaris from soils labeled for several years with ^{15}N.*New phytologist* 134.

Jabaji- Hare S. (1998). Lipid and profiles of some vesicular arbuscular mycorrhizal fungi: Contribution to taxonomy. *Mycologia* 80: 622-629.

Jackson I, Rosendahl L. (1990). Carbon flow into soil and external hyphae from roots of mycorrhizal cucumber plants. *New phytol.*115: 77-83.

Jacobsen DJ, Beurkensk, Klomparens KL. (1998). Microscopic and Ultrastructural examination of vegetative incompatibility in partial diploids heterozygous at heterozygous loci in *Neurospora crasa, Fung Genet Biol.*23: 45-46.

Jakobsen I. (1995). Transport of phosphorus and carbon in VA mycorrhizas. In Mycorrhiza: Structure, Function, Molecular Biology and Biotechnology. (eds A Varma, B Hock), Springer-Verlag, Berlin, pp. 297-323.

Jensen A and Jakobsen I. (1980). The occurance of vesicular-arbuscular mycorrhiza in barley and wheat grow in some Danish soils with different fertilizer treatments, *Plant soil.* 55: 403-414.

Joner EL and Levyal C. (1997). Uptake of ^{109}cd by roots and hyphae of a Glomus mosseae/Trifolium subterranean mycorrhiza frm soil amended with high and low concentrations of cadmium. *Phytol.* 135: 353-360.

Jones MD, Durall DM, Tinker PB. (1998). Comparison of arbuscular and ectomycorrhizal *Eucalyptus coccifera*: Growth response, phosphorous uptake efficiency and external hyphal production. *New Phytol* 140: 125-134.

Kahiluoto H, Ketoja E and Vestberg M, Saarela I. (2001). Promotion of AM utilization through reduced P fertilization Z. Field studies. *Plant Soil* 231: 65-79.

Kahiluoto H, Vestberg M, Olesen JE, Eltun R, Gording MS, Jensen ES and Kopke U. (1999). Impact of cropping system of mycorrhizae. In: *Designing and Testing Crop Rotations for Organic Farming.* Proceedings from an International Workshop Danish Centre for Organic Farming (DAECOF). 305-309 DAECOF.

Kellam MK and Schenck NC. (1980). Interaction between a vesiculsr arbuscular mycorrhizal fungus and root knot nematode on soyabean. *Phytopathology* 70: 293-296.

Khaossad T, Garcia-Garrido JM, Steinkelner S, Vierheilig. (2007). Take all disease is systemically reduced in roots of mycorrhizal barley plants. *Soil Biol. Biochem.* 39: 727-734.

Koide RT, Goff MD, Dickie IA. (2000). Component growth efficiencies of mycorrhizal and non-mycorrhizal plant. *New Phyto.* 148: 163-168.

Koide RT, Schreiner RP. (1992). Regulation of the vesicular-arbuscular mycorrhizal symbiosis. *Annu Rev. Plant Physiol Plant Mol Biol* 43: 557-581.

Kothari SK, Marschner H, Romheld V. (1990). Direct and Indirect effects of VAMF and rhizospheric-microorganism on acquisition of mineral nutrients by maize (*Zea mays L.*). in calcareous soil. *New Phyt*ol. 116: 637-645.

Krishna KR and Bagyaraj DJ. (1983). Interaction between Glomus -fasisculatum and Sclerotium-rolfsii in peanut. *Can.J.Bot.*61: 2349-2351.

Kruger NJ, Ratcliffe RG, Roscher A. (2003). Quantitative approaches for analyzing fluxes through plant metabolic networks using NMR and stable isotope labeling. *Phytochemistry Reviews* 2: 17-30.

Kumar P, Duschenkov V, Motto H and Raskin I. (1995). Phytoextraction: the use of plants to remove heavy metals from soils. *Environmental Science and Technology* 29: 1232-1238.

Lambert DH, Baker DJ, Code H (1979). The role of mycorrhize in the interactions of phosphorous with Zn, Cu and Other elements. *Soil Sci. Am. J.* 43: 976-980.

Lammers PJ, Jun J, Abubaker J, Arreola R, Gopalan A, Bago B, Hernandez-Sebastia C, Allen JW, Douds DD, Pfeffer PE. (2001). The glyoxylate cycle in an arbuscular mycorrhizal fungus: gene expression and carbon flow. *Plant Physiol* 127: 1287-1298.

Lanfranco L, Gabella S, Bonfante P. (2000). EST as a useful tool for studying gene expression in arbuscular mycorrhizal fungi.In: Procedings the third International Congress on Symbiosis. Marburg.

Lanfranco L, Novero M, Bonfante P. (2005). The mycorrhizal fungus *Gigaspora margarita* possesses a CuZn superoxide dismutase that is up-regulated during symbiosis with legume hosts. *Plant Physiol.* 137: 1319-1330.

Lerat S, Gauci R, Catford JG, Vierheilig H, Pichey Y, Lapointe L. (2002). C-14 transfer between the spring epehemeral Erythronium americanum and sugar maple saplings via arbuscular mycorrhizal fungi in natural strands. *Oceologia.* 132: 181-187.

Lerat S, Gauci R, Catford JG, Vierheilig H, Pichey, Lapointe L. (2002). C-14 transfer between the spring ephemeral Erythronium americanum and sugar mapl Saplings via arbuscular mycorrhizal fungi in natural sands. *Oecologia;* 132: 181-187.

Lewis JD and Koide RT. (1990). Phosphorous supply mycorrhizal infection and plant offspring vigour. *Functional Ecology* 4: 695-702.

Leyval C, Turnau K and Haselwandter K. (1997). Effect of heavy metal pollution on mycorrhizal colonization and function: physiological, ecological and applied aspects, *Mycorrhizae* 7: 139-153.

Leyval C, Turnau K and Haselwandter K. (2002). Potential of arbuscular mycorrhizal fungi for bioremediation. In: *Mycorrhiza technology in agriculture from genes to bioproducts* (eds. Gianinazzi S, Schuepp H, Barea JM, Haselwandtark). Basal, Switzerland: Birkhauser Verlag, pp. 175-186.

Li X-L, George E, Marschner H. (1991). Extension of the phosphorous, depletion zone in VA-mycorrhizal white clover in calcareous soil. *Plant and Soil* 136: 41-48.

Linderman RG. (1994). Role of VAM fungi in biocontrol. In: *Mycorrhizae and plant health.* (Eds. Pfleger FL, Linderman RG.). St Paul: APS Press, pp. 1-25.

Liu J, Blaylock LA, Van den, Bosch KA, Endre G, Cho J, Harrison MJ. (2003). Transcript profiling coupled with spatial expression analyses reveals genes involved in district developmental stages of an arbuscular mycorrhizal symbiosis. *Plant cell.* 15: 21016-21023.

Macaskie LE, Dean ACR. (1990). Metal-sequestering biochemicals. In: *Biosorption of Heavy Metals* (Ed., Volesky, B.), CRC Press, Boca Raton, Florida, pp. 200-248.

Mada RJ, Bagyaraj DJ. (1993). Root exudation from *Leucaena leucocephala* in relation to mycorrhizal colonization. World *Journal of Microbiology and Biotechnology.* 9: 342-344.

Maldnado-Mendoja IE. (2001). A phosphate transporter gene from the extraradical mycelium of an arbuscular–mycorrhizal fungus Glomus intraradices is regulated in response to phosphate in the environment. Mol. *Plant* Microbe *Interact.* 14: 1140-1148.

Marschner H. (1991). Mechanism of adaptation of plants toacid soils. *Plant and soil* 134: 1-20.

Marulanda A, Azcon R, Ruiz-Loza JM. (2003). Contribution of six arbuscular mycorrhizal fungal isolates to water uptake by *Lactuca sativa* plants under drought stress. *Physiologia- Plantarum*119: 1-8.

Mastubar AY, Ohba N and Fukui H. (2001). Effect of arbuscular mycorrhizal fungus infection on the incidence of *Fusarium* root rot in asparagus seedlings. *Journal of Japanese Society of Horticultural Sciences* 70: 202-206.

Mastubara Y, Kayukawa Y, Yano M, Fukui H. (2000). Tolerance of asparagus seedlings infected with arbuscular mycorrhizal fungus to violet root rot caused by *Helicobasidium mompa. J. Japn. Hortic. Sci.* 69: 552-556.

Melo IS, Costa CP and Silviera APD. (1985). Effect of vesicular arbuscular mycorrhizae on aubergine wilt caused by verticillium albo-atrum Reinke and Berth. *Summa Phytopathologia*. 11: 173-179.

Miller RM and Jastraw JD. (2004). Mycorrhizal fungi influence soil structure. In: kapulink Y, Douds DD, Arbuscular mycorrhizas-*Physiology and function*. Dordrecht: Kluwer Academic Publishers.3-19.

Miller RM and Jastrow JD. (1992). The role of mycorrhizal fungi in soil conservation. In: GJ Bethlenfalvay, RG Linderman (eds.), Mycorrhizae in sustainable agriculture. ASAspec. Publ. No. 54 American society of agronomy, Madison WI.pp. 29-44.

Miller RM and Jastrouw JD. (2000). Mycorrhizal fungi influence soil structure. In *Arbuscular Mycorrhiza: Physiology and Function*, 4-8, Kluwer Academic Publications.

Millner PD and Kitt DG. (1992). The Beltsville methord for soilless production of vesicular arbuscular-mycorrhizal fungi. *Mycorrhiza* 2: 9-15.

Mishra M, Dubey A, Singh P and Vyas D. (2006). VAM association in *Catharanthus roseu.J.Basic.Appl.Mycol*. 5(I and II): 57-59.

Mohammad MJ, Malkwai HI, Shibli. (2003). Effects of mycorrhizal fungi and phosphorous fertilization on growth and nutrient uptake of barley grown on soils with different levels of salts. *J. Plant Nuter*. 26: 125-137.

Monzon A and Azcon R. (1996). Relevance of mycorrhizal fungal origin and host plant genotype to inducing growth and nutrient uptake in *Medicago Species. Agric. Ecosyst. Envion*. 60: 9-15.

Mosse B (1973). Advances in the study of vesicular arbuscular mycorrhizal fungi; *Annu. Rev. Phytopathol*. 11: 171-196.

Munkvold L, Kjoller R, Vestberg M, Rosendahl S, Jakobsen I. (2004). High functional diversity with in species of arbuscular-mycorrhizal fungi, *New phyto*. 164: 357-364.

Nichols K. (2003). Characterization of Glomalin-A Glycoprotein Produced by Arbuscular- mycorrhizal fungi. PhD Dissertation, University of Maryland, College Park, Maryland.

Nichols K, Wright S, Schmidt W, Cavigelli M, Dzantor E. (2002). Carbron contribution and Characteristics opf humid acid, fulvic acid, particulate organic matter, and glomalin in ecosystems. In: *Proceedings of Humic Substances: Nature's most versatile materials*, International Humic Substances Society, Boston Massachusetts, pp. 365-367.

Nicoloson TH (1975). Evolution of vesicular-arbuscular mycorrhizas In: SandersE, MosseB, Tinker PB, *Endomycorrhizas*. landon: Academic press. p. 25-34.

Nurlaeny N, Marschner H, George E. (1996). Effects of liming and mycorrhizal colonization on soil phosphate depletion and phosphate uptake by maize (*Zea mays* L.). and soyabean (*Glycine max* L.) grown in two tropical soils. *Plant and Soil* 181: 275-285.

Oades JM and Waters AG. (1991). Aggregate hierarchy in soils. *Aust. J. Soil. Res.*, 29: 815-828.

Ocampo JA and Azcon R. (1985). Relationship between the concentration of sugars in the roots and VA mycorrhizal infection. *Plant and Soil* 86: 95-100.

Ojala JC and Linderman RG. (2001). Preinoculation of Lettuce and onio with VA mycorrhizal fungi reduces deleterious effect of soil salinity. *Plant and Soil*.223: 269-281.

Olivera AAR and Zambolim L. (1987). Interacao entro o fungo endomicorrizicio *Glomus facicculatum* e o nematoide de galhas Meloidogyne javanica em feijoeiro com raiz partida. *Fitopathol. Bras.*12: 222-225.

Orlowska E, Zubek SZ, Jurkiewic ZA, Szarek- Lukaszewska G. (2002). Influence of restoration on arbuscular mycorrhiza of *Biscutella laevigata L.* (Brassicaceae). and *plantago lanceolata L.* (Plantaginaceae) from calamine spoil mounds. *Mycorrhiza* 12: 153-160.

Owusu-Bennoah E, Wild A (1979). Autoradiography of the depletion zone of phosphate around onion roots in the presence of vesicular-arbuscular mycorrhiza. *New Phytologist* 82: 133-140.

Pawloska TEJ, Blaszkowski and Riihling A. (1996). The mycorrhizal status of plants colonizing a calamine spoil mound in southern Poland. *Mycorrhiza* 6: 499-505.

Pfeffer PE, Douds DD, Becard G, Shachar-Hill Y. (1999). Carbon uptake and the metabolism and transport of lipids in and arbuscular mycorrhiza. *Plant Physiol* 120: 587-598.

Pfeiffer CM and Bloss HE. (1988). Growth and nutrition of guayule (*Parthenium argenatum*) in a saline soil as influenced by esicular-arbuscular mycorrhiza and phosphorous fertilizer. *New phytologist* 108: 315-321.

Rancadori RW and Hussey RS (1977). Interaction of the endomycorrhizal fungus *Gigaspora-margarita* and root knot nem atode on cotton. *Phytopathology* 67: 1507-1511.

Raticliffe RG and Shachar Hill. (2006). Measuring multiple fluxes through plant metabolic networks. *Plant journal* 45: 495-511.

Ratnayake M, Leonard RT, Menge JA (1978). Root exudation in relation to supply of phosphorus and its possible relevance to mycorrhizal formulation. *New Phytologist* 81: 543-552.

Redecker D, Kodner R, and Graham LE. (2000). Glomalean fungi from Ordovician. *Science* 289: 1920-1921.

Regvar M, Vogel K, Irgel N, Wraber T, Hildebrandt U, Wilde P, Bothe H. (2003). Colonization of pennycresses (Th laspi spp.) of the Brassicaceae by arbuscular mycorrhizal fungi. *Journal of Plant Physiology* 160: 615-626.

Remy W, Taylor TN, Hass H, Kerp H. (1994). Four hundred–million year–old vesicular arbuscular mycorrhizae. *Proceedings of the National Academy of Sciences*, USA 91: 11841-11843.

Repett O, Bestel-Corre G, Dumas Gaudot E, Berta G, Gianinazzi-PearsonV, Gianinazzi S. (2003). Targeted proteomics to identify cadmium induced protein modification in *Glomus–mosseae* pea roots.*New phytol*. 157: 555-567.

Requena N, Mann P, Hampp R, Franken P. (2002). Early development regulated genes in the arbuscular mycorrhizal fungus *Glomus mosseae*: Identification of GmGINI, aC-terminus of metazoan hedgehog proteins. *Plant soil* 244: 129-139.

Rhodes H and Gerdemann JW (1975). Phosphate uptake zones of mycorrhizal and non-mycorrhizal onions. New Phytologist 75: 555-561.

Rilling MC, Field CB, Allen MF. (1999). Soil biota responses to long term atmospheric CO_2 enrichment in two Califorina annual grasslands. *Oceologia* (Berlin). 119: 572-577.

Rilling MC, Wright SF, Nichols KA, Schmidt WF, Torns MS. (2001). Large contribution of arbuscular mycorrhizal fungi to soil carbon pools in tropical forest soils. *Plant soil* 233: 167-177.

Rilling, MC, Ramsey PW, Morriis S, Paul EA. (2003). Glomalin, an arbuscular-mycorrhizal fungi soil protein, respond to land use change. *Plant and Soil*, 253: 293-299.

Rozema J, Arp W, Vandiggelen J,Vanesbroek M,Broekman R, Punte H. (1986). Occurrence and ecological significance of vesicular arbuscular mycorrhizae in the salt Marsh environment. *Acta Botanica Neerlandica* 35: 457-467.

Saleh H and Sikora RA. (1984). Relationship between *lomus facicculatum* root colonization of cotton and its effect on *Meloidogyne incognita. Nematologica* 30: 230-237.

Salt DE, Smith RD and Raskin I. (1998). Phytoremediation. Annual Review of Plant *Physiology and Plant Molecular Biology* 49: 643-668.

Samara A, Dumas- Gaudot E, Gianinazzi S. (1997). Detection of symbiosis-related polypeptides during the early stages of the establishment of arbuscular mycorrhiza between *Glomus-mosseae* and *Pisum-sativum* roots. New phytol.135: 711-722.

Samara A, Dumas-Gaudot E, Gianinazzi-Pearson V, Gianinazzi S. (1996). Soluble proteins and polypeptide profiles of spores of arbuscular mycorrhizal fungi. Interspecific variability and effect of host (myc+). and non-host (myc-). *Pisum sativum* root exudates. *Agronomie* 16: 709-719.

Sanders FE and Sheikh NA. (1983). The development of vesicular-arbuscular mycorrhizal in plant root systems. *Plant and Soil* 71: 223-246.

Sanders IR and Fitter AH. (1992). The ecology and functioning of vesicular arbuscular mycorrhizas in coexisting grassland species I. Seasonal patterns of mycorrhizal occurrence and morphology. *New Phytologist* 120: 517-524.

Sauer U. (2004). High-throughput phenomics: experimental methods for mapping fluxomes. *Current Opinion in Biotechnology* 15: 58-63.

Sauer U, Lasko DR, Flaux J, Hochuli M, Glaser R, Szyperski T, Wuthrich K, Bailey JE. (1999). Metabolic flux ratio analysis of genetic and environmental modulations of *Escherichia coli* central carbon metabolism. *Journal of Bacteriology* 181: 6679-6688.

Schenck NC. (1981). Can mycorrhiza control root disease? *Plant Dis. Rep.* 65: 230-234.

Schenck NC, Ridings WH and Cornell JA (1977). Interaction of endomycorrhizal fungi and *Phytophthora parasitica* of two citrus root stocks, in *Proceedings of the third North American Conference on Mycorrhizae* (Oregon: Corvallis). 9.

Schoenbeck F (1979). Endmycorrhizas in relation to plant diseases.In soil-borne plant pathogens (B. Schippers and W. Gam, eds).Academic press, New York pp. 271-280.

Schoenbeck F and Dehne HW. (1981). Mycorrhiza and Plant Health, *Gesunde Pflanzen.* 33: 186-190.

Schonbeck F. (1980). Endomycorrhiza: Ecology, function and phytopathological aspects: *Forum Microbial* 3: 90-96.

Schwab SM, Leonard RT, Menge JA. (1984). Quantitative and qualitative comparison of root exudates of mycorrhizal and nonmycorrhizal plant species. C*anadian Journal of Botany* 62: 1227-1231.

Schwab SM, Menge JA, Leonard RT. (1983). Quantitative and qualitative effects on phosphorus on extracts and exudates of sudangrass roots in relation to vesicular-arbuscular mycorrhiza formation. *Plant Physiology* 73: 761-765.

Schwender J, Goffman F, Ohlrogge JB, Shachar-Hill Y. (2004a). Rubisco without the Calvin cycle improves the carbon efficiency of developing green seeds. *Nature* 432: 779-782.

Shachar-Hill Y, Pfeffer PE, Douds DD, Osman SF, Doner LW, Ratcliffe RG. (1995). Partitioning of intermediary carbon metabolism in vesicular-arbuscular mycorrhizal leck. *Plant Physiology* 108: 7-15.

Sidhu OP and Behl HM. (1997). Response of three *Glomus* species on the growth of *Prosopis Juliflora* Qwartz at high pH levels. *Symbiosis* 23: 23-24.

Sikora RA and Schonbeck F (1975). Effect of vesicular–arbuscular mycorrhiza (*Endogone mosseae*) on the population dynamics of the root knot nematode (Meloidogyne–incognita and Meloidogyne hapla). Proceedings of VIII International congress protection. 5: 158-166.

Simoneau P, Louisy-Lois N, Plenchettec, Strullu DG. (1994). Accumulation of new polypeptides in Ri-tdna-transformed roots of tomato (*Lycopersicon-esculentum*) during the development of vesicular-arbuscular mycorrhizae. Appl. *Environ Microbiol* 60: 1810-1813.

Simoneau P, Viemont JD, Moreau JC, Strulu DJ. (1993). Symbiosis is related polypeptides associated with the early stages of ectomycorrhiza organogenesis in birch (*Betula pendula* Roth). *New Phytol* 124: 495-504.

Sin H. (2004). Phosphate transport in Arabidopsis: pht1: and pht1;4 play amajor role in phosphate acquisition from both low and high phosphate environments. *Plant J*. 39: 629-642.

Singh P and Vyas D. (2008). To study microbial interaction of below ground organism with special reference to *Fusarium* wilt of Chickpea. Ph.D. Thesis. Dr. H.S.G.University, Sagar.

Smith FA and Smith SE. (1997). Structural diversity in (vesicular)-arbuscular mycorrhizal symbiosis. *New Phytologist*. 151: 469-475.

Smith GS, Hussey RS and Roncadori RW. (1986). Penetration and postinfection development of *Meloidogyne- incognita* on cotton as affectd by *Glomus intraradices* and phosphorous.*J.Nematology*. 18: 429-435.

Smith SE and Read DJ. (1997). Mycorrhizal symbiosis. Academic Press, London.

Solaimain MD, Satio M. (1997). Use of sugars by intraradical hyphae of arbuscular mycorrhizal fungi revealed by radiorespirometry. *New phytol*. 136: 533-538.

Soni P and Vyas D. (2008). Studies on some medicinal herbs with special reference to nutrient uptake by VAM fungi. Ph.D. Thesis. Dr. H.S.G. University, Sagar.

Sorensen N, Larsen J, Jakobsen I. (2005). Mycorrhiza formation and nutrient concentration in looks (*Allium porrum*) in relation to previous crop and cover crop management on high P soils. *Plant soil* 273: 101-114.

Srivastava AK, Singh S, Marathe RA. (2002). Organic citrus, soil fertility and plant nutrition. *Sustai.agric*19: 5-29.

Stanley MR, Koide RT, Shumway DL. (1993). Mycorrhizal symbiosis increases growth, reproduction and recruitment of Abutilon theophrasti Medicin the field. *Oecologia* 94: 30-35.

St-Arnaud M, Hamel C, Vimard B,Caron M, Fortin A. (1996). Enhanced hyphal growth and spore production of the arbuscular mycorrhizal fungus Glomus intraradices in an vitro system in the absence of host roots. *Mycol. Res.* 100: 328-332.

Stommel M, Mann P, Franken P. (2001). Construction and analysis of an EST library using RNA from dormant spores of the arbuscular mycorrhizal fungus *Gigaspora rosea. Mycorrhiza* 10: 281-285.

Subramanian KS, Charest C, Dwyer LM, Hamilton RI. (1997). Effects of arbuscular mycorrhizae on leaf water potential, sugar content and phosphorous content during drought and recovery of maize. *Canadian journal of Botany*.75: 1582-1591.

Suresh CK and Bagyaraj DJ. (1984). Interaction between a vesicular-arbuscular and a root-knot nematode and its effecton growth and chemical composition of tomato. *Nematol.* Medit. 12: 31-39.

Swaki H and Satio M. (2001). Expressed genes in the extraradical hyphae of an arbuscular mycorrhizal fungus, *Glomus intraradices* in the symbiotic phase. FEMS. *Microbiol Lett.* 195: 109-113.

Tamasloukht M, Sejalon-Delmas N, Kluever A, Jauneau A, Roux C, Becard G, Franken P. (2003). Root factors induce mitochondrial related gene expression and fungal respiration during the devlopment switch from asymbiosis to presymbiosis in the arbuscular mycorrhizal fungus *Gigaspora-rosea. Plant physiology*, 131: 1468-1478.

Tarkka MT, Nyman TA, Kallkinen N, Raudaskoski M. (2000). Scots pine expresses short-root specific peroxidases during development. *Eur.J.Biochem.* 267: 1-8

Thingstrup I, Rubaek G, Sibbesen E, Jakobsen I. (1998). Flax (*Linum uritatiusim* L.). depends on arbuscular mycorrhizal fungi for growth and P uptake at intermediate but not high soil P levels in the field. *Plant soil.* 20: 37-46.

Thomas RS, Dakessian S, Ames RN, Brown MS, Bethlenfalvay GJ. (1986). Aggregation of a silty clay loam soil by mycorrhizal onion roots. Society of America, Journal 50: 1494-1499.

Thompson JP. (1987). Decline of vesicular arbuscular mycorrhizae in long fallow disorder of field crops and its expression in phosphorus deficiency of sunflower, *Aust. J. Agric. Res.* 38: 847-86.

Thompson JP. (1994). Inoculation with vesicular-arbuscular mycorrhizal fungi from cropped soil overcomes long-fallow disorder of linseed (*Linum usitatissimum L.*). by improving P and Zn uptake, *Soil Biol. Biochem.* 26: 1133-1143.

Thompson JP. (1991). Improving the mycorrhizal condition on the soil through cultural practices and effects on growth and P uptake in plants. In: *Phosphorous Nutrition of Grain Legumes in the Semi Arid Tropics*, (eds C. Johansen, Lee, K.K and Sahrawat, K.). International crops Research institute for semi arid Tropics, Andhra Patancheru, India pp. 117-137.

Tisdall JM and Behl HM. (1997). Organic matter and water stable aggregates in soils. *Journal of soil science.* 33: 141-163.

Tisdall JM and Oades JM (1979). Stabilization of soil aggregates by the root system rye grass. *Australian journal of soil Research* 17: 429-441.

Turman W, Bennett MH, Kubigsetelting I, Turnbull C, Grant M. (2007). Arabidopsis systemic immunity uses conserved defense signaling pathways and is mediated by Jasmonates. *Proc. National Acad. Sci. USA.* 104: 1075-1080.

Turnau K, Jurkiewicz A, Lingua G, Barea JM, Gianinazzi-Pearson V(2005). Role of arbuscular mycorrhiza and associated microorganisms in phytoremediation of heavy metal polluted sites. *Trace element in the environment biochemistry, biotechnology and bioremediation*. CRC Press/Lawis Publishers (in press).

Vallorani L, Bernardini F, Sacconic C, Pierleoni R, Pieretti B, Piccoli G, Buffalini M, Stocchi V. (2000). Identification of Tuber *borchii* vittad. Mycelium proteins separated by two dimensional polyacrylamide gel electrophoresis using amino acid analysis and sequence tagging. *Electrophoresis* 21: 3710-3716.

Van der Heijden. (2002). Arbuscular mycorrhizal fungi as determinant of plant diversity, in search for underlying mechanisms and general principles. In: *Mycorrhizal Ecology*. (eds. MGA Van der Heijdenand IR Sanders), *Ecological studies*. 157. Springer Verlag, Berlin, Germany, 243-265.

Van der Heijden MGA, Moutoglis P, Streitwolf, Klironomos JN, Ursic M, Engel R, Boller T, Wiemken A. (1998). Mycorrhizal fungal diversity determines plant biodiversity, ecosystem variability and productivity. *Nature*. 396: 69-72.

Van der Heijden, MGA, Wiemken A, Sanders IR. (2003). Different arbuscular mycorrhizal fungi alter coexistence and resource distribution between co-occurring structure. *Ecology*.79: 2082-2091.

Vyas D, Mishra M, Singh P, Soni P. (2006). Studies on mycorrhizal association in wheat.*Indian phytopath.* 59(2): 174-179.

Vyas D and Dwiedi OP. (2002). Effect of potassium on the occurrence of VAM fungi.*J. Basic.Appl.Mycol*1(2): 233-235.

Vyas D and Soni P. (2007). Arbuscular mycorrhizal fungi associated with important medicinal plants of Sagar. *Indian phytopathology* 60(1): 52-57.

Vyas D, Dubey A, Singh P. (2006). VA Mycorrhizal Fungi in tropical monsoonic grassland. *J.Basic. Mycol.* 5(I and II): 78-81.

Vyas D, Dubey A, Soni A, Mishra M and Singh P. (2007). Arbuscular mycorrhizal fungi in early land plants. *Mycorrhiza News* 19(2).

Vyas D, Soni A, Singh P. (2007). Differential effects of pesticides on occurrence of Vam fungi associated with some leguminous plants. *J.Basic Appl. Mycol.* 6(I and II): 143-150.

Watkins NK, Fitter AH, Graves JD, Robinson D. (1996). Carbon transfer between C_3 and C_4 plants linked by a common mycorrhizal network, quantified using stable carbon isotopes. *Soil Biol Biochem*. 28: 471-477.

Wellings NP, Wearing AH, Thompson JP. (1991). Vesicular-arbuscılr mycorrhizal (VAM) improve phosphorous and zinc nutrition and growth of pigeonpea in vertisol. *Austt J. Agric Res.* 42: 835-845.

Whipps JM. (2004). Prospects and limitation for mycorrhiza in biocontrol of root pathogen. *Can J. Bot.* 82: 1198-1227.

Wilcox HE. (1991). Mycorrhizae. In: Waisel Y, Eshel A, Kafkafi U. *The Plant Root*, The Hidden Half. New York: Marcel Dekker. 731-765.

Wright SF and Upadhayaya A. (1996). Extraction of an abundant and unusual protection from soil and comparison with hyphal protection of arbuscular mycorrhizal fungi. *Soil Sci.* 161: 575-586

Wright SF, Upadhyaya A. (1998). A survey of soil for aggregate stability and glomlin, a glycoprotein produced by hyphae of arbuscular-mycorrhizal fungi. *Plant and Soil* 1: 97-107.

Yao MK, Desilets, Charales MT, Boulanger R and Tweddell RJ. (2003). Effect of mycorrhization on the accumulation of rishitin and *solavetivone* in potato plantlets challenged with *Rhizoctonia solani. Mycorrhiza* 13: 333-336.

Zambolim L and Schenck NC. (1983). Reduction of the effects of pathogenics root-infecting fungi on soyabean by the mycorrhizal fungus. *Glomus mosseae. Phytopathology* 73: 1402-1405.

Microbial Biotechnology and Ecology (2011) *Pages* **256–267**
Editors: **Deepak Vyas, G.S. Paliwal, P.K.Khare and R.K Gupta**
Published by: **DAYA PUBLISHING HOUSE, NEW DELHI**

Chapter 14

Cumulative Effect of VAM Fungi

☆ ***O.P. Dwivedi, Meenakshi Mishra, Pradeep K. Singh, Pramod Kumar Richhariya, Prashant Soni and Deepak Vyas***

Lab of Microbial Technology and Plant Pathology, Department of Botany, Dr. H.S. Gour University, Sagar – 470 003, M.P.

ABSTRACT

The studies on effect of chemical fertilizer, VAM and other biofertilizer (*viz.* Farm Yard Manure (FYM), Phosphate Solubilizing Bacteria (PSB), *Pseudomonas* and *Azotobacter*, etc.), individually and in combination on the growth responses in wheat Cv. C-306 were carried out. For the present study, two experiments were conducted; (1) field experiments with VAM and chemical fertilizer; (2) field application of VAM and other biofertilizers. Results revealed that chemical fertilizer, VAM and other biofertilizers inoculation greatly influence the growth parameter i.e. germination, heading, maturity, plant height and yield as compared to controlled wheat (Cv. C-306). As far as the growth parameter is concerned in both experiments, VAM inoculation was found to be more effective in comparison to other inoculants and chemical fertilizers. Thus it may be concluded that VAM has greater impact on the growth and yield of wheat Cv. C-306 in the soils, which are already saturated with chemical fertilizer. So, there is no need to add any more chemical fertilizer in these soils. Use of VAM and phosphobacterin should be increased, because these organisms are not only responsible for the soil health but also are responsible for the good growth and better grain yield of wheat crop. Out of all the selected biofertilizers VAM was found best for good growth and higher grain yield of wheat.

Introduction

Phosphorus plays a key role in the balanced nutrition of plants; however, the native soil phosphorus is mostly unavailable because of its low solubility. It's deficiency in soil is met by the addition of phosphatic fertilizers but the efficiency of utilization of the added phosphorus by plants is very low. Microorganisms play an important role in mineralization and solubilization of phosphorus in different environments.

In recent past, the use of phosphatic fertilizers has increased to a very great extent. However, due to their heavy cost and pollution problems associated with them, their use especially in developing countries is loosing its relevance. Under the circumstances, availability of a system which can improve the fertilizer efficiency will be a great asset to the agriculture in these countries. According to Mosse (1973) 75 per cent of the phosphorus applied to the crops is not utilized by them but gets converted in to forms unavailable to plants. It has been estimated that in soils of high pH, a major portion of the fertilizers applied becomes non-usable via chemical reactions. VAM fungi have been found to be very effective under such conditions, because of their ability to make use of extremely small quantities of fertilizer.

That is the reason why VAM fungi are being regarded as biofertilizers and their use in agriculture is being encouraged. These fungi have been reported from almost all the important agricultural crops of the tropical countries. Mycorrhizal symbiosis may play an important role in the tropical agriculture because in the tropics, the soils are phosphorus deficient as well as phosphorus fixing (Dobin, 1980).

During last twenty years, much attention has been paid to VAM fungi as a tool for improving the growth of agricultural crops and horticultural plants (Tinker, 1978; Gianinazzi *et al.*, 1989, 1990a, b). The symbiotic system of these fungi has also been exploited to save the costly phosphatic fertilizers (Abbott and Robson, 1982 a, b). Their importance in natural ecosystem (Koske, 1981) and in revegitation of the disturbed lands has also been recognized (Reeves *et al.*, 1979). There is growing evidence that VAM can increase plant growth, especially in infertile soils (Bowen, 1978; Azcon-Aguilar *et al.*, 1982; Santhi and Kothandaraman, 1995) and that such growth increases are the result of an enhanced ability of the infected roots to absorb more nutrients. The uptake of phosphorus from rock phosphate and phosphatic fertilizers has been increased in plants by the inoculation of soils with mycorrhizal fungi, if the number of mycorrhizae in the soil is initially very low (Kucey, 1987).

Researches in the last few decades have established that VAM and phosphate solubilising bacteria (PSB) are the two groups of soil microorganisms associated with phosphorus (P) nutrition of plants. VAM fungi or obligate symbiotic association with plant roots and increase P availability by mobilizing the P with the help of their extramatrical hyphae, particularly in soil with less available P (Mosse, 1973). On the other hand, PSB live freely in soil and solubilise insoluble form of P with the help of different organic acids, secreted by them and thus increase the quantity of available P in soil for absorption by plant roots (Banik and Dey, 1962). Growth of wheat has been increased by inoculating VAM in sterilised soils (Thompson, 1990). Similarly, inoculation with PSB increased growth of different crops, particularly when rock phosphate and PSB were applied together (Gaur, 1987). However, the magnitude of plant growth may vary depending on the type of VAM, PSB strain, crop, amount of P present in soil and presence of coinoculant. Improved effects of *Rhizobium* as a nitrogen fixing agent have been achieved when it was used in certain cases along with *Azotobacter* (Rawat and Sanoria, 1976, 1977; Tosh and Sanoria, 1978). The role of *Azotobacter* in stimulating the crop growth appears to be a controversial issue. *Azotobacter* spp. produces auxins or hormones which accelerate the plant development and are also antagonistic to soil borne pathogens. Since the favorable response has been obtained only under the condition of high fertility (Mehrotra and Lehri, 1971). Allison (1947) referred to the positive response observed by several Russian and other workers in the crop yield due to *Azotobacter* inoculation. The subject of bacterial fertilizers should not be neglected and their value should not be dismissed as negligible. According to Alexander (1961), it is conceivable that nitrogen fixation takes place in the root zone, a region of intense microbiological activity and an area in which carbohydrate from root excretions and decomposition are abundant.

Strain variation, soil condition such as moisture, organic matter, phosphate content, pH and soil type also influence the result of bacterial fertilizers (Sundara Rao *et al.*, 1963). The combined inoculation of PSB and VAM has given encouraging results in many crop plants (Raj *et al.*, 1981).

Wheat is vital to the health of people and animals in a predominantly vegetarian population. Therefore the experiment were carried out to ascertain the effects of inoculated bioagents (*viz.* VAM, PSB, *Pseudomonas, Azotobacter*), farm yard manure (FYM) and chemical fertilizer (N, P, K) on growth and yield of wheat cultivar C-306.

Materials and Methods

The efficacy of selected combination of bioagents including VAM fungi and chemical fertilizer in improving the growth and yield of wheat (Cultivar C-306) was evaluated under field conditions. The field experiments were carried out at departmental Botanical Garden, Sagar University, Sagar on $1m^2$ micro-plots laid out in a randomized block design during crop seasons.

In the present study two experiments were conducted; (1) field experiment with VAM and chemical fertilizer, (2) field application of Bioagents including VAM fungi.

Mineral Manuring

For the chemical treatment, doses of nitrogen was applied in the form of urea (NH_2CONH_2), phosphorus in the form of rock phosphate (P_2O_5) and potash applied in the form of Potassium oxide (K_2O) as chemical fertilizer in test micro-plots. Table 14.1 gives a summary of the amount of the mineral fertilization.

Table 14.1: Amount of Chemical Fertilizers Used in Test Microplot for Wheat Cultivar C-306

Fertilizer	*Amount (Kgha^{-1})*
N (NH_2CONH_2)	60
P (P_2O_5)	60
K (K_2O)	100

Inoculation Procedure of Bioagents for Field Experiment

For the experiment, inoculation procedure of bioagents is given below:

VAM Fungal Inoculation

The VAM inoculum containing *Glomus mosseae* (20 spore/gm soil), which was consisted of infected roots and soil from pot culture on wheat, was uniformly spread over the soil @ 500 gm/micro-plot.

FYM Treatment

Sufficient steam sterilized form yard manure (FYM) (500 gm/micro-plot) was applied uniformly to all the micro-plots before mycorrhizal inoculation.

PSB Inoculation

The carrier based inoculant culture containing *Bacillus subtilis* was used as a source of PSB.

Pseudomonas Inoculation

The charcoal based inoculum of fluorescent *Pseudomonas* (GRP_3) was used as a source of *Pseudomonas*.

Azotobacter Inoculation

The peat based effective mutant of *Azotobacter chroococcum* was used as a source of *Azotobacter*. For all the micro-plots 15gm. of wheat (Cv. C-306) seeds were used for the sowing. In the case of bacterial treatment, seeds were treated with 2.5gm inoculant of all three bacterial cultures (*viz.* PSB,

Pseudomonas, Azotobacter) by preparing a slurry of the culture. Seeds of wheat were uniformly sprayed with a suspension of bacterial culture.

Treatments were done just before sowing, and sowing was done in row. Colonization of bioagents were studied in non-sterile soil. Along with each treatment series, control was maintained. All these bioagtents except VAM fungi were obtained from J.N.K.V. Field Station Ratouna, Sagar for present study. For each treatment there were three replications. The micro-plots were irrigated with equal amount of water as and when required. Observations on germination, heading, maturity, plant height, yield and physico-chemical properties of rhizosphere soil were recorded.

Physico-chemical Analysis of Soil

The soils were analysed for their nitrogen (A.O.A.C., 1965), potassium (Jackson, 1973) and phosphorus by the method of Jackson (1967).

Statistical Analysis

The data were statistically analysed and the minimum difference required for significance (C.D.) at 5 per cent level of probability was calculated and recorded (Gupta and Kapoor, 1997).

Results

Physico-chemical Properties of Soil

Nitrogen (N)

In experiment 1, the available soil N was maximum in chemical fertilizer treated micro-plot (536 kgha^{-1}) followed by control micro-plot (426.75 kgha^{-1}) and minimum (Table 14.2) in VAM inoculated micro-plot (380 kgha^{-1}) whereas, in experiment 2, the maximum N was recorded in FYM + PSB + *Pseudomonas* treated micro-plot (610.50 kgha^{-1}) followed by FYM + PSB and FYM + *Azotobacter* + PSB treated micro-plot (594 kgha^{-1}) then FYM and FYM + *Pseudomonos* treated micro-plot (585.75 kgha^{-1}), FYM + *Azotobacter* treated micro-plot (528 kgha^{-1}), FYM + VAM inoculated micro-plot (426.75 kgha^{-1}) and minimum was recorded (Table 14.4) in control micro-plot (420.51 kgha^{-1}).

Table 14.2: Effect of Chemical Fertilizer and VAM on Nutrient (N-P-K) in the Rhizosphere Soil of Wheat Cultivar C-306 Cultivated at Departmental Botanical Garden

Sl.No.	Treatment	Nitrogen (kgha^{-1})	Phosphorus (kgha^{-1})	Potassium (kgha^{-1})
1.	Control (Soil alone)	426.75	14.8	260.0
2	Chemical fertilizer	536.00	12.8	472.0
3	VAM inoculum	380.00	6.4	172.0

Phosphorus (P)

In the experiment 1, maximum soil phosphorus was recorded with control micro-plot (14.8 kgha^{-1}) followed by chemical fertilizer treated micro-plot (12.8 kgha^{-1}) and minimum was recorded (Table 14.2) with VAM inoculated micro-plot (6.4 kgha^{-1}) whereas, in experiment 2, Table 14.4 shows the maximum soil P with FYM + *Azotobacter* treated micro-plot (16 kgha^{-1}) followed by control micro-plot (13.7 kgha^{-1}) then FYM + PSB + *Pseudomonas* treated micro-plot (12 kgha^{-1}), FYM + *Pseudomonas* treated micro-plot (10 kgha^{-1}); FYM + PSB treated, FYM alone and FYM + *Azotobacter* + PSB treated micro-plot (9.6 kgha^{-1}) and minimum was recorded with FYM + VAM inoculated micro-plot (7.4 kgha^{-1}).

Potassium (K)

In experiment 1, the maximum soil potassium was recorded with chemical fertilizer treated micro-plot (472 $kgha^{-1}$), followed by control micro-plot (260 $kgha^{-1}$) and minimum (Table 14.2) was recorded with VAM inoculated micro-plot (172 $kgha^{-1}$).

In experiment 2, the maximum soil K was recorded with FYM + *Pseudomonas* treated micro-plot (312.6 $kgha^{-1}$) followed by control micro-plot (312 $kgha^{-1}$) then FYM treated micro-plot (308 $kgha^{-1}$), FYM + PSB + *Pseudomonas* treated micro-plot (291.2 $kgha^{-1}$), FYM + PSB treated micro-plot (240.8 $kgha^{-1}$), FYM + *Azotobacter* +PSB treated micro-plot (205 $kgha^{-1}$), FYM + *Azotobacter* treated micro-plot (145.6 $kgha^{-1}$) and minimum was recorded (Table 14.4) with FYM+VAM inoculated micro-plot (121 $kgha^{-1}$).

Growth Parameters of Wheat (Cv. C-306)

Germination

In experiment 1, the highest per cent germination was recorded with VAM inoculated plants (79 per cent) followed by chemical fertilizer treated plants (64 per cent) and lowest per cent germination was recorded (Table 14.3) with control plants (55 per cent).

Table 14.3: Effect of Chemical Fertilizer and VAM Inoculum on the Growth Parameter and Yield of Wheat Cultivar C-306 Cultivated at Departmental Botanical Garden

Sl.No.	Treatment	Germination (per cent)	Heading (Days)	Maturity (Days)	Plant Height (cm)	Yield (kg ha^{-1})
1.	Control (Soil alone)	55.0	74	128	37.74	232.1
2	Chemical fertilizer	64.0	77	132	60.49	625.0
3	VAM inoculum	79.0	81	137	86.13	725.0
	CD (P<0.05)	3.84	ND	ND	5.16	48.67

In experiment 2, the highest germination was recorded with FYM + VAM inoculated plant (81 per cent), followed by FYM + *Azotobacter* (75 per cent), FYM + *Azotobacter* + PSB treated plant (72 per cent), FYM + PSB + *Pseudomonas* treated plants (69 per cent), FYM + *Pseudomonas* and FYM alone treated plant (65 per cent) and lowest was recorded (Table 14.5) with control plant (52 per cent).

Heading

In experiment 1, the heading appeared after 81 days with VAM inoculated plants which was higher time period followed by chemical fertilizer treated plants (77d), whereas, control plants required lesser time period *i.e.* 74 days for the appearance of headings (Table 14.3).

The experiment 2, revealed that headings appeared after higher time period *i.e.* 84 days with FYM + *Azotobacter* and FYM + *Azotobacter* + PSB treated plants followed by FYM + VAM inoculated plant (83d) then FYM + PSB treated plant (80d), FMY + *Pseudomonas* treated plants (78d), FYM + PSB + *Pseudomonas* treated plants (76d), FYM treated plant (74d); whereas, control plant require lesser time period *i.e.* 71 days for the appearance of headings (Table 14.5).

Maturity

In experiment 1, the rate of maturity was achieved with VAM inoculated plant after 137 days in maximum time period followed by chemical fertilizer treated plant (132d) and with control plants rate of maturity was achieved after 128 days which was minimum time period in comparison to other *i.e.* VAM inoculated and chemical fertilizer treated plants respectively (Table 14.3).

In experiment 2, the rate of maturity was achieved with FYM + VAM inoculated plant, FYM + *Azotobacter* treated plants, FYM + *Azotobacter* + PSB inoculated plants after 138 days, which was maximum time period followed by FYM + PSB treated plant (137d) then FYM + PSB + *Pseudomonas* treated plant (136d), FYM alone treated plant (134d), control plant (132d) and minimum time period of 130 days was required to achieve maturity with FYM + *Pseudomonas* treated plants (Table 14.5).

Table 14.4: Effect of Bioagent on Nutrient (N-P-K) in the Rhizosphere Soil of Wheat Cultivar C-306 Cultivated at Departmental Botanical Garden

Sl.No.	*Treatment*	*Nitrogen (Kg ha^{-1})*	*Phosphorus (Kg ha^{-1})*	*Potassium (Kg ha^{-1})*
1.	FYM	585.75	9.6	308.0
2.	FYM + VAM	426.75	7.4	121.0
3.	FYM + PSB + *Pseudomonas*	610.50	12.0	291.2
4.	FYM + *Pseudomonas*	585.75	10.0	312.6
5.	FYM + PSB	594.00	9.6	240.8
6.	FYM + *Azotobacter*	528.00	16.0	145.6
7.	FYM + PSB + *Azotobacter*	594.00	9.6	205.0
8.	Control (Soil alone)	420.51	13.7	312.0

Table 14.5: Effect of Bioagent on Growth Parameter and Yield of Wheat Cultivar C-306 Cultivated at Departmental Botanical Garden

S.No.	*Treatment*	*Germination (per cent)*	*Heading (Days)*	*Maturity (Days)*	*Plant Height (cm)*	*Yield (Kgha^{-1})*
1.	FYM	65.0	74	134	61.2	717
2.	FYM + VAM	81.0	83	138	101.4	1350
3.	FYM + PSB + *Pseudomonas*	69.0	76	136	70.4	1200
4.	FYM + *Pseudomonas*	65.0	78	130	87.3	1283
5.	FYM + PSB	70.0	80	137	84.2	1250
6.	FYM + *Azotobacter*	75.0	84	138	98.7	1317
7.	FYM + PSB + *Azotobacter*	72.0	84	138	94.1	1125
8.	Control (Soil alone)	52.0	71	132	40.7	472
	CD ($P < 0.05$)	3.86	ND	ND	4.55	57.33

Plant Height

In experiment 1, the tallest plant was recorded in VAM inoculated pot (86.13cm.) followed by chemical fertilizer treated plant (60.49 cm.) and shortest plant was recorded (Table 14.3) with control (37.74 cm.).

However, in experiment 2, plant showed tallest height with FYM + VAM inoculated plant (101.4 cm.), followed by FYM + *Azotobacter* treated plant (98.7 cm.), FYM + *Azotobacter* + PSB treated plant (94.1 cm.), FYM + *Pseudomonas* treated plant (87.3 cm.), FYM + PSB treated plant (84.2 cm.), FYM + PSB

+ *Pseudomonas* treated plant (70.4 cm.), FYM treated plant (61.2 cm.) and shortest height was recorded with control plant (40.7 cm.) (Table 14.5).

Grain Yield

For the experiment 1, the maximum grain yield was recorded with VAM inoculated plant (725 $kgha^{-1}$), followed by chemical fertilization plant (625 $kgha^{-1}$) and minimum was obtained (Table 14.3) with control plants (232.1 $kgha^{-1}$).

In experiment 2, the maximum yield was recorded with FYM + VAM inoculated plant (1350 $kgha^{-1}$), followed by FYM + *Azotobacter* treated plant (1317 $kgha^{-1}$), FYM + *Pseudomonas* treated plant (1283 $kgha^{-1}$), FYM + PSB treated plant (1250 $kgha^{-1}$), FYM + PSB + *Pseudomonas* treated plant (1200 $kgha^{-1}$), FYM + *Azotobacter* + PSB (1125 $kgha^{-1}$), FYM treated plant (717 $kgha^{-1}$) and minimum grain yield was obtained (Table 14.5) with control plant (472 $kgha^{-1}$).

Discussion

Decreasing yields in continuous wheat mono-culture can be compensated only to a limited extent by agronomic practices such as regular supply of straw and green manure (Kurten and Range, 1980). This problem of continuous cropping of winter wheat is documented in diverse investigations (Debruck, 1974; Diereks *et al.*, 1980; Gutser *et al.*, 1981; Heyland, 1975; Pommer *et al.*, 1979). The activity of soil microorganism in continuous wheat mono-culture is limited. According to Beck (1974) the reduced microbial soil activity in continuous wheat mono-culture might result in a smaller N-supply by mineralization and thus in an insufficient N-supply for the plants.

Despite the fact that the favourable influence of VAM on the nutrient uptake and drought resistance of plants is generally accepted, relatively little is known about the occurrence and importance of these fungi in intensive agriculture, although several investigation have already been performed (Baltruschat and Dehne, 1982; Black and Tinker, 1979; Hayman, 1975; Jensen and Jacobsen, 1980; Ruissen, 1982; Schenck and Kinloch, 1980).

The results of present study indicate that, the rhizosphere soils of micro-plots are saturated with chemical substances particularly N-P-K, therefore addition of more N-P-K was not found as effective as it was expected. However, the rhizosphere soils were supplemented with VAM fungi (*Glomus mosseae*) inspite of that presence of indigenous VAM population, identified as species of *Glomus*. The addition of *G. mosseae* in the rhizosphere soils of wheat plant did not only develop intensive colonization but also helped in the nutrient uptake, resulting in to better growth of the plant and higher grain yield.

The role of VAM fungi in mineral nutrition has been discussed in depth in recent past (Rhodes and Gerdemann, 1980; Smith, 1980; Bowen and Smith, 1981). It is now well established that mycorrhizae can improve P nutrition of a host and it is likely that they can also assist in the uptake of other ions.

However, evidences to suggest that VAM affect the nitrogen nutrition of plants directly and cause an increased uptake resulting in higher N content in them are also available (Bowen and Smith, 1981; Ames *et al.*, 1983; Jensen, 1982).

The yield and uptake of nitrogen and phosphorus was substantially increased due to use of inoculants (Kundu and Gaur, 1980c). In non-sterilized soil, the highest increase in grain yield was recorded with FYM + VAM inoculated plants followed by FYM + *Azotobacter* treated plants. Mixed inoculation yielded better results than single inoculant. The becterization effect was well marked when the soil was amended with FYM. The better response in sterilized soil may be due to lack of competition and availability of more nutrients to the introduced PSB. It has been established that application of organic matter improves the physical, chemical and biological properties of soil (Gaur, 1982; Gaur *et al.*, 1984). However, other combination fails to gave high yield which may be attributed to the competition for the growth among the microbes or antagonistic activity between/among them. Pavlovich (1959) reported an adverse effect of *Bacillus subtilis* and *B. mesentericus* and a beneficial effect of *B. megaterium* on *Azotobacter* growth. Chan *et al.* (1970) observed inhibition of *Azotobacter* by *Pseudomonas putida* and the inhibition of *Azotobacter* was attributed to their sensitivity to the acidity produced. The antagonism of *Pseudomonas* sp. to *Azotobacter* (Chan *et al.*, 1963) and that of *Bacillus circulans* to fungi such as *Alternaria solani, Helminthosporium oryzae, Rhizoctonia solani, Fusarium udam* (Vasantharajan, 1964) were reported.

The phosphorus solubilising bacteria have the capacity to dissolve the insoluble phosphatic compounds present in soil in the form of tricalcium, aluminium and iron phosphates and also solubilize rock phosphate, bone meal and basic slag. The increases in phosphorus uptake by plants have been made possible by combining the abilities of the phosphorus solubilising microorganisms and the efficient P uptake mechanisms of the VAM fungi (Azcon *et al.*, 1976; Raj *et al.*, 1981; Kucey, 1987).

Increase in yield and phosphate uptake by wheat crops inoculated with phosphobacterin were reported by several workers (Arao *et al.*, 1956; Panova, 1956; Andronova, 1958; Kudzin and Yaroshevich, 1958; Afanaseva and Andronova, 1959; Timoriu *et al.*, 1964). Besides increase in yield, the increase in protein content has also been reported (Kudashev, 1956; Ivchenko, 1961). The increase in gliadin/gluten ratio (Pinevich, 1956) improved quality of grains, and increased gluten content (Ivchenko, 1961), better growth and germination (Mishustin and Naumova, 1956) have been observed. Smallii (1958) reported increased P_2O_5 uptake by wheat plants and grain yield by inoculation with *Pseudomonas. Bacterium glutinsus* and *Bacillus magaterium.* On the other hand, some workers did not get any response of wheat crop to phosphobacterin inoculation (Bystrova, 1958; Lauzne, 1960; Smith *et al.*, 1961).

The combined impact of inoculation of all bioagents tested in the present study on growth and yield response of wheat Cv. C-306 has not so far been found in the literature.

Conclusion

It is concluded here that VAM has greater impact on the growth and yield of wheat Cv. C-306 in the soils, which are already saturated with chemical nutrients. This is suggested here that there is no need to go on pouring chemical fertilizer in the soils, which instead of making the soil more fertile forced it to become barren.

Use of VAM and phosphobacterin should be increased, because these organisms are not only responsible for the soil health but also responsible for the good growth and better yield of wheat.

References

A.O.A.C. (1965). *Official Methods of Analysis of the Association of Official Agricultural Chemists.* 8th (ed.) Vol. I. Minnesota. U.S.A.: 523.

Abbott, L.K. and Robson, A.D. (1978). Growth of subterranean clover in relation to the formation of endomycorrhiza by introduced and indigenous fungi in field soil. *New Phytol.* 81: 575-585.

Afanaseva, A.L. and Andronowa, T.M. (1959). Experiment on use of phosphobacterin on the soils of the Omek region. *Udobr. Urozh.* 5: 44-47.

Alexander, M. (1961). *Introduction to Soil Microbiology.* John Wiley and Sons, New York and London.

Allison, F.E. (1947). *Azotobacter* inoculation of crops (1) *Historical. Soil Sci.* 64: 413-429.

Ames, R., Reid, C., Porter, L. and Cambardella, C. (1983). Hyphal uptake and transport of nitrogen from two 15 N-labelled sources by *Glomus mosseae*, a vesicular-arbuscular mycorrhizal fungus. *New Phytol.* 95: 381.

Andronova, T.M. (1958). Effectiveness of Phosphobacterin. Bull. nauchtech, Inform. Sibir.Nauchissled. *Inst. Sel. Khoz.* 2: 14-19.

Arao, I., Kan, Y.S. and Sihe, T.L. (1956). Bacterial transformation of insoluble organic and inorganic phosphorus compounds in to soluble phosphate in soils. Part II. Results obtained in pot and field experiments to test the practical value of inoculating wheat with *Bacillus megatherium* var. *phosphaticum. Kungchuling Acta Pedol. Sir.* 4: 179-184.

Azcon, R., Barea, J.M. and Hayman, D.S. (1976). Utilization of rock phosphate in alkaline soils by plants inoculated with mycorrhizal fungi and phosphate solubilizing bacteria. *Soil Biol. Biochem.* 8: 135-138.

Azcon-Aguilar, C., Barea, J. M., Azcon, R. and Olivares, J. (1982). Effectiveness of *Rhizobium* and VA-mycorrhiza in the introduction of *Hedysarum coronarium* in a new habitat. *Agric. Environ.* 7: 199-206.

Baltruschat, H. and Dehne, H.W. (1982). Zum Auftreten der endotrophen mycorrhizen in verschiedenen Getreidefruchtfolgen und Dungung- ssystemen. *Med. Fac. Landbouww. Rijksuniv. Gent*, 47:831-839.

Banik, S. and Dey, B.K. (1962). Plant soil. 69: 353.

Beck, T. (1974). Der Einfluβ langjahriger Monokultur auf die Bodenbelebung im Vergleich zur Fruchtfolge. Landw. Forschg. 31. *Sonderheft*. II: 268-276.

Black, R.L.B. and Tinker, P.B. (1979). The development of endomycorrhizal root systems. II. effect of agronomic factors and soil conditions on the development of vesicular–arbuscular mycorrhizal infection in barley and on spore density. *New Phytol.* 83: 401-413.

Bowen, G.D. and Smith, S.E. (1981). The effects of mycorrhizas on nitrogen uptake by plants. *Ecol. Bull. (Stockholm)*. 33: 237.

Bystrova, N.A. (1958). The effect of phosphobacterin on the development of brown rust and increase in grain yield of winter wheat. *Trudv. vesesovuz Inst. Zashch. Rest.* 13: 68-70.

Chan, E.C.S., Basavanand, P. and Liivak, T. (1970). The growth inhibition of *Azotobacter chroococcum* by *Pseudomonas* sp. *Can. J. Microbiol.* 16: 9-16.

Chan, E.C.S., Rouatt, J.W. and Ketznelson, H. (1963). The influence of soil and root extracts on the associative growth of selected soil bacteria. *Can. J. Microbiol.* 9: 187.

Debruck, J. (1974). Intensiver Weizenbau-Zu Fragen der Fruchtfolge und Pflanzenges-undheit. Kali-Briefe. 6. *Folge*. 114.

Diercks, R., Bachthaler, G. and Pommer, G. (1980). Langjahrige Auswirkungen unterschiedlicher Fruchtfolge und Anbausysteme auf Ertrag und schaderregerbefall von winterweizen und sommergerste. *Z. Acker und Pflanzenbau*. 149: 454-471.

Dobin, R. (1980). Phosphorus deficiency in tropical soil as a constraint on agricultural output. In: Priotities for Alleviatting soil related constraints to food production in the Tropics. *IRRI:* 217-232.

Gaur, A.C. (1982). *A Practical Manual of Rural Composting*. Food and Agriculture Organization of United Nations: 102.

Gaur, A.C. (1987). In: *Mycorrhiza Round Table*. (eds.) A.K.Verma, K.J. Mukerji, K.V.B.R. Tilak and J. Raj. Proceedings of a National Workshop, J.N.U., New Delhi: 505.

Gaur, A.C., Neelakantan, S. and Dargan, K.S. (1984). *Organic Manures*. ICAR. New Delhi: 159.

Gianinazzi, S., Gianinazzi-Pearson, V. and Trouvelot, A. (1990a). Potentialities and procedures for use of endomycorrhizas with special emphasis on high value crops. In: *Biotechnology for fungi for improving plant growth*. (eds.) J.M. Whipps and B. Lumsden. Cambridge University Press. Cambridge U.K.: 41-54.

Gianinazzi, S., Trouvelot, A. and Gianinazzi-Pearson, V. (1989). Conceptual approaches in agriculture for the rational use of VA-endomycorrhizae in agriculture: Possibilities and limitations. *Agric. Ecosys. and Environments*. 29: 153-161.

Gianinazzi, S., Trouvelot, A. and Gianinazzi-Pearson, V. (1990b). Role and use of mycorrhizas in horticultural crop production. *Plenary lecture at the XXIII International Horticultural Congress*, I.S.H.S. Italy. (1990: 25-30.

Gupta, S.C. and Kapoor, V.K. (1997). *Fundamentals of applied statistics* (III ed.) Sultan Chand and Sons. New Delhi: 6.1-6.113.

Gutser, R., Amberger, A. and Hoffmann, G.M. (1981). Gesundung einer Winter-weizen- Monokultur durch dungung und pflanzenschutz. Landw. Forsch, Sonderheft. 38: 693-708.

Hayman, D.S. (1975). The Occurrence of Mycorrhiza in crops as affected by soil fertility. In *Endomycorrhizas*. (eds.) F.E. Sanders, B. Mosse and P.B. Tinker. Academic Press. London: 495-509.

Heyland, K.U. (1975). Uber den Einfluβ der zunehmenden sommerweizen-Monokultur auf den kornertrag und die kornertragsstruktur. *Z. Acker und Pflanzenbau*. 140: 117-129.

Ivchenko, N.P. (1961). Effect of fertilizers on the quality of the grain of spring wheat in the ural zone. *Agrobiologiya*. 2: 293-295.

Jackson, M.L. (1967). *Soil Chemical Analysis*. Prentice Hall of India (Ltd.) New Delhi: 428.

Jackson, M.L. (1973). *Soil Chemical Analysis*. Prentice Hall of India (Pvt. Ltd.) New Delhi.

Jensen, A. (1982). Influence of four vesicular-arbuscular mycorrhizal fungi on nutrient uptake and growth in barley (*Hordeum vulgare*). *New Phytol*. 90: 45-50.

Jensen, A. and Jacobsen, I. (1980). The occurrence of vesicular-arbuscular mycorrhiza in barley and wheat grown in some Danish soils with different fertilizer treatments. *Plant and Soil*. 55: 403-414.

Koske, R.E. (1981). A preliminary study of interaction between species of vesicular-arbuscular fungi in a sand-dune. *Trans. Br. Mycol. Soc*. 76: 411-418.

Kucey, R.M.N. (1987). Increased phosphorus uptake by wheat and field beans inoculated with a phosphorus solubilizing *Penicillium bilaji* strain and with vesicular-arbuscular mycorrhizal fungi. *Appl. Env. Microbiol*. 53: 2699-2703.

Kudashev, I.S. (1956). The effect of phosphobacterin on the yields and protein content in grains of autumn wheat, maiz and soyabean. *Dokl. Akad. Skh. Nauk*. 8: 20-23.

Kudzin, Y.K. and Yaroshevich, T.V. (1958). The use of phosphobacterin for winter wheat on chernozems. *Udobr. Urozh*. 9: 19-20.

Kundu, B.S. and Gaur, A.C. (1980c). Establishment of nitrogen fixing and phosphate dissolving bacteria in rhizosphere and their effect on yield and nutrient uptake of wheat crop. *Plant and Soil*. 57: 223-230.

Kurten, P.W. and Range, W. (1980). Results of an 8 years fertilization comprising winter wheat and winter barley in cereal rotation and one-crop system. *Landw. Forsch*. 33: 385-407.

Lauzne, E. (1960). Inter-relation of phosphorus bacteria and some cultivated plants. *Trudv. Inst. Microbiol. Akad. Nauk. Latv. SSR*. 11: 153-167.

Mehrotra, C.L. and Lehri, L.K. (1971). Effect of *Azotobacter* Inoculation on crop yields. *J. Indian Soc. Soil. Sci*. (19): 243-248.

Mishustin, E.N. and Naumova, A.N. (1956). The use of bacterial fertilizers in sowing vegetable seeds in to peat manure nutrient cubes. *Mikrobiologiya*. 25: 41-48.

Mosse, B. (1973). Advances in the study of vesicular-arbuscular mycorrhiza. *Annu. Rev. Phytopathol*. 11: 171-194.

Panova, A.V. (1956). Trials with bacterial fertilizers. *Semledelie*. 12: 85-86.

Pavlovich, D.Y. (1959). Interrelations of *Azotobacter* with other groups of soil microorganisms. Trudy. Inst. Mikrobiol. *Akad. Nauk. Latv. SSR*. 8: 127-143.

Pinevich, V.V. (1956). The effect of granular phosphorus fertilizers and phosphobacterin on the composition of wheat grain. *Dokl. Akad. Nauk*. 108: 157-159.

Pommer, G., Oppitz, K. and Fink, K. (1979). Winterweizensorten in Fruchtwechsel und Daueranbau-Ertagsrelationen und Einfluβ produktionstechnischer MaBnahmen. *Z. Acker-und Pflanzenbau*. 148: 214-229.

Raj, J., Bagyaraj, D.J. and Manjunath, A. (1981). Influence of soil inoculation with vesicular-arbuscular mycorrhiza and a phosphate dissolving bacterium on plant growth and ^{32}P uptake. *Soil Biol. Biochem*. 13: 105-108.

Rawat, A.K. and Sanoria, C.L. (1976). Effect of *Rhizobium*, *Azotobacter* and *Bejerinckia* inoculation on *Cicer arietinum* var. type I. *Curr. Sci*. 45: 665-666.

Rawat, A.K. and Sanoria, C.L. (1977). Influence of seed bacterization on nodulation, yield and amino acid composition of used protein of *Cicer arietinum* var. type I. *Curr. Sci*. 46: 373-375.

Reeves, F.B., Wagner, D., Moorman, T. and Kiel, J. (1979). The role of endomycorrhizas in revegetation practices in the semi-arid west. I. A comparison of incidence of mycorrhizae in severely disturbed and natural environments. *Am. J. Bot*. 66: 6-13.

Rhodes, L.H. and Gerdemann, J.W. (1980). Nutrient translocation in vesicular–arbuscular mycorrhizae, in cellular interactions in symbiosis and parasitism. (eds.) C.B. Cook, P.W. Pappas and E.D. Rudolph. The Ohio State University Press, *Columbus:* 173.

Ruissen, M.A. (1982). The development and significance of vesicular-arbuscular mycorrhizas as influenced by agricultural practices. *Thesis*, Agricultural University, Waageningen. The Netherlands: 111.

Santhi, R. and Kothandaraman, G.V. (1995). Effect of endomycorrhizal colonization and phosphorus sources on the phosphorus recovery, nutrient uptake and growth of green gram. *Indian J. Agric. Res*. 29: 209-214.

Schenck, N.C. and Kinloch, R.A. (1980). Incidence of mycorrhizal fungi on six field crops in monoculture on newly cleared woodland site. *Mycologia*. 72: 445-456.

Smallii, V.T. (1958). The effect of rhizosphere bacteria on the growth and productivity of wheat. Akad. Nauk. Ukrain, SSR. *Kiev:* 153-159.

Smith, J.H., Allison, F.E. and Soulides, D.A. (1961). Evaluation of Phosphobacterin as a soil inoculant. *Soil Sci. Soc. Am. Proc.* 25: 109-111.

Smith, T.F. (1980). The effect of season and crop rotation on the abundance of spores of vesicular-arbuscular (VA) mycorrhizal endophytes. *Plant and Soil*. 57: 475-479.

Sundara Rao, W.V.B., Bajpai, P.D., Sharma, J.P. and Subbaiah, B.V. (1963). Solubilization of phosphates by phosphorus solubilizing organism using P^{32} as tracer and the influence of seed bacterization on the uptake by the crop. *J. Indian Soc. Soil. Sci.* 11: 209-219.

Thompson, J.P. (1990). *Soil Biol. Biochem*. 22: 229.

Timoriu, G., Rosu, G. and Ciobana, V. (1964). Contribution to the study of the influence of bacterial fertilizers on the yield of certain varieties of autumn wheat. Inst. Agron. "I. Ionescu de la Brad". Iasi Luc Stiint. 2: 67-72.

Tinker, P.B. (1978). Effect of vesicular–arbuscular mycorrhizas on plant nutrition and plant growth. *Physiol. Veg*. 16: 743-749.

Tosh, B.N. and Sanoria, C.L. (1978). Combined effect of *Rhizobium* and *Azotobacter* on soil properties and yield of gram (*Cicer arietinum* L.) Varieties. *Fert. Technol*. 15: 35-37.

Vasantharajan, V.N. (1964). Inhibition of plant pathogenic fungi by *B. circulance* solubilizing phosphorus. *Indian J. Microbiol*. 4: 27.

Microbial Biotechnology and Ecology (2011) *Pages* **268–274**
Editors: **Deepak Vyas, G.S. Paliwal, P.K.Khare and R.K Gupta**
Published by: **DAYA PUBLISHING HOUSE, NEW DELHI**

Chapter 15

Some Additions to the Foliicolous Fungi from the Forest Flora of Madhya Pradesh, India

☆ ***P. Chauksay, A.N. Rai* and Naveen Verma***

Department of Botany, Dr. H.S. Gaur University, Sagar – 470 003, M.P.

ABSTRACT

During frequent surveys for phytoparasitic foliicolous microfungi, two interesting specimens were collected from Sagar Forest Circle of Madhya Pradesh, which upon detailed examination proved to be undescribed taxa of *Cytoplea palmacearum* sp.nov., and *Diplodia zizyphiae* sp.nov. infecting *Phoenix sylvestris* Roxb. (Palmaceae) and *Zizyphus oenoplia* Mill. (Rhamnaceae). These are illustrated, described and compared with closely related species in the genera.

Cytoplea palmacearum Chauksay *et al.*, sp. nov. (Figure 15.1)

Maculae amphigenosae, irregulares, disperseae per totam superficiem folii, atro brunneae. Coloniae, pleraeque epiphyllosae, raro hypogenae, atro. Mycelium hypharum immersum, ramosum, septatum, brunneae. Conidiomata immersum et demum erumpentia, subepidermalis, subglobosa vel irregularis, pallide brunneae, usque 550 µm diam. Ostiolum et conidiophora absentia. Conidiogenosae, ampulliformes, hyallina vel subhyllina, laevia, 2.5-8 × 3.5-6 µm. Conidia simplicia, solitaria, aseptata, ovalis vel fusiformia vel ellipsoiformia, laevia, tenuibus parietibus eguttulate, pallide olivacea, 2.5-13 × 1.5-5.

* E-mail: anrai_mycology@yahoo.com.

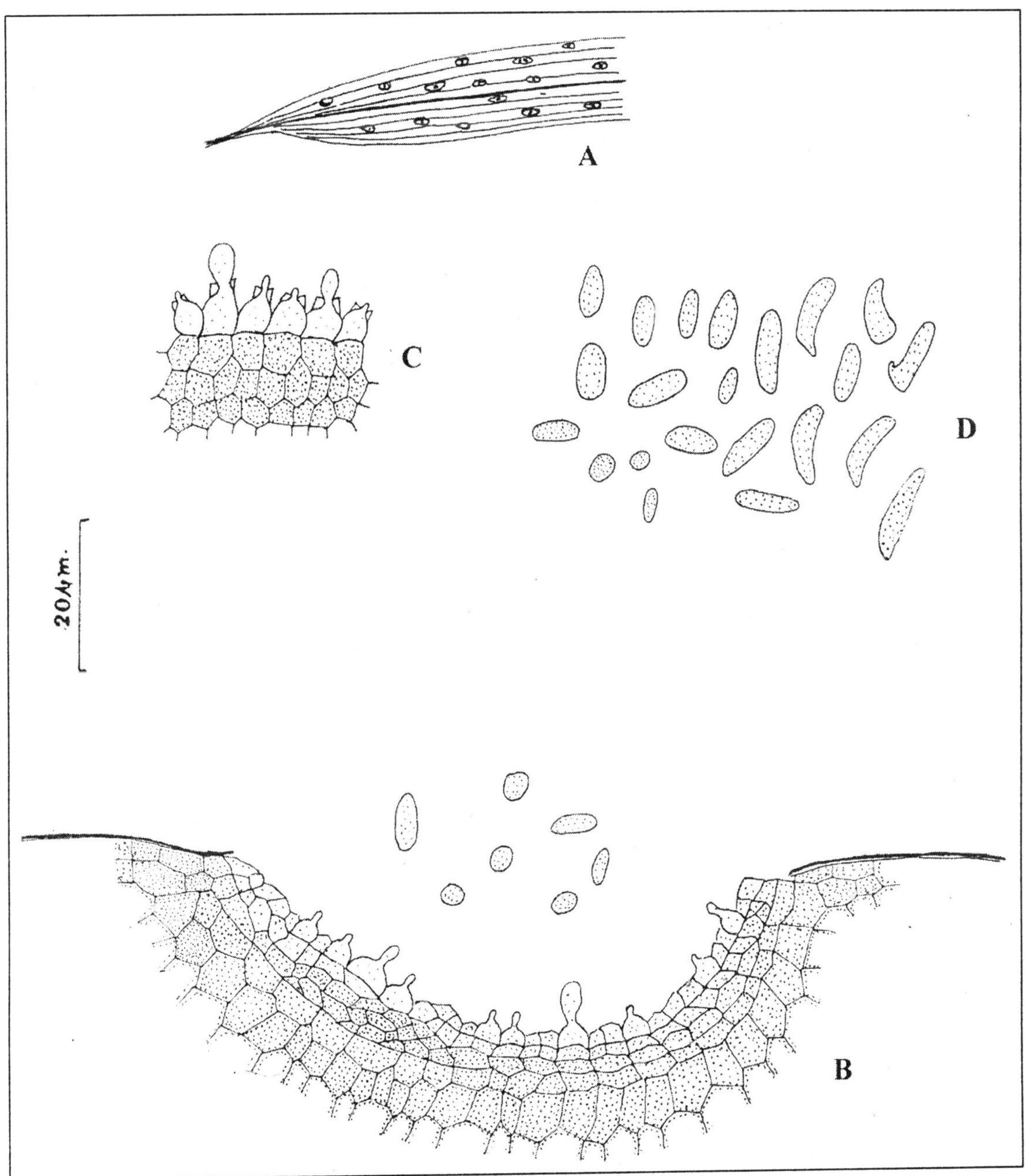

Figure 15.1: *Cytoplea palmacearum* sp.nov.
A: Symptom; B: Conidiomata; C: Conidiogenous cells; D: Conidia

Hab. In foliis vivis *Phoenix sylvestris* Roxb. (Palmaceae), October 1988 Gopalpura (South Sagar Forest Division), leg. M. Gupta. RG 52, typus, IMI 333066.

Lesions amphigenous, irregular, distributed all over the leaf surface, blackish brown. Colonies predominantly epiphyllous, rarely hypophyllous represented by very hard and warty dots, black. Mycelium of hyphae immersed, branched, septate, brown. Conidiomata immersed and strongly erumpent, subepidermal, subspherical to irregular light brown, up to 550 µm in diam. Ostioles absent, dehiscence by irregular fissured, rupturing in the central region of the upper wall. Conidiophores absent. Conidiogenous cells enteroblastic discrete, determinate, ampulliform, hyaline to subhyaline, smooth, 2.5-8 × 3.5-6 µm. Conidia simple, solitary, aseptate, oval to fusiform to ellipsoidal, smooth, thin walled, eguttulate, light olivaceous, 2.5-13 × 1.5-5 µm (Figure 15.1).

Only a few species of *Cytoplea* have been described so far, the only full treatment of *Cytoplea* is given by Petrak and Sydow (1927), and the most authoritative and detailed work is presented by Sutton (1980). Dr. E. Punithalingam of C.A.B. International Mycological Institute, in his expert opinion reported it *Cytoplea* sp. near *C. orientalis* Sutton (Sutton, 1980). Thus for convenience the proposed species is compared with *C. orientalis* Sutton (Table 15.1).

Table 15.1: Comparative Account *C. palmacearum* sp. nov. with Related Species

Species	*Spot and Colonies*	*Conidiophores*			*Conidia*		
		Structure	*Colour*	*Size (µm diam)*	*Structure*	*Colour*	*Size (µm)*
C. orientalis	Amphigenous, lenticular to ellipsoid, seprate, grayish brown with a paler brown centre.	Eustromatic, immersed to strongly erumpent, epidermal, lenticular to pulvinate, multilocular, wall thin and dark, ostiole absent, dehiscence by irregular breakdown of upper wall.	Dark brown	750	Fusiform, aseptate, verruculose, thin walled.	Pale brown	9-11 x 3-4.
C. palmacearum sp. nov.	Amphigenous, irregular blackish brown. Colonies epiphyllous, rarely hypophyllous, hard and warty dots, black	Immersed to strongly erumpent, sub epidermal, sub spherical to irregular ostiole absent, dehiscence by irregular fissure in the central region of the upper wall.	Light brown	Upto 550	Oval to fusiform to ellipsoid, thin walled, aseptate, eguttulate, smooth.	Light olivaceous	2.5-13 x 1.5-5.

A critical look to the table 1 shows that the authors' collection resembles a little bit to *C. orientalis* in infection spots and structure of conidomata while it is quite dissimilar in other morphological characters of taxonomic values. *C. palmacearum* is at large variance in having epiphyllous, hard and warty black colonies, light coloured, conidiomata with smaller diameter and oval to fusiform to ellipsoid, smooth walled, light olivaceous, larger and thicker conidia as against *C. orientalis* having amphyllous, rarely hypophyllous colonies with dark coloured and large diameter of conidiomata and fusiform, verruculose, pale brown comparatively smaller and thinner conidia. The forgoing discussion, therefore, concludes that authors' taxon has its own identity and merits description and illustration as a new species.

Diplodia zizyphiae Chauksay, *et al.*, sp. nov. (Figure 15.2)

Maculae, epigenosae, parvae circulares vel irregulares, interdem carbonaceous, dispersae per totam superficiem folii, brunneae atro. Mycelium hypharum immersum vel partim superficiale, globosa, unilocularis, fusce parietibus, extra laminae fusce brunneae, fusce parietibus sclerotiodeis formatis, medio laminae tenuibus parietibus hyaline cellulae et interius laminae tenuibus parietibus hyaline cellulae, 800 µm dimetro, ostiolata singularis, circularis, simplicia, centralis. Conidiophori cylindreta, formatus interius cellulae pycnidial parietibus, eramosa, septati, usque. 1-3 transverse septati, leavibus parietibus, erecta vel suberecta, hyalinae vel pallide olivacea, 26-75 × 5-8.5 µm. Conidiogenosae cellulae holoblastae, integratae, cylindratae, laevia, formatus singula apicale conidium, hyalinae vel pallide olivacea. Conidia simplicia, solitaria, aseptata, laevia, intio hyaline quam fusco brunneae et modreta 1 euseptata, fusce parietibus, subglobosa vel ovalis vel oblonga vel ellipsoiformia, apices et bases obtuse, 5-34.5 × 4.5-26 µm

Hab. In foliis vivis *Zizyphus oenoplia* Mill. (Rhamnaceae), January, 1989, Gopalpura (South Sagar Forest Division), leg. M. Gupta, RC 57, typus, IMI 333075.

Lesions epigenous, small circular to irregular, coal-tar like, distributed all over the leaf surface, brownish black, colonies epiphyllous, conferred to the center of the spot, represented by very fine dots, black. Mycelium of hyphae immersed branched, septate, brown. Conidomata pycnidial, immersed to partly superficial, globose to sub-globose, unilocular, thick walled, outer layer dark brown thick walled textura angularis, median layer light brown of thin walled cells and inner layer thin walled, hyaline cells, 800 µm in diam., ostiole single, circular, simple, central. Conidiophores cylindrical, formed from the inner cells of pycnidial wall, unbranched, septate, upto 1-3 transversely septate, smooth walled, erect to sub-erect, hayaline to light brown. Conidia simple, solitary, aseptate, smooth, at first hyaline then dark brown and medially 1 equiseptate, thick walled, subglobose to oval to oblong to ellipsoidal, apex and base obtuse, 5-34.5 × 4.5-26 µm (Figure 15.2)

Hab. on living leaves of *Zizyphus oenoplia* Mill. (Rhamnaceae), January, 1989, Gopalpura (South Sagar Forest Division), leg. M. Gupta, RC 57, type, IMI 333075.

Petrak and Sydow (1927) placed *Shaeria malorum* Berk. synonymy of *Botryodiploadia malorum* (Berk.) Petrak and Sydow but these names are regarded as synonyms of *Diplodia mutila* by Stevens (1933) who quoted an extensive synonymy. Shoemaker (1964) has clarified the identity of certain *Botryodiploadia* spp. in which *S. stenvensii* Shoem., was regarded as the ascomycetous state of *D. mutila*. Zambettakis (1954) in a reassessment of generic concepts in the didymosporous sphaeropsidales erroneously adopted *D. conigena* Desm. as the type for *Diplodia* and referred *D. mutila* to the genus *Metadiplodia* Syd., the genus is need of further revision. A number of *Diplodia* species are reported from different host families but for convenience the authors' collection is compared with *D. mutila* Fr. apud Mont. (Sutton, 1980) in Table 15.2.

A critical analysis of the Table 15.2 shows that the proposed species resembles *D. mutila* in a few characters such as structure of conidiomata, conidiophores and conidia while it is drastically dissimilar from *D. mutila* (*D. zizyphiae* has larger diam. of conidiomata, unbranched, longer, thicker and comparatively dark coloured conidiophores, conidia subglobose to oval to oblong to ellipsoid with obtuse base and apex having comparatively longer but considerably wider (almost just double) conidial dimensions as against *D. mutila*) so much so that it needs its description and illustration as a new species.

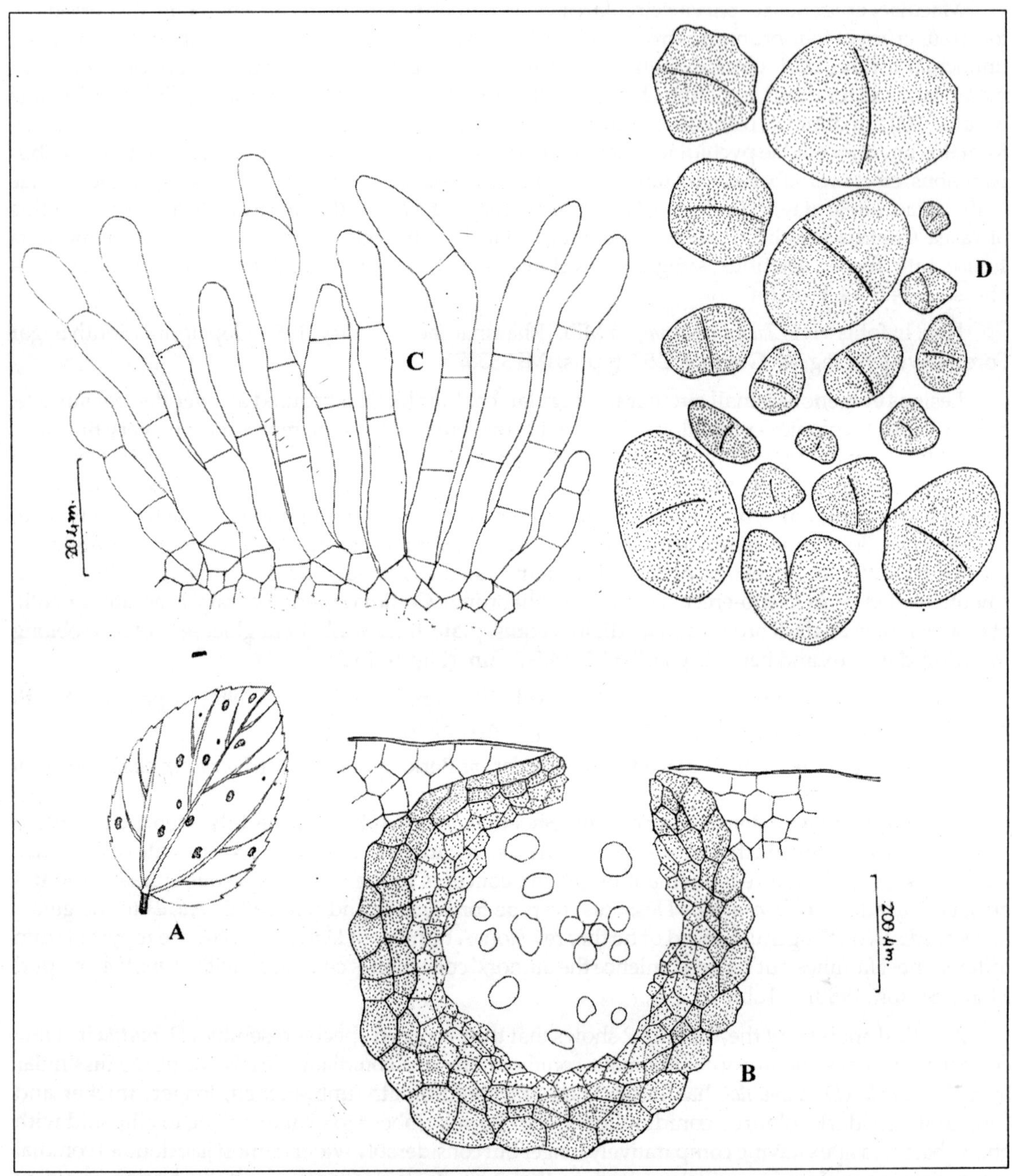

Figure 15.2: ***Diplodia zizyphiae*** **sp.nov.**

A: Symptom; B: Conidiomata; C: Conidiophores; D: Conidia

Table 15.2: Comparative Account *D. zizyphiae* sp. nov. with Related Species

Species	*Spot and Colonies*	*Conidiomata*			*Conidiophores*			*Conidia*		
		Structure	*Colour*	*Size (μm diam.)*	*Structure*	*Colour*	*Size (μm diam.)*	*Structure*	*Colour*	*Size (μm)*
D. mutila	–	Pycnidial, immersed, separated to aggregate, globose, unilocular, thick walled, single ostiole, papillate.	Dark brown to black	Upto 600	Cylindrical, branched, septate, smooth	Hyaline	45 x 3-5	Aseptate, centrally guttulate, thick walled, smooth, medianly 1 euseptate, apex obtuse and bases tr.	First hyaline then dark brown	27-31 x 12-13.5.
D. zizyphiae sp. nov.	Epigenous, circular to irregular, coaltar like, brownish black. Colonies epiphyllous black.	Pycnidial immersed to partly superficial, globose to subglobose, unilocular, thick walled, single ostiole	Dark brown	Upto 800	Cylindrical, unbranched, erect to sub erect, 1-3 trans. Septate, smooth.	Hyaline to light olivaceous	26-75 x 5-8.5.	Sub globose to oval to oblong to ellipsoid, aseptate but medianly 1 euseptate, thick walled, smooth, apex and base obtuse.	First hyaline then dark brown.	5-34.5 x 4.5-26.

Acknowledgements

The authors are grateful to the Director, International Mycological Institute, Kew, (U.K.) for the accession of the deposited fungal specimens and the Head, Department of Botany, Dr. H.S. Gour University, Sagar for providing facilities. The financial assistance from UGC Research Award Scheme to ANR is thankfully acknowledged.

References

Petrak, F. and Sydow, H. (1927). Die Gattungen der Pyrenomyzeten, Shaerospideen und Melanconieem. *Beih. Rep. Spec. nov. Regni Veg.*, 42: 1-551.

Sutton, B.C. (1980). *The Coelomycete.* Fungi Imperfecti with Pycnidia, Acervuli and Stromata. C.M.I., Kew, England.

Stevens, N.E. (1933). Two apple black rot fungi in the United States. *Mycologia*, 25: 536-548.

Shoemaker, R.A. (1964). Conidial state of some *Btryosphaeria* species on *Vitis and Quercus*. *Can. J. Bot.*, 42: 1297-1301.

Zambettakis, E.C. (1954). Recherches sur ia systematique des "Sphaeropsidales-Phaeodidymae". *Bull. Soc. Mycol. Fr.*, 70: 219-350.

Microbial Biotechnology and Ecology (2011) *Pages* **275–292**
Editors: Deepak Vyas, G.S. Paliwal, P.K.Khare and R.K Gupta
Published by: DAYA PUBLISHING HOUSE, NEW DELHI

Chapter 16

Current Status of Sesame and Niger Diseases and Their Management

☆ *Sushma Nema*[1], *T.S. Rajpurohit*[2] *and M.N. Khare*[3]

[1]*Senior Scientist, Plant Pathology, AICRP (S&N) JNKVV, Jabalpur*
[2]*Pathologist, Oilseeds (Rajasthan Agricultural University), Agricultural Research Station, Mandor, Jodhpur*
[3]*Ex. Dean and Professor Emeritus, Plant Pathology*

Both Sesame and Niger suffer due to diseases caused by fungi, bacteria, viruses, nematodes and phytoplasma making the host weak resulting in losses both in quantity and quality. The pathogens are both seed borne and soil borne. The important diseases of sesame are damping off (*Pythium aphanidermatum, Thielavia terricola var. minor*); foot rot (*Sclerotium rolfsii*); wilt (*Fusarium oxysporum* f. sp. *sesami*); root rot, stem rot, charcoal rot, blight, seedling rot [(*Rhizoctonia bataticola*) (*Macrophomina phaseolina*)]; Phytophthora blight (*Phytophthora nicotianae var. parasitica*); Alternaria blight (*Alternaria sesami*); Cercospora leaf spot (*Cercospora sesami* and *C. sesamicola*); Corynespora blight (*Corynespora cassicola*); Botryosphaeria blight (*Botryosphaeria ribis*); *Cylinderosporium* leaf spot (*Cylinderosporium sesami*); anthracnose (*Colletotrichum* sp.); powdery mildew (*Leveillula taurica, Oidium* sp., *Sphaerotheca fuliginea*); Phoma leaf blight, blight, stem black (*Phoma sesamina, P. variosporeae*); bacterial leaf spot (*Pseudomonas syringae pv. sesami*); bacterial blight (*Xanthomonas campestris pv. sesami*) Leaf curl (*Nicotiana virus* 10); Phyllody (Phytoplasma) etc. Several other microorganisms have also been found associated with sesame seeds.

The incidence of important diseases vary from state to state based on agroclimatic situations. The diseases of sesame and Niger and their management are summarised below:

Diseases of Sesame

Fungal Diseases

About 72 fungi are responsible for causing diseases in sesame. Several such fungi have been observed associated with seed and soil which play a vital role in disease cycle.

Damping Off [*Pythium aphanidermatum* (Eds.) *Fitz.; Thielavia terricola* var. *minor* Rayss and Borut.]

Damping off of seedlings is important under high soil moisture both at pre and post emergence. The radicle and plumule get infected before emergence and no seedlings are formed. At post-emergence stage, the stem close to the soil becomes water soaked, shrinks, rots and the seedling topples down. The pathogens are soil borne *T. terricola* also causes root rot.

Foot Rot (*Sclerotium rolfsii* Sacc.)

Mishra and Khare (1970) first reported the disease from Jabalpur. The disease has been observed at different sesame growing areas. The basal part of the stem develops brown to black lesion due to necrosis of tissues. The affected stem shrivels and the plant dies. White mycelium is seen around the diseased part which develops mustard like sclerotia. The disease is severe under high humidity and high temperature. Leaf infection has also been observed.

Wilt [*Fusarium oxysporum f. sp. sesami (Zapro.) Castellani*]

The disease was first reported by Butler (1918). The disease is common in all the sesame growing areas. Loss upto 20 per cent has been observed due to wilt. As the diseased plants die before maturity heavy losses are possible. The leaves of diseased plants turn yellowish, droop down and dry. The vascular bundles turn brown and this brown discolouration starts from roots and gets extended upto the tip.

The fungus is soil borne as well as seed borne. The seed borne inoculum leads to infection of seedling at very early stage, resulting in mortality, depending upon the inoculum potential. The soil borne inoculum attacks and enters through finer roots.

Root Rot, Stem Rot, Charcoal Rot, Blight, Seedling Rot (*Macrophomina phaseolina* (Maubl.) Ashby (Pycnidial stage); *Rhizoctonia bataticola* Taub. Butler) (Mycelial and Sclerotial Stage)

These diseases are very important as infection occurs from seed germination and emergence to adult plant stage. The losses incurred are even upto 100 per cent. Murugesan *et al.* (1978) observed 1.8 kg yield loss per hectare at every one per cent increase in disease intensity. *M. phaseolina* causes seedling rot, stalk rot, root rot, charcoal rot and blight in sesame (Ali Ahmad and Saidawi, 1998). It is of major importance in West Bengal (Anonymous, 2001). The infected seeds are discoloured, on germination, seed rot occurs or the seedlings get damaged and dry. Brown dark spots develop on the stem which turn into lesions. The stem breaks. A number of pycnidia are formed in the lesion on the stem. Sclerotia develop in the tissues of diseased root and stem. On splitting it appears as if charcoal powder has bean sprinkled on the tissues, hence the disease is called charcoal rot. Black spots of various sizes are formed on the leaves which coalesce. The infected leaves are dropped off. Similar spots are also formed on capsules and sclerotia as well as pycnidia develop on them. Blackish hyphae are seen on the seed surface, associated with seed coat.

The pathogen is both seed and soil borne. The sclerotia survive for many years in soil. The seed borne infection is both externally and internally associated. Soil and seed borne inoculum is responsible for recurrence of the disease and seed borne inoculum helps in long distance transmission. The spread of the disease is through movement of workers, animals, water and equipments used in cultural management in the field. Seed to plant infection is systemic as well as local through seed borne inoculum and infected inert matter. Plant to seed transmission is through capsule. The pathogen has a very wide host range. High temperature and humidity favour the disease development. Phosphorus in soil checks the disease severity. Appressoria formation has bean observed on the epidermis of infected seedlings which helped the mechanical and chemical penetration. The hyphae extend inter and intracellularly from roots to stem, fruits and seeds. Gupta (1992) negatively correlated the production of volatile aldehyde compounds with the extent of seed infection. The infection of sesame plants was positively correlated with percentage of infected seeds. Singh and Singh (1990) examined sesame seed samples from 18 districts of Rajasthan and found 108 samples to be infected with 1-67 per cent incidence. Microsclerotia of the pathogen were present in the seed. Gupta and Cheema (1990) positively correlated the number of microsclerotia on sesame seeds with plant infection and negatively with seed germination, dry matter production and root and shoot length of seedlings. Kushi and Khare (1979) examined several seed samples of 21 sesame varieties and found 17 fungi associated of which *M. phaseolina* was the most important along with *Corynespora cossicola* and *A. sesami*. Karunanithi *et al.* (1999) established three groups of *M. phaseolina* isolates based on colony characters and virulence.

Phytophthora Blight (*Phytophthora nicotianae var. parasitica* Dastur)

The disease was first observed by Dastur in India. It is the most serious disease in northen India described by Butler (1918). High humidity and heavy rains increase the disease severity resulting in even 80 per cent seedling mortality (Singh *et al.*, 1976). The plants get diseased at all stages of crop growth. The disease starts from the base of the plants and gradually moves up covering the stem which turns black; Infloresence, flowers and fruits are also attacked by the fungus. The first symptom of the disease appears as brown, water soaked spots on leaves and seedlings in very early stage. In old plant, leaves develop water soaked spots which coalesce and give blight appearance. Many times the disease is so severe that nothing is left in the field if attack is at seedling stage and continuous rains occur for about a week. The partially affected plants produce shrivelled smaller seeds with brown discolourations, severely infected plants dry up.

The pathogen survives in soil during unfavourable period in the form of dormant mycelium and or in the form of chlamydospores/oospores. It is seed borne, the mycelium remains in embryo. The recurrence of the disease is through these two sources. Once the plants are attacked, sporangia are produced by the mycelium which spread the disease. Zoospores are formed in the sporangium, which are oozed out and infect the host plants. High humidity and 28-30°C temperatures favour the disease spread. Heavy soil and severe rains are responsible for high disease intensity low lying fields with poor or no drainage get the disease with very high severity.

The disease is both seed and soil borne, hence effective sanitation, rotation with other suitable crops and seed treatment are essential. Resistant sources are also available. In Sri Lanka, Pathirana (1992) obtained a high yielding mutant tolerant to Phytophthora blight by Gamma irradiation of 450 and 600 Gy.

Alternaria Blight (*Alternaria sesami* Zimm.)

The disease was first reported by Mohanti and Behera (1958) in Orissa, now the disease is prevalent in all sesame growing states in the country. Both typical leaf spot and blight symptoms are produced by the fungus. Losses upto 50 per cent have been reported due to this disease. The disease occurs at all the stages of crop growth however, Ojiambo *et al.* (1999) observed the plants to be least susceptible at 4 weeks and most susceptible at 8-10 weeks age. Dark brown spots develop on cotyledons. Water soaked, circular or irregular brown spots develop on leaf. Brown stripes are formed on stem. Capsules are also infected resulting in seed infection.

The pathogen is seed borne and the fungus survives in seed coat as well as in embryo. The recurrence of the disease is due to this inoculum. The cotyledons are infected on which conidia are produced which attack the foliage of other plants through air and the disease gets spread. The pathogen also survives in crop residues in soil and helps in disease recurrence. Temperature 20-30°C and pH 5-7 favour the disease development. *A. sesami* produced PGTE, PTE, PG enzymes in vitro (Rajpurohit and Prasad, 1982). Cultural studies *viz:* effect of different media, temperature, level of pH, Effect of Carbon and Nitrogen on growth and sporulation of *A. sesami* were carried out in detail (Rajpurohit and Prasad, 1982; Rajpurohit *et al.*, 1983). The possibility of races has been expected by some workers. A description of morphology and taxonomy of Sesamum Alternaria given by Rajpurohit (1981).

For the detection of *A. sesami* associated with seed, oat meal agar medium is the best. The seed infection has been observed from 9 to 25 per cent. Seed to plant transmission of the pathogen is important as 8 per cent infected seeds resulting in high incidence of the disease in field. According to Ojiambo *et al.* (2000) the tolerance level should be less than 2 per cent. In Karnataka it causes yield loss of 0.1 to 5.7 g seed per 100 capsules (Siddaramaiah, 1981). Seed infection reduces viability of seeds.

Rao and Vijayalakshmi (2000) tested nutritional requirements of *A . sesami* and its ability to produce phytotoxic and antibacterial metabolites. Chloroform extracts of the fungus exhibited antibacterial activity. The culture filtrate contained tenuazonic acid.

The pathogen survives in seeds as well as in soil on residues for more than one year as mycelium or chlamydospores. Excessive rainfall favours occurrence and spread of the disease (Maiti *et al.*, 1988) Cumulative rains, rainy days and relative humidity for many days positively correlated whereas maximum and minimum temperature had negative co-relation with Alternaria leaf spot (Naik *et al.*, 2003). The time of plant to seed infection has been determined by Ojiambo *et al.* (1999) in Kenya, which was maximum in plants inoculated between 8–10 weeks age and least when inoculated at 4, 6 and 12 weeks age.

Cercospora Leaf Spot (*Cercospora sesami* Zimm. and *C. sesamicola*)

The disease is prevalent in all sesame-growing areas but more severe and important in Madhya Pradesh, Uttar Pradesh, Orissa, Tamil Nadu and Karnataka. Losses upto 60 per cent have been reported due to the disease. *C. sesami* produces conidia which attack both the sides of leaves by forming water soaked spots which later become circular or irregular. Initially the leaf spots are whitish to light brown, later turning dark brown. The leaf spots coalesce and occupy a large area of lamina giving blight appearance. The infected leaves dry and drop off. The disease spread to petioles, stem and pods on which linear, dark coloured, deep-seated lesions are formed. *C. sesamicola* produces brown angular spots (Mohanti, 1958).

The pathogen is both seed and soil borne survives in the plant debris in soil as well as in and on seed for more than one year and acts as primary inoculum in the recurrence of the disease. The secondary invasion or spread of the pathogen is through conidia from plant to plant and field to field by wind. Plant to seed infection is through capsule.

Corynespora Blight [*Corynespora cassiicola* (Berk. and Curt.) Wei]

The disease was first observed at Bhubaneshwar. It has been reported from different sesame growing areas in this country. All the plant parts except root are attacked but stem and leaves are badly affected. On leaves brown specks are formed which later turn into large spots. At advanced stage of infection the leaves curl and drop off. On stem, purple brown specks develop which turn into elongated, scattered, irregular lesions, which enlarge at both the ends. Lesions turn into canker with straw coloured central area surrounded by dark brown margin. The infected stem bends and cracks. When both stem and leaves get infected plant dies prematurely. On capsules circular to elongate, minute, sunken, black spots develop which cover the whole surface. The infected seeds turn brown and become light. The disease reduces the yield. Low temperature and high humidity favour the disease development.

The pathogen is seed and soil borne. It is internally and externally seed borne. The fungus survives in soil in infected crop residues. Both the sources are responsible for recurrence of the disease. The spread occurs through conidia formed after the primary inoculum infects plants, gets established and produces conidia. The pathogen has several other hosts like pulses, tomato etc. also on which it causes diseases, survives and attacks sesame. *C. cassicola* is highly seed borne. In seed stored at 26± 2°C and 50 per cent RH, the infection decreased from 89.8 to 8 per cent in seven months and in ten months the fungus was fully inactive (Navas and Subero, 1995).

Botryosphaeria Blight [*Botryosphaeria ribis* (Gross) Duggar]

The disease was first observed by Shukla and Vyas (1977) at Jabalpur. The disease appears towards crop maturity and causes heavy losses in yield. All above ground plant parts are infected and brownish specks are formed which later become irregular lesions. They coalesce and enlarge 2-25 mm in length. On leaves the infection starts from the margin, the spots are brown but later the central part turns black. The spots even cover the whole leaf. On capsules small, black sunken spots appear which increase under high humidity and temperature. The seeds inside the capsule get infected and turn brown.

The disease is both soil borne and seed borne. The pathogen survives on diseased plant refuge in soil and is associated with seed externally and internally. These sources act as primary inoculum for recurrence of the disease. Ascospores and conidia formed on diseased parts spread the disease through air.

Cylindrosporium Leaf Spot (*Cylindrosporium sesami* Hansford)

The disease has been reported in 1965 from Gujarat. Water soaked spots are formed on leaves which later become darker and angular limited by veins. Necrosis occurs. Black acervuli of the fungus are formed on the upper surface in these spots and conidia are formed in large number. For the growth of the fungus 27°C temperature is the best. Sclerotia are formed which get mixed with the seed as inert matter and are responsible for recurrence of the disease alongwith those present in the infected crop residues in soil. The spread of the disease is through conidia formed on infected plant parts of the standing crop.

Anthracnose (*Colletotrichum* sp.)

Anthracnose has been reported from several sesame growing countries. In India, it was first reported from Uttar Pradesh in 1953. Infection occurs at all stages of crop growth and all the above ground parts attacked. Water soaked spots appear which turn brown and enlarge irregularly. The margins are dark brown. Black acervuli develop on the diseased portions. Stem also develops symptoms. The cortex is separated and woody part gets exposed. The infected plants dry. Capsules are either not formed on diseased plants or they are very few. The pathogen is seed borne and also survives in infected plant parts in soil and they help in recurrence of the disease. The spread is through conidia.

Powdery Mildew (*Leveillula taurica, Oidium* sp., *Sphaerotheca fuliginia*)

Powdery mildew is an important in all the sesame growing areas. The disease is severe under dry conditions. Small circular areas with whitish powder appear on leaves, later stem, leaves and capsules get fully covered with whitish powdery mass. The leaves start drying and fall off. The seeds produced from diseased plants are small and wrinkled. The disease is not seed borne. The pathogen has a wide host range and is always present in nature.

Rajpurohit (1993) has reported powdery mildew caused by *Erysiphe orontii* from Rajasthan. Ganesh *et al.* (1992) have found *Erysiphe cichoracearum* D.C. to be the casual fungus of powdery mildew in Tamil Nadu.

Phoma Leaf Blight and Black Stem (*Phoma sesamina* Sacc., *Phoma variosporeae* Shreemali)

Shreemali (1978) has reported *P. variosporeae* and *P. sesamina* from various places in India. The ashy spots surrounded by brown margin are formed on the leaf margins, which later cover entire leaf. The stem also develop similar symptoms. Black pycnidia are formed on the infected portions.

Bacterial

Bacterial Leaf Spot (*Pseudomonas syringae* pv. *sesami* Malkoff.)

The disease occurs in all the sesame growing areas of the world. In India the disease was first reported by Durgapal and Rao (1967) and is prevalent in Rajasthan, Uttar Pradesh, Madhya Pradesh, Tamil Nadu, Andhra Pradesh etc. The disease is also called black rot. The pathogen is seed borne. The pathogen has two physiological races. The most suited temperature for the growth is 30°C. Seed to plant transmission of the pathogen is systemic as well as local. Stomata and wounds are the entry points for the bacterium in disease spread. High temperature and frequent rain showers favour the disease development.

The crop is attacked at all stages of crop growth but it is more devastating at seedling stage. The disease starts from petiole, moves to leaf blade and small angular brown to black spots with dark margins are formed. They are confined by the veins. Bacterial exudates can be observed on the lower surface of the leaf. Under high humidity and temperature, the spots increase and coalesce. The diseased leaves drop off. On stem, black lesions are formed which girdle the whole stem and the plant dies. The capsules become black and seeds are not formed in them, but seeds, are formed in partially infected capsules which are discarded. The pathogen is internally and externally seed borne. Pandya *et al.* (2000) observed a decrease in N,P,K, Ca and increase in Mg content in infected leaves as disease intensity increased.

Bacterial Blight (*Xanthomonas campestris* pv. *sesami* Sabet and Dowson)

Sabet and Dowson (1960) reported the disease from Sudan first. At Jabalpur 10-25 per cent plants were found diseased in local and exotic varieties. The pathogen is highly seed borne and the recurrence of the disease is through infected seeds. The seed to plant transmission is both systemic and local. The spread of the disease is through air borne inoculum and rain splashes.

When infected seeds are sown, the colyledonary leaves exhibit small water soaked spots on the lower surface. These spots turn black. Under severe infection, the cotyledons dry and drop off. Typical dark brown to black angular spots appear on leaves which coalesce and give blight appearance. Bacterial ooze comes out from the affected parts under favourable conditions. Stem is also infected forming chlorotic spots which later turn dark brown and exude bacterial ooze. Capsules also develop redish brown raised spots (Wasnikar *et al.*, 1991). The bacterium also attacks certain weeds on which it survives till next season. Younger leaves are more susceptible. High humidity and 20-26°C temperature favour the disease. Higher dose of N increases the disease severity. Poor seed germination and damping off have been observed in Assam due to the bacterium by Phookan and Hazarika (1994).

Viral

Leaf Curl (Nicotiana Virus 10)

Leaf curl is a very harmful disease of sesame occurring in many sesame growing countries and sesame growing regions in India. As the diseased plant dies before flowering, 60-100 per cent losses have been observed. The virus has several hosts like tomato, tobacco, papaya etc. and is transmitted by white fly (*Bemisia tabaci* Gen.) hence the recurrence and spread of the disease take place through white fly obtaining the virus from such sources.

MLO

Phyllody (*Mycoplasma Like Organism- Phytoplasma*)

Phyllody is one of the most serious and wide spread disease of sesame and occurs in sesame growing states, Rajasthan, Madhya Pradesh, Tamil Nadu, Orissa, Maharashtra, Uttar Pradesh, Gujarat, Andhra Pradesh, Haryana, Punjab every year. The disease incidence ranges 1 to 100 per cent. Considerable losses are caused due to the disease. The disease was earlier considered to be due to physiological and genetic disorder, then due to virus and finally MLO. Murugesan *et al.* (1978) reported 8.36 kg/ha loss in yield on each one per cent increase in disease incidence. No capsules are formed on severely infected plants.

The disease symptoms of phyllody get manifested at flowering which get changed in leafy structures with abundant vegetative growth. Petals enlarge and turn green. The filaments of stamens are flattened and become green. Anthers also turn green and have no functional pollen. Ovules in the ovary get small petiole like growth. The diseased plants develop more branches with smaller leaves with clear veins.

The disease is transmitted by leaf hopper *Orosius albicinctus*, it has 15-23 day incubation period. The MLO survives in the leaf hopper throughout its life. It attacks various crops as well as weeds (82 plant species) throughout the year and is transmitted to sesame plant as the leaf hopper is also present. The MLO is transmitted fast by the leaf hopper at 25-40°C. Increased Indole Acetic Acid (IAA) due to infection is responsible for proliferation of vegetative and reproductive parts.

Application of N (15-45 kg/ha) imparted resistance to phyllody when coupled with medium dosage of P (15-30 kg/ha) (Borkar and Krishna, 2000).

Other Diseases

Besides above diseases, there are many other diseases which are not of great importance at present but close eye is needed so that they do not become limiting factor in sesame production.

Choanophora Wet Rot (*Choanephora cucurbitarum* Thax.)

The disease becomes severe in heavy rains. Small water soaked spots are formed on leaves which coalesce. Under high humidity whitish hyphae cover the diseased parts.

Drechslera Blight [*Drechslera sesami* (Miyake) Richa and Frasier]

The disease is prevalent in all the sesame growing areas. Small brownish elongated spots (0.2 × 2.0 cm) are formed on leaves and (1x4 cm) on stem. Capsules are also infected in which the seeds get spoiled. The spots are of V shape and later give blight appearance. *D. sesami* is seed borne.

Myrothecium Leaf Spot (*Myrothecium roridum* Tode ex Fries)

Small light brown circular spots are formed with darker margin and ashy central portion. Black spordochia are formed in the centre of the spot. The diseased portion is blown off by wind and shot hole symptoms develop. The pathogen is seed borne.

Synchytrium Gall Disease (*Synchytrium sesamicola*)

The disease has been reported from Bihar and Uttar Pradesh. Galls are formed due to hypertrophied host tissues.

Cyst Nematode Disease (*Heterodera* sp.)

The diseased plants remain stunted and roots do not develop fully. Capsules are either not formed or if formed, they remain small with small shrivelled seeds. The disease was first reported from Rajasthan.

Seed-borne Microorganisms

Several scientists (Kushi and Khare, 1979; Singh and Singh, 1990; Mahatma *et al.*, 2001) have examined the sesame seeds of different varieties and locations and observed the following fungi and bacteria associated with seeds. They are internally seed borne, externally seed borne, extraembryal, intraembryal, concomitant contaminant, mixed with the seed as inert matter or associated with inert matter *viz.*

Alternaria alternata, A. longissima, A. sesami, A. sesamicola, Aspergillus flavus, A. niger, A. ochraceus, A. tamarii, A. terreus, Beltrama rhombica, Botrytis cinerea, Cercospora sesami, C. sesamicola, Chaetomium globosum, Cladosporium herbarum, Colletotrichum dematium, Corynespora cassicola, Curvularia lunata, Cylindrosporium sesami, Drechslera hawaiensis, D.sesami, Epicocum nigram, Fusarium moniliforme, F. oxysporum, F.semitectum, F.solani, Macrophomina phaseolina, Mucar haematis, Myrothecium roridum, Penicillium chrysogenum, P. citrinum, P. purpurogenum, Phoma sp., Phytophthora parasitica, Pleospora infectoria, Pseudomonas syringae, Rhizopus nigricans, R. oryzae, R. stolonifer, Setophaeria sp., *Stemphylium* sp., *Syncephalasturm racemosum, Trichoderma hamatum, T. viride, Ulocladium* sp., *Xanthomonas campestris* etc.

Management

Cultural Practices

It is necessary to follow suitable phytosanitary measures, crop rotations in endemic areas, proper date of planting, integrated fertilizer management, application of required micro nutrients, desired plant population, removal of weeds etc. Sesame grown as mixed or inter cropped with moth bear or green gram 1:1 gave less incidence of Macrophomina stem and root rot of sesame (Rajpurohit, 2003).

Chemical Control

Seed treatment with suitable chemicals like Thiram (3g/kg), Bavistin (2g/kg), Captan (3g/kg), Thiram + Bavistin (2g + 1g) should be done before planting (Rajpurohit, 2005). Foliar fungal diseases can be checked by the spray of Mancozeb (0.2 per cent), Zineb (0.2 per cent), Copper oxychloride (0.2 per cent). Soil treatment with Benlate or Rizolax-T (0.04-0.1 per cent) has been recommended (Gabr *et al.*, 1998). Powdery mildew can be checked by spraying sulfex (0.3 per cent) (Rajpurohit, 1993). Efficacy of plant product and new chemicals against *A. sesami* reported by Rajpurohit (2004).

To control bacterial diseases seed, treatment with Streptocycline (250-1000 ppm) is recommended. For hot water treatment, seeds are dipped in water at 51°C for 10 minutes then dipped for 6-9 hours in water having 0.025 per cent Agrimycin 100. The foliar infection can be checked by spraying streptocycline.

For the control of leaf curl white fly needs to be checked by the application of 0.1 per cent metasystox as spray or any other suitable insecticide. Foliar spray of Mancozeb + Methyl demeton reduced Alternaria blight, Phyllody and leaf curl diseases of sesame (Rajpurohit, 2004). Spray of 0.05 per cent. Dimethoate, Fenthion and Monocrotophos has been recommended to control *Orosius albicinctus* the transmitting insect of phyllody MLO. Soil application of Phorate granules 11kg/ha combined with 0.03 per cent Dimethoate spray checks the disease. Management of Macrophomina stem and root rot through fungicidal seed treatment and varietal resistance reported by Rajpurohit (1997).

Integrated Disease Management

Integrated disease management module comprised seed treatment with Thiram 0.2 per cent + Carbendazim 50 WP 0.1 per cent + foliar spray of Mancozeb 0.2 per cent + Endosulfan 0.07 per cent at 30-45 DAS and 45-55 DAS reduced Macrophomina stem and root rot from 24.54 to 11.93 per cent, Alternaria leaf spot 41.73 to 10.76 per cent, Phyllody from 3.20 to 0.64 per cent, Leaf curl 3.3 to 0.47 per cent. This module recorded seed yield of 693 kg/ha with 2.92 BC ratio (Rajpurohit and Bishnoi, 2004).

Biological Control

Three isolates of *Bacillus subtilis* suppressed wilt and root rot diseases when applied in artificially infested soil (Gabr *et al.*, 1998). Seed treatment with *Trichoderma viride* (0.4 per cent) was effective in checking *M. phaseolina* (Rajpurohit, 1995). Application of phosphorus solublizing bacteria (PSB) alongwith neem cake or 50 per cent NPK + FYM or NPK + PSB reduced phytopthora blight (Verma and Bajpai, 2001).

From the experiments conducted under All India Coordinated Project on Sesame during the last three years, it was inferred that seed treatment with *T. viride* or *T. harzianum* (0.4 per cent) and Carbendazim 25 SD (0.25 per cent) + Thiram (0.15 per cent) minimized the incidence of Macrophomina stem and root rot; Seed treatment with *Pseudmonas fluorescens* (0.4 per cent) and Contaf (0.05 per cent) effectively managed Cercospora leaf spot incidence (Anonymous, 2001). Soil amendment with neem cake @ 500 kg/ha+ seed treatment with *I. viride* (0.47 per cent) + soil application of *T. viride* @ 2.5 kg/ha was found highly effective for the management of soil borne diseases.

Resistance

Resistance source is the most important to control the diseases. Selim *et al.* (1976a) have reported susceptibility in mature plants to *M. phaseolina* to be dominant over tolerance, controlled by 1, 2 or 3 pairs of genes. Selim *et al.* (1976 b) have reported that in mature plants the tolerance to wilt (*F. oxysporium* f. sp. *sesami*) is governed by 1 or 2 dominant pairs of genes and in one cross it was governed by 3 pairs of genes. Tolerance was recessive. The resistance to powdery mildew (*Erysiphe cichoracearum*) is controlled by two major complimentary genes (Krishnaswami *et al.*, 1983). Mishra *et al.* (1994) while studying the inheritance of leaf curl disease observed both additive × additive and/or additive x dominance types of gene interaction. The resistance to phyllody disease in *Sesame alatum* is due to insect resistance (Parani *et al.*, 1996). The available genotypes resistant to single disease is given in Table 16.1 and to multiple diseases in Table 16.2.

Abd El, Moneem *et al.* (1997) evaluated 112 somaclones obtained from epicotyl segments of variety Giza 25 grown in tissue culture. S_2 clones had higher resistance to root rot, charcoal rot and wilt diseases. The resistance is attributed to increased contents of either peroxidase or phenolic compounds in roots.

Table 16.1: Varieties/Lines of Sesame Resistant to Different Diseases

Disease	*Resistant Varieties/Lines*	*Reference*
Wilt	JT-7, N-32, MB-12	Vyas *et al.* (1981)
Macrophomina diseases	AT-9, HT-16, RT-46, ST-58, Gwalior-5, ES-25, ES-105, ES-124, IS-156, IS-190	Gupta (1995)
	Line-144, 885,	Saharan and Chand (1988)
	BAG-59, 21, 65, 9, 5, 11	Li *et al.* (1991)
	RT-46, JTS-8, SI-249, SI-254-1	Arriel *et al.* (1998)
	EC-370932, EC-370929, EC-351832, ES379-3-84, IS-97, IS-100 B, IS-646-1	Anonymous (2001) Rajpurohit *et al.* (2003)
Phytophthora blight	75A/1-1/2-1	Gemawat and Prasad (1964)
	M-3-1, M-3-2, No.2-39, No.66-193	Saharan and Chand (1988)
	Spring borok	Sasikumar and Sardana (1988)
Alternaria blight	No.-2, No.-4, J-77, E-8	Saharan and Chand (1988)
	EC-370929, EC-370932	Rajpurohit and Solanki (2002)
Cercospora leaf spot	IS-4, 14, 15, 21, 29, No.-41, No.-41A, No.-41B, No-128, No.128A	Kushwaha and Kaushal (1970), Vyas *et al.* (1981)
	L-36, L-45, RSB-1, HT-1, SI-2373, SI-1501, SI-1032, X-79-6, TMV-6, S-1683,	Saharan and Chand (1988)
	BIC-7-2, Sidhi-54, Rewa-114, Seoni Malwa	Tripathi *et al.* (1994)
	65B58, 60/2/3-1-8B, 69B-392, 73A-96B	Poswal and Misari (1994)
Powdery mildew	CO-1, BS-129, BS-518-6G, X-74-24, SI-3170, 59-1-1, IS-401	Ganesh *et al.* (1992) Shadakshari *et al.* (1981)
	OMT 30 and DORS 101	Rajpurohit (1993)
Synchytrium gall	JT-66-276, SP-70-23	Variar *et al.* (1981)
Bacterial leaf spot	Maporal, Ajimo Atar S-5, Morada, Almora white, C-24, C-87, C-96, M-31, NP-8, NP-23, Punjab-1, SSM-34, SSM-44, SSM-49, EC-4094, EC-13536, EC-14536, EC-20783, EC-20785, EC-20787, N-63-177-74-145, TC-325, T-58	Urdaneta and Mazzani (1976) Duragapal *et al.* (1969)
Bacterial blight	T-58	Saharan and Chand (1988)
	Tozi-3, S-76F2-22, K-112	Abdal Rahim and Adam (1990)
Phyllody	RT-46, RT-54, RT-103, RT-125, VRI-1	Anonymous (2001)

Diseases of Niger and their Management

Niger is a crop of dry areas grown mostly by tribals in interior places due to which desired attention has not been given on the biotic and abiotic stresses. Now the crop is gaining importance and studies are being made on disease aspects. The diseases observed are given herewith. The important diseases of niger are ozonium wilt (*Ozonium texanum* var. *parasiticum*); collar rot (*Sclerotium rolfsii*); Macrophomina rot and blight (*Macrophomina phaseolina*); Cercospora leaf spot (*Cercospora guizoticola*), powdery mildew (*Sphaerotheca* sp.); rust (*Puccinia guizotiae*); Bacterial leaf spot (*X. campestris pv guizotiae*) and Cuscuta as *Phanerogamic* parasite.

Table 16.2: Sesame Varieties/Lines Resistant to Multiple Diseases

Disease	*Resistant Varieties/Lines*	*Reference*
Phyllody + wilt	Mulayanum	Mehetre *et al.* (1994)
Powdery mildew + Bacterial leaf spot	ES-277	Shadakshari *et al.* (1989)
Phytophthora blight + Alternaria blight	Suwonkkae	Lee *et al.* (1992)
Phytophthora blight + Alternaria blight + Cercospora blight	Sesame radiatum	Malaguti (1973)
Fusarium wilt + Macrophomina rot + Rhizoctonia solani root rot	87-AN, Golmarmara, Muganli, Ozberk-82, 9/10-1-2, 1/10-2-1	Alac *et al.* (1994)
Powdery mildew + Bacterial wilt + Cercospora blight + Fusarium stem rot	RAU-8817-4, CO-1, AT-6	Ram *et al.* (1995)
Macrophomina rot + Bacterial spot + Phyllody + Powdery mildew	Rajeshwari	Gangakishan *et al.* (1989)

Ozonium Wilt (*Ozonium texanum* var. *parasiticum* Thirum.)

The disease was reported by Rao and Pavgi (1975) around Varanasi where it appeared in great severity. Heavy losses are incurred as the diseased plants dry. Necrotic lesions develop on stem of well grown plants near the soil level, which gradually extend upwards. Whitish fungal mycelium grows on these necrotic areas under high humidity. The branches, leaves, inflorescence etc. become soft and start rotting. The diseased stem breaks. The mycelium grows on dead plants if enough moisture is present. Root rot is also commonly observed.The fungus forms rhizomorphs and sclerotia. The sclerotia are oval, grey to dark brown. The recurrence takes place through soil borne sclerotia and mycelium.

Collar Rot (*Sclerotium rolfsii* Sacc.)

The disease was first reported from Dharwad (Karnataka) by Siddarmaiah *et al.* (1979). The tissues of collar region become soft and depressed. White fungus grows on the diseased part and forms mustard seed like sclerotia. The diseased plants turn yellow and dry. The perfect stage of the fungus is *Corticium rolfsii*. The disease is soil borne. As the plant number is reduced, the disease causes yield losses.

Macrophomina Rot and Blight [*Macrophomina phaseolina* (Maubl.) Ashby]

The sclerotial stage of the fungus is *Rhizoctonia bataticola*. It is seed and soil borne. Typical root rot, stem rot, charcoal rot, leaf blight symptoms are produced. The recurrence of the disease takes place through seed and soil borne inoculum, later spread is through workers, tools and insects like *Melanoagromyza* stem borer.

Damping Off, Root Rot (*Rhizoctonia solani*)

The fungus attacks stem of the seedling at ground level and makes it water soaked soft and incapable of supporting the seedling, which falls over and dies. On older seedling elongated brownish black lesions appear which increase in length and width girdling the stem often the roots are blackened due to the fungal attack resulting in root rot. The disease is favoured by cold and wet weather.

Cercospora Leaf Spot (*Cercospora guizoticola*)

The disease was reported by Rao (1962). This disease is prevalent in all the niger growing areas and caused yield reduction. The disease is severe under warm and humid weather. Small straw coloured to brownish spots are formed on both the leaf surfaces. Later the spots increase in number and size and cover the entire lamina and the leaves start dropping off. Elongated dark brown spots are produced on the stem. The capsules are also affected.

The pathogen is seed and soil borne. The primary infection occurs through seed borne inoculum as well as the inoculum present on diseased plant left over in the soil. The spread of the disease is through conidia formed on infected plant parts. The fungus is active throughout the year where niger is grown in *rabi* and *kharif* seasons. The pathogen remains active on other collateral hosts also.

Alternaria Leaf Spot (*Alternaria* sp.)

Spots are brown to blackish, with grey centre circular to irregular with concentric rings on leaf. If floral buds are affected, they become black and fails to open. The pathogen is seed and soil borne.

Curvularia Leaf Spot (*Curvularia lunata*)

Small circular to irregular brown to reddish brown spots are formed on leaves, which later coalesce to form larger spots. The leaf turn yellow, dries and defoliates. The pathogen is seed borne and survives in plant debris.

Powdery Mildew (*Sphaerotheca* sp.)

The disease occurs in *rabi* as well as *kharif* season but it is more severe in *rabi*. The yield loses are due to early defoliation as a result of the disease. All the aerial parts may be affected. Small cottony spot develops on the leaves, which gradually covers the whole lamina. The diseased leaves turn yellow and drop off. The seed formed on diseased plants are small and shrivelled.

Rust (*Puccinia guizotiae*)

Rust was first reported from Ethiopia (Yirgu, 1964 a). Brown coloured pustules are formed on the lower leaf surface and the corresponding upper surface becomes chlorotic. Later teletospores are formed.

Bacterial Leaf Spot (*Xanthomonas campestris* pv. *guizotiae*)

This disease was first reported from Ethiopia by Yirgu (1946 b). Small brownish spots are formed on leaves which are surrounded by yellow halo. Most of the spots are on the leaf margin. The spots increase, coalesce and give appearance of blight. Under severe condition all the leaves get destroyed.

Cuscuta (*Cuscuta hyalina* and *C. chinensis*)

Cuscuta, a phaneroganic plant parasite has been observed to attack Niger badly. The plants remain stunted, pale yellow and bear a very small number of flowers and capitula due to the association of Cuscuta. It is a total stem parasite depending for shelter and food totally on the host. The food is obtained through haustoria from the host. Usually the Cuscuta seed gets mixed with Niger seed and such mixtures are planted. The Cuscuta seeds can be removed by sieving.

Seed Borne Microorganisms

Several fungi have been reported seed borne like *Alternaria* sp., *Aspergillus flavus*, *A. niger*, *Rhizopus nigracans*, *Cercospora guizoticola*, *M. phaseolina*, *R. batalicola* etc. (Siddarmaiah *et al.*, 1980 a, b). Besides fungi, bacteria like *Xanthomonas campestris* are also seed borne.

Management

(i) Cultural Practices

Sl.No.	Practice	Diseases Managed
1.	Pathogen free site	All diseases
2.	Deep ploughing in summer	Collar rot, root rot, wilt
3.	Pathogen free seed	Seed borne diseases
4.	Manipulation in planting	
	(a) Shallow planting (1")	Diseases caused by *Rhizoctonia solani* and *R.bataticola*
	(b) Space Planting 30 x 10 cm (3 lakh plants/ha)	– do –
5.	Irrigation whenever necessary to avoid stress condition	*Rhizoctonia bataticola*
6.	Mixed cropping with Kodo, Kutki, Mung	*Cercospora, Curvularia, Alternaria* leaf spot, powdery mildew and rust
7.	Hot water treatment at 52° for 10 minutes	Bacterial leaf spot
8.	Proper and timely rouging, uprooting and destruction of diseased plant	Root rot, collar rot, phyllody
9.	Clean cultivation, destruction of collateral host plant debris	All diseases
10.	Sieving of seed before sowing	Cuscuta
11.	Removal of Cuscuta infested niger seedlings	Cuscuta

(ii) Use of Resistant Varieties

Variety	Resistant to	
	Alternaria Leaf Spot	Cuscuta
IGP-76	+	-
Deomali	+	-
GA-11	+	-
ONS-8	+	+ (Moderately susceptible)

(iii) Chemical Protection from Pathogen

Disease	Chemical	Mode of Application
Root rot and wilt	Thiram (0.15 per cent) + Captan (0.15 per cent) in 1:1 + Urea (2 per cent)	2-3 times soil drenching, in infected area and one meter around, along with the plant using sprayer without nozzle from the initiation of disease at 7 days interval
Leaf spots caused by *Alternaria Cercospora* and *Curvularia*	Zineb (0.25 per cent) or Mancozeb (0.25 per cent) or Topsin-M (0.1 per cent) or Bavistin (0.1 per cent)	3 sprays as and when disease appear at 15 days interval

Contd...

(iii)–Contd...

Disease	Chemical	Mode of Application
Bacterial leaf spot	Agrimycin 100 (250 ppm) or Streptocycline (500ppm) or plantomycin (100 ppm)	– do –
Powdery mildew	Sulfex (0.3 per cent)	2 sprays starting from the initiation of disease at 10 days interval
Phyllody	Phorate 10 G (10 kg/ha)	Soil application
	Dimethoate (0.3 per cent) or Monocrotophos (0.3 per cent)	2-3 foliar sprays at 45, 60, 70 days after sowing
Cuscuta	Pendemethlene	Pre-emergence soil application

References

Abd El Moneem, K.M.H., El Farash, E.M. and Fahmy, F.G. (1997). In vitro selection for higher yielding somaclones resistant to charcoal rot and wilt disease complex in sesame. *Assiut Journal of Agricultural Sciences* 28: 201-224.

Abdel Rahim, A.M. and Adam, F.S. (1990). Some etiological characteristics of *Xanthomonas campestris pv. sesami* and disease reaction of different sesame cultivars. *Journal of Phytopathology* 129: 165-169.

Al Ahmad, M. and Saidawi, A. (1998). Macrophomina (charcoal) root rot of sesame in Syria. *Arali Journal of Plant Protection* 6 (2): 88-93.

Anonymous. (2001). Annual Progress Report Sesame and Niger 2000-2001. All India Coordinated Research Project (Sesame and Niger), J.N. Agricultural University Campus, Jabalpur, M.P. pp. 152.

Arriel, N.H.C., Moreira, J. de, A.N., Guedes, A.R., Costa, I.T., Da, Tarso, F.P. de, da Costa, I.T. and da, Tarso, F.P. (1998). Agronomic and botanical evaluation of the live collection of sesame germplasm at Embrapa Algodao. Pesquisa em Andamento, Embraba Algodao. No. 91 pp. 9.

Atac, A., Cetin, V. And Ipkin, B. (1994). Studies on root and crown rot disease of sesame. Bitki Koruma Bulletin 34: 43-54.

Borkar, S.G. and Krishna, A. (2000). Effect of fertilizers on development of phyllody in Sesame. *Indian Journal of Mycology and Plant Pathology*. 30: 422-423.

Butler, E.J. (1918). Fungi and Disease in Plants. Thaker Spink and Co. Calcutta. pp. 547.

Durgapal, J.C. and Rao, Y.P. (1967). Bacterial leaf spot of *Sesamum orientale in India. Indian Phytopath.* 20: 178-179.

Durgapal, J.C., Patel, P.N. and Rao, Y.P. (1969). Resistance in crops to bacterial diseases in India. Evaluation of Sesame for resistance to bacterial leaf spot incited by *Pseudomonas sesami. Indian Phytopathology*. 22: 292-294.

Gabr, M.R., Hussein, N.A., Saleh, O.I. and Khalil, M.A. (1998). Susceptibility of certain varieties and genotypes and control of wilt and root rot diseases of sesame attributed to *Fusarium oxysporum* f. sp. *sesami* and *Macrophomina phaseolina. Egyptian Journal of Microbiology* 33: 403-428.

Ganesh, S.K., Kandasamy, G., Kousalya, G., Sivarman, M.R. and Gangadharan, K. (1992). Field evaluation of (*Erysiphe cichoracearum* D.C.). *Madras Agric.* 79: 115-117.

Gangakishan, A., Jagadishwar, K., Raju, C.S. and Sudarshanum, A. (1989). Rajeshwari- a high yielding white seeded variety of sesame for Andhra Pradesh. *Indian Farming* 39(3): 7-8.

Gemavat, P.D. and Prasad, N. (1964). Further studies on Phytophthora blight of Sesame. *Indian Phytopathology*. 17: 273-283.

Gupta, I.J. and Cheema, H.S. (1990). Effect of microsclerotia of *Macrophomina phaseolina* and seed dressers on germination and vigour of sesame seed. *Seed Research* 18: 169-172.

Gupta, L.J. (1992). Change in the production of volatile aldehyde compounds in Macrophomina infected sesame (*Sesamum indicum*) seed. *Seed Research* 20: 27-30.

Gupta, R.B.L. (1995). Evaluation of sesame genotypes for resistance to root rot and oozing. *Indian Phytopathology* 48; 194-195.

Karunanithi, K. Muthusamy, M. and Seetharaman, K. (1999). The cultural and pathogenic variability among the isolates of *Macrophomina phaseolina* causing root rot of sesame. *Plant Disease Research* 14: 113-117.

Krishinaswami, S., Rao, A.V., Appadurai, R. and Venkatarao, A. (1983). A preliminary study on the inheritance of powdery mildew disease in Sesame. Proc. National Seminar on breeding crop plants for resistance to pests and diseases. TNAU, Coimbatore.

Kushi, K.K. and Khare, M.N. (1979). Seed borne fungi of sesame and their significance. *Seed Research* 7: 48-53.

Kushwaha, U.S. and Kaushal, P.K. (1970). Reaction of Sesame varieties to Cercospora leaf spot in M.P. *Mysore Journal of Agricultural Sciences*. 4: 228-230.

Lee, J.I., Kang, C.W., Lee, B.H. and Park, R.K. (1992). A nonbranching good quality and high yielding sesame variety 'Suwonkkae'. Research Report R.D.A.U. and I.C. 34: 91-96.

Li, L.L., Wang. S.Y., Fang, X.P., Hyang, Z.H., Wang, S.T., Li, M.L. and Cui, M.Q. (1991). Identification of *Macrophomina phaseolina* resistant germplasm of sesame in China. *Oil crops of China*. No. 1: 3-6.

Mahatma, L., Singh, S.D. and Lodha, P.C. (2001). Pathogenic seed mycoflora of sesame (*Sesamum indicum L.*) *Journal of Mycol. Pl. Pathol.* 31: 377-379.

Malaguti, G. (1973). Leaf diseases of sesame (*Sesamum indicum L.*) in Venezuela. Rev. de la Fac. de. *Agronomia* 7: 109-125.

Mahetre. S.S., Ghatge, R.D. and Lad, S.K. (1994). Wild *Sesame mulayanum*: a source of multiple disease resistance. *Annals of Agricultural Research* 15: 243-244.

Mishra, A.K., Tiwari, R.C., Pathak, K.N., Ali, S.A. and Ghuraya, R.S. (1994). Inheritance of leaf curl disease in *Sesamum indicum* L. *Crop Research* Hisar 8: 131-136.

Mishra, R.P. and Khare., M.N. (1970). A sclerotial leaf and stem rot of mesta. *Indian Phytopath.* 23: 706-708.

Mohanti, N.N. (1958). Cercospora leaf spot of sesame. *Indian Phytopathology*. 11: 186-187.

Mohanti, N.N. and Behera, B.C. (1958). Blight of sesame (*Sesame orientale* L.) caused by *Alternaria sesami* (Kawamara) Comb. *Current Science* 27: 492-493.

Murugesan, M., Shanmugam, N., Menon, P.P.V., Arokiaraj, A., Dhamo, K.P. and Kochubabu, M. (1978). Statistical arrangement of yield loss of Sesame due to insect pests and diseases. *Madras Agric.* J. 65: 290-295.

Navas, M. and Subero, L.J. (1995). Survival of *Corynespora cassicola* in sesame seeds under two storage temperatures. *Anales de Botanica Agricola* 2: 16-19.

Ojiambo, P.S., Ayiecho, P.O. and Nyabundi, J.O. (1999). Effect of plant age on sesame infection by Alternaria leaf spot. *African Crop Science Journal* 7: 91-96.

Ojiambo, P.S., Ayiecho, P.O., Narla, R.D. and Mibey, R.K. (2000). Tolerance level of *Alternaria sesami* and the effect of seed infection on yield of sesame in Kenya. *Experimental Agriculture* 36: 335-342.

Pandya, R.K., Triphathi, M.L., Reetu Singh and Singh, R. (2000). Change in mineral contents in sesame leaves infected by *Pseudomonas syringae* pv. *sesami* (Malkoff). *Crop Research*- Hisar 20: 140-144.

Parani, M., Singh, K.N., Rangasamy, S.R.S. and Ramalingam, R.S. (1996). A study on mechanism of phyllody disease resistance in *Sesame alatum* Thonn. *Current Science* 70: 86-89.

Pathirana, R. (1992). Gamma ray induced field tolerance to Phytophthora blight in sesame. *Plant Breeding* 108: 314-319.

Phookan, A.K. and Hazarika, R. (1994). Damping off of Sesame caused by *Xanthomonas campestris* pv. *sesami* in Assam. *Indian Phytopathology*. 47: 249-250.

Poswal, M.A.T. and Misari, S.M. (1994). Resistance of sesame cultivars to Cercospora leaf spot induced by *Cercospora sesami* Zimin. *Discovery and Innovation* 6: 66-70.

Rajpurohit, T.S. (1981). Morphology and taxonomy of sesamum Alternaria. Madras Agricultural Journal. 68(10): 696-697.

Rajpurohit,T.S. and Prasad, N. (1982). Effect of different media, temperature and levels of pH on the growth and sporulation of *Alternaria sesami.Geobios* Vol.9(3)142-144.

Rajpurohit, T.S. and Prasad, N. (1982). Production of pectinolytic enzymes by *Alternaria sesami* in vitro. *Indian Journal of Mycology and Plant Pathology*.Vol 12(2): 220-221.

Rajpurohit, T.S.N. Prasad and Gemawat, P.D. (1984). Evaluation of fungicides against *Alternaria sesami* in vitro. Pesticides special issue on fungicides Jan.: 57.

Rajpurohit, T.S. (1993). Occurrence, varietal reaction and chemical control of new powdery mildew (*Erysiphe orontii* Cast) of sesame. *Indian Journal of Mycology and Plant Pathology*. 23: 207-209.

Rajpurohit,T.S. (1997). Management of Macrophomina stem and root rot of sesame through fungicidal seed treatment and varietal resistance *Indian Journal of Mycology and Plant Pathology*. 27: 98.

Rajpurohit,T.S. (1998). Integrated management of Phytophthora blight, Cercospora leaf spot and Alternaria leaf spot of sesame. *Indian Journal of Mycology and Plant Pathology*. 28: 68.

Rajpurohit, T.S. (1999). *Trichoderma viride* Biocontrol agent effective against Macrophomina stem and root rot of sesame. 4th Agricultural Science Congress, Feb. 21-24, Jaipur. Abstract P.297.

Rajpurohit,T.S and Solanki, Z.S. (2002). Identification of resistance sources of Alternaria leaf spot of sesame. *Asian congress of Mycology and Plant Pathology*. Oct. 1-4, University of Mysore.Page : 207.

Rajpurohit, T.S., Solanki, Z.S. and.Ahuja, D.B. (2003). Screening of promising sesame genotypes against stem and root rot (*Macrophomina phaseolina*) under sick plot. National Seminar on Strees management in oilseeds for attaining self reliance in vegetable oils, Indian Society of Oilseeds Research, DOR Hyderabad. 28-30, Jan. 2003.

Rajpurohit, T.S. (2002). Influenced of intercropping and mixed cropping sesame with pearl millet, greengram and mothbean on the incidence of stem and root (*Macrophomina phaseolina*) of sesame *Sesamum* and *Safflower News letter*. No.-17: 40-41.

Rajpurohit, T.S. (2003). Studies on fungicides plant products and bioagents as spray in sesame disease management. *Journal of Eco-physiology* 6(3-4): 87-88.

Rajpurohit, T.S. (2004). Studies on plant products and new chemicals as spray against Alternaria blight of sesame. Geobios, 31: 64-65.

Rajpurohit, T.S. (2004). Efficacy of foliar spray on incidence of diseases of sesame. *Sesamum* and *Safflower News letter*. No.-19: 67-69.

Rajpurohit, T.S. (2004). Evaluation of plant products and fungicides and insecticides against Alternaria blight, Phyllody and leaf curl diseases of sesame. Indian *Phytopathology*. 57: 340-341.

Rajpurohit, T.S. and Bishnoi, H.R. (2004). Integrated disease management in sesame (*Sesamum indicum* L.). Paper presented in 26 Annual Conf. and Symposium. ISMPP. Goa University, Goa, 7-9 Abstract. pp. 144-145.

Rajpurohit, T.S. (2005). Seed treatment and Bioagent for the management of stem and root rot of sesame. *Sesamum* and *Safflower* News letter. (Under publication)

Ram, T., Ansari, M.M. and Gangwar, B. (1993). Evaluation of sesame varieties in rainfed conditions for better yield and resistance to diseases in a rice based cropping system. In Proceedings of Symposium on farming systems for sustained productivity in humid tropics. Ed. Rao, G.C., Central Agricultural Research Institute, Port Blair. pp. 119-122.

Rao, N.R. and Vijayalakshmi, M. (2000). Studies on *Alternaria sesami* pathogenic to sesame. *Microbiological Research* 155: 129-131.

Rao, R. and Pavgi, M.S. (1975). Two sclerotial diseases of crops in Varanasi. *Indian Phytopathology*. 28: 401-404.

Sabet, K.A. and Dowson, W.J. (1960). Bacterial leaf spot of sesame (*Sesame orientale* D.). *Phytopath. Z.* 37: 252-258.

Saharan, G.S. and Chand, J.N. (1988). Tilhani Faslon ke Rog. Commission for Scientific and Technical Terminology, Government of India, New Delhi. pp. 47-83.

Siddarmaiah, A.L., Kulkarni, S. and Basavarajaiah, A.B. (1979). Occurrence of a new collar rot disease of Niger (*Guizotia abyssinica* Cass.) in India. *Current Science* 18: 174.

Siddarmaiah, A.L., Desai, S.A., Hegde, R.K. and Kulkarni, S. (1980a). Seed mycoflora of *Guizotia abyssinica* Cass. and their control. *Mysore Journal of Agricultural Sciences*. 14: 334-336.

Siddarmaiah, A.L., Desai, S.A., Hegde, R.K. (1980b). Effect of seed mycoflora of Niger on seed germination and oil content under different moisture levels. *Mysore Journal of Agricultural Sciences*. 14: 497-499.

Sasikumar, B. and Sardana, S. (1988). Siping borok (Jhum til). Source of some valuable genes. *Journal of Oilseeds Research* 5: 183-184.

Selim, A.K., Serry, M.S., Omran, A.O. and Satour, M.M. (1976a). Breeding for disease resistance in Sesame, *Sesamum indicum* L. II. Inheritance of resistance to root and stem rot disease caused by *Sclerotium bataticola* Taub. *Egyptian Journal of Phytopathology* 8: 15-18.

Selim, A.K., Serry, M.S., Satour, M.M. and Al Ahmar, B.A. (1976b). Breedidng for disease resistance in sesame, *Sesamum indicum* L. III Inheritance of resistance to *Fusarium oxysporum* Schlecht. *Egyptian Journal of Phytopathology* 8: 19-24.

Shadakshari, Y.G., Virupakshappa, K. and Siddaramaiah, A.C. (1989). Reactions of Sesame genotypes against powdery mildew and bacterial leaf spot. *Current Research* 18: 4-5.

Shreemali, J.L. (1978). Two new species of Phoma from India. *Indian Journal of Mycology and Plant Pathology*. 8: 220-221.

Shukla, B.N. and Vyas, S.C. (1997). Two new diseases of Sesame (*Sesamum indicum* L.). J.N.K.V.V. Research Journal, 11: 142-143.

Singh, B.P., Shukla, B.N. and Kaushal, P.K. (1976). Evaluation of Sesame varieties for their susceptibility to *Phytophthora parasitica* Dastur at Jabalpur, M.P. J.N.K.V.V. Research Journal, 10: 76-77.

Singh, T. and Singh, D. (1990). Incidence of *Macrophomina phaseolina* (*Tassi*) Goid in sesame seeds of Rajasthan. *Indian Journal of Mycology and Plant Pathology*. 20: 111-114.

Tripathi, S.K., Tiwari, K.L. and Patel, R.P. (1986). Assessment of stability in resistance to Cercospora leaf spot in Sesame. *Agricultural Science Digest Karnal*, 16: 233-236.

Urdaneta, U.R. and Mazzani, B. (1976). Varietal differences in susceptibility to bacteriosis in sesame (*Sesamum indicum L.*) in Venezuela. *Agronomia Tropical* 26: 311-320.

Variar, M., Pavgi, M.S. and Variar, M. (1981). Varietal reaction of sesame to Synchytrium gall disease. *Indian Phytopathology*. 34: 430-433.

Verma, M.L. and Bajpai, R.P. (2001). Effect of bio-inoculants on phytopthora blight and Macrophomina root/stem rot of Sesame (*Sesamum indicum* L.). National Symposium on plant protection strategies for sustainable Horticulture Society at Plant Protection Science. SKAUT, Jammu, 12-13 Oct. pp: 113.

Vyas, S.C., Prasad, K.V.V. and Khare, M.N. (1981). Diseases of Sesame and Niger and Their Control. Department of Plant Pathology, J.N.K.V.V, Jabalpur, M.P. Bull. pp.16.

Wasnikar, A.R., Khare, M.N., Deshmukh, M.R. and Yasin, M. (1991). Bacterial blight of sesame. *Current Research* 20: 183.

Yirgu, D. (1964a). Some diseases of *Guizotia abyssinica* in Ethiopia. *Plant Disease Reporter* 48: 672.

Yirgu, D. (1964b). *Xanthomonas guizotia* sp. nov. on *Guizotia abyssinica*. *Phytopathology* 54: 1490-1491.

Microbial Biotechnology and Ecology (2011) Pages 293–302
Editors: Deepak Vyas, G.S. Paliwal, P.K.Khare and R.K Gupta
Published by: DAYA PUBLISHING HOUSE, NEW DELHI

Chapter 17

Integrated Disease Management of *Piper betle*

☆ *Deepak Vyas*[1]* *and Rajesh Yadav*[2]

[1]*Lab of Microbial Technology and Plant Pathology*
Department of Botany, Dr. H.S. Gour University, Sagar – 470 003, M.P.
[2]*ABR PG College, Anpra, Sonbhadra, U.P.*

ABSTRACT

The present investigation deals with the study on disease management of Pan caused by *Phytophthora parasitica* var. *piperina*. The result reveals that when the different control agents such as Ofloxacin (antibiotic), Calc. sulph (homoeodrug), Fytalon (fungicide), *Allium sativum* (botanical), *Trichoderma* sp. (biocontrol agent), *Microcystis* cell extract (Algal bloom), are used in higher concentration, they all shows complete killing of pathogen but when they used in lower concentration they show variable inhibitory effect against the pathogen. Different combination of control agents under *in vitro* and *in vivo* condition showed variation in the inhibitory action against the pathogen. When 100 ppm of ofloxacin combined with 10 per cent plant extract of *Allivum sativum* produces best result and shows 100 per cent killing of pathogen *in vitro* and *in vivo* condition.

Introduction

The Concept of integrated disease management (IDM), which is derived from integrated pest management, is being considered quite important in relation to disease management. Integrated pest management; aims at keeping population below the level of economic injury using best combination of various components of management. FAO has defined IPM as a pest management system that in the context of associated environment and the population dynamics of the pest species, utilizes all suitable

* E-mail: dvyas64@yahoo.co.in.

techniques and methods, in as compatible manner as possible and maintains the pest populations at levels below those causing economic injury. This new concept actually, describes what the farmers were doing before chemical pesticides came in vogue. In IPM, various components of management are tailored so as to get cost-effective control without any adverse effect on environment and ecosystem. IPM or IDM relied more on non-toxic means but does not intend to keep pesticides at bay from the management system; rather ecosystem advocates minimal or requisite use of pesticides as may be appropriate to make disease management not only effective but non-hazardous and environment friendly. IDM or IPM thus rules out total reliance on pesticides, which by and large is used as the strongest weapon against pests.

An effective IDM system aims at minimising crop losses due to diseases through efficient management of soil, water, nutrient and plant by integrating cultural and agronomic practices, chemical application, host plant resistance, biological agents and by the application of physical, mechanical and regulatory control methods.

Integrated disease management (IDM) as practiced in the developed countries is a sophisticated technology achieving a computerised on line service. Practical IDM methods have been suggested for less developed countries or traditional agro-ecosystems. It is based on efficacy, ecology and economics employing routine and supervisory practices with minimum use of agrochemicals being backed by epidemiology and management science without using computers. Disease management has to be integrated with total crop management.

Disease management strategy largely depends upon the stage/form of pathogen responsible for carrying over a particular disease from one season to another and role of various agencies such as soil, stubbles and crop debris play important role in the spread of pathogen. Thus, to evolve a suitable and efficient system for disease control, prerequisite is availability/generation of information on various aspects such as diagnosis, measurement and appraisal *i.e.* economic significance epidemiology and influence of cultural practices on intensity of disease initiation and development. Several workers have reported the integrated management of various crop diseases (Kumar and Dubey, 2001; Dohroo, 1995; Vyas, 1994; Vadhera *et al.*, 2001; Koshy *et al.*, 2002 and Dubey, 2002). Srivastava (2000) recommended integrated plant disease management for sustainable agriculture. According to Ahuja and Kandhari (2000) integrated disease management has been adopted in rice crop.

Over the years people have been trying to control pan disease by using single drug (fungicide, homoeopathic drug, antibiotic, plant extract, etc.) against test pathogen but recurrence of diseases again and again reflects that no single drug can control the disease until and unless it is used in high concentration. The existing methods for disease control of pan mainly aim for the management of individual disease through different practices. Cultural practice/chemical and plant products together and their use for control measures come under IDM. Though not impossible but cumbersome is the task to combine high level of resistance in a genotype with desirable attributes. Therefore it would be worth-while to integrate available compatible control practices to develop viable and economic management strategies against diseases particularly for the genotype which possess desirable attributes with high yield and low level of resistance to diseases.

The aim of present study is to follow the integrated approach or combination of various drugs and other agents. Thus the attempts have been made to control the leaf rot of pan caused by *P. parasitica* var. *piperina* by integrated disease management system.

Materials and Methods

In vitro Effect of Various Combinations on Mycelial Growth of *P. parasitica* var. *piperina*

In the present study the drugs and organisms were selected and tested on the basis of their earlier good performance. These include Ofloxacin, Calc sulph, Fytalon, extract of *Allium sativum*, biocontrol agents *Trichoderma* sp. and *Microcystis* cell extract (CELk). The selected drugs and organisms were taken into different combination *viz.* double and triple and their approx LD-50 doses were selected for this study. The different combinations of Ofloxacin (100 ppm), Calc sulph (30 potency), Fytalon (200 ppm), *Allium sativum* (10 per cent), CELk (100 mgl^{-1}) and *Trichoderma* sp. were taken. For double combination, 1:1 v/v ratio was used and is case of *Trichoderma* sp. dual culture method was used. In triple combination 1:1:1 v/v/v ratio was followed. The various combination of drugs mixed in oat meal agar medium before pouring except *Trichoderma* sp. Then plates were inoculated with disc of test pathogen and *Trichoderma* sp. Plates were incubated at 27±1°C for 144 hours. Plates without having any drug served as control. Each experiment was designed in triplicate form. Data were taken after 144 hours. From this, mycelial growth and percent inhibition of test pathogen were calculated.

The Effect of Various Combinations on the Leaf Rot of Pan

Healthy betelvine leaves were collected from natural habitat (bareja) and washed with running tap water and followed by sterilized distilled water. Then leaves were dipped in each combination for an hour, these were inoculated with disc of test pathogen. Before inoculation leaves were injured with sterilized needle at centre of leaves. Each experiment was performed in triplicate with suitable control. In case of *Trichoderma* sp. suspension was prepared and mixed with double combination in 1:1 v/v ratio and triple combination in 1:1:1 v/v/v ratio respectively. Then plates were incubated at 27±1°C for 144 hours. The rotten area of leaf was measured and from this growth and percent inhibition were recorded.

Result

Table 17.1 shows that drug Ofloxacin caused 33.4 per cent inhibition of mycelial growth at 100 ppm concentration; however 200 ppm concentration of this drug caused complete killing of the test pathogen. Calc sulph caused 37.5 per cent reduction of mycelial growth at 30 potency and it's 200 potency was found to suppress the growth of test pathogen completely. Fytalon, a fungicides at 200 ppm concentration caused 54.5 per cent inhibition however its 500 ppm caused complete suppression of mycelial growth of test pathogen. Extract of *A. sativum* caused 80 per cent reduction in mycelial growth at 10 per cent concentration and at 20 per cent concentration it inhibited the growth of test pathogen completely. It was found that fungal bio-agent *Trichoderma* spp. reduced 66.7 per cent mycelial growth when used as dual culture. Cyanobacterial extract CELk showed 51.2 per cent inhibition of mycelial growth at 100 mgl^{-1} whereas the complete killing of fungal growth of test pathogen was observed at 400 mgl^{-1} concentration.

Table 17.2 showed that Ofloxacin + *A. sativum* combination cause complete suppression of mycelial growth under *in vitro* and *in vivo* condition followed by Fytalon + CELk combination which caused 93.1 per cent reduction and 88.4 per cent reduction under both *in vitro* and *in vivo* condition respectively. Combination of *Trichoderma spp.* + Calc sulph caused 77.8 per cent reduction in mycelial growth *in vitro* and 80.7 per cent reduction *in vivo* condition. Trichoderma sp. + Fytalon combination showed 66.6 per cent inhibition of mycelial growth under *in vitro* condition and 65.4 per cent inhibition under *in vivo* condition.

Table 17.1: Comparison of Highly Effective Control Agents of *P. parasitica* var. *piperina*

Treatments	LD-50		LD	
	Inhibition (%)	*Concentration*	*Inhibition (%)*	*Concentration*
Ofloxacin	33.4	100	100	200 ppm
Calc. sulph	37.5	30 potency	100	200 potency
Fytalon	54.5	200 ppm	100	500 ppm
A. sativum	80.0	10 per cent	100	20 per cent
Trichoderma spp.	66.7	-	-	-
CELk	51.2	100 mgl^{-1}	100	400 mgl^{-1}

Table 17.2: Integrated Effect of Different Control Agents Against *P. parasitica* var. *piperina*

Treatments	In vitro		In vivo	
	Growth (mm)	*Inhibition (%)*	*Growth (mm)*	*Reduction (%)*
Control	90	00	52	00
Ofloxacin + *A. sativum* (100 ppm) (10 per cent)	00	100	00	100
Fytalon + CELk (200 ppm) (100 mgl^{-1})	06	93.1	06	88.4
Trichoderma sp. + Calc sulph (30 potency)	20	77.8	10	80.7
Trichoderma sp. + Fytalon (200 ppm)	30	66.6	18	65.4
CD (P = 0.05)	ND	1.35	ND	1.77

ND: Not detected.

Table 17.3 shows that combination of Ofloxacin and Fytalon caused 93.1 per cent and 88 per cent inhibition of mycelial growth of test pathogen under *in vitro* and *in vivo* condition respectively, and this was followed by the combination of Ofloxacin + CELk which caused 91.2 per cent *in vitro* and 84 per cent reduction *in vivo* condition. Combination of *A. sativum* and *Trichoderma* sp. caused 88.9 per cent reduction of mycelial growth under *in vitro* and 80 per cent inhibition under *in vivo* condition. Combination of CELk and Calc sulph caused 75.5 per cent and 70 per cent reduction of mycelial growth of test pathogen under in vitro and *in vivo* conditions.

Table 17.4 shows that Fytalon and *A. sativum* combination caused complete suppression of mycelial growth under *in vitro* condition. Interestingly the same combination of the drugs was not so much effective and caused only 88.4 per cent reduction of mycelial growth of test pathogen under *in vivo* condition. This is followed by the combination of *Trichoderma* sp. and CELk which caused 73.4 per cent reduction of mycelial growth under *in vitro* and 71.2 per cent under *in vivo* condition. When Fytalon used with Calc sulph it caused 71.2 per cent reduction of mycelial growth under *in vitro* condition and 65.4 per cent reduction *in vivo* condition. The combination of *Trichoderma* sp. + Ofloxacin exhibited 71.2 per cent and 69.2 per cent reduction under *in vitro* and *in vivo* conditions respectively.

Combination of Ofloxacin and Calc sulph was found less effective and caused only 62.2 per cent and 65.4 per cent inhibition of growth under *in vitro* and *in vivo* condition respectively.

Table 17.3: Integrated Effect of Different Control Agents against *P. parasitica* var. *piperina*

Treatments	*In vitro*		*In vivo*	
	Growth (mm)	*Inhibition (%)*	*Growth (mm)*	*Reduction (%)*
Control	90	00	50	00
Ofloxacin + Fytalon (100 ppm) (200 ppm)	06	93.1	06	88
A. sativum + *Trichoderma* sp. (10 per cent)	10	88.9	10	80
CELk + Calc sulph (100 mgl^{-1}) (30 potency)	22	75.5	15	70
Ofloxacin + CELk (100 ppm) (100 mgl^{-1})	08	91.2	08	84
CD (P = 0.05)	ND	3.06	ND	3.95

ND: Not detected.

Table 17.4: Integrated Effect of Different Control Agents against *P. parasitica* var. *piperina*

Treatments	*In vitro*		*In vivo*	
	Growth (mm)	*Inhibition (%)*	*Growth (mm)*	*Reduction (%)*
Control	90	00	52	00
Fytalon + *A. sativum* (200 ppm) (10 per cent)	00	100	06	88.4
Ofloxacin + Calc sulph (100 ppm) (30 potency)	34	62.2	18	65.4
Trichoderma spp + CELk (100 mgl^{-1})	24	73.4	15	71.2
Fytalon + Calc sulph (200 ppm) (30 potency)	26	71.2	18	65.4
Trichoderma spp + Ofloxacin (100 ppm)	26	71.2	16	69.2
CD (P = 0.05)	ND	2.47	ND	3.82

ND: Not detected.

Table 17.5 shows that combination of Ofloxacin, Fytalon and Calc sulph proved highly effective among the other tested combinations. It caused 93.1 per cent reduction in mycelial growth under *in vitro* and 88 per cent under *in vivo* condition. This was followed by the combination of *A. sativum* + *Trichoderma* sp. + Calc sulph which caused 88.9 per cent and 84 per cent of mycelial growth of test pathogen under *in vitro* and *in vivo* condition respectively. Combination of *A. sativum* + CELk + Ofloxacin was also found very inhibitory causing 86.6 per cent and 80 per cent reduction of mycelial growth under *in vitro* and *in vivo* condition respectively. The combination of *A. sativum* + CELk +

Trichoderma sp. appeared to be less effective and caused 77.8 per cent reduction in mycelial growth under *in vitro* condition and 70 per cent under *in vivo* condition.

Table 17.5: Integrated Effect of Different Control Agents against *P. parasitica* var. *piperina*

Treatments	In vitro		In vivo	
	Growth (mm)	Inhibition (%)	Growth (mm)	Reduction (%)
Control	90	00	50	00
A. sativum and Trichoderma spp. + Calc sulph (10 per cent) (30 potency)	10	88.9	08	84
Ofloxacin + Fytalon + Calc sulph (100 ppm) (200 ppm) (30 potency)	06	93.1	06	88
A. sativum + CELk + Ofloxacin (10 per cent) (100 mgl^{-1}) (100 ppm)	12	86.6	10	80
A. sativum + CELk + *Trichoderma* sp. (10 per cent) (100 mgl^{-1})	20	77.8	15	70
CD (P = 0.05)	ND	2.03	ND	4.47

ND: Not detected.

For comparative study of control measures used against test pathogen are presented in Table 17.6.

Table 17.6: Comparative Analysis of Control Measures Used against *P. parasitica* var. *piperina*

Source	Easily Available (M/L)	Eco-friendly (Yes/No)	Effective (Yes/No)	Economically Viable (Yes/No)
ANTIBIOTICS				
Acyclovir	M,L	Yes	Yes	Yes
Amoxycillin	M,L	Yes	No	Yes
Ampicillin	M,L	Yes	Yes	Yes
Azithromycin	M,L	Yes	No	No
Cefadroxil	M,L	Yes	No	Yes
Cefixime	M,L	Yes	No	No
Cefpodoxime	M,L	Yes	Yes	No
Cefuroxime	M,L	Yes	Yes	No
Cephalexin	M,L	Yes	No	Yes
Clarithromycin	M,L	Yes	Yes	No
Clomiphene	M,L	Yes	Yes	Yes
Cloxacillin	M,L	Yes	Yes	Yes
Ofloxacin	M,L	Yes	Yes	Yes
Roxithromycin	M,L	Yes	No	Yes
Sparfloxacin	M,L	Yes	Yes	Yes
Amoxycillin + Clavulanate	M,L	Yes	No	No

Contd...

Table 17.6–Contd...

Source	*Easily Available (M/L)*	*Eco-friendly (Yes/No)*	*Effective (Yes/No)*	*Economically Viable (Yes/No)*
Amoxycillin + Carbocisteine	M,L	Yes	Yes	Yes
Ampicillin + Cloxacillin	M,L	Yes	No	Yes
Ciprofloxacin + Tinidazole	M,L	Yes	Yes	Yes
Ofloxacin + Tinidazole	M,L	Yes	Yes	Yes
FUNGICIDES				
Thiram	M,L	No	No	Yes
Bavistin	M,L	No	No	No
Fytalon	M,L	No	Yes	No
HOMOEOPATHIC DRUGS				
Kali Sulph	M,L	Yes	No	Yes
Calc Sulph	M,L	Yes	Yes	Yes
Nat Sulph	M,L	Yes	Yes	Yes
PLANT EXTRACTS				
Allium sativum	L	Yes	Yes	Yes
Allium cepa	L	Yes	Yes	Yes
Azadirechta indica	L	Yes	Yes	Yes
Cinnamomum camphora	L	Yes	Yes	Yes
Lantana camara	L	Yes	Yes	Yes
Mentha spicata	L	Yes	No	Yes
Ocimum sanctum	L	Yes	Yes	Yes
Zingiber officinale	L	Yes	Yes	Yes
BIOCONTROL AGENTS				
Trichoderma sp.	M,L	Yes	Yes	Yes
Penicillium sp.	L	Yes	No	Yes
Aspergillus sp.	L	Yes	No	Yes
MICROCYSTIS EXTRACT				
CELk	L	Yes	Yes	Yes
CELb	L	Yes	No	Yes

L: Lab; M: Market.

Discussion

To control the leaf rot of pan caused by *P. parasitica* var. *piperina* many control measure such as antibiotics, fungicides, homoeopathic drugs, plant extracts, biocontrol agents have been tried. For the purpose of IDM the best drug, plant extract, bio agents which were showing greater inhibitory activity against test pathogen were selected. Drugs, fungicides, plants extracts and bioagents were randomly selected for preparing different combinations. For avoiding unnecessary use of fungicides and antibiotics only those concentrations of these drugs were choosen which had shown 50 per cent reduction of mycelial growth when used separately.

Results obtained from the present study suggest that when chemical agents such as fungicide Fytalon was used with *A. sativum* in combination, the complete killing of the test pathogen was seen under *in vitro* condition. *A. sativum* contains allylopropyl disulphide, diallyl disulphide and two more sulphur compound including which are known to be fungitoxic in nature, allicin (Chopra *et al.*, 1956, 1969). Fytalon is a copper oxychloride and copper compounds are well known antifungal agents. Chandel and Katoch (2001) have also reported chemical control of *Fusarium oxysporum*, an incitant of carnation wilt with Fytalon. Here it appears that both fungicide and plant extract caused synergestic effect due to which test pathogen could not grow. Under *in vivo* condition however, the combination caused 88.4 per cent reduction which may also be considered a quite significant. The differential behaviour of the Fytalon and *A. sativum* under *in vitro* and *in vivo* condition is the subject of further work. Management of Tikka leaf spot of ground nut by spraying potash and Neem seed extract has been reported by Chandrasekar *et al.* (1994).

Almost similar results were obtained when Ofloxacin and *A. sativum* were used together, the only difference here was that this combination caused complete inhibition under both *in vitro* and *in vivo* conditions.

Combined effect of Ofloxacin and Fytalon showed 93.1 per cent and 88 per cent reduction of mycelial growth of test pathogen respectively. Since both antibiotic and fungicide were found to be more effective in concentration, it appears as if both induced synergestic effect against test pathogen.

However, when Fytalon was used with Calc sulph no satisfactory result could be obtained. The poor inhibitory action of this combination might be due to lower concentration of the drug or it might be quite possible that Calc sulph becomes ineffective when used in combination.

Interestingly when CELk was used in combination with Fytalon and antibiotic it reduced more or less 90 per cent mycelial growth under *in vitro* and *in vivo* conditions but when it was used in combination with Calc sulph its inhibitory activity was affected adversely and it could cause only 75 per cent reduction of the mycelial growth of test pathogen.

When *Trichoderma* sp. was used with Calc sulph it caused only 77.8 per cent and 80.7 per cent and when it was used with CELk it caused 73.4 per cent and 71.2 per cent reduction in mycelial growth under *in vitro* and *in vivo* conditions respectively. Almost similar results were obtained when *Trichoderma* sp. was used with Ofloxacin showing 71.2 per cent and 69.2 per cent reduction; when used with Fytalon it caused 66.6 per cent and 65.4 per cent reduction under both *in vitro* and *in vivo* conditions. The lesser efficacy of this combination may be attributed to the detrimental affect of all the drugs on *Trichoderma* sp. resulting poor growth of the fungal antagonist. Klassen (1981) observed the opposite result when he used *Trichoderma* sp. with (PCNB) fungicide. Pant and Mukhopadhyay (2001) reported the maximum control of seed and seedling rot complex of soyabean by using *T. harzianum* and Vitavax (fungicide). According to Sharma and Mishra (1995) *Trichoderma* sp. gained considerable importance either alone or when integrated with lower dose of fungicides for the management of soil-born plant pathogens. Dubey (2002) also reported the similar result with the combination of Thiram and *T. viride* against collar rot of french bean.

In contrast, combination of plant extract of *A. sativum* and *Trichoderma* sp. was found more effective by causing 88.9 per cent and 80 per cent reduction in the mycelial growth of test pathogen in both *in vitro* and *in vivo* conditions. This is an interesting finding because it would be expected that presence of many sulphur containing substances in *A. sativum* will inhibit the growth of *Trichoderma* spp. and it would not cause significant harm to *Phytophthora* but the result of present study suggest that the plant extract of *A. sativum* was so powerful that it not only restricted the growth of *Trichoderma* but also reduced the growth of test pathogen. Since this combination is a purely of origin. It is also a ecofriendly and highly effective. Use of this combination certainly reduces he unnecessary load of chemical drugs, which are not only hazardous to plants but also to human beings.

No triple combination was found to cause complete reduction of the growth of *Phytophthora*. Among he tested combinations best effective against test pathogen was Ofloxacin + Fytalon + Calc sulph which caused 93 per cent and 88 per cent reduction under both conditions, then followed by *A. sativum* and *Trichoderma* sp. and Calc sulph 88.9 per cent and 84 per cent suppression of pathogen; and least effective combination was *A. sativum* + CELk + Calc Sulph with 77.8 per cent and 70 per cent reduction of mycelial growth under *in vitro* and *in vivo* conditions. As such it may be summarised from these results that combination of only two, one chemical control agent and one plant extract are two drugs or two botanical agents were more effective measure for IDM. Thus on the basis of these results it may be we recommended that Ofloxacin + *A. sativum*, Fytalon + *A. sativum*, Fytalon + CELk and *A. sativum* + *Trichoderma sp.* may be successfully used for the control of betelvine *Phytophthora*. The present findings are supported by other workers who have also achieved success on integration of biological agents with fungicides to get significantly higher disease control in several crops than that obtained by either biocontrol agent or fungicide alone (Henis *et al.*, 1978; Upadhyay and Mukhopadhyay, 1983; Mukhopadhyay and Kaur, 1990; Sawant and Mukhopadhyay, 1990; Vyas, 1994; Dubey *et al.*, 1996; Dubey, 1997). Obviously if the disease can be controlled by two drugs in their low concentration then there is not need of using higher concentration. This is the only way by which practical viability of IDM can be achieved. This practice will help to avoid the anticipated environmental pollution due to the sole use of chemicals for disease management and also will nullify the probable development of fungicide resistant strains in pathogen if any, arising out of the repeated use of some fungicides for disease management.

References

Ahuja, S.C. and Kandhari, J. (2000). Integrated disease management in Rice crop. In: *Glimpses in Plant Sciences* (Eds. Aneja, K.R., Charaya, M.U., Aggarwal, A., Hans, D.K. and Khan, S.A.) Pragati Prakashan, Meerut. 153-160.

Chandel, S.S. and Katoch, R. (2001). Chemical control of *Fusarium oxysporum f.sp. dianthi* an incitant of carnation wilt. *Indian J. Microbiol.* 41: 135-137.

Chandrasekar, V., Narayanaswami, R. and Ramabardran, R. (1994). Effect of foliar spray of potash and neem seed extract on the Tikka leaf spot of groundnut. *Indian Phytopatho.* 47: 188-189.

Chopra, R.N., Nayar, S.L. and Chopra, I.C. (1956). *Glossary of Indian Medicinal Plants*. Publications and Information Directorate. C.S.I.R. New Delhi.

Correa, F. and Zeigler, R. (1991). Integrated management of rice blast disease (*P. oryzae*). *Fitopathologia Colombiana*. 15: 35-37.

Dohroo, N.P. (1995). Integrated management of yellows of ginger. *Indian Phytopath.* 48: 90-92.

Dubey, S.C. (1997). Biological control of web blight of groundnut caused by *Thanatephorus cucumeris*. *Golden Jubilee International Conference of IPS* at IARI, New Delhi. p. 194.

Dubey, S.C. (2002). Bio-agent based integrated management of collar rot of french bean. *Indian Phytopath.* 55: 230-231.

Ghewande, M.P., Desai, S., Prem Narayan and Ingle, A.P. (1991). An integrated approach to the management of foliar diseases of groundnut (*Arachis hypogea L.*). *Poster Abstract, Second Inter. Groundnut Workshop*, ICRISAT, Patancheru, A.P. India.

Henis, Y., Ghaffar, A. and Baker, R. (1978). Integrated control of *Rhizoctonia solani* of radish: Effect of successive plantings, PCNB and *Trichoderma harzianum* on pathogen and disease. *Phytopathol.* 69: 1164-1169.

Hooda, K.S. and Srivastava, M.P. (1995). Efficacy of different fungitoxicant and neem products in the control of rice blast. *Pestology*. 19: 41-44.

Khurana, S.M.P., Garg, I.D. Singh, B.P. and Gadewar, A.V. (1998). Major disease of potato and their management. *Integrated pest and disease management* (Eds.) Upadhyay, R.K., Mukerji, K.G., Chamola, B.P., and Dubey, O.P.. APH Publishing Corporation, New Delhi. 11-64.

Koshy, P.K., Kumar, Y., Jayasree, D., Joseph, V. and Sosamma, V.K. (2002). Integrated management of leaf rot diseases and insect pests on coconut. *Indian Phytopath*. 55: 545-56.

Kumar, D. and Dubey, S.C. (2001). Management of collar rot of pea by the integration of biological and chemical methods. *Indian Phytopath*. 54: 62-66.

Mukhopadhyay, A.N. and Kaur, N.P. (1990). Biological control of chickpea wilt complex by *Trichoderma harzianum Proc. Third Intr. Conf. on plant protection in the tropics*. Malaysia, 1990.

Mukhopadhyay, A.N., Shrestha, S.M. and Mukherjee, P.K. (1992). Biological seed treatment for control of soil born plant pathogens. *FAO Plant Prot. Bull.* 40: 21-30.

Pun, K.B., Doraiswamy, S. and Jeyarajan, R. (2000). Screening of virus inhibitory chemicals and neem products against okra yellow vein mosaic virus. *Indian Phytopath*. 53: 95-96.

Rajappan, K., Ramaraj, B. and Natarajan, S. (2000). Field evaluation of fungicides and neem formulations against bacterial blight of French bean. *Indian Phytopath*. 53: 303-304.

Sharma, S.D. and Mishra, A. (1995). Tolerance of *Trichoderma harzianum* to agrochemicals. *Indian J. Mycol. Pl. Pathol.* 25: 129.

Srivastava, M.P. (2000). Integrated plant disease management for sustainable agriculture. *Glimpses in Plant Sciences* (Eds.) Aneja, K.R., Charya, M.U., Aggarwal, A. Hans, D.K. and Khan, S.A. Pragati Prakashan, Meerut. 77-81.

Tondon, J.P. (1998). Research development and management for production of wheat. *Integrated pest and disease management* (Eds.) Upadhyay, R.K., Mukerji, K.G., Chamola, B.P. and Dubey, O.P. A.P.H. Publishing Corporation, New Delhi. 131-144.

Upadhyay, J.P. and Mukhopadhyay, A.N. (1983). Effect of non volatile and volatile antibiotics of *Trichoderma harzianum* on growth of *Sclerotium rolfsii*. *Indian J. Mycol. Pl. Pathol.* 13: 232-233.

Vadhera, I., Tiwari, S.P. and Shukla, B.N. (2001). Estimation of yield losses in tomato and integrated management of root-knot nematode. *Indian Phytopath*. 54: 495-496.

Vyas, S.C. (1994). Integrated biological and chemical control of dry root rot of Soyabean Indian *J. Mycol. Pl. Pathol.* 24: 132-134.

Microbial Biotechnology and Ecology (2011) *Pages* 303–319
Editors: Deepak Vyas, G.S. Paliwal, P.K.Khare and R.K Gupta
Published by: DAYA PUBLISHING HOUSE, NEW DELHI

Chapter 18

Thermophilic Fungi: Occurrence, Characteristics and Enzymatic Potential

☆ *Naveen Kango**

Department of Applied Microbiology and Biotechnology
Dr. H.S. Gour University, Sagar – 470 003, M.P.

ABSTRACT

A heterogeneous group of high temperature loving molds is commonly referred as thermophilic fungi. The biotechnological potential of thermophilic molds stems from their inherent ability to utilize complex organic matter including lignocelluloses for their growth by virtue of their extracellular thermostable hydrolytic enzymes. About 30 such fungal species that infringe the upper temperature limit of eukaryotes deserve special attention. These fungi are naturally bestowed with the ability to produce several thermostable bioactive molecules. Thermostable enzymes are of special interest in industries as higher operational temperature allows better solubility of the substrate and undesirable contaminations are avoided. The present article takes a glance at the occurrence, properties and enzymatic potential of this interesting group of molds.

Introduction

Temperature is one of the key environmental variables that profoundly affects survival, growth and distribution of microorganisms in nature. Hence, temperature relationship of microorganisms is an important criterion used for their assortment to different groups namely mesophiles, psychrophiles and thermophiles. Most microorganisms are mesophilic and grow in the temperature range of 10-

* E-mail: nkango@gmail.com

45°C. Those growing at lower temperatures between 0-20°C are referred as psychrophiles while thermophilic microorganisms have ability to survive and proliferate in the habitats of high temperature regimes (45-100°C) such as hot springs, composts, geothermal soils, storages, bird's nests, woodchip piles etc. Extreme thermophily is witnessed in eubacteria or archaea, some of which are able to grow near or above 100°C in thermal springs, solfatara fields, or hydrothermal vents (Tansey and Brock, 1978; Brock, 1995; Blochl *et al.*, 1997). Among fungi, only a few species have the ability to thrive at temperatures between 45-55°C. Such fungi comprise thermophilic and thermotolerant forms, which are arbitrarily distinguished on the basis of their minimum and maximum temperature of growth (Cooney and Emerson, 1964). Thermophilic fungi have a growth temperature maximum at or above 50°C and a minimum at or above 20°C while thermotolerant fungi are distinguished from the above on the basis of their lower temperature limit of growth, allowing them to grow below 20°C. Considering that the vast majority of eukaryotes cannot survive prolonged exposure to temperatures above 45°C, the ability of some fungal species to infringe this upper temperature limit is an important phenomenon (Alexandrov, 1977; Maheshwari *et al.*, 2000). Thermotolerant fungi are the chief components of the microflora that develops in heaped masses of plant material, piles of agricultural and forestry products, and other accumulations of organic matter wherein the self-heating, aerobic and organically rich conditions provide a conducive atmosphere for the development of thermophilic mycoflora in succession (Allen and Emerson, 1949; Cooney and Emerson, 1964). High temperature loving fungi constitute a

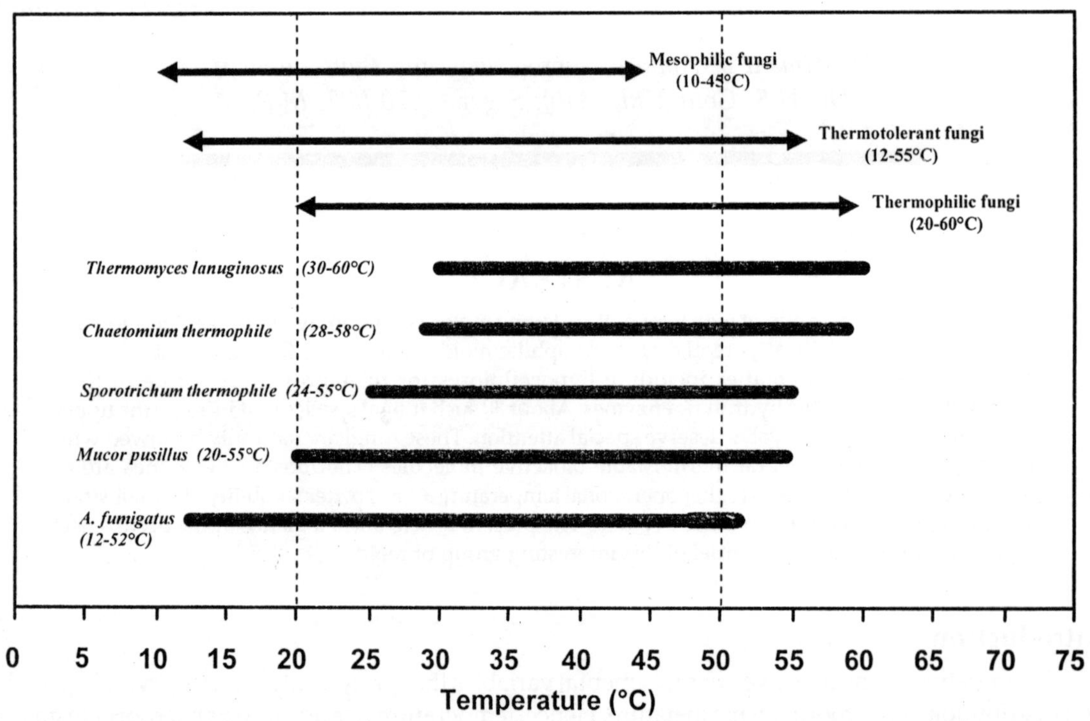

Figure 18.1: Range of Growth Temperature of Various Groups of Fungi and Some Typical Thermophilic and Thermotolerant (*A. fumigatus*) Forms (Modified from Cooney and Emerson, 1964).

heterogeneous group of moulds consisting of a large number of morphologically and physiologically different forms including representatives from zygomycetes, ascomycetes, basidiomycetes and fungi imperfecti, having in common certain biochemical and ecological characteristics associated with their ability to grow at elevated temperatures (Mouchacca, 1997). Figure 18.1 shows range of temperature for growth of mesophilic, thermophilic and thermotolerant fungi. True thermophilic molds fail to grow below 20°C while *A. fumigatus*, being thermotolerant, is able to grow at 12°C. Over the years different workers have proposed terminologies and definitions to express temperature relations of high temperature loving fungi. Some of these are as follows:

Thermophilic Fungi

La Touche (1950) suggested this term to designate those fungi that can grow and reproduce between 40-50°C. Cooney and Emerson (1964) used this term for fungi that have maximum growth temperature at or above 50°C and minimum at or above 20°C while Crisan (1973) considered all those forms growing above 40°C as thermophilic. Abdel-Hafez *et al.* (1983) included all those fungi in this category that could grow in temperature range of 45-60°C with optimum growth at 45°C.

Thermotolerant Fungi

This term was used by Cooney and Emerson (1964) for fungi with maximum temperature limit for growth at or above 50°C but could grow below 20°C.

Transition Thermophiles

Apinis and Pugh (1967) applied this term to the fungi that have ability to grow below 20°C but can also withstand high temperatures approaching 40°C.

Eurythermal Fungi

These include fungi that have 50°C as optimum growth temperature while their minimum lies between 28-40°C (Henssen, 1957).

Sterothermal Fungi

Moulds that have an optimum growth temperature at 50°C but can also grow well at higher temperatures (Henssen, 1957).

Thermophilous Fungi

Johri (1980) while enumerating fungi living at high temperature has used this term to include both thermophilic and transitional mesophilic moulds.

Although breaching of defined temperature limits, specially with changing nutritional conditions, has been observed in many cases, the definition of thermophilic moulds as given by Cooney and Emerson (1964) provides a good working basis and holds appropriate to most fungi thriving at high temperatures (Cole, 1980).

Prevalence of these moulds is anticipated in habitats where temperature regime approaches their optimum and higher *i.e.* 45-60°C. Early reports of their occurrence were made from composts wherein the daily temperature during the peak heating hours reaches 65-70°C (La Touche, 1950; Fergus, 1964; Fergus and Sinden, 1969; Chang and Hudson, 1967; Hayes, 1969; Jodice *et al.*, 1975; Moubasher *et al.*, 1982; Satyanarayana and Johri, 1983). Stored grains likewise provide an environment where internal heating leads to regular appearance of thermophilic moulds (Flanningan, 1969, Mulinge and Apinis, 1969; Wallace *et al.*, 1986; Jain, 1999).

Occurrence of Thermophilic Fungi

Isolation of thermophiles from soil was reported as early as 1939 and it still remains to be an ideal niche for thermophilic moulds (Waksman and Cordon, 1939; Waksman *et al.*, 1939). Sun-heated soils remain insolated during day hours and this causes rise in its temperature. Tansey and Jack (1977) have reported isolation of thermophilic moulds from sun heated soils whereas other soils including hot spring soils (Tansey and Brock, 1971; Tansey and Brock, 1972), tropical and subtropical soils (Eggins *et al.*, 1972; Udagawa *et al.*, 1973; Morgan-Jones, 1974, Tansey and Jack, 1977; Rajasekaran and Maheshwari, 1993), coal mine soils (Thakre and Johri, 1976), pasture soils (Eggins and Malik, 1969) and those of temperate and cold regions are also known to lodge a good number of these moulds (Ellis, 1980).

Bird nests act as incubators providing ambient temperature for thermophilic moulds (Apinis and Pugh, 1967; Tansey, 1973; Satyanarayana *et al.*, 1977). Stored peat and oil palm kernels have also been reported to harbor a variety of these moulds (Eggins and Coursey, 1964; Kuster and Locci, 1964). Retting guayule (Cooney and Emerson, 1964), industrial wood chip piles (Hajny, 1966; Ofosu-Asiedu and Smith, 1973; Greaves, 1971), moldy hay (Gregory *et al.*, 1963), sugarcane bagasse (Lacey, 1974), litter (Johri, 1980), saw dust (Singhai and Jain, 1992) etc. are certain more habitats in which thermophilic moulds proliferate and play important role. Kango *et al.* (2003a) have reported occurrence of 48 fungal forms belonging to 13 different genera and 18 species of thermophilic and thermotolerant fungi from soil, wheat straw, compost, wood chips, litter, bird nesting materials and storage seeds.

The ubiquitous nature of thermophilic moulds is well established as evidenced by numerous reports of their occurrence from different parts of the world. Subrahmanyam (1999) has reviewed the ecology of thermophilic moulds and has given distribution of more than ninety species belonging to forty-two genera of such moulds over 18 countries including Africa, Antarctica and sub-Antarctica, Australia, Germany, Poland, India, Indonesia, Italy, Japan, The Netherlands, New Zealand, Malaysia, Pakistan, Republic of Honduras, Saudi Arabia, United Kingdom, USA and Russia. Amongst documented species, a maximum of 52 have been found in India and it seems to have more diversity of these moulds in comparison to other countries. Other countries having relatively more accounts of isolation of different thermophilic moulds include USA, UK and Africa with reports of harboring a total of 37, 33 and 25 species, respectively. *Aspergillus fumigatus, Chaetomium thermophile, Humicola insolens, Malbranchea pulchella* var. *sulfurea, Mucor pusillus, Sporotrichum thermophile, Talaromyces emersonii, Thermoascus aurantiacus, Thermomyces lanuginosus* are relatively more prevalent thermophilic moulds than others (Subrahmanyam, 1999). On behalf of high temperature requirement of these moulds it is anticipated that they must be more prevalent in tropics. However, several records of thermophilic fungi from colder areas including Arctic and Antarctic regions indicate their surprisingly successful survival in extreme cold. Moreover, soil samples from Brazil, Honduras and Costa Rica and those of USA and UK are reported to contain more or less similar thermophilic mycoflora.

Growth Requirements

Most of the thermophilic fungi can grow on simple media containing carbon and nitrogen sources with few mineral salts (Cooney and Emerson, 1964; Rosenberg, 1975; Deploey, 1976; Sahm and

Chapman, 1976; Satyanarayana and Johri, 1984) while many of these have been found to grow on a wide range of carbon sources including simple sugars, organic acids and complex polymers such as starch, cellulose, hemicellulose, lignin and pectin (Subrahmanyam, 1980; Satyanarayana and Johri, 1984; Satyanarayana *et al.*, 1992; Gupta and Maheshwari, 1985). They proliferate in decaying organic matter during high-temperature phase succeeding mesophilic generation (Hedger and Hudson, 1974). At this point of time, initially available simple C-sources are depleted and the C-source available for the growth of thermophilic fungi is mainly polysaccharide component of lignocellulosic biomass. Interestingly, many compost fungi such as *Thermomyces lanuginosus, Talaromyces duponti, Mucor pusillus, Melanocarpus albomyces* etc. are reported to be non-cellulolytic. These species grow commensally by utilizing sugars produced by cellulolytic partners *e.g. Chaetomium thermophile* (Hedger and Hudson, 1974). Some of thermophilic fungi, namely *T. lanuginosus, Humicola insolens* etc. rapidly utilize xylan as an accessible C-source (Chang, 1967) while some cellulolytic thermophiles such as *Sporotrichum thermophile* could utilize cellulose as efficiently as glucose (Gaikwad and Maheshwari, 1994). Concurrent utilization of mixed C-substrates has also been indicated in *T. lanuginosus* and *Penicillium duponti* (Maheshwari and Balasubramanyam, 1988).

Simple N-sources such as nitrates and asparagine support good growth of these moulds (Satyanarayana and Johri, 1984) while protein hydrolysis by growing cultures of some thermophilic moulds, as monitored by pulse-labeled protein, has been reported to be twice that of mesophilic fungi suggesting high turnover of soluble protein in cultures of thermophilic fungi (Rajasekaran and Maheshwari, 1990).

Thermophilic fungi inhabiting different environmental conditions in different habitats may show a great variation in their temperature requirement for their optimum growth. Whether different geographical isolates of same fungal species inhabiting different habitats possess same temperature growth relations is a subject of active interest and enquiry. It has been suggested that subtropical strains of a particular fungus, may have higher optimum growth temperatures than strains from temperate regions and hence geographical isolates of the same species may differ in their temperature-growth relationships and possibly other physiological aspects (Maheshwari *et al.*, 2000). Thermostability in enzymes of thermophilic moulds is an important characteristic and most of them have optimal activity between 40-55°C (Liu *et al.*, 1974; Somkuti and Babel, 1968a, b; Ogundero, 1980; Craveri *et al.*, 1974). Enzymes with carbohydrate moiety (glycoproteins) *e.g.* xylanases and cellulases have been found to have temperature optima in the range of 50-70°C (Matsuo *et al.*, 1977; Margaritis and Creese, 1981; Vandamme *et al.*, 1982) and removal of carbohydrate residue reduces their thermal stability suggesting important role played by carbohydrate moiety in stabilizing their conformation at elevated temperatures.

Enzymatic Potential

The desire of identifying fungi capable of secreting high levels of thermostable enzymes with high temperature optima and a long shelf life has stimulated many workers to explore thermophilic moulds for industrial usage. The adaptability of thermophilic moulds to various habitats heterogeneous in terms of temperature, nutrients, gases, water activity (a_w) and saprophytic microbiota indicates their potentiality desirable in industrial strains. Thermophilic moulds possess a comprehensive range of extracellular enzymes as evidenced by their growth in plant organic matter where they degrade complex polymers such as starch, protein, pectin, hemicellulose and lignin (Emerson, 1968; Johri and Satyanarayana, 1986; Maheshwari *et al.*, 2000).

Several enzymes from these moulds including protease, lipase, α-amylase, glucoamylase, cellulase, cellobiose dehydrogenase, glucuronidase, pectinase, lactase, laccase, phytase have been found to exhibit better thermal stabilities as compared to their mesophilic counterparts (Berka *et al.*, 1997; 1998). However, their thermostability is much lower to that of enzymes from hyperthermophilic bacteria (Adams, 1993) but the optimal temperature of enzymes from hyperthermophilic bacteria is too high to suit realistic operational temperature range in industries *i.e.* 50-65°C (Maheshwari *et al.*, 2000).

Proteases have long been used in food, dairy, detergent and leather industries. A variety of thermophilic moulds have been reported to produce thermostable proteases. These include *Mucor pusillus* (Arima *et al.*, 1967; Somkuti and Babel, 1968a), *M. miehei* (Ottesen and Rickert, 1970), *Penicillium duponti* (Hashimoto *et al.*, 1972), *Malbranchea pulchella* var. *sulfurea* (Ong and Gaucher, 1976) and *Humicola lanuginosa* (Shenolikar and Stevenson, 1982).

Lipases (EC 3.1.1.3) catalyzing hydrolysis of triacylglycerides are also used in laundry detergents where they are expected to remain active in presence of surfactants at 30-60°C. These have been characterized from *Mucor pusillus, Humicola lanuginosa, Rhizomucor miehei* (Somkuti and Babel, 1968b; Arima *et al.*, 1972; Huge-Jensen *et al.*, 1989). *H. lanuginosa* lipase (Lipolase, Novo industries) is being used in detergent formulations in conjunction with other microbial enzymes. A recombinant plasmid containing the cDNA for *R. miehei* lipase was successfully expressed in *Aspergillus oryzae* and large amounts of this enzyme without any alteration in thermal properties could be produced (Huge-Jensen *et al.*, 1989). Similarly, *H. lanuginosa* lipase gene has also been cloned in *A. oryzae* (Arima *et al.*, 1972).

Enzymatic hydrolysis of glycosidic linkages of starch using amylases finds main application in food and textile industries. α-Amylase (EC 3.2.1.1) have been produced from several thermophilic moulds *viz. Rhizomucor pusillus, H. lanuginosa* (Adams, 1994), *Mucor pusillus, M. miehei* (Adams and Deploey, 1976), *Humicola* sp. (Barnett and Fergus, 1971), *Talaromyces emersonii* (Bunni *et al.*, 1989), *Thermoascus aurantiacus* (Jaychandran and Ramabadran, 1970) and *Myceliophthora thermophila* D14 (Sadhukhan *et al.*, 1992) while strains of *T. lanuginosus* have been shown to produce both α-amylase and glucoamylase (EC 3.2.1.3) (Rao *et al.*, 1979; Arnesen *et al.*, 1998).

Enzymatic conversion of cellulose into glucose using fungal cellulases (EC 3.2.1.4) has multifarious prospects since glucose is the most readily utilized source of energy and carbon. Several thermophilic moulds used as source of this enzyme include *Sporotrichum thermophile* (Coutts and Smith, 1976), *Talaromyces emersonii* (Folan and Coughlan, 1978), *Thermoascus aurantiacus* (Kawamori *et al.*, 1987), *Humicola insolens* (Hayashida and Yoshioka, 1980) and *Humicola grisea* var. *thermoidea* (Yoshioka *et al.*, 1982). Pectin hydrolyzing enzyme, polygalactouronase (EC 3.2.1.15) cleaves α-1,4 linkages of pectin. Among all pectinases, polygalactouronase of *T. aurantiacus* has been found to be most stable exhibiting a temperature optima of 65°C and a half life of 20 minutes at 55°C (Inamdar, 1987).

Laccase (EC 1.10.3.2) activity is believed to be significant in polymerization of phenolic substrates to humic substances. Laccase catalyze oxidation of phenolic compounds coupled with reduction of oxygen to water. Among thermophilic moulds laccase has been characterized from *Myceliophthora thermophila* (Berka *et al.*, 1997) and *Chaetomium thermophilum* (Chefetz *et al.*, 1998). The gene encoding laccase of *M. thermophila* was cloned and expressed in mesophilic *A. oryzae*. Laccase from *C. thermophilium* was found to have half-life of 12 hours at 50°C and was active over broad pH range of 5-12.

Table 18.1: Characteristics of Some Industrially Important Thermostable Glycosidases Produced by Thermophilic Fungi

Thermophilic Fungi		*M(r) kDa*	*Optimum*		*Reference*
			pH	*T (°C)*	
		Endo-glucanase (EC 3.2.1.4)			
Chaetomium thermophile var. coprophile		36	6.0	60	Ganju *et al.*, 1990.
Humicola grisea var. thermoidea		63	5.0	–	Hayashida and Mo, 1986
Myceliophthora thermophila		100	4.8	65	Roy *et al.*, 1990
Thermoascus aurantiacus		32	2.9	76	Khandke *et al.*, 1989
		β-glucosidase (EC 3.2.1.21)			
Sporotrichum thermophile		240	5.4	65	Bhat and Bhat, 1997
Humicola grisea var. thermoidea		156	4.0-4.5	60	Filho, 1996
Humicola insolens		250	5.0	50	Hayashida *et al.*, 1988
Humicola lanuginosa		110	4.5	60	Anand and Vithayathil, 1989
Thermoascus aurantiacus		15.1	4.2	71	Khandke *et al.*, 1989
		α-amylase (EC 3.2.1.1)			
Thermomyces lanuginosus			4.6-5.2	60	Jensen and Olsen, 1992
Scytalidium sp.		87	6.5	50	Odibo *et al.*, 1992
Rhizopus		64	4.0-6.0	60-65	Siqueria *et al.*, 1997
		Glucoamylase (EC 3.2.1.3)			
Humicola lanuginosa		–	4.9-6.6	65, 70	Taylor *et al.*, 1978
Thermomyces lanuginosus		37	–	70	Rao *et al.*, 1981
		Xylanase (EC 3.2.1.8)			
Humicola insolens		6, 21	6-6.5	55-60	Rana *et al.*, 1996
Malbranchea pulchella var. *sulfurea* No. 48		---	6-6.5	70	Matsuo and Yasui, 1985
Melanocarpus albomyces		24, 38	5.6, 6.6	65	Prabhu and Maheshwari, 1999
Paecilomyces variotii		20	4	50	Kelly *et al.*, 1989
Thermomyces lanuginosus SSBP		23.6	6.5	70-75	Lin *et al.*, 1999
Thermomyces lanuginosus		25.5	7	60-70	Cesar and Mrsa, 1996
Thermomyces lanuginosus		32	5.1	80	Gomes *et al.*, 1993
Chaetomium thermophile	Xyl I	26	4.8-6.0	70	Ganju *et al.*, 1989
	Xyl II	7	5.4-6.0	60	

Spurt of interest in identifying thermostable xylanases for biobleaching of pulp in paper industries to reduce the burden of residual organochloro compounds due to chemical bleaching has lead many workers to investigate thermophilic moulds (Kango and Jain, 2005). Xylanolytic enzymes include endoxylanase, β-xylosidase, arabino-furanosidase, acetyl xylan esterase, glucuronidase and exo-xylanase. Among these, endoxylanase (EC 3.2.1.8) is understood to be the chief enzyme hydrolyzing the backbone of xylan macromolecule and therefore plays a central role in xylan depolymerization. Applications of xylanases include saccharification of lignocelluloses, clarification of fruit juices and wines, enhancement of quality and nutritional value of feed, fibre upgradation etc. (Kango, 2007). Biobleaching using microbial xylanases that replaces toxic chlorine has been realized as a major application of these enzymes. Development of an efficient process for xylan hydrolysis using microbial xylanases opens up novel prospects for xylan utilization where the hydrolysate can be utilized for the production of fuel, SCP and other value-added products. *Humicola insolens*, a thermophilic mould, secreted two xylanases of molecular weight equal to 6 kDa and 21 kDa (Dusterhoft *et al.*, 1997). Similarly, *H. grisea* var. *thermoidea* also secreted two xylanases having different low molecular weights *i.e.* 13 kDa and 73 kDa (Rana *et al.*, 1996). Two different strains of *Melanocarpus albomyces* have been shown to produce thermostable xylanases with distinct characteristics (Prabhu and Maheshwari, 1999; Saraswat and Bisaria, 2000). Strains of *Thermomyces lanuginosus*, a potent xylanolytic fungi elaborating high levels of thermostable xylanase have been shown to produce single form of xylanase in the range of 20-30 kDa (Lin *et al.*, 1999) while *T. lanuginosus* BS1 strain has been reported to secrete two xylanases of 25 kDa and 54 kDa (Chadha *et al.*, 1999). *E. nidulans* NK-62 and *T. lanuginosus* NK-2 have been reported to produce higher titres of thermostable xylanase, 362 U/ml and 1418 U/ml, respectively utilizing wheat bran (Kango *et al.*, 2003b; Kango *et al.*, 2006).

Along with the above said secretory enzymes, many useful intracellular enzymes have also been noticed in thermophilic moulds. Characterization of intracellular pentose phosphate pathway enzyme, glucose-6-phosphate (EC 1.1.1.49) has been done from *Penicillium duponti* (Broad and Shepherd, 1970) while malate dehydrogenase (TCA cycle) could be isolated from *H. lanuginosa* and *M. pusillus* (Yang *et al.*, 1997). Intracellular trehalose (EC 3.2.1.28) acts upon trehalose, which is believed to provide stability to membranes and enzymes against drying and thermal denaturation (Crowe *et al.*, 1984; Colaco *et al.*, 1992), has been isolated from *T. lanuginosus* (Prasad and Maheshwari, 1978), *H. grisea* var. *thermoidea* (Cardello *et al.*, 1994) and *Scytalidium thermophilum* (Kadowaki *et al.*, 1996). Endocellular invertase and phosphodiesterase have also been characterized from thermophilic *T. lanuginosus* and *T. duponti*, respectively (Fontana *et al.*, 1974; Maheshwari *et al.*, 1983). Other intracellular enzymes of thermophilic moulds include aminopeptidase (Chapuis and Zuber, 1970), ATP sulfurylase (Renosto *et al.*, 1985), galactosidases (Arnaud *et al.*, 1976; Fischer *et al.*, 1995), β-D-xylosidase (Almeida *et al.*, 1995) etc.

Enzymes having high temperature optima and thermostability, as in case of thermophilic moulds, are better suited to industrial applications. This fact is substantiated by a number of available patents disclosing classified applications of enzymes from thermophilic moulds (Fangerstrom *et al.*, 1997; Bruins *et al.*, 2001). Looking at their ubiquity, ease of isolation and culture, minimal growth requirements and broad spectra of thermostable enzymes, thermophilic moulds appear to be good candidates for potential biotechnologies.

References

Abdel-Hafez, S.I.I., Aboel-Hafez, A.H. and Abdel-Kader, M.I.A. (1983). Composition of fungal flora of Syrian-soils 4. Thermophilic fungi. *Mycopathol.* 81: 177-182.

Adams, M. W. W. (1993). Enzymes and proteins from organisms that grow near and above 100°C. *Annu. Rev. Microbiol.* 47: 627-658.

Adams, P. R. (1994). Extracellular amylase activities of *Rhizomucor pusillus* and *Humicola lanuginosa* at initial stages of growth. *Mycopathol.* 128: 139-141.

Adams, P. R. and Deploey, J.J. (1976). Amylase production by *Mucor miehei* and *M. pusillus. Mycologia* 68: 934-938.

Alexandrov, V. Y. (1977). *Cells, Molecules and Temperature.* Translated from the Russian by V. A. Bernstam. Springer-Verlag KG, Berlin, Germany.

Allen, P. J., and Emerson, R. (1949). Guayule rubber, microbiological improvement by shrub retting. *Ind. Eng. Chem.* 41: 346-365.

Almeida, E. M. de, Lourdes, M. de, Polizeli, T. M., Terenzi, H. F. and Jorge, J. A.(1995). Purification and biochemical characterization of β-xylosidase from *Humicola grisea* var. *thermoidea. FEMS Microbiol. Lett.* 130: 171-176.

Anand, L. and Vithayathil, P. J. (1989). Purification and properties of β-glucosidase from a thermophilic fungus *Humicola lanuginosa* (Griffon and Maublanc) Bunce. *J. Ferment. Bioeng.* 67: 380-386.

Apinis, A.E. and Pugh, G. J. F. (1967). Thermophilic fungi of bird's nest. *Mycopathol. Mycol. Appl.* 33: 1-9.

Arima, K., Iwasaki, S. and Tamura, G. (1967). Milk clotting enzyme from microorganisms I. Screening test and the identification of the potent fungus. *Agric. Biol. Chem.* 31: 540-545.

Arima, K., Liu, W.H. and Beppu, T. (1972). Studies on the lipase of thermophilic fungus *Humicola lanuginosa. Agric. Biol. Chem.* 36: 893-895.

Arnaud, N., Bush, D. A. and Horisberger, M. (1976). Study of an intracellular α-galactosidase from the thermophilic fungus *Penicillium duponti. Biotechnol. Bioeng.* 18: 581-585.

Arnesen, S., Eriksen, S.H., Olsen, J. and Jensen, B. (1998). Increased production of α-amylase from *Thermomyces lanuginosus* by the addition of Tween 80. *Enzyme Microb. Technol.* 23: 249-252.

Barnett, E. A. and Fergus, C. L. (1971). The relation of extracellular amylase, mycelium, and time, in some thermophilic and mesophilic *Humicola* species. *Mycopathol. Mycol. Appl.* 44: 131-141.

Berka, R. M., Schneider, P., Golightly, E. J., Brown, S. H., Madden, M., Brown, K. M., Halkier, T., Mondorf, K. and Xu, F. (1997). Characterization of the gene encoding an extracellular laccase of *Myceliophthora thermophila* and analysis of the recombinant enzyme expressed in *Aspergillus oryzae. Appl. Environ. Microbiol.* 63:3151–3157.

Berka, R. M., Rey, M. W., Brown, K. M., Byun, T. and Klotz, A. V. (1998). Molecular characterization and expression of a phytase gene from the thermophilic fungus *Thermomyces lanuginosus. Appl. Environ. Microbiol.* 64: 4423-4427.

Bhat, M. K., and Bhat, S. 1997. Cellulose degrading enzymes and their potential industrial applications. *Biotechnol. Adv.* 15: 583-620.

Blochl, E., Rachel, R., Burggraf, S., Hafenbradl, D., Jannasch, H. W. and Stetter, K. O. (1997). *Pyrolobus fumarii*, gen. and sp. nov., represents a novel group of archaea, extending the upper temperature limit for life to 113°C. *Extremophiles* 1: 14-21.

Broad, T. E. and Shepherd, M. G. (1970). Purification and properties of glucose-6-phosphate dehydrogenase from the thermophilic fungus *Penicillium duponti. Biochim. Biophys. Acta* 198: 407-414.

Brock, T. D. (1995). The road to Yellowstone and beyond. *Annu. Rev. Microbiol.* 49: 1-28.

Bruins, M.E., Janssen, A.E.M. and Boom, R.M. (2001). Thermozymes and their applications-A review of recent literature and patents. *Appl. Biochem. Biotechnol.* 90: 155-186.

Bunni, L., McHale, L. and McHale, A. P. (1989). Production, isolation and partial characterization of an amylase system produced by *Talaromyces emersonii* CBS 814.70. *Enzyme Microb. Technol.* 11: 370-375.

Cardello, L., Terenzi, H. F. and Jorge, J. A. (1994). A cytosolic trehalase from the thermophilic fungus *Humicola grisea* var. *thermoidea. Microbiology* 140:1671-1677.

Cesar, T. and Mrsa, V. (1996). Purification and properties of the xylanase produced by *Thermomyces lanuginosus. Enzyme Microb. Technol.* 19: 289-296.

Chadha, B.S., Jaswinder, K., Rubinder, K., Saini, H.S. and Singh, S. (1999). Xylanase production by *Thermomyces lanuginosus* wild and mutant strains. *World J. Microbiol. Biotechnol.* 15: 217-221.

Chang, Y. (1967). The fungi of wheat straw compost. II. Biochemical and physiological studies. *Trans. Br. Mycol. Soc.* 50:667–677.

Chang, Y. and Hudson, H.J. (1967). Fungi of wheat straw compost I. Ecological studies. *Trans. Br. Mycol. Soc.* 50: 649-666.

Chapuis, R. and Zuber, H. (1970). Thermophilic aminopeptidases: AP I from *Talaromyces duponti. Methods Enzymol.* 19: 552-555.

Chefetz, B., Chen, Y. and Hadar, Y. (1998). Purification and characterization of laccase from *Chaetomium thermophilium* and its role in humification. *Appl. Environ. Microbiol.* 64: 3175-3179.

Colaco, C., Sen, S., Thangavelu, M., Pinder, S. and Roser, B. (1992). Extraordinary stability of enzymes dried in trehalose: simplified molecular biology. *Biotechnol.* 10: 1007-1011.

Cole, A.L.J. (1980). Thermophilic fungi. In: *Recent advances in Biology of Microorganisms* (Bilgrami, K.S. and Vyas, K.M., Eds.) Bishen Singh Mahendrapal singh, Dehradun, pp. 113-118.

Cooney, D. G. and Emerson, R. (1964). *Thermophilic Fungi: An Account of Their Biology, Activities and Classification*. W. H. Freeman and Company, San Francisco, p188.

Coutts, A. D. and Smith, R. E. (1976). Factors influencing the production of cellulases by *Sporotrichum thermophile. Appl. Environ. Microbiol.* 31: 819-825.

Craveri, R., Manachini, P.L. and Aragozini, F. (1974). Thermostable and alkaline lipolytic and proteolytic enzymes produced by a thermophilic mold. *Mycopathol. Mycol. Appl.* 54: 93-204.

Crisan, E.V. (1973). Current concepts of thermophilism and thermophilic fungi. *Mycologia* 63: 1171-1198.

Crowe, J. H. Crowe, L. M. and Chapman, D. (1984). Preservation of membranes in anhydrobiotic organisms: the role of trehalose. *Science* 223: 701-703.

Deploey, J.J. (1976). Carbohydrate nutrition of *Mucor miehei* and *Mucor pusillus*. *Mycologia* 68: 190-194.

Dusterhoft, E.M., Linssen, V.A.J.M., Voragen, A.G.J. and Beldman, G. (1999). Purification, characterization and properties of two xylanases from *Humicola insolens*. *Enzyme Microb. Technol.* 20: 437-445.

Eggins, H.O.W. and Coursey, D.G. (1964). Thermophilic fungi associated with Nigerian oil palm produce. *Nature* 203: 1081-1084.

Eggins, H.O.W. and Malik, K.A. (1969). The occurrence of thermophilic and cellulolytic fungi in pasture land soil. *Antonie Van Leeuvenhoek* 354 : 178-184.

Eggins, H.O.W., Szilvinyi, A. and Allsopp, D. (1972). The isolation of actively growing thermophilic fungi from insolated soils. *Int. Biodet. Bull.* 8: 53-58.

Ellis, D.H. (1980). Thermophilous fungi isolated from some Antarctic and sub-Antarctic soils. *Mycologia* 72: 1033-1036.

Emerson, R. (1968). Thermophilic fungi. In: *The Fungi*, Vol 3. (Anisworth, G.C. and Sussman, A.S., Eds.), Academic Press, New York. pp. 105-128.

Fangerstrom, R., Paloheimo, M., Lantto, R., Lahtinen, T. and Suominen, P. (1997). *Novel xylanases and their uses*. (Assignees: Primalco, Finland) Patent No. WO 9722691.

Fergus, C.L. (1964). Thermophilic and thermotolerant moulds in mushroom compost during peak heating. *Mycologia* 56: 267-284.

Fergus, C.L. and Sinden, J.W. (1969). A new thermophilic fungus from mushroom compost *Thielavia thermophila* sp. Nov. *Can. J. Bot.* 47: 1635.

Filho, E. X. F. (1996). Purification and characterization of a β-glucosidase from solid-state cultures of *Humicola grisea* var. *thermoidea*. *Can. J. Microbiol.* 42:1-5.

Fischer, L., Scheckermann, C. and Wagner, F. (1995). Purification and characterization of a thermotolerant β-galactosidase from *Thermomyces lanuginosus*. *Appl. Environ. Microbiol.* 61: 1497-1501.

Flanningan, B. (1969). Microflora of barley grains. *Trans. Br. Mycol. Soc.* 53: 371-379.

Folan, M. A. and Coughlan, M. P. (1978). The cellulase complex in the culture filtrate of the thermophilic fungus, *Talaromyces emersonii*. *Int. J. Biochem.* 9: 717-722.

Fontana, A., Boccu', E. and Veronese, F. M. (1974). Purification of a phosphodiesterase from the thermophilic fungus *Talaromyces duponti*. Hoppe-Seyler's Z. *Physiol. Chem*. 355: 1436-1442.

Gaikwad, J. S. and Maheshwari, R. (1994). Localization and release of b-glucosidase in the thermophilic and cellulolytic fungus, *Sporotrichum thermophile*. *Exp. Mycol*. 18: 300-310.

Ganju, R. K., Vithayathil, P. J. and Murthy, S. K. (1989). Purification and characterization of two xylanases from *Chaetomium thermophile* var. coprophile. *Can. J. Microbiol*. 35: 836-842.

Ganju, R. K., Murthy, S. K. and Vithayathil, P. J. (1990). Purification and functional characteristics of an endocellulase from *Chaetomium thermophile* var. *coprophile*. *Carbohydr. Res*. 197: 245-255.

Gomes, J., H. Purkarthofer, M. Hayn, J. Kapplmuller, M. S. and Steiner W. (1993). Production of a high level of cellulase-free xylanase by the thermophilic fungus *Thermomyces lanuginosus* in laboratory and pilot scales using lignocellulosic materials. *Appl. Microbiol. Biotechnol*. 39: 700-707.

Greaves, H. (1971). Biodeterioration of tropical hardwood chips in outdoor storage. *TAPPI* 54: 1128-1133.

Gregory, P.H., Lucey, M.E., Festenstein, G.N. and Skinner, F.A. (1963). Microbiological and biochemical changes during molding of hay. *J. Gen. Microbiol*. 33: 147-174.

Gupta, S. D. and Maheshwari, R. (1985). Is organic acid required for nutrition of thermophilic fungi? *Arch. Microbiol*. 141: 164-169.

Hajny, G.J. (1966). Outside storage of pulp wood chips, a review and bibliography. *TAPPI*. 49: 97-109.

Hashimoto, H., Iwaasa, T. and Yokotsuka, T. (1972). Thermostable acid protease produced by *Penicillium duponti* K1014, a true thermophilic fungus newly isolated from compost. *Appl. Microbiol*. 24: 986-992.

Hayashida, S. and Yoshioka, H. (1980). Production and purification of thermostable cellulases from *Humicola insolens* YH-8. *Agric. Biol. Chem*. 44: 1721-1728.

Hayashida, S. and Mo., K. (1986). Production and characteristics of aviceldisintegrating endoglucanase from a protease-negative *Humicola grisea* var. *thermoidea* mutant. *Appl. Environ. Microbiol*. 51:1041-1046.

Hayashida, S., K. Ohta, and Mo. K. (1988). Cellulases of *Humicola insolens* and *Humicola grisea*. *Methods Enzymol*. 160: 323-332.

Hayes, W. A. (1969). Microbiological changes in composting wheat straw horse manure mixtures. *Mush. Sci*. 7: 173-186.

Hedger, J. N. and Hudson, H. J. (1974). Nutritional studies of *Thermomyces lanuginosus* from wheat straw compost. Trans. *Br. Mycol. Soc*. 62: 129-143.

Henssen, A. (1957). Uber die Bedeutung der thermophilen Mikro-organismen fur die Zersetzung des Stallmistes. *Arch. Mikrobiol*. 27: 63-81.

Huge-Jensen, B., Andreasen, F., Christensen, T., Christensen, M. Thim, L. and Boel, E. (1989). *Rhizomucor miehei* triglyceride lipase is processed and secreted from transformed *Aspergillus oryzae*. *Lipids* 24: 781-785.

Inamdar, A. (1987). Polygalacturonase from *Thermoascus aurantiacus*: isolation and functional characteristics. *Ph.D. thesis*. Indian Institute of Science, Bangalore, India.

Jain, P.C. (1999). Spoilage of stored products. In: *Thermophilic Moulds in Biotechnology* (B.N. Johri, T. Satyanarayana and J. Olsen, Eds.) Kluwer Academic publishers, Dordrecht, pp. 289-316.

Jaychandran, S. and Ramabadran, R. (1970). Production of amylase by *Thermoascus aurantiacus*. *Indian J. Exp. Biol.* 8: 344.

Jensen, B., and Olsen, J. (1992). Physicochemical properties of a purified alpha-amylase from the thermophilic fungus *Thermomyces lanuginosus*. *Enzyme Microb. Technol.* 14: 112-116.

Jodice, F.R., Jole, C.S., Fiusello, N., France, O. and Cantini, G. (1975). Thermophilic fungi I. Contribution to their isolation, metabolism and their ability to degrade organic matter. *Allonia* 20: 53-74.

Johri, B.N. (1980). Biology of thermophilous fungi. In: *Recent Advances in Biology of Microorganisms* (Bilgrami, K.S. and Vyas, K.M., Eds.) Bishen Singh Mahendrapal singh, Dehradun, pp. 265-277.

Johri, B.N. and Satyanarayana, T. (1986). Thermophilic moulds- Perspective in basic and applied research. *Indian Rev. Life Sci.* 6: 75-100.

Kadowaki, M. K., Polizeli, M. L. T. M., Terenzi, H. F. and Jorge, J. A. (1996). Characterization of trehalose activities from the thermophilic fungus *Scytalidium thermophilum*. *Biochim. Biophys. Acta* 1291: 199-205.

Kango, Naveen (2007) Lignocellulose Biotechnology: Harnessing renewable plant materials for energy and chemicals. *Everyman's Science*, XLII (4) 194-197.

Kango, Naveen, Agrawal, S.C. and Jain, P.C. (2006). Production and properties of thermostable xylanase by *Thermomyces lanuginosus* NK-2 grown on lignocelluloses. *Biotechnol.* 5(2): 148-152.

Kango, Naveen and Jain, P.C. (2005). Production and application of fungal xylanases. In: *Fungi: Diversity and Biotechnology* (Rai, M.K. and Deshmukh S.K., Eds.), Scientific Publishers, New Delhi. pp. 251-281. ISBN 81-7233-403-6.

Kango, Naveen, Agrawal, S.C. and Jain, P.C. (2003a). Isolation of thermophilic fungi from soil and decomposing organic matter. *Asian Jr. of Microbiol., Biotechnol. Env. Sci.* 5(4): 445-447.

Kango, Naveen, Agrawal, S.C. and Jain, P.C. (2003b). Production of xylanase by *Emericella nidulans* NK-62 on low-value lignocellulosic substrates. *World J. Microbiol. Biotechnol.* 19 (7): 691-694.

Kawamori, M., Takayama, I. K. and Takasawa, S. (1987). Production of cellulases by a thermophilic fungus *Thermoascus aurantiacus* A-131. *Agric. Biol. Chem.* 51: 647-654.

Kelly, C.T., O'Mahony, M.R. and Fogarty, W.M. (1989). Extracellular xylanolytic enzymes of *Paecilomyces variotii*. *Biotechnol. Lett.* 9: 125-130.

Khandke, K. M., P. J. Vithayathil, and S. K. Murthy. (1989). Purification of xylanase, β-glucosidase, endocellulase, and exocellulase from a thermophilic fungus, *Thermoascus aurantiacus*. *Arch. Biochem. Biophys*. 274: 491-500.

Kuster, E. and Locci, R. (1964). Studies on peat and peat microorganisms II. Occurrence of thermophilic fungi in peat. *Arch. Microbiol*. 48: 319-324.

La Touche, C. J. (1950). On thermophilic species of *Chaetomium*. *Trans. Br. Mycol. Soc*. 33: 94-104.

Lacey, J. (1974). Moulding of sugarcane bagasse and its prevention. *Ann. Appl. Biol*. 76: 63-76.

Lin, J., Ndlovu, L.M., Singh, S. and Pillay, B. (1999). Purification and biochemical characteristics of β-D-xylanase from a thermophilic fungus, *Thermomyces lanuginosus*-SSBP. Biotechnol. *Appl. Biochem*. 30: 73-79.

Liu, W.H., Beppu, T. and Arima, K. (1974). Cultural conditions and some properties of lipase of *Humicola lanuginosa* S-38. *Agr. Biol. Chem*. 36: 1919-1924.

Maheshwari, R. and Balasubramanyam, P.V. (1988). Simultaneous utilization of glucose and sucrose by thermophilic fungi. *J. Bacteriol*. 170: 3274-3280.

Maheshwari, R., Balasubramanyam, P. V. and Palanivelu, P. (1983). Distinctive behaviour of invertase in a thermophilic fungus, *Thermomyces lanuginosus*. *Arch. Microbiol*. 134: 255-260.

Maheshwari, R., Bharadwaj, G. and Bhat, M. K. (2000). Thermophilic fungi: their physiology and enzymes. *Microbiol. Mol. Biol. Rev*. 64: 461-488.

Margaritis, A. and Creese, E. (1981). Thermal stability characteristics of cellulase enzymes of *Sporotrichum thermophile*. *Biotechnol. Lett*. 3: 471-476.

Matsuo, M., and Yasui, T. (1985). Properties of xylanase of *Malbranchea pulchella* var. *sulfurea* no. 48. *Agric. Biol. Chem*. 49:839-841.

Matsuo, M., Yasui, T. and Kobayashi, T. (1977). Purification and some properties of β-glucosidase from *Malbranchea pulchella* var. *sulfurea* no. 48. *Agric. Biol. Chem*. 41: 1593-1599.

Morgan-Jones, G. (1974). Notes on hyphomycetes V. A new thermophilic species of *Acremonium*. *Can. J. Bot*. 52: 429-431.

Moubasher, A.H. Aboel-Hafez, S.I.I., Aboelfattah, M.M. and Moharrarh, A.M. (1982). Fungi of wheat and bean straw composts 2. Thermophilic fungi. *Mycopathol*. 84: 61-72.

Mouchacca, J. (1997). Thermophilic fungi: biodiversity and taxonomic status. Cryptogam. *Mycol*. 18: 19-69.

Mulinge, S.K. and Apinis, A.E. (1969). Occurrence of thermophilic fungi in stored moist barley grain. *Trans. Br. Mycol. Soc*. 53: 361-370.

Odibo, F.J.C., Okafor, N., Tom, M.U. and Oyeka, C.A. (1992). Purification and characterization of β-amylase from *Hendersonula toruloidea*. *Starch* 44: 192-195.

Ofosu-Asideu, A. and Smith, R. S. (1973). Degradation of soft wood by thermophilic and thermotolerant fungi. *Mycologia* 65: 240-244.

Ogundero, V.W. (1980). Lipase activity of thermophilic fungi from mouldy groundnuts in Nigeria. *Mycologia* 72: 118-126.

Ong, P. S. and Gaucher, G. M. (1976). Production, purification and characterization of thermomycolase, the extracellular serine protease of the thermophilic fungus *Malbranchea pulchella* var. sulfurea. *Can. J. Microbiol.* 22: 165-176.

Ottesen, M. and Rickert, W. (1970). The isolation and partial characterization of an acid protease produced by *Mucor miehei*. C. R. *Trav. Lab. Carlsberg* 37: 301-325.

Prabhu, K. A., and Maheshwari, R. (1999). Biochemical properties of xylanases from a thermophilic fungus, *Melanocarpus albomyces*, and their action on plant cell walls. *J. Biosci.* 24: 461-470.

Prasad, A. R. S. and Maheshwari, R. (1978). Growth and trehalase activity in the thermophilic fungus *Thermomyces lanuginosus*. *Proc. Indian Acad. Sci.* 87B: 231-241.

Rajasekaran, A. K. and Maheshwari, R. (1990). Growth kinetics and intracellular protein breakdown in mesophilic and thermophilic fungi. *Indian J. Exp. Biol.* 28: 46-51.

Rajasekaran, A. K. and Maheshwari, R. (1993). Thermophilic fungi: an assessment of their potential for growth in soil. *J. Biosci.* 18: 345-354.

Rana, B.K., Johri, B.N. and Thakur, I.S. (1996). Formation and activities of xylan-hydrolysing enzymes of *Humicola grisea* var. *thermoidea*. *World J. Microbiol. Biotechnol.* 12: 12-15.

Rao, V. B., Maheshwari, R., Sastry, N. V. S. and Subba Rao, P. V. (1979). A thermostable glucoamylase from the thermophilic fungus *Thermomyces lanuginosus*. *Curr. Sci.* 48: 113-115.

Rao, V. B., Sastri, N. V. S. and Subba Rao, P. V. (1981). Purification and characterization of a thermostable glucoamylase from the thermophilic fungus *Thermomyces lanuginosus*. *Biochem. J.* 193: 379-387.

Renosto, F., Schultz, T., Re, E. Mazer, J., Chandler, C. J., Barron, A. and Segel, H. (1985). Comparative stability and catalytic and chemical propertiesm of the sulfate-activating enzymes from *Penicillium chrysogenum* (mesophile) and *Penicillium duponti* (thermophile). *J. Bacteriol.* 164: 674-683.

Rosenberg, S. L. (1975). Temperature and pH optima for 21 species of thermophilic and thermotolerant fungi. *Can. J. Microbiol.* 21: 1535-1540.

Roy, S. K., Dey, S. K., Raha, S. K. and Chakrabarty S. L. (1990). Purification and properties of an extracellular endoglucanase from *Myceliophthora thermophila* D-14 (ATCC 48104). *J. Gen. Microbiol.* 136: 1967-1971.

Sadhukhan, R., Roy, S. K., Raha, S. K., Manna, S. and Chakrabarty, S. L. (1992). Induction and regulation of a-amylase synthesis in a cellulolytic thermophilic fungus *Myceliophthora thermophila* D14 (ATCC 48104). *Indian J. Exp. Biol.* 30: 482-486.

Sahm, D.F. and Chapman, E.S. (1976) Effects of carbon sources on *Papulospora thermophila* at various temperatures. *Mycologia* 68: 168-174.

Saraswat, V. and Bisaria, V.S. (2000). Purification, characterization and substrate specificities of xylanase isoenzymes from *Melanocarpus* albomyces IIS 68. *Biosci. Biotechnol. Biochem.* 64: 1173-1180.

Satyanarayana, T. and Johri, B.N. (1983). Extracellular protease of thermophilic fungi isolated from decomposing paddy straw. *Trop. Plant. Sci. Res.* 1: 137-140.

Satyanarayana, T. and Johri, B.N. (1984). Ecology of thermophilic fungi. In. *Progress in Microbial Ecology* (Mukerjee *et al.*, Eds.) Print House, Lucknow pp. 349-361.

Satyanarayana, T., Johri, B.N. and Klein, J. (1992). Biotechnological potential of thermophilic fungi. In: *Handbook of Applied Mycology*, Vol.4 (Arora, D.K., Elander, R.P. and Mukerji, K.G., Eds.) Marcell Dekker, New York, pp. 729-761.

Satyanarayana, T., Johri, B.N. and Saksena, S.B. (1977). Seasonal variation in mycoflora of nesting materials of birds with special reference to thermophilic fungi. *Trans. Br. Mycol. Soc.* 68: 307-309.

Shenolikar, S. and Stevenson, K. J. (1982). Purification and partial characterization of a thiol proteinase from the thermophilic fungus *Humicola lanuginosa*. *Biochem. J.* 205: 147-152.

Singhai, S. and Jain, P.C. (1992). Thermophilous fungi from decomposing organic matter: compost and sawdust. *Geobios New Reports*. 11: 41-44.

Siqueira, E.M.D., Mizuta, K. and Giglio, J..R. (1979). α-amylase of *Pycnoporus sanguineus*. *Mycol. Res.* 101: 188-190.

Somkuti, G. A. and Babel, F. J. (1968a). Purification and properties of *Mucor pusillus* acid protease. *J. Bacteriol.* 95: 1407-1414.

Somkuti, G.A. and Babel, F.J. (1968b). Lipase activity of *Mucor pusillus*. *Appl. Microbiol.* 16: 617-619.

Subrahmanyam, A. (1980). Studies on *Thermoascus aurantiacus*. *Acta Mycologia* 16: 121-131.

Subrahmanyam, A. (1999). Ecology and Distribution. In: *Thermophilic Moulds in Biotechnology*. (Johri, B.N. Satyanarayana, T. and Olsen, J., Eds.), Kluwer Academic Publishers, Dordrecht, pp. 13-42.

Tansey, M. R. and Brock, T. D. (1972). The upper temperature limit for eukaryotic organisms. *Proc. Natl. Acad. Sci. USA* 69: 2426-2428.

Tansey, M. R. and Brock, T. D. (1978). Microbial life at high temperatures: ecological aspects. In: *Microbial Life in Extreme Environments* (Kushner, D. J., Ed.), Academic Press Ltd., London, pp. 159-216.

Tansey, M.R. (1973). Isolation of thermophilic fungi from alligator nesting material. *Mycologia* 65: 594-601.

Tansey, M.R. and Brock, T.D. (1971). Isolation of thermophilic and thermotolerant fungi from hot spring effluents and thermal soils of yellow stone national park. *Bacteriol. Proc.* p 36..

Tansey, M.R. and Jack, M.A. (1977). Growth of thermophilic fungi in soil *in situ* and *in vitro*. *Mycologia*. 69: 563-578.

Taylor, P. M., Napier, E. J. and Fleming I. D.(1978). Some properties of glucoamylase produced by the thermophilic fungus *Humicola lanuginosa*. *Carbohydrate Research* 61: 301-308.

Thakre, R. P. and Johri, B. N. (1976). Occurrence of thermophilic fungi in coalmine soils of Madhya Pradesh. *Curr. Sci.* 45: 271-273.

Udagawa, S., Furuya, K. and Horie, Y. (1973). Notes on some ascomycetous micro fungi from soil. *Bull. Natl. Sci. Mus.* (Tokyo), 16: 503-520.

Vandamme, E.J., Logghe, J.M. and Geeraerts, H.A.M. (1982). Cellulase activity of a thermophilic *Aspergillus fumigatus* (Fresinius). *J. Chem. Technol. Biotechnol.* 32: 968-974.

Waksman, S.A., and Cordon, T.C. (1939). Thermophilic decomposition of plant residues in composts by pure and mixed culture of microorganisms. *Soil Sci.* 47: 217-225.

Waksman, S.A., Umbreit, W.W. and Cordon, T.C. (1939). Thermophilic actinomycetes and fungi in soils and in composts. *Soil Sci.* 47: 37-61.

Wallace, H.A., Sinha, R.N. and Mills, J.T. (1986). Fungi associated with small wheat bulks during prolonged storage. *Can. J. Bot.* 54: 1332-1343.

Wyss, M., Brugger, R., Kronenberger, A., Re´my, R., Fimbel, R., Osterhelt, G. Lehmann, M. and Van Loon, A. P. G. M. (1999). Biochemical characterization of fungal phytases (myo-inositol hexakisphosphate phosphohydrolase): catalytic properties. *Appl. Environ. Microbiol.* 65: 367-373.

Yang, J., Teplyakov, A. and Quail, J. W. (1997). Crystal structure of the aspartic proteinase from *Rhizomucor miehei* at 2.15 Å resolution. *J. Mol. Biol.* 268: 449-459.

Yoshioka, H., Anraku, S.I. and Hayashida, S. (1982). Production and purification of a novel type of CMCase from *Humicola grisea* var. *thermoidea* YH-78. *Agric. Biol. Chem.* 46: 75-82.

Microbial Biotechnology and Ecology (2011) *Pages* **320–343**
Editors: **Deepak Vyas, G.S. Paliwal, P.K.Khare and R.K Gupta**
Published by: **DAYA PUBLISHING HOUSE, NEW DELHI**

Chapter 19

Biodiversity and Conservation of Mushroom in Chhattisgarh Region

☆ *M.P. Thakur*, C.S. Shukla and V.K. Yadav*

Department of Plant Pathology,
Indira Gandhi Agricultural University, Raipur – 492 006, Chhattisgarh

ABSTRACT

Chhattisgarh State is divided into three agroclimatic zone (Plains of Chhattisgarh, Bastar Plateau, Northern Hill Region) and occupied 135191 sq. km area of which 43.8 per cent area is under forest. More than 80 per cent of the population is engaged in agricultural and forest activities. Among these activities mushrooms are one of the choicest item which are collected and consumed by local people during rainy season. It constitutes an important source of their income. They sold mushroom in local market hats/towns. The survey was conducted for occurrence of naturally growing mushrooms in all districts of Chhattisgarh. The survey for naturally growing mushroom flora was initiated in 1988 and continued till date. In all, 78 mushrooms were collected during rainy season and identified. Among the collected mushrooms, 33 edible, 22 were as non edible, 2 medicinal, 2 poisonous and 19 were unidentified. Maximum number of mushrooms were collected from Bastar Plateau and most of them were consumed by tribals. The most frequent mushrooms observed from different places of Chhattisgarh were *Volvariella volvacea*, *Cantherellus* spp., *Tuber* sp., *Rusula* sp. and *Termitomyces* spp. Some mushrooms like *Termitomyces* spp., *Rusulla* spp., *Volvariella* like and *Ganoderma lucidum* were used as medicine to reduce labour pain, headache, constipation and healing of wounds respectively.

---

* E-mail: mp_thakur@yahoo.com

Introduction

Chhattisgarh State has 135191 sq. km area, which accounts 4.11 per cent of the total geographical area of the country. The state has 43.8 per cent of total geographical area covered by forest and 35 per cent area is under cultivated land. It is located between 17° 48 N and 24 ° 5 N latitude and 80° 15–84° 20E longitude. It is touched with the boundaries of Uttar Pradesh and Jharkhand in North, Orissa in East, Andhra Pradesh in South and M. P., Maharastra in West. Administratively, it is divided into 146 blocks, 97 Tehsils with 16 Districts. According to Census Report of 2001, the total population is about 20795956 of which 16622627 lives in villages and rest in Urban areas. Near about 80 per cent of the population is engaged in agricultural activities. The population is dominated by Schedule Tribe (32 per cent), Schedule Caste (12 per cent) and backward classes. Thus, the weaker section constitute about 44 per cent of the total population. The population density is 154 per sq. km. The state has 28 per cent area under irrigation and paddy is the main crop grown in 80 per cent of the area as rainfed.

The climatic conditions prevailing in Chhattisgarh made the natural habitat for a large number of mushroom flora. The detailed information for the presence of natural agaric flora in different agroclimatic zones of Chhattisgarh was started with the inception of All India Coordinated Mushroom Improvement Project in 1988 at IGAU, Raipur. Prior to 1988, no systematic efforts were made for collection, identification and preservation of fleshy fungi of this state. But, thereafter, the systematic work was started to explore the kind of wild mushroom flora available and exploit their production potential in a commercial scale.

Agroclimatic Zones

Chhattisgarh is divided into 3 agroclimatic zones *i.e.* Plains of Chhattisgarh, Bastar Plateau, Northern Hill Region (Table 19.1). About 74 per cent area of Chhattisgarh Plains, 97 per cent of Bastar Plateau and 95 per cent in Northern Hills are rainfed (Table 19.2). Forest area in Bastar Plateau is highest followed by Northern Hills and Chhattisgarh Plains. The main source of irrigation is canals. The cropping intensity of the region is 121 per cent.

Table 19.1: Area, Classification and Rainfall in Chhattisgarh

Months	*Raipur*				*Jagdalpur*				*Ambikapur*			
	Max. Temp.	*Min. Temp.*	*Rain-fall*	*Relative Humidity*	*Max. Temp.*	*Min. Temp.*	*Rain-fall*	*Relative Humidity*	*Max. Temp.*	*Min. Temp.*	*Rain-fall*	*Relative Humidity*
January	26.8	11.9	026.0	92	25.2	10.8	38.3	94	24	8	28	85
February	28.9	12.3	031.0	88	28.1	12.1	13.6	92	28	11	22	79
March	36.6	17.7	011.6	74	35.0	17.1	6.4	89	31	14	55	63
April	39.9	23.4	004.2	57	36.0	22.9	43.5	84	34	22	26	50
May	41.1	27.9	008.9	48	35.6	23.0	85.6	73	39	23	31.5	50
June	36.0	25.9	252.2	74	30.0	22.3	351.8	84	35	23	300	79
July	31.8	24.3	379.8	92	27.6	22.2	356.3	91	32	21	455	90
August	29.1	24.4	156.6	92	25.9	21.8	308.6	93	32	21	349	89
September	32.2	24.4	136.4	92	29.6	21.9	258.2	93	30	19	310	89
October	30.8	19.3	020.2	93	29.3	19.0	151.4	93	30	19	50	88
November	30.2	13.8	000.0	90	27.1	12.2	7.6	92	28	10	25	87
December	28.1	10.9	000.0	90	26.8	8.0	0.0	94	26	8	22	85

Table 19.2: Details of Agroclimatic Zones of Chhattisgarh

Agroclimatic Zone	Districts	Geographical Area	Area Under Forest (%)	Rainfall	Soil Type
Plains of Chhattisgarh	Raipur, Mahasamund, Dhamtari, Durg, Rajnandgaon, Kawardha, Kanker, Bilaspur, Janjgir, Korba and Raigarh	7493.781 sq km	33.3	900-1000 mm	Antisol (Bhata) Alfisol (Dorsa) Vertisol (Kanhar) Inceptisol (Matasi)
Bastar Plateau Zone	Bastar, Dantewada	3262.626 sq km	65.2	1200-1600 mm	Mollisoils
Northern Hill Region	Sarguja, Korea, Jashpur	2846.954 sq km	43.8	1200-1400 mm	Vertisols Alfisols

Fleshy Fungi of Chhattisgarh

The work on survey, collection, isolation and preservation of naturally growing fleshy fungi during monsoon season was initiated in 1988. The local people of Chhattisgarh do collect and consume some edible mushrooms as well as bring them to the local market for sale during July to October. According to Kumar and Agrawal (1989) nearly 50 tons of naturally growing edible fleshy fungi is collected from Bastar alone during monsoon season. A survey for the presence of naturally occurring fleshy fungi was conducted from 1989 to 1995 (Anonymous, 1989-1995). Shukla *et al*. (2001) surveyed the forest area of Chhattisgarh and collected edible and wild mushrooms. Thakur *et al*. (2005) reported enormous wild mushroom flora existing in Chhattisgarh. They isolated, identified and characterized some of the mushroom flora. Some wild edible mycorrhizal mushrooms of Chhattisgarh were also reported by Shukla (2005). Shukla *et al*. (2001) collected various species of mushroom from Bilaspur division and reported that some mushrooms have antitumour, antibacterial, antifungal and antiviral properties. The species of *Agaricus, Russula, Termitomyces* are being used for treatment of goitre, wound and small pox respectively. During survey, most commonly available mushrooms encountered were *Russula* spp., *Volvariella* spp., *Termitomyces* spp., *Tuber* spp. and *Cantherellus* spp. (Annonymous, 2002, 2003, 2004, Sharma and Samota, 2006). The fleshy fungi collected from different areas of Chhattisgarh with respect to habitat, season, distribution and ethnic information is presented. Most of these fungi were identified using standard monographs (Purkayastha and Chandra, 1985; Pacioni, 1985; Rinaldi and Tyndalo, 1974; Pegler and Spooner, 1997). The details are as under:

Agrocybe erebia

Habit and habitat : Sporophore in groups on ground

Season : Rainy season (June–October)

Distribution : Achanakamar sanctuary area of Bilaspur

Edibility : Non edible

***Agrocybe* sp.**

Habit and habitat : Sporophore in groups or scattered in soil

Season : Rainy season (June–October)

Distribution : From different places of Bilaspur

Edibility : Non edible

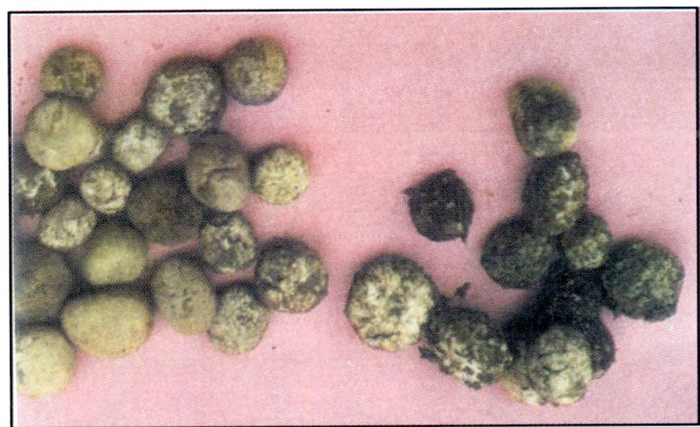

***Tuber* sp.**

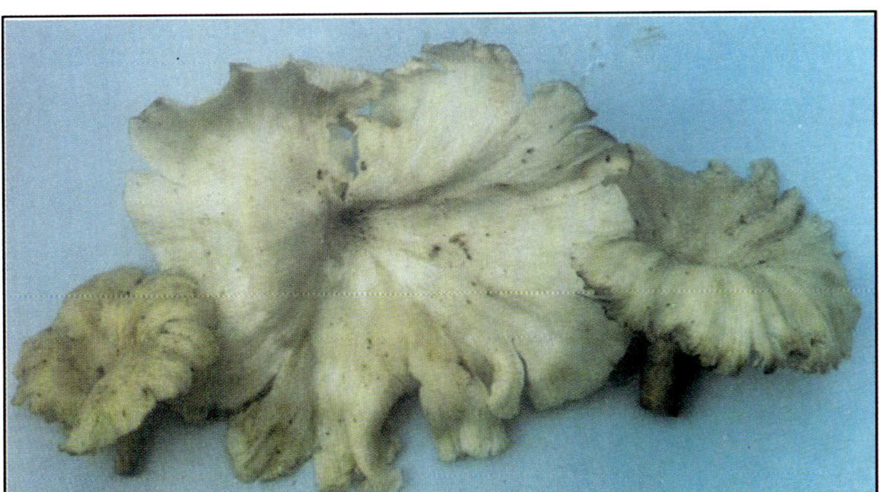

***Cantherellus* sp.**

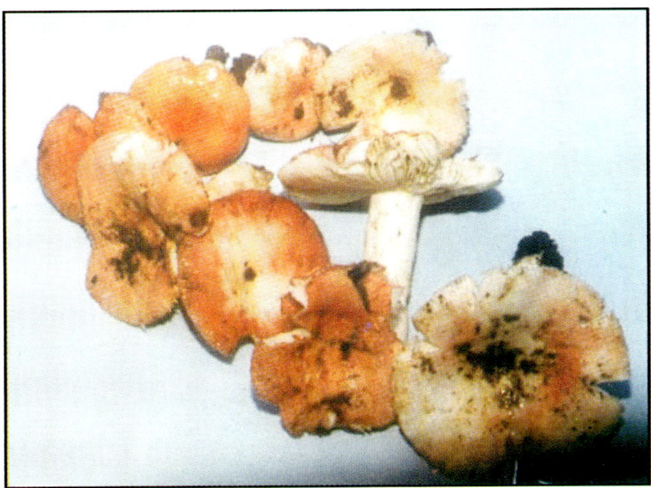

***Russula* sp.**

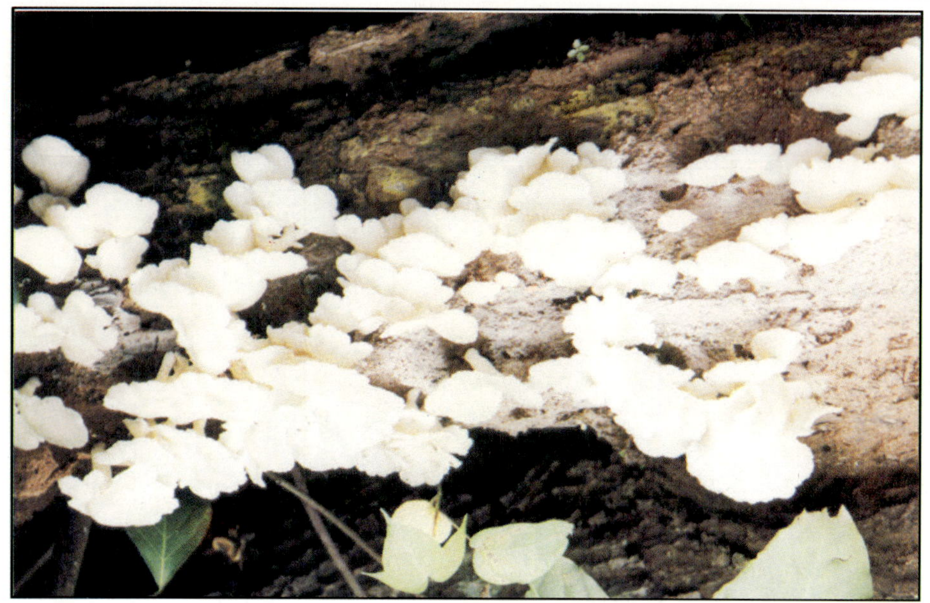

Pleurotus florida

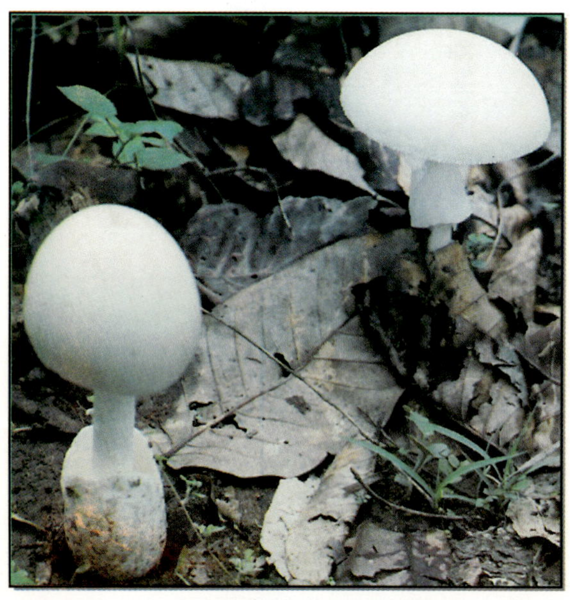

***Amanita* sp.**

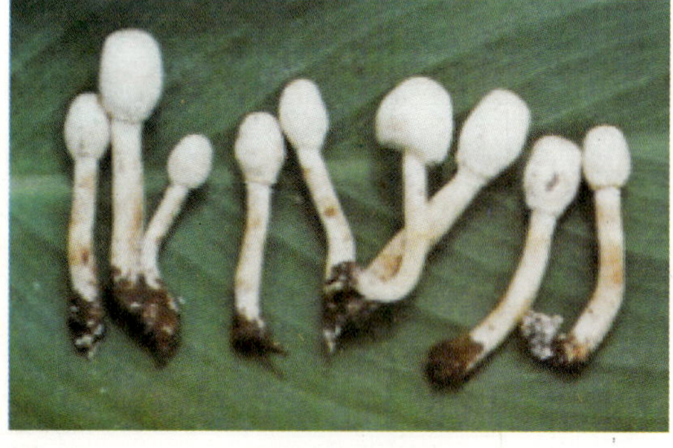

***Coprinus* sp.**

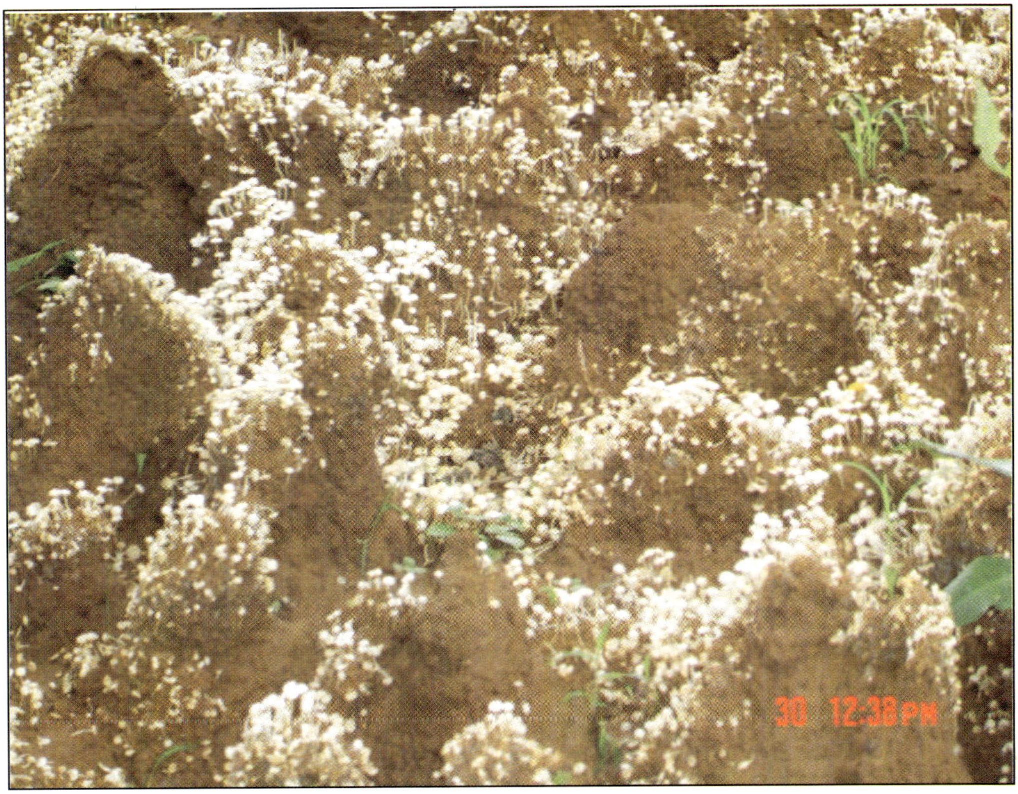

Termitomyces microcarpus

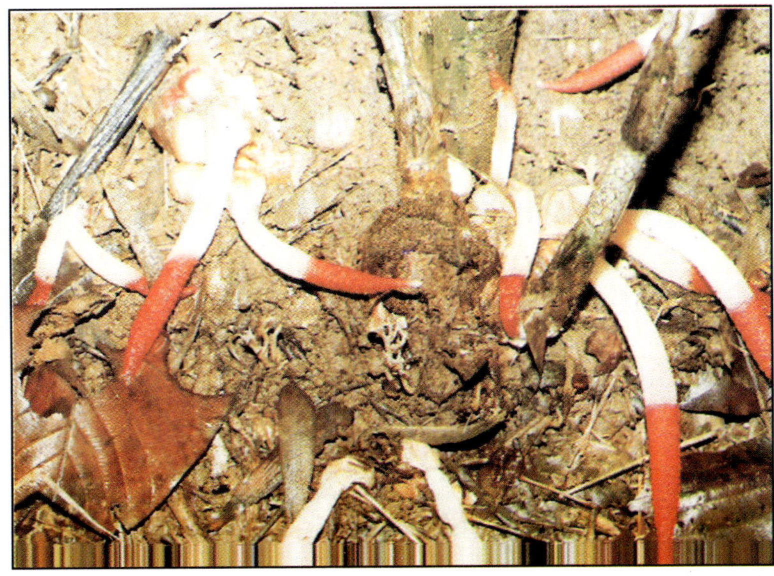

Mutinus **sp.**

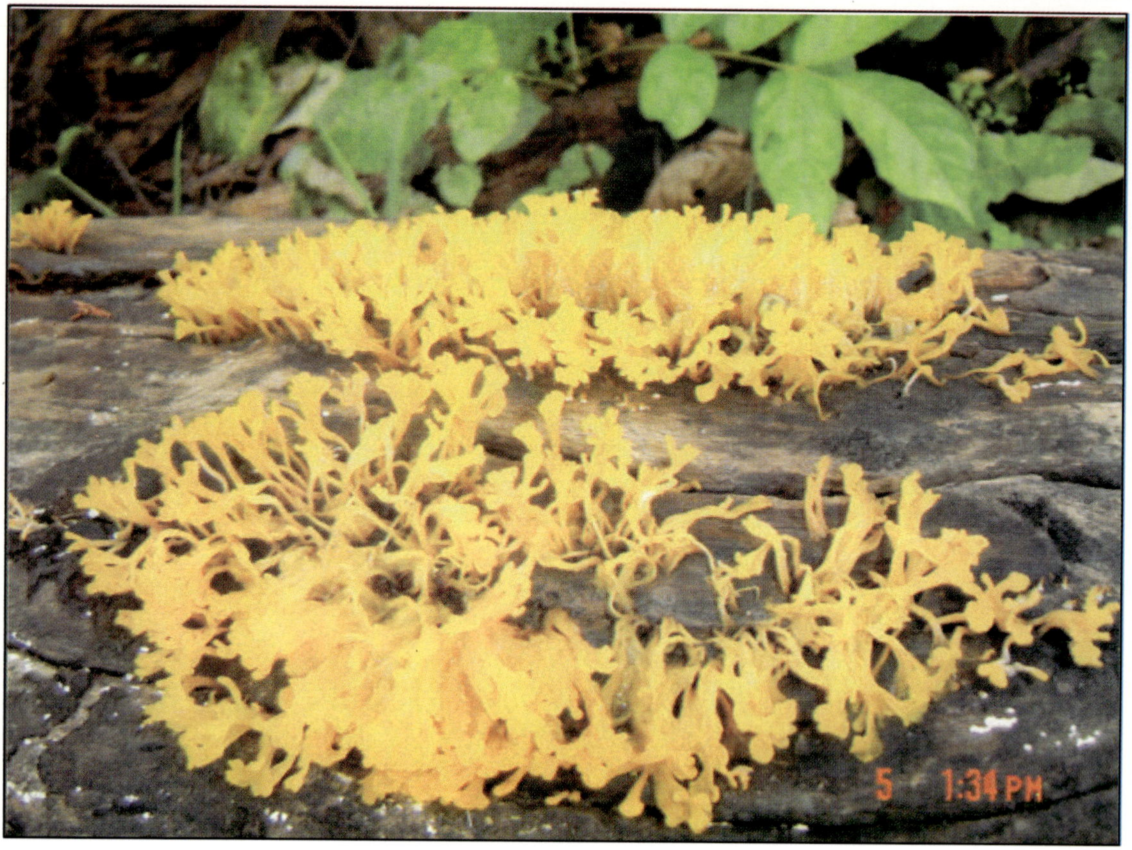

Ramaria **sp.**

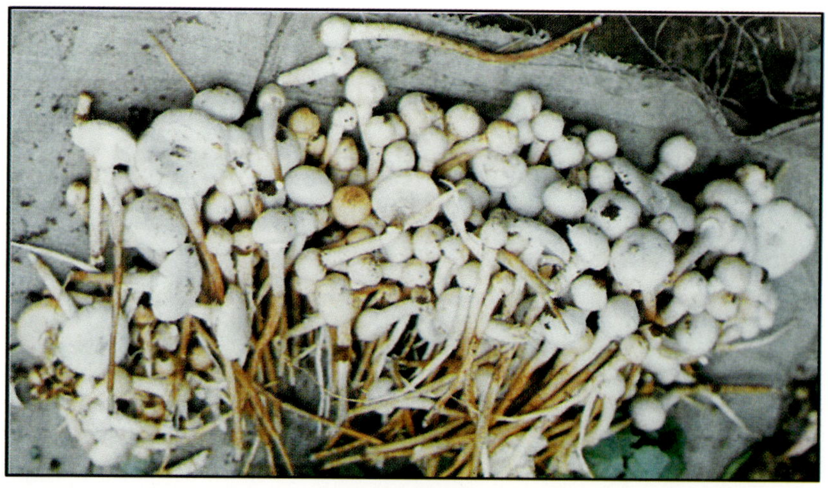

Termitomyces **sp.**

Amanitopsis

Habit and habitat : Growing singly in scattered on leaf litter

Season : Rainy season (August)

Distribution : Barnavapara

Edibility : Edible but consumed by local people

Amanita citrina

Habit and habitat : Under shrubs

Season : Rainy season (June–October)

Distribution : Collected from different places of Bastar forest

Edibility : Poisonous

***Amanita* sp.**

Habit and habitat : Sporophore occurred in scattered on the soil under shrubs

Season : Rainy season (June–October)

Distribution : Collected from different places of Bastar forest

Edibility : Not known

Armillaria mellea

Habit and habitat : Habit and habitat- sporophore growing on deciduous stumps of dead trunk of tree

Season : Rainy season (June–October)

Distribution : Raipur and Bilaspur

Edibility : Non edible

***Astreatus hygrometricus* (Boda)**

Habit and habitat : Scattered on the soil, Hypogeal mycorrhizal association with root of sal tree

Season : Rainy season (June–October)

Distribution : All the forest area of Chhattisgarh

Edibility : Excellent

Auricularia polytricha

Habit and habitat : Solitary or gregarious on dead wood and logs in all region of Chhattisgarh

Season : Rainy season (June–October)

Distribution : All region of Chhattisgarh

Edibility : Edible

***Auricularia* sp.**

Habit and habitat : On dead branches of mango, Custard apple, subabool, gulmohar

Season : Rainy season (June–October)

Distribution : Raipur

Edibility : Edible

***Boletus* sp.**

Habit and habitat	:	Sporophore solitary on sandy soil under dense shrubs on leaf litter
Season	:	After good monsoon rains
Distribution	:	In the area of Uddanti and Barnawapara Wild life Sanctuary of Raipur
Edibility	:	Edible but not consumed by local people

Bovista appendicellata

Habit and habitat	:	Sporophore scattered on leaf litter under the shed of broad leaves trees
Season	:	Rainy season (June–October)
Distribution	:	Bilaspur
Edibility	:	Not known

***Calocybe* sp.**

Habit and habitat	:	Sporophore solitary in soil under broad leaves trees
Season	:	Rainy season (June–October)
Distribution	:	Restricted in few localities of Ambikapur forest
Edibility	:	Edible but not consumed by the local people

Clavatia cyantiformis

Habit and habitat	:	Solitary or in groups on leaf litter of shrubs
Season	:	Rainy season (June–October)
Distribution	:	Forest area of Korea District
Edibility	:	Edible but not consumed by local people

***Cantherellus* sp. (Bans phutu)**

Habit and habitat	:	Sporophore in groups, have with mycorrhizal association with bamboo trees
Season	:	Rainy season during August month near Raksh Bandhan
Distribution	:	In all bamboo growing areas of Chhattisgarh
Edibility	:	Excellent and sold in local market @ 60-80/kg

Clavaria fumosa

Habit and habitat	:	Sporophore grows in groups on the ground on fallen branches
Season	:	Rainy season
Distribution	:	Sitanadi Wild Life Sanctuary
Edibility	:	Not Known

***Clavaria* sp.**

Habit and habitat	:	On wood in scattered
Season	:	Rainy season
Distribution	:	Tirathgarh, Narayanpur
Edibility	:	Not edible

Clitocybe gestrpoa

Habit and habitat	:	Sporophore grows in groups under the shrubs on leaf litter
Season	:	Rainy season
Distribution	:	Tirathgarh, Chitrakut and other places of Bastar
Edibility	:	Poisonous

***Coprinus comatus* (Shaggy cap)**

Habit and habitat	:	Gregarious in grassland and road side
Season	:	Rainy season
Distribution	:	In all districts of Chhattisgarh
Edibility	:	Edible but rarely consumed by local people

***Coprinus* sp. (Ink cap)**

Habit and habitat	:	Sporophore grows solitary or in groups
Season	:	Rainy season
Distribution	:	Cow dung, damp soil, rotten paddy straw in heaps
Edibility	:	Not edible but people in Korea district do eat it before pileus formation.

Coriolus versicolor

Habit and habitat	:	On dead wood
Season	:	Rainy season
Distribution	:	Narayanpur
Edibility	:	Medicinal or therapeutic value

***Crepodorus* sp.**

Habit and habitat	:	Sporophore grows solitary or in groups on dead wood of broad leaves trees
Season	:	Rainy season during August
Distribution	:	Teerathgarh
Edibility	:	Not known

Cyathus limbatus

Habit and habitat	:	Sporophore grows solitary or in groups in open grass and same times in the soil
Season	:	Rainy season
Edibility	:	Not known

Daldinia concentrica

Habit and habitat	:	Dead wood logs or live plants
Season	:	Rainy season
Distribution	:	Teerathgarh, Narayanpur forest area
Edibility	:	Not known

***Flamulina* sp.**

Habit and habitat	:	On dead wood, mainly stumps
Season	:	Rainy season
Distribution	:	Teerathgarh, Barnawapara, Khajuri Nala and Uddanti Sanctuary
Edibility	:	Edible

Ganoderma applanatum

Habit and habitat	:	Sporophore grows solitary or in groups on dead trunk of broad leaves tree
Season	:	Rainy season
Distribution	:	All forest area of Chhattisgarh
Edibility	:	Not edible

Ganoderma lucidum

Habit and habitat	:	Sporophore grows solitary or in groups on dead trunk of broad leaves tree
Season	:	July- October
Distribution	:	All forest area of Chhattisgarh, mainly on live/dead trunk of subabul, gulmohar, babool
Edibility	:	Not edible

Ganoderma suiji

Habit and habitat	:	Sporophore grows solitary or in groups
Season	:	Rainy season
Distribution	:	Ambikapur, Bastar and Bilaspur forest area
Edibility	:	Not edible

***Geastrum fimbriatum* (Earth stars)**

Habit and habitat	:	Sporophore grows solitary or in groups in soil
Season	:	Rainy season
Distribution	:	Labhandi research farm
Edibility	:	Not edible

Hygrocybe marchee

Habit and habitat	:	Sporophore scattered on grass land
Season	:	Rainy season
Distribution	:	Churra, Gariabandh and Manpur area of Raipur
Edibility	:	Not known

Hypholoma udum

Habit and habitat	:	Sporophore grows in groups on the trunk of deciduous tree
Season	:	Rainy season
Distribution	:	Kevnchi, Lormi and Achanakmar forest
Edibility	:	Not known

Hypoxylon fragiformae

Habit and habitat : Normally gregarious on rooting beech, grow on wood, crust like stromata

Season : Rainy season

Distribution : Manpur, Sihava, Gariabandh forest

Edibility : Not edible

Laccaria laccata

Habit and habitat : From soil of mixed forest, sporophore in groups, singly or scattered

Season : Rainy season

Distribution : Chitrakut, Teeratgarh, Narayanpur

Edibility : Edible but not consumed by local people

Lactarius aceverimus

Habit and habitat : Solitary or in groups under broad leaves trees

Season : Rainy season

Distribution : Narayanpur

Edibility : Not known

Lactarius vellereus

Habit and habitat : Sporophore grows singly in scattered form under shrubs of broad leaves

Season : Rainy season

Distribution : Narayanpur

Edibility : Not known

***Lactarius* sp.**

Habit and habitat : Grows singly on leaf litter

Season : Rainy season

Distribution : Narayanpur

Edibility : Not known

***Lentinus* sp.**

Habit and habitat : Sporophore in bunches on dead wood logs.

Season : Rainy season

Distribution : Korea

Edibility : Edible but not consumable by local peoples

Lepista nuda

Habit and habitat : In humus rich ground under broad leaves shrubs

Season : Rainy season

Distribution : Achanakmar (Bilaspur)

Edibility : Good

Lycoperdon maximum

Habit and habitat : Sporophore solitary or scattered in grass land

Season : Rainy season

Distribution : Sandy loam soil

Edibility : Edible

Marasmius oreades

Habit and habitat : Sporophore gregarious in grass land

Season : Rainy season

Distribution : Bastar forest

Edibility : Edible

Melanoleuca alboflavida

Habit and habitat : Sporophore grows in soil or in leaf litter

Season : Rainy season

Distribution : Barnawa forest area

Edibility : Not edible

Microglossum viridae

Habit and habitat : On the ground in grass or woods

Season : Rainy season

Distribution : Narayanpur

Edibility : Not edible

***Mutinus* sp.**

Habit and habitat : Sporophore in group under shade of old bamboo trees

Distribution : Bamboo rhizomes near Bilaspur area

Edibility : Inedible

Panaiolima foenislcic

Habit and habitat : Gregarious in grassy areas

Season : Rainy season

Distribution : Achanakmar, Korea, Bilaspur

Edibility : Not edible

***Phallorina* sp.**

Habit and habitat : Sporophore solitary or in groups on soil under the trees

Season : Rainy season

Distribution : Near guest house of Guru Ghasidas University, Bilaspur

Edibility : Edible but not consume by local people

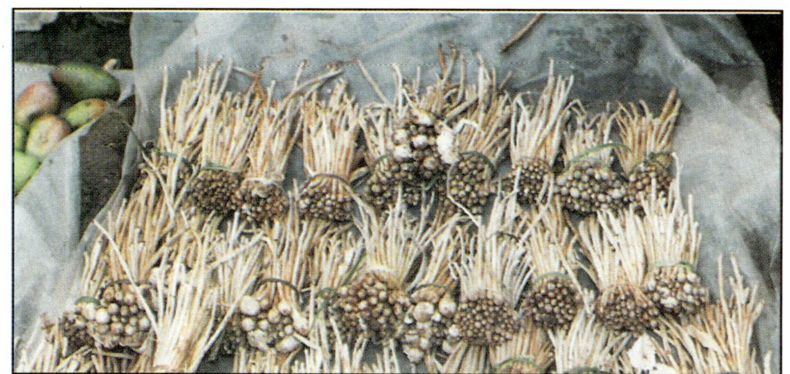

Termitomyces heimii

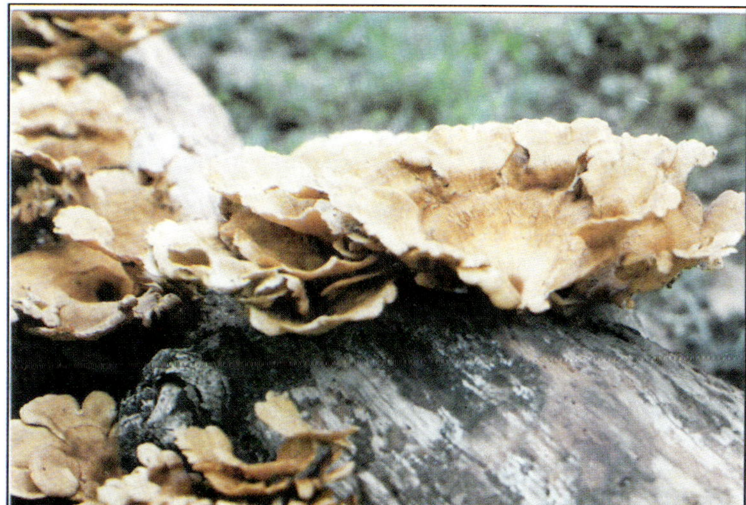

***Polyporus* sp.**

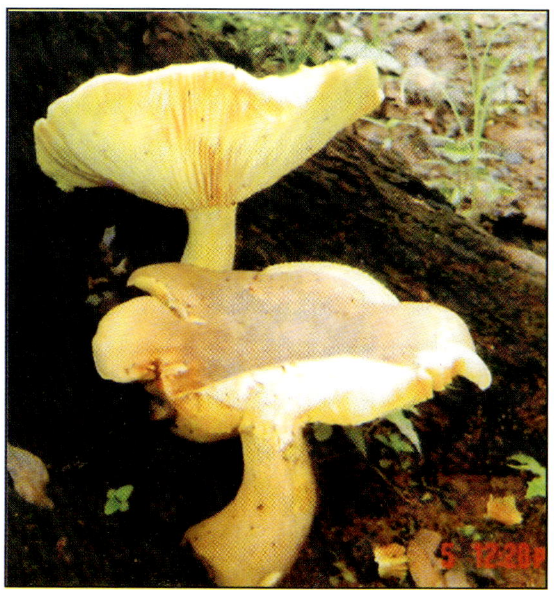

***Tricholoma* sp.**

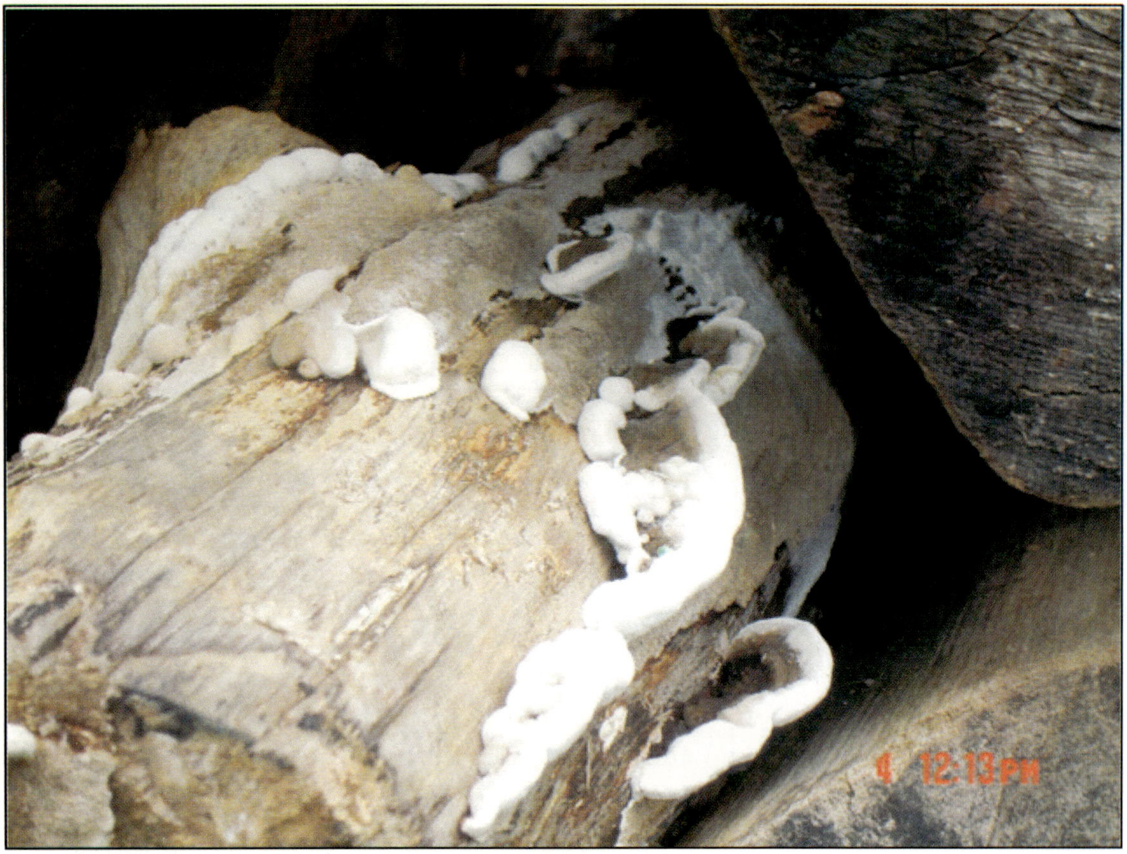

Coriolus versicolor

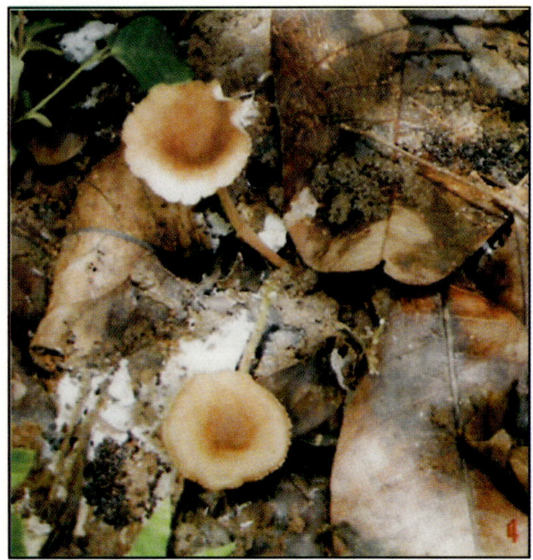

***Lactarius* sp.**

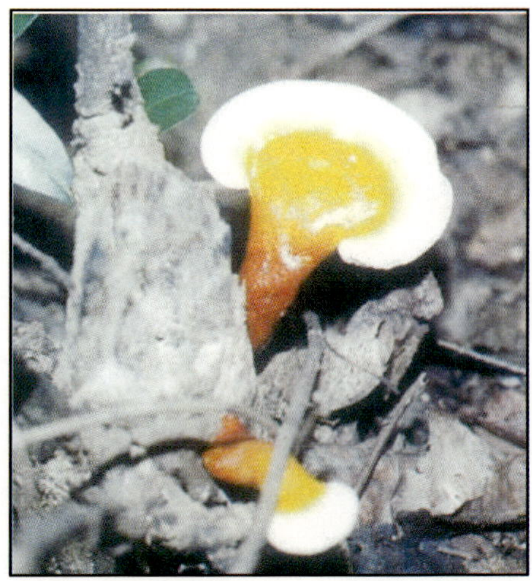

Ganoderma lucidum

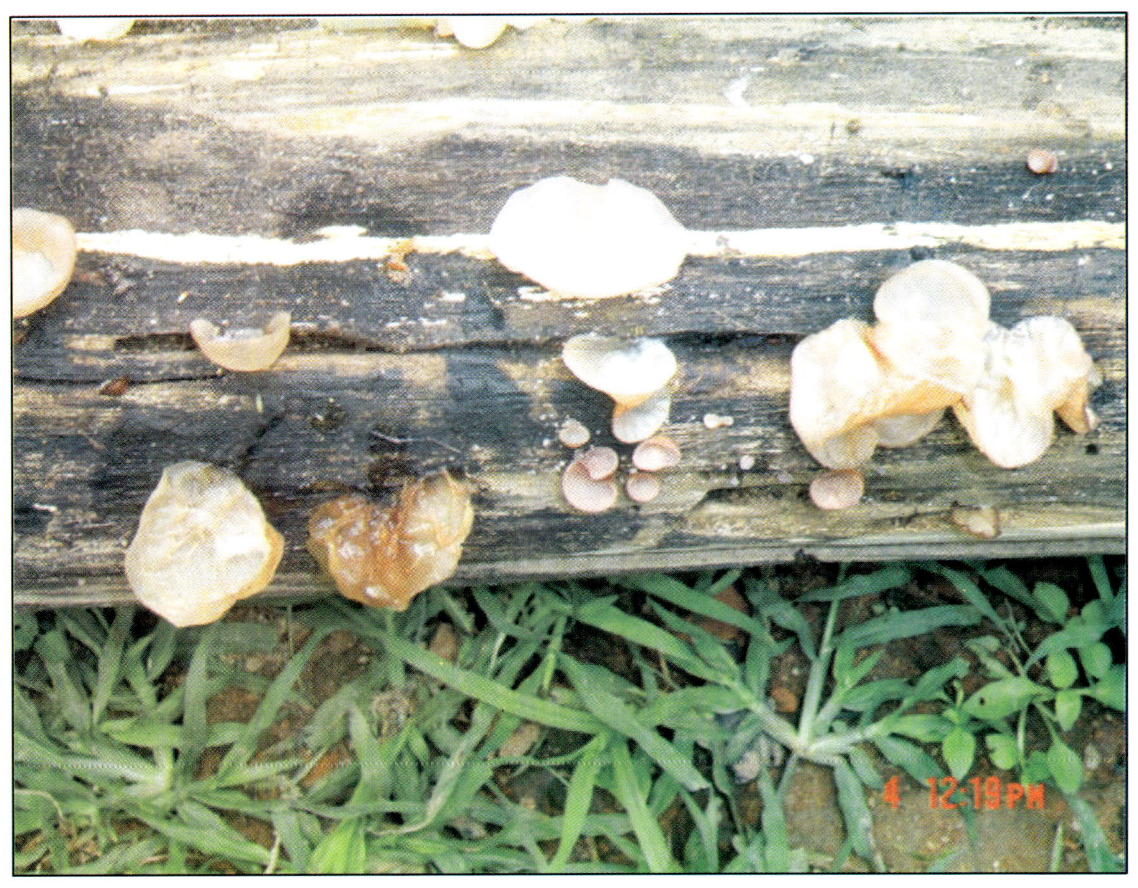

Auricularia polytricha

***Pleurotus florida* (Pihri)**

Habit and habitat	:	Sporophore grows solitary or in groups on mango logs
Season	:	Rainy season
Distribution	:	Narayanpur area
Edibility	:	Edible

Pleurotus sajor caju

Habit and habitat	:	Sporophore in groups on dead wood logs
Season	:	Rainy season
Distribution	:	Branches of mango trees
Edibility	:	Good

Pleurotus stramonius

Habit and habitat	:	Sporophore in groups on dead branches of Mango
Season	:	Rainy season

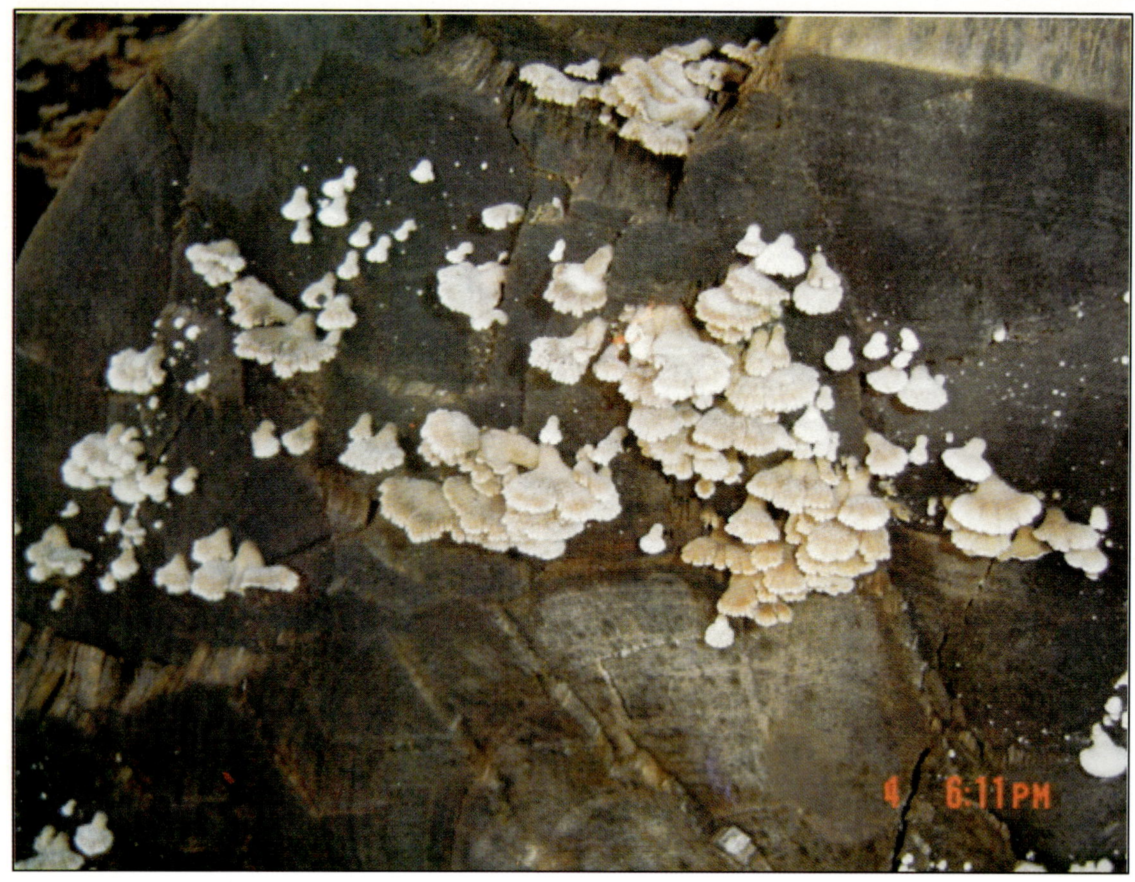

Schizophyllum commune

Distribution : House of C. S. Shukla

Edibility Good

Pleurotus sp.

Habit and habitat : Sporophore in groups on dry wood logs of many trees

Season : Rainy season

Distribution : Bilaspur

Edibility Good

Podbrella microcarpa

Habit and habitat : In soil in singly or groups

Season : Rainy season

Distribution : College campus Nandghat Bilaspur

***Podaxis* sp.**

Habit and habitat	:	Sporophore solitary and grows on sandy soil
Season	:	Rainy season
Distribution	:	Tarra village
Edibility	:	Edible but not consumed by local people

Podoscypha mutzonata

Habit and habitat	:	Sandy loam in singly
Season	:	Rainy season
Distribution	:	Nilanjee
Edibility	:	Non edible

Polyporus varius

Habit and habitat	:	Sporophore in groups on dead wood
Season	:	Rainy season
Distribution	:	All districts of Chhattisgarh
Edibility	:	Not known

Polyporus elegans

Habit and habitat	:	On dead wood
Season	:	All districts of Chhattisgarh
Distribution	:	Bilaspur
Edibility	:	Not edible

Ramaria formosa

Habit and habitat	:	On wood logs of many trees
Season	:	Rainy season
Distribution	:	Narayanpur
Edibility	:	Not edible

Russula delica

Habit and habitat	:	Sporophore grows solitary or in groups and occur on shades of many forest shrubs
Season	:	Rainy season
Distribution	:	All districts of Chhattisgarh
Edibility	:	Good

Russula lepida

Habit and habitat	:	Under broad leaves trees in soil, scattered
Season	:	Rainy season
Distribution	:	All places of Chhattisgarh
Edibility	:	Edible

Russula aeruginla

Habit and habitat : In groups under sal forest

Season : Rainy season

Distribution : All places of Chhattisgarh

Edibility : Edible

Russula atropurpurea

Habit and habitat : Under broad leaves trees specialy in acidic soil

Season : Rainy season

Distribution : Bastar, Bilaspur

Edibility : Edible

Russula mairei

Habit and habitat : Under shrubs or mixed forest

Season : Rainy season

Distribution : Achanakma, Barnawapara

Edibility : Not edible

Russula virginca

Habit and habitat : Under shrubs or mixed forest

Season : Rainy season

Distribution : Achanakma, Barnawapara

Edibility : Edible

Rozites caperata

Habit and habitat : Under broad leaves on leaf litter

Season : Rainy season

Distribution : Korea, Manendragarh

Edibility : Not edible

***Scleroderma verucosum* (Dhela phutu)**

Habit and habitat : Sporophore grows solitary or in groups and occur in laterite soil

Season : Rainy season

Distribution : Labhandi farm

Edibility : Good

***Scleroderma* sp.**

Habit and habitat : Sporophore grows singly or gregarious in the ground

Season : Rainy season

Distribution : Bastar

Edibility : Good

***Stereum* sp.**

Habit and habitat	:	Sporophore on dead wood of broad leaves trees
Season	:	Rainy season
Distribution	:	Korea, Ambikapur, Pendra, Marvahi
Edibility	:	Not edible

Strophoria semiglobata

Habit and habitat	:	Sporophore grows on soil and either solitary or gregarious
Season	:	Rainy season
Distribution	:	Bilaspur, Ratanpur, Pali, Kathghora forest
Edibility	:	Not known

Schizophyllum commune

Habit and habitat		On dead wood
Season		Rainy season
Distribution		Mahasamund
Edibility		Medicinal or therapeutic uses

***Termitomyces clypeatus* (Patera phutu)**

Habit and habitat	:	Sporophore solitary or scattered on the ground
Season	:	Collected from laterite and bunds of ricefield soil after onset of good monsoon
Distribution	:	Associated with termite mounds
Edibility	:	Excellent

***Termitomyces heinii* (Bhado phutu)**

Habit and habitat	:	Sporophore gregarious and grows in large numbers in forest in undisturbed ground. Local people collected for consumption's and sold in local market
Season	:	In the month of September
Distribution	:	All agroclimatic zone of Chhattisgarh
Edibility	:	Excellent

***Termitomyces microcarpus* (Kanki phutu)**

Habit and habitat	:	Sporophore grows in large numbers on the termite mounds
Season	:	After onset of good monsoon
Distribution	:	All agroclimatic zone of Chhattisgarh
Edibility	:	Excellent

***Termitomyces robustus* (Dashara phutu)**

Habit and habitat	:	Sporophore scattered or groups in undisturbed forest area on the ground
Season	:	During September to October

Distribution	:	All agroclimatic zone of Chhattisgarh
Edibility	:	Excellent

Tricholoma sp. (Hardola phutu)

Habit and habitat	:	Sporophore solitary or group in under the shade of broad leaves tree
Season	:	During Rainy season in August and September
Distribution	:	Barnawapara Sanctuary, Achanakmar and forest area of Bastar Plateau
Edibility	:	Good

Tuber sp. (Safed boda)

Habit and habitat	:	Sporophore scattered under soil in mixed forest area
Season	:	During September to October
Distribution	:	Collected from all forest of state
Edibility	:	Excellent

Volvaria umbonata

Habit and habitat	:	Sporophore scattered on the ground
Season	:	Rainy season
Distribution	:	Bastar
Edibility	:	Not known

Volvariella volvacea (Paira phutu)

Habit and habitat	:	Sporophore grows solitary or scattered on paddy straw leaf
Season	:	All the localities of Chhattisgarh state. Local people collected and sold in local market
Distribution	:	All districts of Chhattisgarh
Edibility	:	Excellent

Volvariella like

Habit and habitat	:	Sporophore scattered in leaf litter on living trees
Season	:	After onset of good rains in the during August
Distribution	:	Dense forest area of Pali and Katghora
Edibility	:	Good

Volvariella sp.

Habit and habitat	:	Sporophore scattered or groups on rotten paddy straw
Season	:	During September to October
Distribution	:	All Agroclimatic Zone of Chhattisgarh
Edibility	:	Excellent

***Xylaria* sp.**

Habit and habitat	Sandy loam in groups
Season	Rainy season
Distribution	India
Edibility	Non edible

Xylaria polymorpha

Habit and habitat	Sandy loam in groups
Season	Rainy season
Distribution	Nilanjee
Edibility	Non edible

Future Strategies

- ☆ Intensive survey work needs to be carried out to collect wild and edible mushroom flora from different districts of Chhattisgarh and these should be conserved *in situ* and *ex situ*.
- ☆ Evaluation of locally available mushroom germplasm for cultivation, yield potential, insect pests and diseases resistance, nutritional values, medicinal values, export etc.
- ☆ Multidisciplinary research is required to characterize and study the wild mushroom flora.
- ☆ A need was felt to monitor and map the mushroom diversity of forest ecosystem using Satellite Remote Sensing, GPS and GIS techniques.
- ☆ Isolation, purification, identification and characterization of endangered mushroom and other mushroom species by molecular approaches, community participation and their cataloguing.
- ☆ An efficient, cheap solar dryer with electrical backup needs to be developed for drying of fresh mushrooms.
- ☆ A need was felt to develop different varieties of mushrooms suiting to taste of people and prevailing agroclimatic conditions of Chhattisgarh.
- ☆ An awareness is to be created to grow mycorrhizal mushroom species either by forest departments or by tribals in forest areas in order to conserve these species from deforestation or environmental degradation.
- ☆ To compile ethnic information/traditional knowledge from tribals regarding nutritional and medicinal values of mushrooms.
- ☆ Efforts are to be made to exploit the medicinal values of wild mushrooms (*Ganoderma lucidum*) commonly present in the forest areas of Chhattisgarh.
- ☆ The potential of medicinal mushroom in India is untapped and need to evolve into a successful biotechnological industry for the benefit of the mankind.

References

Annonymous. (1990). *Survey, Collection and idenfification of Mushrooms in Chhattisgarh*. Annual report of AICMIP centre Raipur.

Annonymous. (1991). *Survey, Collection and Identification of Mushrooms in Chhattisgarh*. Annual report of AICMIP centre Raipur.

Annonymous. (1992). *Survey, Collection and Identification of Mushrooms in Chhattisgarh*. Annual report of AICMIP centre Raipur.

Annonymous. (1993). *Survey, Collection and Identification of Mushrooms in Chhattisgarh*. Annual report of AICMIP centre Raipur.

Annonymous. (1994). *Survey, Collection and Identification of Mushrooms in Chhattisgarh*. Annual report of AICMIP centre Raipur.

Annonymous. (1995). *Survey, Collection and Identification of Mushrooms in Chhattisgarh*. Annual report of AICMIP centre Raipur.

Annonymous. (2002). *Survey of Fleshy Fungi of Chhattisgarh*. Annual report of AICMIP centre Raipur.

Annonymous. (2003). *Survey of Fleshy Fungi of Chhattisgarh*. Annual report of AICMIP centre Raipur.

Annonymous. (2004). *Survey of Fleshy Fungi of Chhattisgarh*. Annual report of AICMIP Centre Raipur.

Annonymous (1989). *Survey, Collection and Identification of Mushrooms in Chhattisgarh*. Annual Report of AICMIP Centre, Raipur.

Kumar, S.M. and Agrawal, K.C. (1999). Mushroom a supplement to diet in Chhattisgarh. Paper presented at symposium on Chhattisgarh Agricultural system- Accomplishment, present status and future strategies. Held at IGKV Raipur from 20-23rd January, 1989.

Pacioni, G. (1985). *The Macdonand–Encyclopedia of Mushrooms and Toadstools*. Mac donald and company limited London Sydnee. p. 511.

Pegler, D. and Spooner, B. (1997). *The mushroom identifier*. Leefung- Ascoprinters Limited China. P. 144.

Purkyastha, R. P. and Chandra, A. (1985). *Manual of Indian Edible Mushrooms*. Jagmandar Book Agency, New Delhi. p. 316.

Ramsbottom, J. (1989). *Mushroms and Toadstools*. Willam collins sons and Company Ltd. London. p. 382.

Rinaldi, A. and Tyndalo, V. (1974). *The Complete Book of Mushrooms*. Crown Publishers Inc. Crescent Books, New York. p. 430.

Sharma, S.S. and Samota, R.K. (2006). Tapping into India's mushroom biodiversity: identification, conservation and domestication of wild mushroom flora. In : Compendium of lectures of ICAR short course on "*Emerging Areas in Mushroom Diversity, Production and Postharvest Developments*" at IGAU, Raipur from 9th to 18th January, 2006. pp. 69-84.

Shukla, C.S., Khatri, A.K. and Thakur, M.P. (2002). Fleshy fungi from Chhattisgarh. *Paper presented in National Seminar on Role of Antimicrobials on Sustainable Horticulture* held at IGAU Raipur on 28th January. p.70.

Shukla, R.V., Tiwari, M., and Tripathi, A. (2005). Mushrooms and tribals in sal forest of Chhattisgarh. In National Mushroom Workshop on "*Awareness Creation on Biodiversity and Conservation of Mushrooms*" organized by IGAU, Raipur from December 1-2, 2005. p 5.

Shukla, R.V. (2005). Wild edible mycorrhizal mushrooms of Chhattisgarh. In: National Mushroom Workshop on "*Awareness Creation on Biodiversity and Conservation of Mushrooms*" organized by IGAU, Raipur from December 1-2, 2005. p 4.

Thakur, M.P., Shukla, C.S. and Yadav, V.K., 2005. Mushroom wealth of C. G., their conservation and exploitation. In National Mushroom Workshop on "*Awareness Creation on Biodiversity and Conservation of Mushrooms*" organized by IGAU, Raipur from December 1-2, 2005, p.3.

Microbial Biotechnology and Ecology (2011) *Pages* **344–352**
Editors: **Deepak Vyas, G.S. Paliwal, P.K.Khare and R.K Gupta**
Published by: **DAYA PUBLISHING HOUSE, NEW DELHI**

Chapter 20

Mushrooms: A Nutritive Food for Human Beings

☆ ***Poonam Dehariya*, Anjuli Chaubey and Deepak Vyas***

Lab of Microbial Technology and Plant Pathology,
Department of Botany, Dr. H.S. Gour University, Sagar – 470 003, M.P.

Introduction

Mushrooms have played an important role in the diet of many people for thousands of years. Ancient Egyptian hieroglyphics reveal that mushrooms were thought to bring immortality. Many later cultures believed that eating mushrooms could endow them with super-human strength. Give them clairvoyance in locating lost objects and lead the soul to reside with the gods (Ingramm, 2002). Mushrooms were believed by the Greeks to give strength to the warriors while Romans regarded them as the 'Food for the Gods'. The Chinese prized mushrooms as health food, the 'elixir of life'. The mushrooms were worshipped and consumed as hallucinogens by the Mexican Indians.

In the era of 'healthy eating' by cutting down the calories, saturated fat and cholesterol, mushrooms were bound to attract the attention. Mushrooms have long been considered, especially in the orient, to have medicinal values (King, 1993). Due to unique chemical composition, mushrooms are suited to the specific groups suffering with some ailments. As a low calorie-high protein diet with almost no starch and sugars mushrooms are the 'delight of the diabetic'. Due to high K: Na ratio, few calories and low fat, mushrooms are the choice of the dietician for those with obecity, hypertension and atherosclerosis (heart disease). Alkaline ash and high fibre contents make them suitable for those suffering from hyperacidity and constipation (Rai and Sohi, 1988).

---

* E-mail: poonam.dehariya@yahoo.com

Mushrooms are good source of high quality proteins and are rich in vitamins and minerals. They contain 20-35 per cent protein which is higher than in vegetables and fruits and is a superior quality. They are rich in lysine and tryptophan the two essential amino acids that are deficient in cereals. They contain good amount of vitamin C and B complex (thiamine, riboflavin and niacin), potassium, phosphorus and sodium, also low but available form of iron. In mushrooms, potassium, sodium ratio is very high which is ideal for patients of hypertension. They are low caloric food with very little fat and sugars and without starch and cholesterol (Pathak, Yadav and Gour, 2000).

Nutraceuticals, Nutriceuticals and Pharmaceuticals

The term Nutraceutical is proposed by DeFelice in 1979 and quoted by Brower in 1988 and reported by Chang and Miles (1992). These are often referred as phytochemicals or functional foods. These are natural, bioactive, chemical compounds that have health-promoting, disease-preventing or medicinal properties.

Chang and Buswell in 1996 have coined the term 'mushroom nutriceuticals', is a refined/partially defined extractive which is consumed in form of capsules or tablets as a dietary supplement (not a food) and which has potential therapeutic applications increases resistance to diseases and causes regression in disease state.

Pharmaceuticals are defined chemical preparations, specifications for which are listed in a pharmacopoeia and are mainly used therapeutically; they have high potency, chances of overdose and toxicity are there thus needing regulation by the authorities.

Table 20.1

	Composition	*Usage/Activity*	*Mode of Delivery*	*Accessibility*
Nutraceutical	Modified/enriched food material	Maintenance of healthy diet low potency	Consumed as part of normal diet	Readily available from general retail outlets
Nutriceutical	Refined/partially defined food extractives	Dietary supplements, Medicinal properties, use primarily prophylactic but with potential therapeutic usage	Capsules/tablet low toxicity little scope for overdose	Comparable with over the counter medicines
Pharmaceutical	Almost invariably a defined chemical preparation with medicinal properties. Specification listed in a pharmacopoeia	Specific medical treatment, mostly therapeutic usage.	Oral administratio/ inhalation/topical/ injection High potency, Toxic potential	Range from over the counter medicines to strictly controlled dangerous drugs

Nutritive Contents of Mushrooms

Protein

Protein is one of the most important food factors. The sufficiency of protein in a diet is an important measure of its adequacy and quality. Mushrooms due to high quantity and quality of protein have been recognized by the Food and Agriculture Organization as food contribution to the protein nutrition of the countiers depending largely on cereals (Geda and Joshi, 2006).

On a dry weight basis, mushrooms normally contain 19-35 per cent protein, as compared to 7.3 per cent in rice,13.2 per cent in wheat, 39.1 per cent in soybean, and 25.2 per cent in milk. Therefore in amount of crude protein, mushrooms rank below most animal meats but well above most other foods, including milk, which is an animal product. Jandaik (1974) from Solan reported 33.5 per cent protein in *P. sajor-caju*. Protein content of mushrooms has also been reported to vary from to flush (Crisan and Sands, 1978) and also with the cultivation substrate (Bano and Rajarathanam, 1982). Chang and Miles (1989) have suggested that total protein content of 3.5-4 per cent in commercial edible mushrooms may be more representative. Quality of mushroom protein is far superior to the vegetables proteins, amino acids (Crisan and Sands, 1978; Bano and Rajarathanam, 1982; Chang and Miles, 1989).

Essential amino acids-proteins are made up from over 20 amino acids in varying amounts, they are quantitatively different. The human body can convert some of these amino acids into others, but there are nine essential amino acids (lysine, methionine, tryptophane, threonine, valine, leucine, histidine, and phenylalanine). Table 20.3 shows that for all mushrooms listed in table, the most abundant essential amino acid is lysine, and the lowest levels among the essential amino acids are those of tryptophane and methionine.

Pleurotus flabelltus (Bano *et al.*, 1963) and *P. sajor-caju* (Jandaik and Kapoor, 1976) have been reported to contain seventeen to eighteen amino acids respectively including all the essential amino acids as well as most commonly occurring non-essential amino acids and amides.

Table 20..2: Essential Amino Acid Comparison of Edible Mushrooms

Amino Acids	*Agaricus bisporus*	*Lentinula edodes*	*Pleurotus ostreatus*	*Pleurotus sajor-caju*	*Volvariella volvacea*	*Hen's egg*
Leucine	7.5	7.9	6.8	7	4.5	8.8
Isoleucine	4.5	4.9	4.2	4.4	3.4	6.6
Valine	2.5	3.7	5.1	5.3	5.4	7.3
Tryptophan	2	nd	1.3	1.2	1.5	1.6
Lysine	9.1	3.9	4.5	5.7	7.1	6.4
Threonine	5.5	5.9	4.6	5	3.5	5.1
Phenylalnine	4.2	5.9	3.7	5	2.6	5.8
Methionine	0.9	1.9	1.5	1.8	1.1	3.1
Histidine	2.7	1.9	1.7	2.2	3.8	2.4
Total essential amino acids	38.9	36	33.4	37.6	32.9	47.1

Source: Chang and Miles, 2004.

Carbohydrate and Fiber

According to Crisan and Sands (1978), pentose, methylpentoses, hexoses, as well as disaccharides, amino sugars, sugar alcohols, and sugar acids are constituents of mushroom carbohydrate. *Pleurotus* species contain carbohydrates, ranging from 46.6 to 81.8 per cent (as compared to 60 per cent in *A. bisporus* on a dry weight basis). Fiber is considered to be an important ingredient in a balanced and healthy diet. The fiber content ranges from 7.4 to 27.6 per cent in *Pleurotus* species (as compared to 10.4 per cent in *A. bisporus*, and 4 to 20 per cent in *V. volvacea*).

Minerals

Mushrooms are good source of minerals. In general, mushrooms contain significant quantities of phosphorus, potassium, and copper, *Agaricus bisporus* being especially high in these minerals. A serving of white mushrooms has more potassium than a tomato.

Mushrooms are rich in minerals as may be evident from their ash content 8-10 per cent in *A. bosporus*, 5-15 per cent in *Pleurotus* spp., 11.5 per cent in *V. volvacea* and 7.0 per cent in *Lentinus edodes* mineral of higher content is potassium (45 per cent of total ash content) followed by phosphorus, sodium, magnesium and calcium which together constitute about 56-70 per cent of total ash content (Chang and Miles, 1989). Potassium and phosphorus are the main constituents of ash of *Pleurotus* species also (Bano and Rajarathanam, 1982) iron are present in appreciable amount in *Pleurotus* species.

Vitamins

There are many essential vitamins required daily in the diet. The fruit body of a mushroom is an excellent source of B-complex vitamins including riboflavin (B 2), niacin, pantothenic acid, thiamine (B1) biotin, folate and vitamin B12. Mushrooms are a particularly rich source of riboflavin. Mushrooms are unique in that they contain Vitamin B12, something that vegetables can't produce at all (Ingramm, 2002).

Riboflavin content was 5 mg in *A. bosporus*, 4.9mg in *L. edodes* and 1.63 to 2.98 mg in *V. volvacea* (Chang and Miles, 1989). Folic acid and vitamin B12, which are generally absent in plant foods, are present in mushrooms, although in small quantities. Mushroom also contain vitamin C (Crisan and Sands, 1978; Bano and Rajarathanam, 1982). On fresh weight basis *A. bisporus* contains about 3 mg ascorbic acid (Beelman and Edwards, 1989).

Fat

In general the crude fat of mushrooms has representatives of all classes of lipid compounds including free fatty acids, monoglycerides, diglycerides, triglycerides, sterols, sterol esters, and phospholipids.The values for saponifiable lipid range from 78.1 per cent in *Auricularia auricula* to 58.8 per cent in *Volvariella vovacea*. The low percentage of saponifiable lipid found in *Volvariella volvacea* is mainly due to the presence of unusually high contents of provitamin D2 and ergosterol. Saturated fatty acid found in *Volvariella volvacea* is 14.6 per cent, *Lentinula edodes* 19.9 per cent, *Agaricus bisporus* 19.5 per cent, *Pleurotus sajor caju* 20.7 per cent, *Auricularea auricula* 25.8 per cent, *Tremella fusiformis* 22.8 per cent.

The unsaturated fatty acid found in *Volvariella volvacea* is 85.4 per cent, *Lentinula edodes* 80.1 per cent, *Agaricus bisporus* 19.5 per cent, *Pleurotus sajor-caju* 20.7 per cent, *Auricularea auricula* 25.8 per cent, *Tremella fusiformis* 22.8 per cent (Chang and Miles, 2004).

Moisture

Generally the moisture of fresh mushrooms ranges from 85-95 per cent on an average; the fresh mushroom contains approximately 90 per cent moisture. But it varies from 78.3-90.5 per cent in *Agaricus bisporus*, 89.7 per cent in *Agaricus campestris*, 89.1 per cent, *Auricularia* sp., 87.3 per cent in *Boletus edodes*, 89.2 per cent in *Flammulina velutipes*, 90.0-91.8 per cent in *Lentinula edodes*, 92.2 per cent in *Pleurotus eous*, 91.5 per cent in *Pleurotus florida*, 73.7-90.8 per cent *Pleurotus ostreatus*, 90.1 per cent in *Pleurotus sajor-caju*, 90.4 per cent in *Volvariella diplasia*, 89.1 per cent in *Volvariella volvace* (Chang and Miles, 2004)

Table 20.3: The Nutritive Content of some Mushrooms

	Agaricus bisporus	*Lentinus edodes*	*Pleurotus sajor-caju*	*Pleurotus ostreatus*
Calories	355	356	300	360
Protein g/100g	34.44	32.93	26.6	27.25
Fat g/100g	3.10	3.73	2.0	2.75
Carbohydrate g/100g	47.38	47.60	50.7	52.76
Dietary fiber g/100g	20.90	28.90	13.3	43.80
Vitamin A 1U/100g	0	0	–	0
Thiamine (B1) mg/100g	0.27	0.25	–	0.26
Riboflavin (B2 mg/100g	4.13	2.30	–	2.45
Niacin (B3) mg/100g	69.20	20.40	–	65.80
Pantothenic acid (B5)mg/100	12.70	11.6	–	33.20
Vitamin C mg/100g	0	0	–	0
Vitamin D 1U/100g	235	110	–	136
Calcium mg/100g	23	23	20	5
Copper mg/100g	4.33	1.23	12.2	1.61
Iron mg/100g	2.1	5.5	12.4	11
Potassium mg/100g	4500	2700	3260	4600
Sodium mg/100g	52	18	60	13
Selenium mg/100g	0.415	0.076	–	0.175

Source: Stemet, 2005.

Nutritional Index

Crisan and Sands in 1987 proposed the use of a nutritional index calculated as follows.

$$\text{Nutritional index} = \frac{(\text{EAA Index} \times \text{Percentage protein})}{100}$$

The essential amino acid index (EAA) is measured according to dietary protein in terms of an essential amino acid pattern based on known adult human dietary requirements. The amino acid score (chemical score) is the amount of the most limiting amino acid in the food protein expressed as a percentage of the same amino acid present in the reference protein. The EAA Indexes, amino acid scores, and nutritional indexes for various mushrooms and other foods are shown in Table 20.4. In terms of EAA Indexes and amino acid scores, the most nutritive mushrooms rank alongside meat and milk in potential nutritive value and considerably higher than most legumes and vegetables. The least nutritive mushrooms rank appreciably lower but are still comparable to some common vegetables (Chang and Miles, 2004).

Essential Amino Acid index (EAA Index) was proposed by Oser (1951) reported by Chang and Miles (2004) to evaluate the quality of dietary protein in terms of the ratio of the essential amino acids contained in a food, relative to the essential amino acid content of a highly nutritive reference protein.

Oser (1951) has used whole egg protein as his reference protein.

$$\text{EAA Index} = n\sqrt{\frac{\text{Lysine P}}{\text{Lysine S}}\ \frac{\text{Tryptophane P}}{\text{Tryptophane S}}\ \frac{\text{Histidine P}}{\text{Histidine S}}}$$

P: Food protein; S: Standard (egg); n: The number of amino acids.

Chemical Score or Amino Acid Score is another estimate of nutritive value used by some investigators (FAO, 1968). The Chemical Score is based on the amount of the most limiting amino acid present in the reference protein (egg) and is calculated using the following formula (FAO, 1968).

$$\text{Chemical Score} = \frac{\text{Grams essential amino acid in test protein}}{\text{Total essential acids in test protein}} \times \frac{\text{Total essential amino acids in egg}}{\text{Grams essential amino acids in egg}} \times 100$$

The Chemical Score reflects the 'percentage of adequacy' of the protein and approximates the probable efficiency of utilization of test protein in children (FAO, 1993). By calculating a factor equal to 100 times the reciprocal of the amino acids scores one can determine the present in the reference protein (Crisan and Sands, 1978).

The Chemical Score is also calculated by using FAO reference protein (FAO, 1973) with the help of the following formula.

$$\text{Amino Acid Score} = \frac{\text{Mg of amino acid in 1 g test protein}}{\text{Mg of amino acid in 1 g - reference protein}} \times 100$$

Table 20.4: Comparison of Nutritive Value of Mushrooms with Various Foods

Essential Amino Acid Indexes		*Amino Acid Sources*		*Nutritional Indexes*	
100	Pork; chicken; beef	100	Pork	59	Chicken
99	Milk	98	Chicken; beef	43	Beef
98	Mushrooms (high)	91	Milk	35	Pork
91	Potatoes; kidney beans	89	Mushrooms (high)	31	Soybeans
88	Corn	63	Cabbage	28	Mushrooms (high)
86	Cucumbers	59	Potatoes	26	Spinach
79	Peanuts	50	Corn	25	Milk
76	Spinach; soybeans	46	Kidney beans	21	Kidney beans
72	Mushrooms (low); cabbage	42	Cucumbers	20	Peanuts
69	Turnips	33	Turnips	17	Cabbage
53	Carrots	32	Mushrooms (low)	14	Cucumbers
44	Tomatoes	31	Carrots	11	Corn
		28	Spinach	10	Turnips
		23	Soybeans	9	Potatoes
		18	Tomatoes	8	Tomatoes
				6	Carrots
				5	Mushrooms (low)

Source: Chang and Miles, 2004.

Delicious Recipies of Mushrooms

Mushroom Pakoras

Ingredients

- ☆ Small size mushroom (only the pileups part, 200g)
- ☆ Onion -100g
- ☆ Basan -100g
- ☆ Baking powder-1 tsp.
- ☆ Chilli powder -1/2 tsp.
- ☆ Egg -1
- ☆ Salt to taste
- ☆ Mustard oil/butter-1 tsp.

Method

- ☆ Beat the eggs and add flour, salt, chilli powder, baking powder.
- ☆ Make dough of 25g each. Make a hole on a dough.
- ☆ Stuff the hole with mushroom.
- ☆ Roll the doughs in bread crumbs.
- ☆ Fry the doughs with oil or butter till they become brown.

Button Mushroom fry

Ingredients

- ☆ 100gms button mushroom
- ☆ 1 tsp. chilli powder
- ☆ 1/3 tsp. salt
- ☆ 2 gm cumin seeds
- ☆ Oil required quality.

Method

- ☆ Wash mushroom and place it on Blotting/Old news paper.
- ☆ Heat oil on a tawa. When the oil heats up add the mushrooms.
- ☆ Fry the mushrooms for 2 minutes. Add all the other ingredients and fry for 3 minutes.

Mushroom Sandwich

Ingredients

- ☆ Mushroom-100gm
- ☆ Onion-2 small bulbs
- ☆ Tomato-1
- ☆ Green coriander leaves
- ☆ Green-chilli-2

- ☆ Red chilli powder as required.
- ☆ Salt to taste
- ☆ Butter-25 gm.

Method

- ☆ Wash mushrooms and cut into pieces.
- ☆ Cut onion into small pieces.
- ☆ Put the pieces of onion and mushroom on a pan, add butter and heat gently.
- ☆ In a separate pan, put tomato, pieces of green chilli, green coriander leaves.
- ☆ Add salt and other spices, fry for 10 minutes.
- ☆ Put baked mushroom with onion pieces in the pan.
- ☆ Add few drops of Onion juice and heat gently with butter for 2-3 minutes.
- ☆ Remove from the fire.
- ☆ Put the prepared material into the pieces of bread.

Mushroom Starter

Ingredients

- ☆ Button mushroom-1 packet
- ☆ Butter-250gm.
- ☆ Parsley 1 bunch chopped finely
- ☆ Bread pieces.
- ☆ 1 tps of Garlic paste.

Method

- ☆ Mix butter with finely chopped parsley and garlic paste, remove stem from the mushrooms.
- ☆ Fill the mushroom caps with the herbed butter, in a oven proof dish and grill for 15 min or till the mushrooms are nicely coated with the butter.
- ☆ Serve hot with small bread pieces.

Mushroom Soup

Ingredients

- ☆ Mushroom-250 gm.
- ☆ Butter -25 gm.
- ☆ White flour-one tsp
- ☆ Black peeper-1/2 tsp
- ☆ Ground spices (Chilli, black pepper, cardamom etc.)-3g
- ☆ Milk 1-2 litre

Method

- ☆ Wash and cut mushrooms into very small pieces.

- ✰ Put pressure to remove water from mushrooms
- ✰ Fry mushrooms with butter in a pan.
- ✰ Add milk and boil for 5-7 minutes.
- ✰ A suspension of water and flour is added to the milk for make it thick.
- ✰ Boil the liquid for 5-10 minutes.
- ✰ Add the spices and salt to make it more tasty.

References

Bano, Z., Srivastava, K. S., and Srivastava, H.C. (1963). Amino acid composition of the protein from a mushroom. (*Pleurotus* sp.). (Later on identified as *Pleurotus flabellatus*.). *Appl. Microbiol.*, 11(12): 363-365.

Bano, Z. and Rajarathanam, S. (1982). *Pleurotus* mushroom as nutrition food. In: *Tropical Mushrooms-Biological Nature and Cultivation Methods* (Chang, S. T. and Quimio, T. H., Eds). The Chinese University Press, Hong Kong. 363-382.

Beelman, R.B. and Edwards, C.G. (1989). Variability in the composition and nutritional value on the Cultivated Mushroom, *Agaricus bisporus*. *Mushroom News*, 37: 17-26.

Chang, S. T. and Miles, P.G. (1989). *Edible Mushrooms and their Cultivation*. CRC Press, Boca Raton, pp. 345.

Chang, S.T. and Miles, P.G. (2004). *Mushrooms: Cultivation, Nutritional Value, Medicinal Effect and Environmental Impact*, 2nd edn. CRC Press, p. 28-30.

Chang, S.T. and Buswell, J.A. (1996). Mushroom nutriceuticals. *World J. Microbiol. Biotechnol.*, 12: 473-476.

Crisan, E. V. and Sands, A. (1978). Nutritional value. Un: *The Biology and Cultivation of Edible Mushrooms*, Chang, S.T. and Hayes, W. A., Eds., Academic Press, New York, 137-168.

Food and Agriculture Organisation (FAO) (1968). *Amino acid content of Foods and Biological Data on Proteins*. Food Agric. Organ., U.N., Rome.

Geda, A.K. and Joshi, P. K. (2006). Nutritional qualities of Mushrooms. *Compandium of Lectures-Emerging Areas in Mushroom Diversity, Production and postharvest Developments*, pp. 53-68.

Ingramm, S. (2002). The real nutritional value of fungi. NUTRITIONAL_VALUE.htm.

Jandaik, C.L. and Kapoor, J.N. (1976). Studies on *Pleurotus sajor-caju* (Fr) Singer. *Mushroom Sci.*, 9: 667-672.

King, T.A. (1993). Mushrooms: The ultimate health food but little research in US to prove it. *Mushroom News*, 41(2): 46-29.

Pathak, V. N., Yadav, N. and Gour, M. (2000). *Mushroom Production and Processing Technology*. Agrobios, India.

Rai, R.D. (1997). Medicinal mushrooms. *Advances in Mushroom Biology and Production*, (Rai, Dhar and Verma, eds.) MSI Solan.

Rai, R.D. and Sohi, H.S. (1988). How protein rich are mushrooms. *Indian Horticulture*, 33(2): 2-3.

Stemets, P. (2005). Notes on Nutritional properties of culinary-medicinal mushrooms. *International Journal of Medicinal Mushrooms*, 7: 103-110.

Microbial Biotechnology and Ecology (2011)
Editors: Deepak Vyas, G.S. Paliwal, P.K.Khare and R.K Gupta
Published by: DAYA PUBLISHING HOUSE, NEW DELHI

Pages 353–376

Chapter 21

Mushroom: The Beneficial Fungi

☆ *Anjuli Choubey*[1]*, *Deepak Vyas*[1], *Poonam Dehariya*[1], *A.K. Pandey*[2] and *D.C. Atri*[1]

[1]*Lab of Microbial Technology and Plant Pathology, Department of Botany, Dr. H.S. Gour University, Sagar – 470 003, M.P.*
[2]*Chairman, Madhya Pradesh Private University Commission, Bhopal, M.P.*

ABSTRACT

Mushrooms are the fruiting bodies of macrofungi. They include both edible/medicinal and poisonous species. Mushroom farming is both science and art. The science is developed through research, the art is perfected through curiosity and practical experience. Present review article has studied under following heads:

- ☆ First of all ecological description and taxonomic position of the mushrooms have been described on the basis of their spore production method and their properties.
- ☆ Second, cultivation technology of some mushrooms have been described. Mushroom cultivation is friendly to the environment and helpful in bioconversion/bioremediation of environment adulterants and maintenance of balanced ecosystem.
- ☆ Third, the major attributes of mushrooms, their medicinal properties, has also been drawn to our attention for study *e.g.* immunomodulatory, antitumour activity, hypotensive etc.
- ☆ Forth heading highlights the nutraceutical value of the mushrooms because they are rich in crude fibre and protein. Infact, mushrooms also contain low fat, low calories and good vitamins.
- ☆ Last step of this article is marketing of the mushrooms, which is equally important with the production of the crop. The development of a crop like mushroom depends on its efficient

* E-mail: anjuli83@yahoo.co.in

marketing. The efficiency of mushroom marketing is crucial in determining the profit of the producer on one hand and the level of satisfaction of the consumer on the other. So it is important to throw some light on this aspect with specific objective: to examine the existing marketing pattern of mushroom strategies in order to improve the marketing of mushroom.

Biodiversity of Mushroom

Everyone has had some encounter with mushrooms whether on a walk through the woods, strolling through the park or just finding them in our lawns and gardens. Mushrooms are phenomenon of the nature that is hard to overlook. Mushrooms have been objects of much curiosity and speculation since times immemorial. They are an important component of the forest ecosystem. Their edibility, poisonous nature, psychotropic properties, mycorrhizal and parasitic association with the forest trees make them economically important and interesting to study (Lakhanal, 1996).

India is one of the top ten megadiversity centres and has ample species of wild mushrooms which occur during rainy season. There are at least 12,000 species of fungi that can be considered as mushrooms with at least 2,000 species showing various degrees of edibility (Chang, 1999). Furthermore, over 200 species of mushroom have been collected from the wild and utilized for various traditional medicinal purpose in the far east. Mushrooms are a macrofungi belong to ascomycotina and basidiomycotina. They are achlorophyllous and saprophytic. They absorb their nutrients with the help of very fine thread like structures called mycelium which penetrate into substrate and forms fruiting body that is called mushroom. The fruiting body of the mushroom may be fleshy, subfleshy or sometimes leathery and umbrella like or the various other shapes, size and colour. Generally mushrooms consists a pileus or cap, a long stalk or stipe and gills but some have additional structures like a veil, or annulus, a cup or volva.

Table 21.1: Ascomycotina

Sl.No.	*Group*	*Botanical Name*	*Common Name*	*Morphological Description*	*Ecology*
1.	Cup shaped mushroom	*Aleuria aurantia*	(Orange peel)	Bright orange 2-10 cm wide shallow saucer shaped cup made of brittle flesh. Its outer surface is lighter and often slightly hairy with the inner surface a smooth bright orange that fades to an orange yellow with age.	A very common mushroom found in disturbed areas. They are found in groups or clusters in hard soils on roadsides and in newly disturbed soil.
		Chlorociboria aeruginascens	(Black rubber cup)	A very small (usually to 0.5 cm) blue green cup that leaves a green stain on the rotting logs and barkless wood it grows on.	It is found from june to November on rotting logs and barkless wood.
2.	Morels	*Gyromitra infula*	(Saddle shaped false morel)	This mushroom has a 3-10 cm wide cap that is brownish and saddle shaped with interior chamber and brittle flesh and has 1-5 cm. long stalk is 2 cm thick and whitish or buff in colour. It is hollow and has no ridges.	Found on rotten wood or on the ground in woody debris.

Contd...

Table 21.1–Contd...

Sl.No.	Group	Botanical Name	Common Name	Morphological Description	Ecology
		Helvella lacunose	(Fluted black helvella)	A dark saddle shaped 1-5 cm wide cap that is lobed and wrinkled above but smooth below. It is dark brown or grey to grey-black in colour. It has a 4-10 cm. long deeply fluted or ribbed stalk with interior chambers. It is greyish in color.	It is found on the ground or on decaying wood in coniferous and deciduous woods. It found from September-November.

Table 21.2: Basidiomycotina

Sl.No.	Group	Botanical Name	Common Name	Morphological Description	Ecology
1.	Toad stools (All fleshy gill bearing fungi)	*Amanita phalloides*	Death cap	Pileus 3-3.5 inches across, rounded at first them more or less flattened, variable in color, but usually greenish or yellowish-olive and streaked with fine, darker fibrils in early stages a few large white patches of the volva adhere to the cap.	Grows in mixed deciduous woodland particularly in association with oak. The season is early summer to quite autumn.
		Volvariella volvacea	Paddy straw mushroom	It is a dark species of warm countries, which is occasionally found on decaying vegetable matter in hot houses.	Grows solitary or gregarious on rotten paddy straw mushroom. It found from April–September.
		Lepiota procera	Parasol mushroom	Pileus upto 8 inches across, dull brown or greyish brown, covered with shaggy scales, at first somewhat rounded or oval, so that the young plant has the appearance of a drum stick, later becoming bell shaped and finally expanded and with a prominent umbo, the margin thin, usually turning downwards and fringed.	Grows in small troops among leaf litter or short grass often at the edge of woods.
		Agaricus bisporus	White button mushroom	The fruiting body of this mushroom has a stipe and an umbrella shaped cap. on the under side of the pileus gills are present. When the fruiting body is young the gills are enclosed by a membrane that extends from	It grows on compost heaps, in garden waste and beside roads. Occasionally on the edges of hedges.

Contd...

Table 21.2–Contd...

Sl.No.	Group	Botanical Name	Common Name	Morphological Description	Ecology
				the margin of the pileus to the stipe. This membrane is called veil. It is torn around the margin of the pileus. When the pileus expands but it remains as a ring called annulus.	
2.	Bracket fungi	*Ganoderma applanatum*	Artist's conk	A woody often horney, flat to hoof shaped, grey to brownish, stalkless cap with a white pore surface that bruises readily, hence the other common name is "Artist's conk" because a drawing can be made on the surface. The cap is 5-50 cm wide with 0.5-5cm thick brown flesh.	Grows year round on dead wood, particularly deciduous, but has been found on conifers and living trees as well.
3.	Jelly fungi	*Tremella mesenterica*	Witches butter	2.5 cm. wide globular or brain like or lobed, orange yellow to clear yellow in colour, turns orange red on drying.This one looks a lot like Orange jelly (*Dacrymyces palamatus*) but it lacks a stem.	It grows year round on deciduous wood.
4.	Polypores	*Tramates versicolor*	Turkey tail	An overlapping or rosette forming stalkless polypore with thin leathery kidney or spoon shaped, multicolored caps that may be flat or wavy silky, hairy or velvety with alternate smooth zones.	Found on dead woods or wounds in living trees
		Pleurotus ostreatus	Oyster mushroom	A broad fleshy, white, grey or brown cap with broad whitish or yellow tinged gilles. Cap is 15-20 cm. wide, oyster shaped semicircular to elongated margin lobe is wavy, pleasant odour, thick, white flesh, stalk is short or absent.	Usually grows in clusters on dead tree trunks or branches and rarely on living trees. It grows year round in favourable condition.
		Pycnoporus cinnabarinus	*Cinnabar red polypore*	A 2-12 cm. wide semicircular or kidney shaped flattened stalkless polypore. The cap is cinnabar-red to orange, rough and slightly hairy but with age becomes warty and wrinkled.	Found in all seasons on dead deciduous and occasionally aged coniferous wood.

Contd...

Table 21.2–Contd...

Sl.No.	Group	Botanical Name	Common Name	Morphological Description	Ecology
5.	Coral fungi	*Clavularia cristata*	Crested coral	A many branched whitish, crested coral with characteristic tooth like jagged tips color is whitish but becomes yellowish to ochare with age. It grows 2-3 cm wide and about 2-8 cm high.	Found growing on the ground in wooded areas from August to November.
		Lentaria bysiseda	Cotton based coral	A creamy or pinkish tan coloured branched coral mushroom with characteristic pliant-tough flesh. It grows 1-6 cm. high and about as wide, it has short and thick stalk rising out of hairy white mycelial patch, though the stalk is not always present.	This is very common coral mushroom on twigs, leaves and cones or rotten wood of both coniferous and deciduous trees. It can be found in season anywhere from August–November depending on the conditions.
6.	Puff balls	*Lycoperdon perlatum*	Gem studded puffball	A whitish tan coloured round or turban shaped mushroom with an stalk like base. It is covered with detachable long and short spines. It develops a pore in the center and has white flesh that becomes greenish-brown with the age.	Often found growing in moist lowland forests sometimes on rotten wood.
		Pseudohydnum gelatinosum	Jelly tooth	A whitish translucent tongue like jelly with gelatinous flesh, occasionally with brownish or grayish tones. It has tooth like white spines on its underside.	Found on rotting woods in coniferous or mixed forest.
7.	Slime fungi	*Lycogala epidendrum*	Wolf's milk slime	A pinkish or reddish massed that produces small (0.3–0.5 cm wide and high) rounded cushions that may be pink, orange, grey or brownish and exude a pinkish paste when squeezed.	A common mushroom from June-November found scattered or clustered on dead logs
		Physarum polycephalum	Yellow slime	A sheet like yellowish expanding and contracting slimy mass roundish heads on unbranched stalks.	Found from June-October on dead wood and fleshy fungi.

Table 21.3: Edible Mushrooms

Sl.No.	Common Name	Botanical Name
1.	Button mushroom or champignon	*Agaricus bisporus*
2.	Oyster mushroom	*Pleurotus ostreatus*
3.	Pig mushroom or stone mushroom	*Boletus edulis*

Contd...

Table 21.3–Contd...

Sl.No.	Common Name	Botanical Name
4.	Cauliflower mushroom	*Sparassis crispa*
5.	Birch bolete	*Leccinum scabrum*
6.	Saffron milk	*Lactarius deliciosus*
7.	Sweet tooth fungus	*Hydnum repandum*
8.	Chicken mushroom	*Laetiporous sulphureus*
9.	Shimji or beech mushroom	*Hysizygus tessulatus*
10.	Snow fungus	*Tremella fuciformins*
11.	Tooth fungus	*Hericium erinaceus*
12.	Tree ear fungus	*Auricularia polytincha*
13.	Winter mushroom or Enokitake	*Flammulina velutipes*
14.	Chanterelle or Girolle	*Cantharellus cibarius*
15.	Pig's ear gomphus	*Gomphus clavatus*
16.	Wood blewit	*Lepista nuda*
17.	Golden-spotted waxy cap	*Hygrophorus chrysodons*
18.	Trumpet clitocybe	*Clitocybe geotropa*
19.	Silky grey tricholoma	*Tricholoma portentosum*
20.	Wood wooly foot	*Collybia peronata*

Table 21.4: Poisonous Mushrooms

Sl.No.	Common Name	Botanical Name
1.	Herald of the winter	*Hygrophorus hypothejus*
2.	Common funnel cap	*Clitocybe infundibuliformis*
3.	Yellow brown tricholoma	*Tricholoma fulvum*
4.	Blackening lyophyllum	*Lyophyllum fumato fotens*
5.	Collybia confluens	*Tufted collybia*
6.	The stainer	*Mycena crocata*
7.	Tall amanita	*Amanita excelsa*
8.	Garlic mushroom	*Marasmius alliaceus*
9.	Red gilled agaric	*Melanophyllum echinatum*
10.	Safron parasol	*Cystoderma aminthinum*
11.	Glistening ink-cap	*Coprinus micaceus*
12.	Fringed crumble cap	*Psathyrella candolleana*
13.	Scaly crumble cap	*Psathyrella squamosa*
14.	Verdigris agaric	*Stropharia aeruginosa*
15.	Scaly psilocybe	*Psilocybe squamosa*
16.	Fruity cortinarius	*Cortinarius amoenolens*

Contd...

Table 21.4–Contd...

Sl.No.	Common Name	Botanical Name
17.	Slimy banded	*Cortinarius collinitus*
18.	Fleecy milk cap	*Lactarius vellereus*
19.	Golden false pholiota	*Phaeolepiota aurea*
20.	Blood red Cortinarius	*Dermocybe sanguinea*

Table 21.5: Fungi with Conflicting Reports on Edibility

Binomial	Notes
Agaricus arvensis	Reported mostly as edible and eaten in some parts of the world; also said to be a gastrointestinal irritant (Lincoff and Mitchel, 1977).
Agaricus semotus	Said to be edible from Hong Kong (Chang and Mao, 1995).
Amanita flavoconia	Conflicting accounts from Mexico: one report says it is edible, the other that it is poisonous.
Coprinus atramentarius	Edible if eaten in the absence of alcohol; this produces an unpleasant effect if imbibed at the same time, hence remarks that it is potentially poisonous (Lincoff and Mitchel, 1977).
Gyromitra esculenta	In Finland it is a delicacy (Härkönen, 1998) and it is also widely eaten in the Russian Federation and neighbouring regions. In other countries it is said to be poisonous and can kill when raw (Hall *et al.*, 1998a). The toxic properties are mitigated by suitable preparation prior to eating.
Helvella lacunosa	Widely eaten but also reported as toxic if eaten raw (Lincoff and Mitchel, 1977).
Lampteromyces japonicus	A common cause of poisoning in Japan (Hall *et al.*, 1998a) but also has medicinal properties (Hobbs, 1995).
Morchella esculenta	Like other morels said to be poisonous if eaten raw (Lincoff and Mitchel, 1977). Edible and good when cooked.
Tricholoma pessundatum	Edible in Hong Kong (Chang and Mao, 1995) but *T. pessundatum* var. *montanum* reported as poisonous elsewhere (Lincoff and Mitchel, 1977).
Tricholoma sulphureum	All records say it is poisonous apart from an account from India that says it is edible (Purkayastha and Chandra, 1985).

Cultivation Technology of Mushroom

Mushroom cultivation is completely different from growing green plants. Mushroom do not contain chlorophyll and therefore depend on other plant material (the substrate) for their food. A mushroom cultivar should be thoroughly familiar with the life cycle of fungi. Mushrooms can also be grown in lawns, polytonal, vegetable garden, woodlands and in permaculture design (Edwards, 2000).

Mushrooms can be cultivated through a variety of methods. Some methods are extremely simple and demand little or no technical expertise on other hand, cultivations which require aspects of sterile handling technology are much more technically demanding (Chang and Miles, 1989). Mushroom cultivation involves several different operations.

Each of which must be performed properly if the enterprise is to be successful. Failure of any phase will result in a decreased harvest or total loss.

Steps for Mushroom Cultivation

1. Selection of mushroom spores or strains
2. Maintenance of mycelial culture
3. Development of spawn/inoculum
4. Preparation of growing medium
5. Spawn inoculation and colonization of substrate

Mushroom can easily grow on different substrates for instances on domestic, industrial or agricultural wastes, such as paddy straw, cotton waste, jute waste, palm bunch waste, banana leaves, sugarcane waste, water hyacinth, paper waste, sawdust, wood etc.

Cultivation Technology of *Pleurotus* Mushroom

Common Name–Oyster mushroom

Indian Name–Dhingri

Substrate

Wheat/paddy straw, soybean straw or other agricultural wastes can be used as a basal substrate. The straw should be fresh, dried and stored in proper conditions. The substrate should be free from diseases, contaminants and other plant material. For substrate preparation, wheat straw is chemically sterilized/soaked in water 18-24 hours and dipped in hot water for 2-3 hours at 60°C. Excess water is drained off. Polythene bags may be used as containers.

Supplementation

For substrate supplementation, supplements rich in N_2 are added. Soybean meal, Gram powder, Ground nut powder may be used as supplements.

Spawning

For spawning, 18-20 day old spawn is used, very old spawn develops clumps and results into proper mycelial growth. Spawning is done in 3 layers with 40 per cent of grain spawn. The straw are taken in polythene bags and seeded with wheat grain spawn. The spawn layer is covered with wet straw. Two per cent vent area recommended for polythene bags to prevent spoilage of the substrate.

Fruiting

After19 days of spawning, mycelia run through the substrate now polythene bags is removed. Watering is done almost every day. Pinheads are generally appeared after 23 days of spawning. Some of these develop into mature fruit bodies within another 3-4 days. These are picked up and sold in the markets either in fresh conditions or after drying.

Harvesting

First flush occurs 3-4 weeks of spawning. Usually matured ones are picked up gently without disturbing the smaller ones. After first harvest the bed are kept as such for another one week or so and are watered as and when necessary in order to provide appropriate moisture. Yield of second flush is much less than that of first one.

Risk Factors

Tricholoma spp., *Aspergilus* spp., and *Rhizopus* spp. are commonly observed on the substrate during spawn run. These can be avoided by good hygeine.

Cultivation Technology of *Calocybe* Mushroom

Common Name–White milky mushroom

Indian Name–Dudhchatta, Kuduk

Other Name–Saint George's mushroom

Substrate

Wheat/paddy straw can be used as a basal substrate. The straw should be fresh, dried and stored in proper conditions. The substrate should be free from diseases, contaminants and other plant material. For substrate preparation, wheat straw is chemically sterilized/soaked in boiled water for 2-3 hrs. And used for seeding the beds. Polythene bags may be used as containers. Two percent vent area recommended for polythene bags to prevent spoilage of the substrate.

Supplementation

For substrate supplementation, supplements rich in N_2 are added. Soybean meal, may be used as supplements.

Spawning

For spawning, 18-20 day old spawn is used. Very old spawn develops clumps and results into proper mycelial growth. Spawning is done in 3 layers with 40 per cent of grain spawn.

Casing

After completion of mycelial growth the casing is done with two year old cow dung patties of size (1-2") or garden soil, coirdust and farm yard manure (FYM). The thickness of casing should be kept 1".

Fruiting

After 10-12 days of casing, fruit primordia are formed with in 5-6 days, mature fruit bodies of the mushroom become ready for harvest. The bags should not be opened before the mycelial growth completion. The bags can be arranged on alluminium racks at a distance of 5-10cm. The cropping room should be properly ventilated and adequately lighted.

Risk Factors

Due to poor hygenic conditions, many competitor moulds and fungi may develop and hamper the mycelial growth. *Tricholoma* spp., *Aspergilus* spp., and *Rhizopus* spp. are commonly observed on the substrate during spawn run. These can be avoided by good hygeine.The ink caps (*Coprinus* spp.) in the spawned bags can be removed by hand picking or by reducing the humidity of cropping room below 90 per cent. The disease can be reduced by avoiding excess moisture and providing proper aeration.

Harvesting

The right stage for picking can be judged by the size of fruit body. The fruit bodies should be harvested before spore release by twisting so that the stubs are not left on the straw. It is better to pick all the mushroom in the bag at a time and then irrigate them.

The spent straw from *Calocybe indica* can be used for biogas production. The spent substrate can also be used as manure.

Cultivation Technology of *Lentinus edodes*

Common Name–Shittake

Indian Name–King or monarch of mushroom

Other Name–Xiang gu

Substrates

There is good development and high production only with rich sources of wood. The substrate usually comprises a mixture of wood chips, cereal bran and millet. Wood chips from hardwood species are usually preferred, although a small proportion of Softwood species may be mixed with the hardwoods. A formula of sawdust (80 per cent), wheat bran (10 per cent) can also be used. After mixing the drying ingredients by hand or with a mechanical mixer, water is added to the mixture so that the final moisture content of the substrate is between 55 and 68 per cent. Depending on the capacity of the sawdust to absorb water. The ingredients are then packed into autoclavable polypropylene or high density polyethylene bags. After the bags have been filled (1.5 to 4 kg wet wt.) The neck of the bag is fitted with a plastic collar and plugged with a cottonwool stopper.

After filling the bags with either noncompacted or compacted nutrient supplemented sawdust, the substrate is heat–treated to kill unwanted competitive microorganisms. Heat treatment may carried out in an autoclave at 121°C for 1 hr or in a brick or cement lined tower at 90-95°C for 5-7 hr.

Supplementation

Some growers use feather meal, mineral and vitamin supplements.

Spawning

After cooling, the substrate is inoculated with spawn. Inoculation is usually performed in a laminar flow. Spawn run (the time required for the mycelium to colonize the substrate) may range from 18-30 days. During this period, the bags are usually incubated in a 4hr/20hr light/dark cycle at 23-25°C. The substrate may lose 5-10 per cent of its dry weight and may subsequently have a higher moisture content. With longer spawn runs (over 40 days), The surface of the colonized substrate may begin to turn brown. Some exudates may be produced and drain to the bottom of the plastic bag. At the end of the spawn run the plastic bag is cut away and the synthetic logs are subjected to production conditions. The wood chips are held together by the fungal mycelium. In some cases, Portions of the bag may be left on the synthetic logs to retain moisture. Misting be provided daily by overhead nozzles controlled automatically. Relative humidity is often maintained at 85 per cent. Temperature range of 14-16°C optimum for most lines of Shiitake.

Fruiting

Fruiting is near when rings of white mycelia appear on the bags.

Harvesting

Mushroom should be harvested when their caps are about two-third open. Mushrooms may be stored in a cardboard box for up to a month at 36-41°F.

Mushrooms may also be dried whole or sliced before marketing.

Risk Factors

Many competitor moulds, pests, insects may be develop due to poor hygenic conditions. In which *Hypoxylon coccineum*, *Merulius tremellosus*, *Monilia* spp., *Poria vaporaria*, *Achorute* spp., *Lepidocyrtus spp.* are included.

Cultivation Technology of *Ganoderma lucidum*

Common Name–Lingzhi

Indian Name–Reishi

Other Name–Mannentake

Reishi often is associated with health and recuperation, longevity, wisdom, and happiness (Stamets 1990, 1993). It is believed that certain triterpenes and polysaccharides may account for the multiple activities of Reshi. Thus, considerable time and effort has gone into the isolation and characterization of these compounds. About 100 triterpenes have been isolated from either the fruitbodies or mycelium but only a few have been tested for bio-activity (Mizuno *et al.*, 1995).

Substrate

Hardwood sawdust like Oak (*Quercus* spp.), Maple (*Acer* spp.) etc. is the most popular basal ingredient used in synthetic formulation of substrate used to produce reishi (Royse, 1997; Tong and Cheh, 1990; Soto-vela Zco *et al.*, 2002). A very fine grade of saw dust is generally used for cultivation. Other basal ingredients that may be used include wheat straw corn cobs or mixtures paddy straw, bagasse, mixture of saw dust and wheat, paddy etc.

Supplementation

Supplements such as wheat bran, rice bran, millet, rye, corn etc. are added to the mix into the main ingredient. There supplements serve as nutrients to provide an optimum growing medium.

Spawning

For spawning, grain spawn 30-40 g/kg substrate and sawdust spawn 60-80g/kg substrate is used. The inoculated bags are kept in growing houses for approximately 1-1½ months for spawn run. During spawn run, bag should be kept under low light intensity and high humidity with little ventilation. When the spawn run is completed within 30-35 days, the polythene bag cover is removed and the substrate blocks are exposed.

Fruiting

Formulation of young mushroom buttons. 2-expanding (opening) of mushroom caps, colour at the margin is whitish till it grows but turned to red when the fruit body is matured it takes about 20-25 days from the button stage.

Harvesting

Harvesting is done when the edge of mushroom turned to red colour. Harvesting is done by picking the mushroom and holding the mushroom stalk and gently twisting it from the substrate block. Reishi mushroom can be dried. Good yield would be 300 gm reishi per kg dry substrate.

The advantages of mushroom cultivation can be summarized as:

1. Wastes such as cereal straws are largely burnt by the farmers, which causes air pollution. However, these raw materials can actually be used for the cultivation of mushrooms. This kind of bioconversion exercise can greatly reduce environmental pollution.
2. Mushroom cultivation can be a labour intensive activity. Therefore, it will serve as means of generating employment, particularly for rural women and youths in order to raise their social status. It will also provide additional work for the farmers during winter months when the farming schedule is light.
3. It will provide the people with an additional vegetable of high quality, and enrich the diet with high quality proteins, minerals and vitamins which can be of direct benefit to the human health and fitness. The extractable bioactive compounds from medicinal mushrooms would enhance human's immune systems and improve their quality of life.
4. Mushroom is a cash crop. The harvested fruiting bodies can be sold in local markets for additional family income or exported for an important source of foreign exchange that will definitely improve the economic standards of the people

5. Some warm mushrooms, *e.g. Volvariella volvacea* (Straw mushrooms) and *Pleurotus sajor-caju* (Oyster mushrooms) are relatively fast growing organisms and can be harvested in 3 to 4 weeks after spawning. It is a short return agricultural business and can be harvested in 3 to 4 weeks after spawning. It is a short return agricultural business and can be of immediate benefit to the community.

Therapeutic Properties of Mushrooms

There are at least 2000 species of fungi that can be considered as mushroom in which at present 270 species of mushroom that are known to have various therapeutic properties (Ying *et al.*, 1987). The practice of using fungi, especially mushrooms, in chinese herbal medicines has been recordes of the *"Materia medica"*. The earliest book on medicinal materials in China, the *"Shen Noug's Herbal"* (Shen Noug Pen T's ao Jing) (100-200AD) recorded the medicinal effects of several mushrooms including *Ganoderma lucidum, Poria cochos, Tremella fusiformis* and others medicinal mushrooms have become even more widely used as traditional medicinal ingredients for the treatment of various diseases and related health problems largely due to the increased ability to produce the mushrooms by artificial method.

Higher basidiomycetes mushrooms have been used in folk medicine throughout the world since ancient time (Wasser and Weis, 1999). Far from being an outdated curiosity, medicinal mushrooms earn ever growing popularity, stimulated by a high number of scientific studies. The discovery of antibiotics has convinced the public that fungi could produce particularly active substances and that the ancient traditions could have a part of truth. Mushrooms are known to possess all essential amino acids, minerals, vitamins etc., in adequate quantities and low in sugars and such are selective medicinal food for diabetics. Probably this might have captured the attention of F.A.O. for recommending mushrooms as a food especially to the under developed countries where the protein malnutrition has become a real threat to human health.

Mushrooms in Ayurveda

In ayurveda it has been mentioned that mushrooms are body builders, energisers and they cure stomach problems. A special preparation recommended for consumption to tuberculosis patient is mushrooms boiled in milk with sugar. Even though references are lacking in literature, it is a well known belief that "Nilamanga" (*Sclerotium stipipatum*) a rare underground mushroom is supposed to be a valuable natural medicine for a number of common diseases. Ayurvedic medical practitioners accept this as an incomparable medicine for a number of body disorders. Nilamanga are just like a mango in their shape and size and are found underground, usually associated with old termite nests under the soils. They appear singly or in bunches with small stalks. Inner flesh is white and soft when young at maturity it become hard with a thick black outer coating.

It has been reported that a boiled water extract of Nilamanga if consumed will prevent the body dehydration. Boiled Nilamanga extract in *sesamum* oil is a very good medicine for the internal application to cure ear pain in children. A mixture of crushed Nilamanga in butter is very congenial for external application for faster curing of body abscissions. Similarly, extract of crushed "Nilamanga" is reported to be a good remedy for jaundice than any other medicines (Nair *et al.*, 1986).

Mushrooms have various immunological and anticancer properties (Mizuno *et al.*, 1995). They also offer other potentially important therapeutic properties including antioxidant, antihypertensive, cholesterol lowering, liver protection, antifibrotic, anti-inflammatory, antidiabetic, anti-inflammatory, antiviral and antimicrobial (Lakhanpal *et al.*, 2005). Many pharmaceutical companies are viewing the medicinal mushrooms as a rich source of innovative biomedical molecules. Many polysaccharide bound proteins produced by Basidiomycetae fungi have classified as anti-tumour chemicals by the U.S. National Cancer Institute.

Antitumoral

A number of mushroom compounds capable of modifying the biological response of the host by stimulation of the immune system provoking therapeutic effects like inhibition of tumour growth and relief in immunodeficient diseases such as AIDS. Japanese researchers in the 1970's, at a French convention, presented a new type of antitumoral molecule found in a mushroom. This compound, a polysaccharide, does not act on the tumour by direct cytotoxicity like already known substances but acts by stimulation of the immune system (Takashi, 1995). Since then several other substances have been discovered. Several immunotherapeutic drugs have been commercialized in Japan, among them PSK (Krestin) extracted from *Trametes versicolor* mycelium marketed in 1977 to treat digestive organ, lung and breast cancer. About 10 years later was commercialized a similar product, PSP. Lentinan from the *Lentinus edodes* fruit body commercialized in 1985 for stomach cancer, SPG (*Schizophyllan*) from *Schizophyllum commune* put on market 1986 against cervical cancer.

Hypocholesterolemic

The major cause of mortality world is cardiovascular disease. One of the preventive measures against these diseases is to reduce the cholesterol level in the blood. This can be done by diet or by a therapeutical agent, like lovastanin (mevinoline), among Basidiomycetes, *Pleurotus ostreatus* has shown the highest lovastatine content. Other species are active by lowering blood cholesterol *i.e.Pleurotus cornuciopiae, P.eryngii, P. sapidus, Lentinus edodes, Polyporus confluens, Auricularia polytricha, A. auricular-judue, Flammulina velutipes* and *Ganoderma lucidum* (Wasser and Weis, 1999).

Anti-inflammatory Effects

More than half of the people over 65 years old suffer from arthritis. Drugs on the market (aspirin, steroids) are of limited efficiency, because of potential secondary effects. In reason of the long traditional use of *Ganoderma lucidum* in Asia for rheumatism and stiff articulations, several studies have been done on this mushroom seeking a non steroidic drug. The possibility seems to be very promising on developing on an antiinflammtory drug from *Ganoderma* extracts. Some heterogalacton–protein complexes with anti inflammatory and antiallergic functions in *Ganoderma lucidum*. According to Wasser and Weis (1999) anti inflammatory effects can be found in other mushroom products from *Tremella fusiformis, Schizophillum commune, Lentinus edodes, Flammulina velutipes, Marasmius androsaceus.*

Antiviral

Diverse basidiomecetous substances are effective against viral infections including AIDS. These are mostly substances which mobilize the body's humoral defences (Wasser and Weis, 1999) for instances, Lentinane extracted from *Lentinus edodes* suppressed the surface expression of human immunodeficiency virus on T cells when dosed in combination with ayodothymidine (Tochikura *et al.*, 1987). It was also active against vesicular stomatitis virus in mice, encephalitis virus, abelson virus and adenovirus type 12. Other mushrooms like *Grifola frondosa, Tsramates versicolor, Ganoderma lucidum* have antiviral effects too (Wasser and Weis, 1999).

Hypoglycemic

Diabetes is a disease due to the lack of regulation of the blood sugar level due to the malfunction or non function of specialized pancreatic cells. Certain mushrooms could have a positive effect on early stage of type 2 diabetes. For instances Ganoderanes isolated from *Ganoderma lucidum* showed hypoglycemic activity in mice (Hikino *et al.*, 1989). According to Lo *et al.* (2005) *Tremella mesenterica* might be developed as a potential oral hypoglycaemic agent or functional food for diabetic patients and for persons with high risk for diabetes mellitus. *Lentinus edodes* and *calocybe georgii* are two other examples of mushrooms showing hypoglycaemic activity.

Hypotensive

Certain compounds can maintain blood pressure at a normal level (Kabir *et al.*, 1988) showed the effect on blood pressure of a powder prepared from *Ganoderma lucidum* fruit bodies on hypertensive rats. *Grifola frondosa, Lentinus edodes, Auricularia auricular-judae* and *Armellaria mellea* are other mushrooms lowering blood pressure (Wasser and Weis, 1999).

Antifungal

Ecologically the production of antifungal substance is almost surely due to the constant need of the organisms to compete against other fungi. There are indeed a lot of observations of aggressive action of one species towards another. It was 1923 that Falck first recognized such an activity in *Sparassis crispa* (Delmas, 1989).

Miscellanous Activities

Other kinds of activities can be found in Basidiomycetes, *i.e.* Cardiovascular (*i.e. Lentinus edodes, Auricularia auricular-judae, Armellaria mellea, Grifola frondosa, Volvariella volvacea*), Antiallergic (*i.e. Agaricus compestris*), Hepatoprotective (*i.e. Schizophyllum commune, Dendropolyporus umbellatus, Tramates Versicolor, Ganoderma lucidum, Lentinus edodes*).

Table 21.6: Medicinal Mushrooms

Sl.No.	Species	Common Name	Medicinal Value	Key Active Constituents
1.	*Auricularia dimidate*	Jew's ear or wooden ear or tree ear	1. Pile treatment and lowers blood cholesterol 2. Stopping pain and bleeding. 3. Treatment in haemorrhoids and excessive uterine bleeding (ying *et al.*, 1987)	Polysaccharides
2.	*Pleurotus ostreatus*	Oyster mushroom or mushroom of the flower heaven	1. Anticancerous activity 2. Immunomodulating effects. 3. Antiviral, antibiotic and anti-inflammatory activities. 4. Cholestrol lowering ability.	Beta glucans (antitumorous) Lovastatin (Cholestrol lowering)
3.	*Ganoderma lucidum*	Reishi or mannentake or lingzhi or ling chu or ling chin or mushroom of immortality.	1. Treatment of hepatopathy and chronic hepatitis. 2. Treatment of hypertension, arthritis and insomnia. 3. Treatment in asthma, gastric ulcer and bronchitis. 4. Reduce B.P., blood cholesterol and blood sugar levels as well as inhibit platelet aggregations.	Beta and hetro-B-glucans (antitumor, immunostimulating) Lingzhi-8-protein (antiallergenic, immunomodulating). Ganodermatic acids-Triterpenes (antiallergenic agents, cholesterol and B.P. reducing).

Contd...

Table 21.6–Contd...

Sl.No.	Species	Common Name	Medicinal Value	Key Active Constituents
4.	*Lentinus edodes*	Shittake or xiang gu or fragrant mushroom.	1. Treating high blood pressure and lowering blood cholesterol 2. Strenthening health. 3. Anticancerous activity. 4. Enhancing the immune system.	B-D-glucan (lentinan) Heteroglucan protein (LEM). Eritadenine (cholesterol reducing) Ergosterol (Provitamin D-2) RNA fractions (antiviral-nucleic acids)
5.	*Hericium erinaceus*	Monkey head mushroom or hedgehog mushroom	1. Beneficial for heart, Kidney, liver, lung and spleen. 2. To promote digestion and general vigour, strength and general nutrition. 3. The polysaccharide from this mushroom have cytostatic effects on gastric oesophageal hepatic and skin cancers (Mizuno, 1999.)	Beta-D-Glucans (antitumerous) Ergosterol (provitamin D) Cyathane derivatives (nerve growth stimulators)
6.	*Grifola frondosa*	Hen of the woods or sheep's head orfan shaped mushroom	1. Anticancer activity (Hishida *et al.*, 1988, Kurashige *et al.,* 1997) 2. Immunological enhancement together with property of anti HIV, antihypertension, antidiabetic and antiobesity (Zhunang and mizuno,1999) 3. Treatment of flu and common infection (Bacteria and Virus) 4. In diabetes mellitus 5. In hypercholesterolemia 6. In urinary tract infections	1,3, and 1,6 Beta glucans (antitumor and immuno-modulating) commercial product 'Grifolan'.
7.	*Tremella mesenterica*	White auricularia or white jelly fungus	1. Act as immune tonic. 2. For treating debility and exhaustion together with many other ailments including skin 3. Special significance in cosmetic industry.	Acidic polysaccharide-Glucuronoxylomannen (Antitumor, Immunostimulatory, antidiabetic, skin enhancing.)
8.	*Trametes* (*Coriolus*) *versicolor*	Turkey tail	1. Act directly on tumor cells as well as directly in the host to boost cellular immunity (Tsukagoshi,1984) 2. Antiviral activity through stimulation of interferon production. 3. Inhibit HIV-1 (Collins and Ng, 1977).	PSK or "Krestin"- a water soluble protein bound polysaccharide and PSP (direct act on tumour cells)
9.	*Poria cocos*	Wolfiporia cocos	1. Treatment of viral hepatitis. 2. Anticancer activity. 3. Immunomodulatory activities.	Polysaccharide-spachyman and packymaran (antitumour and immunomodulating). Tetracyclic triterpenes (immunomodulation and antiviral).

Contd...

Table 21.6–Contd...

Sl.No.	Species	Common Name	Medicinal Value	Key Active Constituents
10.	*Phellinus linteus*	Meshimakobu or "song gen"	1. "Worked as a miracle medicine" refreshing the human body and prolonging longevity (Ying *et al.*, 1987). 2. Tumour proliferation suppression (Mizuno, 2000). 3. Effects on digestive system cancers *e.g.* gastric, duodenal, colon, rectal and also liver cancer. 4. To treat liver diseases and gastric ulcers. 5. Inhibit the growth of cancers	Beta-glucans marketed as meshima capsules.
11.	*Flammulina velutipes*	Enokitake	1. To treat liver diseases and gastric ulcers. 2. Inhibit the growth of cancers.	Beta glycoprotein-proflamin
12.	*Calocybe indica*	Dudhchhatta	1. Antidiabetic activity	*P. anisaldehyde*
13.	*Agaricus bisporus*	Button mushroom	1. Immune enhancing 2. Antitumour properties.	Proteoglucans Beta (1-6)-D-glucan

Nutritional Value of Mushroom

The greatest difficulty in feeding man is to supply a sufficient quantity of the body-building material – protein. The other three nutritional categories are: the source of energy food-carbohydrates and fats; accessory food factors– vitamins; and inorganic compounds which are indispensable to good health. Of course, water, too, is essential. The moisture content of fresh mushrooms varies within the range of 70–95 per cent depending upon the harvest time and environmental conditions, whereas it is about 10–13 per cent in dried mushrooms. The protein content of the cultivated species ranges from 1.75 to 5.9 per cent of their fresh weight. It has been estimated that an average value of 3.5 to 4.0 per cent would be more representative. This means that the protein content of edible mushrooms in general, is about twice that of onion (1.4 per cent) and cabbage (1.4 per cent), and four times and 12 times those of oranges (1.0 per cent) and apples (0.3 per cent), respectively. In comparison, the protein content of common meats is as follows: pork, 9-1629 per cent; beef, 12-20 per cent; chicken, 18-20 per cent; fish, 18-20 per cent; and milk, 2.9-3.3 per cent. On a dry weight basis, mushrooms normally contain 19-35 per cent protein, as compared to 7.3 per cent in rice, 12.7 per cent in wheat, 38.1 per cent in soybean, and 9.4 per cent in corn. Therefore, in terms of the amount of crude protein, mushrooms rank below animal meats, but well above most other foods, including milk, which is an animal product (Chang and Miles 1989).

Quantitative data relating to the nutritive value of mushrooms is sparse. In the absence of feeding trials, alternative methods have been used to determine or predict the nutritional value of foods based on their content of essential amino acids (Crimson and Sands 1978). The Essential Amino Acid Index (EAA. Index) rates dietary protein in terms of an essential amino acid pattern based on known adult human dietary requirements. The Amino Acid Score (Chemical Score) is the amount of the most limiting amino acid in the food protein expressed as a percentage of the same amino acid present in the reference protein. In an attempt to resolve the difficulties inherent in comparisons between those mushrooms containing small amounts of high quality protein with those containing larger amounts of a protein of lesser nutritional quality, (Crisan and Sands, 1978) proposed the use of a Nutritional Index calculated as:

$$\text{Nutritional index} = \frac{(\text{EAA Index } \times \text{Percentage protein})}{100}$$

Table 21.7: Proximate Composition (Percent fresh weight of cultivated mushrooms)

Mushroom/Vegetable	*Moisture*	*Protein*	*Fat*	*Carbohydrate*	*Fibre*	*Ash*	*Calory*
Agaricus bisporus	90.1	2.9	0.3	5.0	0.9	0.8	36
Pleurotus sajor-caju	90.2	2.5	0.2	5.2	1.3	0.6	35
Cabbage	91.9	1.8	0.1	4.6	1.0	0.6	27
Cauliflower	90.8	2.6	0.4	4.0	1.2	1.0	30
Potato	74.7	1.6	0.1	22.6	0.4	0.6	97

Table 21.8: Essential Amino Acids in Edible Mushroom

Amino Acid	*White Button Mushroom*	*Oyster Mushroom*	*White Milky Mushroom*
Valine	1.63	4.7	2.48
Alanine	2.4	–	1.6
Argenine	1.90	6.7	trace
Aspartic acid	3.14	–	1.00
Metheonine	0.39	1.2	–
Histidine	0.64	2.0	2.4
Tryptophane	3.94	0.89	–
Lysine	1.62	5.0	5.56
Threonine	1.48	4.2	0.52
Phenel alanine	1.55	2.0	–
Cystine	–	–	–
Glutamic acid	7.06	–	2.12
Glycine	1.2	–	10.80
Leucine	2.16	4.4	–
Isoleucine	1.28	5.6	–
References	Hayes and Haddad (1976)	Bano *et al.* (1963)	Purkayastha and Nayak (1981)

The EAA Indices, the Amino Acid Scores, and Nutritional Indices for various mushrooms and other foods, are reported by (Crisan and Sands 1978). EAA Indices and Amino Acid Scores of the most nutritive mushrooms (highest values) rank in potential nutritive value with those of meat and milk, and are significantly higher than those for most legumes and vegetables. The least nutritive mushrooms rank appreciably lower but are still comparable to some of our common vegetables. In addition to their good proteins, mushrooms are a relatively good source of the following individual nutrients: fat, phosphorus, iron, and vitamins including thiamine, riboflavin, ascorbic acid, ergosterine and niacin. They are low in calories, carbohydrates and calcium. It has also been reported that a total lipid content varying between 0.6 and 3.1 per cent of the dry weight, is found in the commonly cultivated mushrooms. At least 72 per cent of the total fatty acids are found to be unsaturated in all the four tested mushrooms (Huang, *et al.*, 1985). It should be noted that unsaturated fatty acids are essential and significant in our diet and to our health. In recent years, there has been a trend toward discovering ways of treating mushrooms so as to give them added value. For example, Wermer and Beelman (2002) have reported on growing mushrooms enriched in selenium. By adding sodium selenite to compost over a range of 30-300 parts per million, they found that the mushrooms increasingly absorbed selenium according to the amount in the compost, so that it is possible to grow mushrooms containing a desired concentration. Selenium is an essential micronutrient that has generated much recent interest in nutritional and medical research–and, more recently, within the food industry (Beelman and Royse, 2006). Selenium has numerous physiological functions, but is best known as necessary 30 cofactor for the glutathione peroxidase enzyme system. This system is responsible for removing free radicals from the body, thus reducing oxidative damage. The desirability of a food product does not necessarily bear any correlation to its nutritional value. However, its appearance, taste, and aroma, sometimes can stimulate one's appetite (preference). In addition to nutritional value, mushrooms have some unique colour, taste, aroma, and texture characteristics, which attract their consumption.

Marketing of Mushrooms

Marketing is the most important consideration for the success of any firm as far as the mushroom's marketing are concerned, if we can't sell our mushrooms at a price that ensures a reasonable profit margin, we don't want to invest in this enterprise. So it is necessary that a good cultivar of mushroom should be well familiar with their marketing management.

"Marketing management is a total system of business activities designed to plan, price, promotion, and distribute want to satisfying products, services and ideas to target markets in order to achieve organizational objectives" (Kotler, 1999).

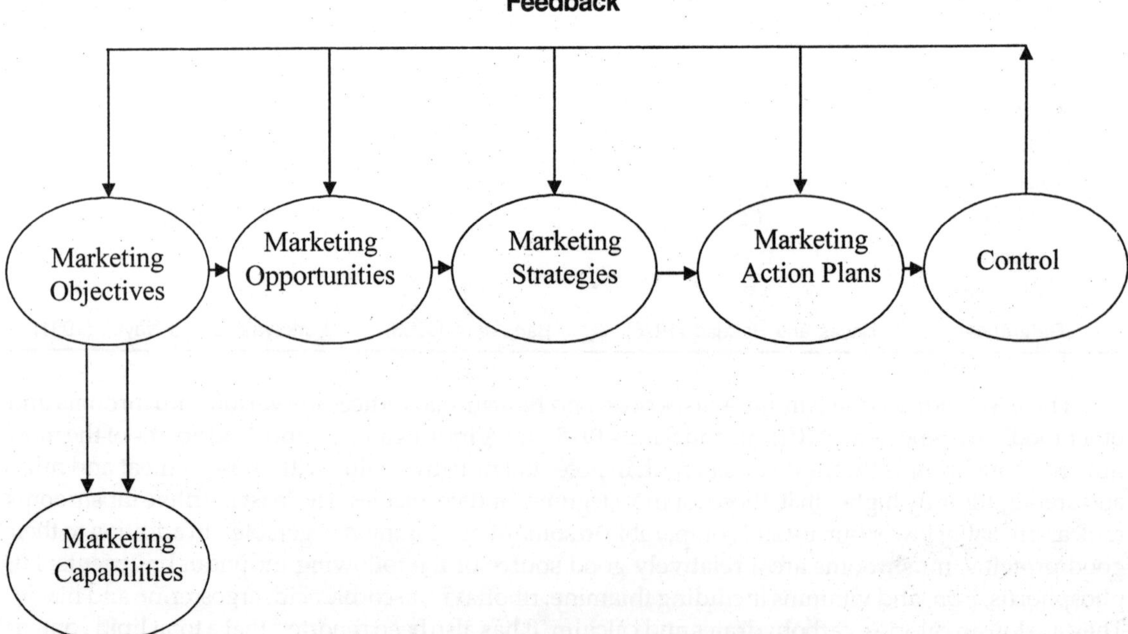

Figure 21.1: Marketing Management Process

Objectives of Marketing Management

- The size, extent and future potential of market.
- The factors governing the purchasing decisions of the consumers.
- The collection of the data about users opinion about the idealness of the product and use this as pointer to the future trend.
- The investigations about the possible new application as of the product.
- The judgement about the threat and its extent of competition and
- The development of optimum effective methods.

These are some techniques which are needed for management of mushroom marketing

- Intellectual skill
- Communication skill
- Organization understanding skill
- Decision making skill
- Motivation skill

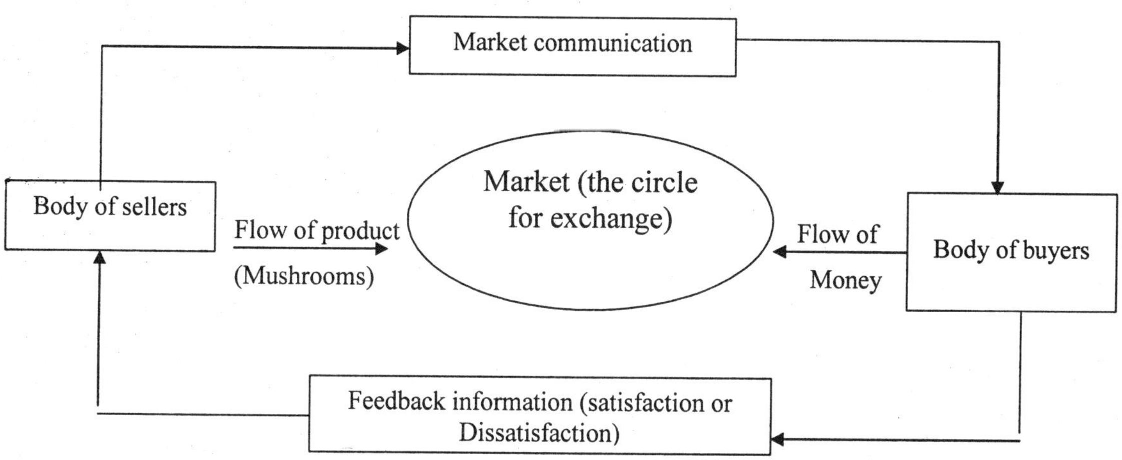

Figure 21.2: A Simple Marketing System

Need of the Mushroom's Marketing

Mushrooms have various nutraceuticals, pharmaceutical, cosmaceutical and medicinal properties. But a number of people of our country are unknown with their health increasing properties. So the main target of mushroom's marketing is may enable to popularize the mushrooms as potential food and medicines. Besides this, their cultivation may be helpful to provide employment and management of organic waste.

Marketing Strategy

Marketing strategy is the set of objectives, policies and rules that guide the firm's marketing efforts. Marketing mix, market segmentation, and distribution strategy are included in it.

Marketing Mix

Marketing mix is a set of numerous tools that the firm or marketers use to elicit desired responses from their target market. These tools classified by McCarthy into four broad groups that he called the 4P's of marketing.

These elements of marketing mix (4P's) discussed below.

Product

It is a bundle of satisfactions, fulfilling the number of needs of targeted customers. The variables are quality, features, brand name, packaging, size etc.

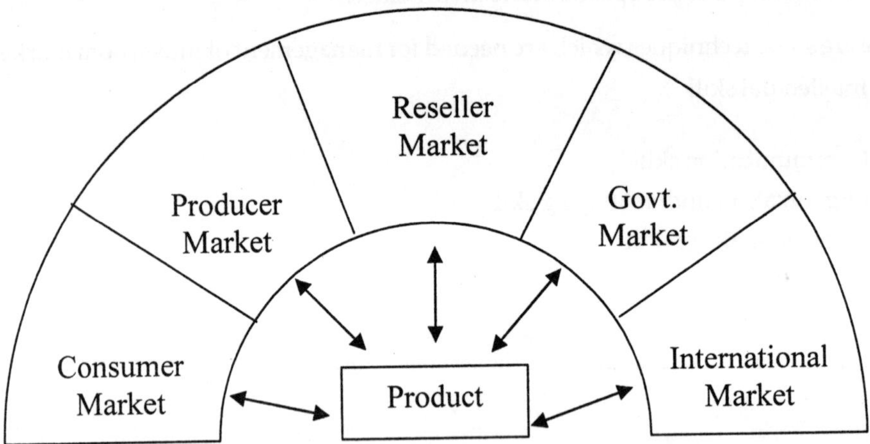

Price Activities

It is the amount which the customer a pay for the product. The deciding factors are target customers, cost, competition etc.

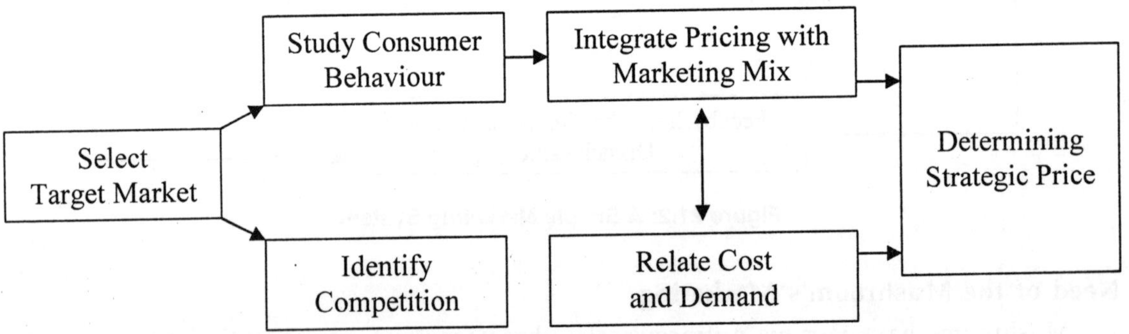

Promotional Activities

Advertisement is the major promotional activity industry. The various sources are sign boards, news papers and periodicals, sponsored programme on radio and T.V.

Place

Place of availability like cooperative stores, nearby shop and general stores in main markets.

R. lanterborn opines that 4P's represent the sellers view of marketing tools to influence buyers. From a buyer point of view, each marketing tool is designed to deliver a customer benefit. He suggest 4P's corresponds to 4C's *e.g.*

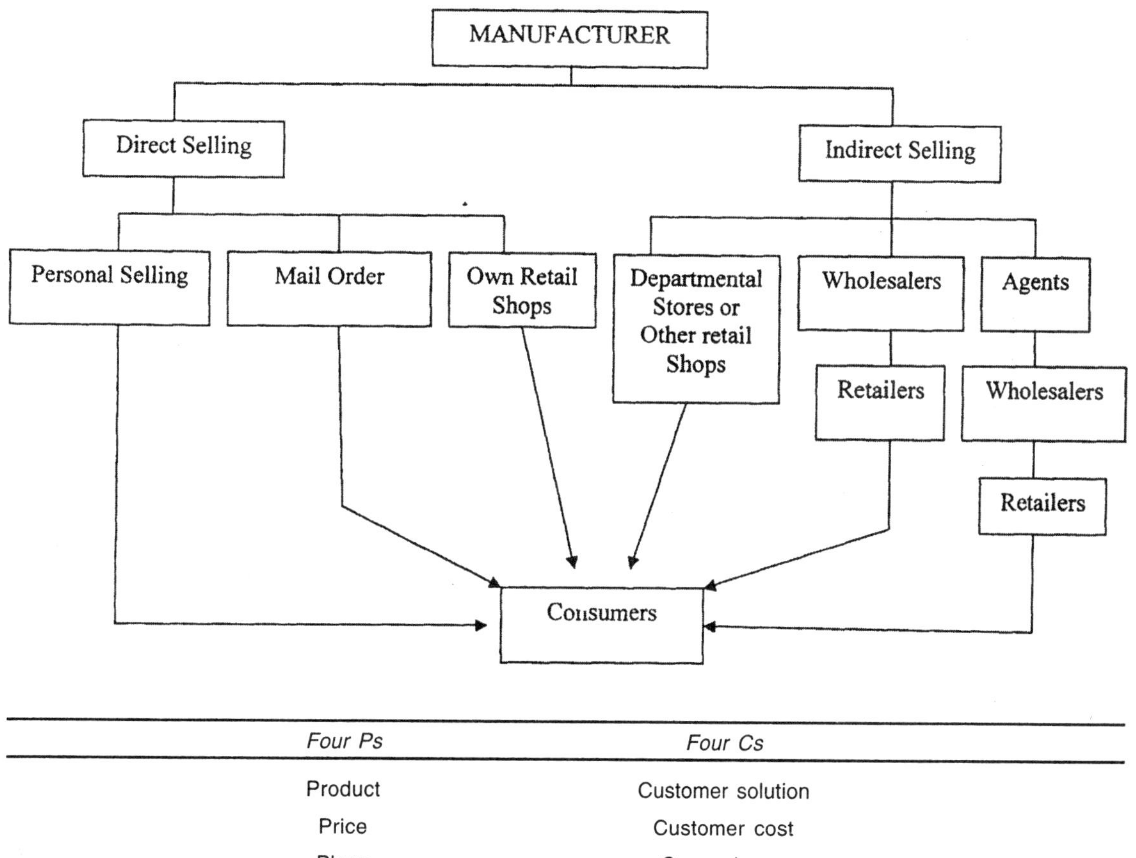

Four Ps	*Four Cs*
Product	Customer solution
Price	Customer cost
Place	Convenience
Promotion	Communication

Market Segmentation

"Market segmentation is the process of identifying group of buyers with different buying desires or requirements."Their conception lies on various base, important one's are listed below.

- ☆ Demographic basis like age, family size, education, occupation etc.
- ☆ Social class source of income, type of house, residential area etc.
- ☆ Family life cycle young, married/unmarried family size, age of youngest child, number of children in family etc.
- ☆ Psychologographic basis mode of living etc.
- ☆ Others like brand loyalty etc.

Goals of the Mushroom Marketing

- ✰ Maximize consumption of the mushrooms.
- ✰ Maximize satisfaction of mushroom's consumers.
- ✰ Maximize choice.
- ✰ Maximize life quality.

References

Adhikari, M.K. and Durrieu, G. (1996). Ethnomycologie nepalise. *Bull soc. Myc. France.* 112: 31-41.

Beelman, R.B., and Royse, D.J. (2006). Selenium enrichment of *Pleurotus cornucopiae* (paulet) Rolland and *Grifola frondosa* (Dicks: fr) S.F.Gray mushrooms. *Int. J. Med. Mush.* 8: 77-80.

Beyer, D. (2005). Spent mushroom substrate (SMS) research in the U.S. AMGA *J. Summer Issue* 31-32.

Chang, S.T. and Buswell, J.A. (1999).*Ganoderma lucidum* (Curt: fr), P.Karst. (Aphyllophoranymycetideae) a mushrooming medicinal mushroom. *Int. J. of Med. Mush.*1: 139-146.

Chang, S.T. and Miles (1989). Recycling of solid wastes with emphasis on organic wastes. *Green Productivity*, March issue 23-26.

Chang, S.T. (1999).World production of cultivated edible and medicinal mushroom in 1997 with emphasis on *Lentinus edodes* (Berk) Sing in China. *Int. J. Med. Mushrooms.*1 (4), 153-167.

Chang, S.T. and Miles, P.G. (2004). *Mushrooms cultivation, Nutritional value, Medicinal effect and Environmental impact*. Second edition.CRC press LLC, Florida.

Chaubey, A., Dehariya, P., Vyas, D. and Jain, A. (2010). Solid waste management by oyster mushroom cultivation. *Biozone International Journal of Life Science*, Vo. 2(1 and 2): 369–372.

Chaubey, A., Dehariya, P. and Vyas, D. (2010). Yield performance of *Calocybe indica* on conventional and non-conventional substrates. *J. of Mycol. and Pl. Pathol.*, 40(2): 176–178.

Collins, R.A., and Ng., T.B. (1987). Polysaccharopeptide from *Coriolus versicolor* has potential for use against human immunodeficiency virus type 1 infections. *Life science* 60, 383-387.

Crisan, E.V. and Sands, A. (1978). Nutritional value. In *"The biology and cultivation of edible mushroom"* edited to S.T.Chang and W.A. Hayes. Academic Press, New York.

Dehariya, P., Chaubey, A., Wagay, J.A. and Vyas, D. (2010). Wild mushrooms of Patharia forest of Sagar. *J. of Mycol. and Pl. Pathol.*, 40(2): 179–186.

Delmas, J. (1989). Les champignons et leur culture. Ed. Flammarion, Paris, 689 pp.

Edwards, R. (2000). The missing link? Mushrooms in permaculture. *Permaculture magazine*. No. 25.p. 37-39.

Hayes, W.A. and Haddad N. (1976). The food value of cultivated mushroom and its importance to the mushroom industry. *The Mushroom Journal* 40: 104-110.

Hikimo, H., Ishiyama, M., Suzuki, Y. and Konno, C. (1989). Mechanisms of hypoglycaemic activity of ganoderan B: a glycan of *Ganoderma lucidum* fruitbodies. *Planta Medica* 55, 423-428.

Hikino, H., and Mizuno, T. (1989). Hypoglycemic actions of some heteroglycans of *Ganoderma lucidum* fruit bodies. *Planta Med Aug.*, 55 (4): 385.

Hobbs,C. (1995). *Medicinal Mushrooms: An Exploration of Tradition, Healing and Culture*. Santa cruz, Botanica press.

Huang, B.H., Yung, K.H., Chang, S.T. (1985). The sterol composition of *volvariella volvacea* and other edible mushrooms. *Mycologia* 77 : 959-963.

Jain, A.K. (2005). *Thesis* on Cultivation technology of *Pleurotus* sp. with special reference to marketing potential in Sagar region.

Kabir,Y., Kimura, S.and Tamura, T. (1988). Dietary effect of *Ganoderma lucidum* mushroom on blood pressure and lipid levelsin spontaneously hypertensive rats (SHR). *J. Nutr. Sci. Vitaminol* (Tokyo). Aug., 34(4): 433-438.

Kotler, P. (1999). *Marketing Management*. The millennium edition. Printice Hall, India, New Delhi.

Kurashige, S., Akuzawa, Y.and Endo, F. (1997). Effect of *Lentinus edodes, Grifola frondosa, and Pleurotus ostreatus* administration on cancer outbreak, and activities of macrophages and immuno pharmacol. *immunotoxicol*. Maym 19(2): 175-183.

Lakhanpal, T. N. (1996). *Mushrooms of India Boletaceae* (eds. Mukherji, K.G.). A.P.H. publishing corporation.Vol. 1.

Lauterborn, Robert (1990). New marketing litany : 4Ps passwords take over, Advertising age,1-26.

Lincoff, Gary, Mitchel, (1977). *Toxic and hallucinogic mushrooms poisoning : A handbook for physians and mushroom hunters*.

Mizuno, T., Satio, H., Nishitoba and kowagishi, H. (1995). Antitumor–active substances from mushrooms. *Food Reviews Internationals* 11: 23-61.

Nair, M.C., and Bhavani Devi, S. (1986). Collection and identification of Agaricales. In beneficial fungi and their utilization. (Eds. Nair, M.C. and Balakrishnan, S.).pp. 25-27.

Noble, R. (2005). Spent mushroom substrate an alternative use. *AMGA J. Summer Issue*, pp. 33-35.

Pathak, V. N., Yadav, N., Gour, M. (1998). *Mushroom Production and Processing Technology*. Agrobios, India.

Purkayastha, R.P.and Nayak, D. (1981). Development of cultivation method and analyses of protein of a promising edible mushroom *Calocybe indica* P and C. *Mushroom Sci.*, 9: 697-713.

Purkayastha, R.P. and Chandra, A. (1985). *Manual of Indian Mushrooms*. 300 pp. New Delhi, India, Today and Tomorrow's printers and Publishers.

Royse, D.J. (1997). Speciality Mushrooms : Consumption, Production and Cultivation. Revista Maxicane *de micologia*, 13 : 1-11.

Soto-velazco, C., Lopez, M.C., Vazquez, E. and Alvarez, I. (2002). Cultivation of *Ganoderma Lucidum* and its effect on the production of lymphocytes in : *Mushroom Biology and Mushroom Products*, Sanchez, J.E., Muerta, G. and Mohtiel, E., Eds., Universities Autonoma Del Estado De Morelos, Mexico, 379-382.

Stamets, P, and Yao, C.C.W. (1998). Mycomedicinals: An informational booklet on medicinal mushrooms. *Mycomedia*, Olympia. 46 pp.

Stamets, P. (1990). A discussion on the cultivation of *Ganoderma lucidum* (Curtis: Fr.) Kar. The reishi of ling zhi mushroom of immortality. *McIlvainea* 9(2): 40-50.

Stamets, P. (2005). *Mycelium running : How mushroom can help save the world*. Ten speed press, Berkeley and Toronto, 574 pp.

Stamets, P. (1993). *Growing Gourmets and Medicinal Mushrooms*. Ted Speen Press. Hong Kong, 551 P.

Stamets, P. (2000). *Growing Gourmets and Medicinal Mushrooms*. Ten Speed Press, Berkely and Toronto, 339 pp.

Thakur, M.P., Shukla, C.S., Saxena, R.,Yadav,V. (2005). Emerging areas in mushroom diversity, production and postharvest developments (compendium of lectures). *IGAU* Raipur.

Tochikura, T.S., Nakashima, H., Kaneko,Y., Kobayashi,. N.(1987). Suppression of human immuno deficiency virus replication by 3-Azido-dexot Hymidine in various human haematopoietic cell lines in vitro. Augmentation by the effect of lentinan. *J. Cancer Res.* (Gann), p. 578-583.

Tong, C. and Z. Chen. (1990). Cultivation of *Ganoderma Lucidum* in Malysia, *Mush J. Tropics*, 10 : 27-30.

Tsukagoshi, N., Sasaki, T., Takemura, T., Ihara, H., Idota, Y., Yamagota, H. and Udaka, S. (1984). Efficient synthesis and secretion of a thermophillic alpha-amylase by protein producing *Bacillus brevis* 47 carrying the Bacillus stearothermophillus amylase gene. *J. Bacteriol.* 164 (3) : 1182-1187.

Tsukagoshi, S. (1984). Krestin (PSK). *Cancer Treatment Reviews* 11,131-155.

Vyas, D., Chaubey, A., Dehariya, P., Wagay, J.A., Bajpay, A., Lodhwal, R.K. (2009). Mushroom cultivation a tool for agripreneurship and rural management. In: *Perspectives on Agripreneurship and Rural Development* (Eds.) Prof. R.K. Pandey, Prof. P.S. Tripathi, Dr. S.K. Dubey, Dr. Ashish Bajpai. Faculty of Studies, BHU, pp. 463–473.

Wang, H.X. and Ng, T.B. (2001). Isolation of pleuriregin, a novel ribosome-inactivating protein from fresh sclerotia of the edible mushroom (*Pleurotus tuber-regium*). Sclerotia. *Int. J. of Biochem. Cell. Biol.*, 33(5): 483-490.

Wasser, S.P. and Weis, A.L. (1999). Therapeutic effects of substances occurring in higher basidiomycetes mushrooms : a modern perspective. *Crit. Rev. Immunol.*, 19(1): 65-96.

Ying, J., Mao.X., Ma, Q., Zhong,Y. and Wen, H. (1987). Icons of medicinal fungi from China. *Science Press*, Beijing, China.

Zhuang, C. and Mizuno,T. (1999). Biological responses from *Grifola frondosa* (Diçk. fr) S..F. gray-maitake. (Aphyllophoranymycetideae). *Int. J. of Med. Mush.* 1: 317-324.

Vyas, D., Jain, A.K., Bajpei, A. (2007). Marketing potential of *Pleurotus* mushroom and management strategies in Sagar region. *J. Bot. Soc. Univ.* Sagar.

Microbial Biotechnology and Ecology (2011) *Pages* 377–390
Editors: Deepak Vyas, G.S. Paliwal, P.K.Khare and R.K Gupta
Published by: DAYA PUBLISHING HOUSE, NEW DELHI

Chapter 22

Trichoderma Species: The History and Evolution of Current Concepts of Biological Control

☆ ***Pradeep Kumar Singh[1]* and Deepak Vyas[2]***

[1]*Government Naveen College, Janakpur, Koriya, CG*
[2]*Department of Botany, Dr. Hari Singh Gour University, Sagar, M.P.*

Introduction

Traditional methods used to protect crops from diseases have been largely based on the use of chemical pesticides. Applications of fungicides and fumigants can have drastic effects on the environment and consumer, and are often applied in greater quantities than herbicides and insecticides in agricultural production. Chemical methods are not economical in the long run because they pollute the atmosphere, damage the environment, leave harmful residues, and can lead to the development of resistant strains among the target organisms with repeated use (Naseby *et al.*, 2000). A reduction or elimination of synthetic pesticide applications in agriculture is highly desirable. One of the most promising means to achieve this goal is by the use of new tools based on biocontrol agents (BCAs) for disease control alone, or to integrate with reduced doses of chemicals in the control of plant pathogens resulting in minimal impact of the chemicals on the environment (Chet and Inbar, 1994; Harman and Kubicek, 1998). To date, a number of BCAs have been registered and are available as commercial products, including strains belonging to bacterial genera such as *Agrobacterium, Pseudomonas, Streptomyces* and *Bacillus,* and fungal genera such as *Gliocladium, Trichoderma, Ampelomyces, Candida* and *Coniothyrium.*

---

* E-mail: pksbotany@gmail.com

Trichoderma spp. are among the most frequently isolated soil fungi and present in plant root ecosystems (Harman *et al.*, 2004). These fungi are opportunistic, avirulent plant symbionts, and function as parasites and antagonists of many phytopathogenic fungi, thus protecting plants from disease. So far, *Trichoderma* spp. are among the most studied fungal BCAs and commercially marketed as biopesticides, biofertilizers and soil amendments (Harman, 2000; Harman *et al.*, 2004; Lorito *et al.*, 2004). Depending upon the strain, the use of *Trichoderma* in agriculture can provide numerous advantages: (i) colonization of the rhizosphere by the BCA ("rhizosphere competence") allowing rapid establishment within the stable microbial communities in the rhizosphere; (ii) control of pathogenic and competitive/deleterious microflora by using a variety of mechanisms; (iii) improvement of the plant health and (iv) stimulation of root growth (Harman *et al.*, 2004).

This review presents a compilation of the most recent advances in understanding the mechanisms involved in the interaction of *Trichoderma* spp. with phytopathogenic fungi and plants. We emphasize the biological and biochemical aspects of this topic, with particular attention paid to the molecular factors involved in the natural crosstalk occurring in soil and root environment. A better understanding of the principles regulating the interaction between fungal pathogens, host plants, and BCAs such as *Trichoderma* would enhance the practical application of these beneficial microorganisms for plant disease control.

Trichoderma–Pathogen Interaction

Trichoderma (teleomorph *Hypocrea*) is a genus of asexual fungi found in the soils of all climatic zones. *Trichoderma* is a secondary opportunistic invader, a fast growing fungus, a strong spore producer, a source of cell wall degrading enzymes (CWDEs: cellulases, chitinases, glucanases, etc.), and an important antibiotic producer. Numerous strains of this genus are 'rhizosphere competent' and are able to degrade hydrocarbons, chlorophenolic compounds, polysaccharides and the xenobiotic pesticides used in agriculture (Harman and Kubicek, 1998; Harman *et al.*, 2004). The main biocontrol mechanisms that *Trichoderma* utilizes in direct confrontation with fungal pathogens are mycoparasitism (Papavizas, 1985; Harman and Kubicek, 1998; Howell, 2003) and antibiosis (Howell, 1998; Sivasithamparam and Ghisalberti, 1998).

Mycoparasitism and Lytic Enzymes

The complex process of mycoparasitism consists of several events, including recognition of the host, attack and subsequent penetration and killing. During this process *Trichoderma* secretes CWDEs that hydrolyze the cell wall of the host fungus, subsequently releasing oligomers from the pathogen cell wall (Kubicek *et al.*, 2001; Howell 2003; Woo *et al.*, 2006). It is believed that *Trichoderma* secretes hydrolytic enzymes at a constitutive level and detects the presence of another fungus by sensing the molecules released from the host by enzymatic degradation (Harman *et al.*, 2004; Lorito *et al.*, 2006; Woo and Lorito, 2007).

The molecular biology of the mycoparasitic interaction between pathogen and antagonist has been studied in detail. The factors activating the biocontrol gene cascade in *T. atroviride* strain P1 mutants containing the green fluorescent protein (*gfp*) or glucose oxidase (*gox*) gene reporter systems controlled by different inducible promoters (*i.e.* from the exochitinase *nag1* gene or the endochitinase *ech42* gene) have been evaluated. Interestingly, the expression of these genes involved in mycoparasitism was induced by the digestion products obtained after treatments of fungal cell walls and colloidal chitin with purified CWDEs or fungal culture filtrates. LC/MS–MS analysis revealed that these novel mycoparasitism related inducers have an oligosaccharide structure (Woo *et al.*, 2004). Recently, the role of *Trichoderma* ABC transporters in both mycoparasitism and nutritional uptake by *Trichoderma* has been investigated (Singh and Vyas, 2008). Unpublished but convincing data demonstrated that culture filtrates or mycelia of numerous plant pathogens induced the expression of specific *T. atroviride* ABC transporter genes, such as *tabc2*. This conclusion was confirmed by producing and analyzing knock-out mutants that showed a slower growth on different culture media or in presence of different fungal pathogens (*Botrytis cinerea, Rhizoctonia solani* and *Pythium ultimum*).

The antifungal arsenal of *Trichoderma* spp. includes a great variety of lytic enzymes (Lorito, 1998; Lorito *et al.*, 1994a, 1996a), most of which play a great role in biocontrol (Harman and Kubicek, 1998; Baek *et al.*, 1999; Carsolio *et al.*, 1999; Woo *et al.*, 1999; Zeilinger *et al.*, 1999; Kullnig *et al.*, 2000; Kubicek *et al.*, 2001). Many CWDEs from different *Trichoderma* strains have been purified and characterized (Lorito, 1998). Interestingly, when tested alone or in combinations, the purified proteins showed antifungal activity towards a broad spectrum of fungal pathogens (*i.e.* species of *Rhizoctonia, Fusarium, Alternaria, Ustilago, Venturia* and *Colletotrichum*, as well as fungus like organisms such as the Oomycetes *Pythium* and *Phytophthora* which lack chitin in their cell walls) (Tronsmo, 1991; Lorito *et al.*, 1993, 1994a).

The direct application of anti-microbial compounds produced by fungal BCAs, instead of the whole "live" organisms, has numerous advantages in industry and agriculture, and may be more amenable to public opinion because of the inability of the agent to reproduce and spread. The selective production of active compounds may be performed by modifying the growth conditions, *i.e.* type and composition of culture medium, temperature of incubation and pH etc. (Lorito and Scala, 1999; Woo and Lorito, 2007). The presence of different carbon sources, such as mono- or polysaccharides, colloidal chitin, or fungal tissues, has been shown to induce the secretion of CWDEs (Mach *et al.*, 1999). Enhanced anti-fungal activity can be obtained by the combined application of *Trichoderma* enzymes with the fungus, different classes of synthetic fungicides, and in particular with compounds that affect the integrity of the cell membrane (Lorito *et al.*, 1994b, 1996a). Moreover, purified mixes of CWDEs with different lytic activities showed improved antifungal effects against various plant pathogens, sometimes comparable to those obtained by using synthetic pesticides alone (Lorito *et al.*, 1994b, 1996a; Baek *et al.*, 1999; Carsolio *et al.*, 1999).

Antibiosis and Secondary Metabolites

Trichoderma produces a plethora of secondary metabolites with biological activity (Ghisalberti and Sivasithamparam, 1991; Sivasithamparam and Ghisalberti, 1998). The term "secondary metabolite" includes a heterogeneous group of chemically different natural compounds possibly related to survival functions for the producing organism, such as competition against other micro- and macroorganisms, symbiosis, metal transport, differentiation etc. (Demain and Fang, 2000). Included in this group are antibiotics, which are natural products able to inhibit microbial growth. Antibiotic production is often well correlated with biocontrol ability, and the application of purified antibiotics was found to show effects on the host pathogen similar to those obtained by using the corresponding living microbe. Ghisalberti *et al.* (1990) demonstrated that the biocontrol efficacy of *Trichoderma harzianum* isolates against *Gaeumannomyces graminis* var. *tritici* is related to the production of pyrone-like antibiotics.

The production of secondary metabolites by *Trichoderma* spp. is strain dependent and includes antifungal substances belonging to a variety of classes of chemical compounds. They were classified by Ghisalberti and Sivasithamparam (1991) into three categories: (i) volatile antibiotics, *i.e.* 6-pentyl-a-pyrone (6PP) and most of the isocyanide derivates; (ii) water-soluble compounds, *i.e.* heptelidic acid or koningic acid; (iii) peptaibols, which are linear oligopeptides of 12–22 amino acids rich in a-aminoisobutyric acid, N-acetylated at the N-terminus and containing an amino alcohol (Pheol or Trpol) at the C-terminus (Le Doan *et al.*, 1986; Rebuffat *et al.*, 1989).

Recently, we isolated and characterized the main secondary metabolites obtained from culture filtrates of two commercial *T. harzianum* strains (T22 and T39), and their production during the antagonistic interaction with the pathogen *R. solani* was also investigated (Vinale *et al.*, 2006). The chemical structures of *Trichoderma* antibiotics may suggest two different mechanisms of action. The production of low molecular weight, non-polar, volatile compounds (*i.e.* 6PP) results in a high concentration of antibiotics in the soil environment that have a relatively long distance range of influence on the microbial community. On the contrary, a short distance effect may be due to the polar antibiotics and peptaibols acting in close proximity to the producing hyphae. Lorito *et al.* (1996b) demonstrated that peptaibols inhibited b-glucan synthase activity in the host fungus, while acting synergistically with *T. harzianum* b-glucanases. The inhibition of glucan synthase prevented the reconstruction of the pathogen cell wall, thus facilitating the disruptive action of b-glucanases. The synergism existing between enzymes and polar antibiotics is strictly related to their mechanism of action (Schirmbock *et al.*, 1994; Lorito *et al.*, 1996a,b; Fogliano *et al.*, 2002). Although the role and the effects of peptaibols are clear, the mode of action of other *Trichoderma* secondary metabolites (*i.e.* pyrones), and their possible synergisms with other compounds have not yet been elucidated (Claydon *et al.*, 1987; Serrano-Carreon *et al.*, 1993; Howell, 1998).

According to the secondary metabolite produced, Howell *et al.* (1993) divided strains of *T. virens* into two groups: the "Q" strains able to produce the antibiotic gliotoxin and the "P" strains that produce a related compound, gliovirin, instead of gliotoxin (Howell and Stipanovic, 1983). Gliotoxin has a broad spectrum of antibiotic activity, while gliovirin is a specific potent inhibitor of Oomycetes and its production was positively correlated with biocontrol efficacy of "P" group strains to control *Pythium* damping-off of cotton (Chet *et al.*, 1997; Howell, 1998). On substrates with high C/N ratios, both "P" and "Q" strains of *T. virens* produce a phytotoxin similar to viridin, that is called viridiol. The viridiol-producing strains may be applied to surface soil as bio-herbicide for weeds, where they do not affect the crop plant that is planted in the treated soil (Howell, 2006). Other observations indicated that the biological control of pre-emergence damping-off by *T. virens* could be also related to its ability to degrade seed-emitted compounds that stimulate pathogen propagule germination (Howell, 2002). On the other hand, the induction of plant defence responses by some strains of *T. virens* plays a pivotal role in successful disease control of *R. solani* on cotton (Howell *et al.*, 2000). In a recent study, Howell and Puckhaber (2005) indicated that "P" strains unable to induce the production of phytoalexins in cotton were ineffective as BCAs and pathogenic to susceptible cultivars. Conversely, "Q" strains inducing high levels of phytoalexin synthesis showed improved biocontrol efficacy and were not pathogenic to cotton roots. Phytoalexin synthesis in cotton is elicited by a protein produced by *T. virens* (Hanson and Howell, 2004), but the exact biochemical processes involved are not yet understood.

Competition with Pathogens and Soil Microbial Community

Competition for carbon, nitrogen and other growth factors, together with competition for space or specific infection sites, may be also used by the BCA to control plant pathogens. *T. harzianum* is able to control *B. cinerea* on grapes by colonizing blossom tissue and excluding the pathogen from its infection site (Gullino, 1992). Sivan and Chet (1989) demonstrated that competition for nutrients is the major mechanism used by *T. harzianum* to control *F. oxysporum* f. sp. *melonis*. Moreover, *Trichoderma* has a strong capacity to mobilize and take up soil nutrients, thus making it more efficient and competitive than many other soil microbes (Benytez *et al.*, 2004).

The biotic components of the soil environment have relevant effects on the biocontrol activity of *Trichoderma* against plant pathogens. Bae and Knudsen (2005), by using a Gfp-tagged mutant, showed that higher levels of microbial soil biomass induced a shift from hyphal growth to sporulation in *T. harzianum*, thus reducing its biocontrol efficacy. This effect may be associated with a phenomenon known as "soil fungistasis", which is largely dependent on the soil microbial community composition (de Boer *et al.*, 2003). In particular, the production of antibiotic compounds and the presence of bacteria belonging to the genus *Pseudomonas* seem to be essential for the development of this phenomenon. In this context a detailed study of the metabolites produced by microorganisms present in the soil environment should be performed in order to avoid the suppression of BCAs.

Trichoderma–Plant Interaction

In addition to the beneficial effects that occur in direct interactions with plant disease agents, some *Trichoderma* species are also able to colonize root surfaces and cause substantial changes in plant metabolism (Harman *et al.*, 2004). It is well documented that some strains promote plant growth, increase nutrient availability, improve crop production and enhance disease resistance (Harman *et al.*, 2004).

Plant Root Colonization

The physical interaction between *Trichoderma* and the plant was observed by electron microscopy to be limited to the first few cell layers of plant epidermis and root outer cortex (Yedidia *et al.*, 1999). The hyphae of the BCA penetrate the root cortex but the colonization by *Trichoderma* is stopped, probably by the deposition of callose barriers by the surrounding plant tissues (Yedidia *et al.*, 1999). It appears that this interaction evolves into a symbiotic rather than a parasitic relationship between the fungus and the plant, whereby the fungus occupies a nutritional niche and the plant is protected from disease. A very active, direct molecular cross-talk occurs between the fungus and the plant. Elicitors from *Trichoderma* activate the expression of genes involved in the plant defence response system, and promote the growth of the plant, root system and nutrient availability. This effect in turn augments the zone for colonization and the nutrients available for the biocontrol fungus, subsequently increasing the overall antagonism to plant pathogens (Yedidia *et al.*, 2003; Hanson and Howell, 2004; Harman *et al.*, 2004).

Plant Growth Promotion

Many BCAs, such as fungi, bacteria and viruses, are not only able to control the pathogens that cause plant disease, but are also able to promote plant growth and development. In greenhouse and field trials, the ability of *T. harzianum* T22 and *T. atroviride* P1 to improve the growth of lettuce, tomato and pepper plants under field conditions was investigated (Vinale *et al.*, 2004). Crop productivity was increased up to 300 per cent, as determined by comparing the treated plots with the untreated controls and measuring fresh/dry root and above ground biomass weights, height of plants, number of leaves and fruits. This study also demonstrated the compatibility of *T. harzianum* T22 and *T. atroviride* P1 with pesticides conventionally used in organic farming by monitoring the effect on mycelia growth in both liquid and solid media. Results indicated a high level of tolerance by *Trichoderma* strains to concentrations of copper oxychloride varying from 0.1 up to 5mM (Vinale *et al.*, 2004). These positive effects of *Trichoderma* may be obtained with different plant species, thus the genetic base of such interactions seems not to be predominant. Conversely, at least in maize the plant growth promotion effect is genotype specific and some inbreds respond negatively to different strains (Harman, 2006).

A yield increase was also observed when plant seeds were exposed to *Trichoderma* conidia that were separated from them by cellophane, suggesting that *Trichoderma* metabolites can influence the plant growth (Benitez *et al.*, 2004). On the other hand, only a few reports deal with the ability of antagonistic fungal strains to produce compounds acting as growth promoting factors. Cutler *et al.* (1986, 1989) reported the isolation, identification and biological activity of secondary metabolites produced by *T. koningii* (koninginin A) and *T. harzianum* (6-pentyl-apyrone) that acted as plant growth regulators. Both metabolites significantly inhibited the growth of etiolated wheat coleoptiles at a relatively high concentration (10^{-3}M), but no effect was registered at lower doses (range from 10^{-4} to 10^{-3} M). It is hypothesized that such Trichoderma secondary metabolites may act as auxin-like compounds, which typically have an optimum activity between at 10^{-5} and 10^{-6}M while having an inhibitory effect at higher concentrations (Thimann, 1937; Cleland, 1972; Brenner, 1981), and/or are involved in the production of auxin inducers. The dose–effect response of such compounds on plant growth and development requires further investigation. *Trichoderma* spp. also produce organic acids, such as gluconic, citric or fumaric acids, that decrease soil pH and permit the solubilization of phosphates, micronutrients and mineral cations like iron, manganese and magnesium, useful for plant metabolism (Benitez *et al.*, 2004; Harman *et al.*, 2004).

Induction of Plant Defence Responses

The induction of plant defence responses mediated by the antagonistic fungus has been well documented (De Meyer *et al.*, 1998; Yedidia *et al.*, 1999; Hanson and Howell, 2004; Harman *et al.*, 2004). Various plants, both mono- and dicotyledonous species, showed increased resistance to pathogen attack when pre-treated with *Trichoderma* (Harman *et al.*, 2004; Singh *et al.*, 2007). Plant colonization by *Trichoderma* spp. reduced disease caused by one or more different pathogens, at the site of inoculation (induced localized acquired resistance, LAR), as well as when the biocontrol fungus was inoculated at different times or sites than that of the pathogen (induced systemic resistance or ISR).

The induction of plant resistance by colonization with some *Trichoderma* species is similar to that elicited by rhizobacteria, which enhance the defence system but do not involve the production of pathogenesis-related proteins (PR proteins) (Van Loon *et al.*, 1998; Stacey and Keen, 1999; Harman *et al.*, 2004). In a recent work Alfano and co-workers (2007) investigated at a molecular level the plant genes involved in *T. hamatum* 382 resistance inductions by using a high-density oligonucleotide microarray approach. Interestingly, *Trichoderma*-induced genes were associated with biotic or abiotic stresses, as well as RNA, DNA, and protein metabolism. In particular, genes that codify for extensin and extensin-like proteins were found to be induced by the BCA, but not those codifying for proteins belonging to the PR-5 family (thaumatin-like proteins), which are considered the main molecular markers of SAR.

During the interaction of *Trichoderma* with the plant, different classes of metabolites may act as elicitors or resistance inducers (Harman *et al.*, 2004; Woo *et al.*, 2006; Woo and Lorito, 2007). These molecules include: (i) proteins with enzymatic activity, such as xylanase (Lotan and Fluhr, 1990); (ii) avirulence-like gene products able to induce defence reactions in plants (Woo *et al.*, 2004); (iii) low-molecular-weight compounds released from fungal or plant cell walls by the activity of *Trichoderma* enzymes (Harman *et al.*, 2004; Woo *et al.*, 2006; Woo and Lorito, 2007). Some of the low-molecular-weight degradation products released from fungal cell walls were purified and characterized, and found to consist of short oligosaccharides comprised of two types of monomers, with and without an amino acid residue (Woo *et al.*, 2006; Woo and Lorito, 2007). These compounds elicited a reaction in the plant when applied to leaves or when injected into root or leaf tissues. Further, they also stimulated the biocontrol ability of *Trichoderma* by activating the mycoparasitic gene expression cascade. Recently, Djonovic *et al.* (2006) identified a small protein (Sm1) elicitor secreted by T. *virens*, and demonstrated its involvement in the activation of plant defence mechanisms and the induction of systemic resistance. In addition to their innate antimicrobial effect, their action may also stimulate the biological activity of resident antagonistic microbial populations or introduced *Trichoderma* strains, and promote an ISR effect in the plant. Other secondary metabolites, like peptaibols, may act as elicitors of plant defence mechanisms against pathogens. In fact, application of peptaibols activated a defence response in tobacco plants (Bený´ tez *et al.*, 2004; Viterbo *et al.*, 2006, personal communication). A peptaibol synthetase from *T. virens* was purified (Wiest *et al.*, 2002), and the achieved cloning of the corresponding gene will facilitate an understanding of the role of this class of compounds in plant defence response.

Influence of Soil Environment on *Trichoderma*–Plant Interaction

The activities of BCAs are also affected by the presence of organic nutrients in soil (Hoitink and Boehm, 1999). Organic matter composition and the associated biotic and abiotic environment can affect the activities of *Trichoderma*, especially in relation to the conduciveness/receptivity of the soil to the strain (Simon and Sivasithamparam, 1989; Wakelin *et al.*, 1999). So far, composts represent an optimal substrate for BCAs, thus encouraging their establishment into the soil environment (Hoitink and Boehm, 1999; Leandro *et al.*, 2007). The mechanisms of action used by *Trichoderma* (competition, antibiosis, parasitism and systemic-induced resistance) are influenced by concentration and availability of nutrients (carbohydrates in lignocellulosic substances, chitin, lipids, etc.) within the soil organic matter (Hoitink *et al.*, 2006). Krause *et al.* (2001) demonstrated that *T. hamatum* inoculation of potting mix with a high microbial capacity, which supported high populations of BCAs, significantly reduced the severity of *Rhizoctonia* damping-off of radish or *Rhizoctonia* crown and root rot of poinsettia. Moreover, *T. hamatum* inoculated into the compost amended potting mix induced systemic acquired resistance on cucumber, reducing the severity of *Phytophthora* leaf blight (Khan *et al.*, 2004). This induction was more effective on plants grown in compost-amended media when compared to lower microbe carrying capacity sphagnum peat media (Hoitink *et al.*, 2006). A better understanding of the activities of *Trichoderma* strains in plant growth media high in organic matter could also help to select strains suitable for multiple acre field conditions associated with stubble retention practices and/or organic farming which are becoming increasingly popular world-wide.

The Three-Way Interaction

Trichoderma–Plant–Pathogen

The three-way interactions involving *Trichoderma*, plant and fungal pathogen have received less attention in comparison to the "simple" two-partner systems (*i.e.* plant–pathogen, plant–antagonist or pathogen–antagonist). There are obvious difficulties in studying such a complex system even if it is reproduced *in vitro*, although it better simulates the natural interactions occurring in soil agro-ecosystems. Recent studies have investigated some of the morphological or molecular aspects involved in plant–pathogen–antagonist interactions by using novel methods such as proteomics (Marra *et al.*, 2006) and gene reporter systems (Lu *et al.*, 2004). The molecular cross-talk taking place during three-way interactions requires experiments that investigate the changes in gene expression occurring in each partner involved, singly and subsequently in all possible combinations. Further, an *in situ* analysis of the compounds implicated when plants are exposed concurrently to different beneficial and/or pathogenic microorganisms could be performed.

Marra *et al.* (2006) studied the three-way interactions of *Trichoderma* with plant and different fungal pathogens by using a proteomic approach in order to analyze the differential proteins produced. Proteins were identified and characterized by using tryptic digestion, mass spectrometry (MS) and in silico analysis. Results indicated that in the plant proteome-specific PR proteins and other disease related factors (*i.e.* potential resistance genes) may regulate the three-way interaction, and that the presence of the antagonist modifies quantitatively and qualitatively the plant response to a pathogen attack. In some cases, the antagonistic fungus reduced production of some defence proteins, but resulted in a higher accumulation of others. These observations suggest that the plant response to a specific BCA depends upon each of the three partners involved. On the microbial side, many differential proteins obtained from the *T. atroviride* interaction proteome showed interesting homologies to those of a fungal hydrophobin and ABC transporters. Virulence factors, like cyclophilins, were also up-regulated in the pathogen proteome during the interaction with the plant alone, as well as with the antagonist.

Gfp-tagged mutants of *T. atroviride* were used to study the *in situ Trichoderma*–plant–pathogen interaction by using different promoters of biocontrol-related genes to drive the expression of the living producer (Lu *et al.*, 2004). In particular, induction of *Trichoderma* genes encoding for different CWDEs in the presence of the soil-borne pathogens *R. solani* and *P. ultimum* was monitored by confocal and fluorescence microscopy. During the three way interaction the transformants were activated by the presence of the host fungal pathogen and purified colloidal chitin chitoligomers, and appeared to fluoresce during the early phases of contact. This approach allowed for the first time a direct visualization of the mycoparasitic gene expression cascade *in vivo*. The authors suggested that specific compounds released by the host cell walls were actively involved in mycoparasitism induction. In addition, the involvement of *T. atroviride* endo- and exochitinases (*nag1* and *chit42*) in the mycoparasitic process other than in the simple host hyphae degradation was also demonstrated.

Further understanding of the mechanisms operating in the interaction between plant and microbes in the soil communities could encourage development of new powerful biotechnologies, useful in the management of fungal diseases and in the improvement of crop production yields.

Conclusions

The success of biocontrol agents is dependant upon the complex interactions that these beneficial microbes establish with pathogens and plants in the soil ecosystem. A better understanding of these processes and of the molecular cross-talk occurring among the participants will not only result in the application of safer and less expensive methods to protect plants and increase crop yield, but also will extend our knowledge of how a disease process develops. Recent advances in modern techniques such as proteomics and metabolomics could provide novel information about the complex tripartite interactions, in particular about the ability of *Trichoderma* to sense the environment, the plant and the microbial community. However, it is clear that different approaches, *i.e.* genetic, molecular, biochemical and ecological, should be integrated to conduct future studies in biocontrol research and development of new technologies. In particular, a modern and more effective use of beneficial microbes such as *Trichoderma* should take into account an actual understanding of the biology and the interaction capabilities of these agents, starting with the implementation of new strain selection protocols that consider the multiple beneficial effects exerted on the colonized plant. Genetic manipulation offers novel opportunity to achieve improved biocontrol efficacy. Brunner *et al.* (2005) by over expressing a glucose oxidase gene from *Aspergillus niger* in *T. atroviride* strain P1 obtained mutants able to control fungal pathogens and induce plant systemic resistance better than the wild-type strain. Finally, the information gathered by fundamental and applied studies conducted with a "wide-view" approach may allow us to overcome in the future, at least in some applications, the difficulties associated with use of living microbes. This can be done by introducing new biopesticides and biofertilizers, *i.e.* based on the metabolites or bioactive compounds responsible for the desired beneficial effects on crops (Singh and Vyas, 2007). The application of *Trichoderma* metabolites for crop protection, such as the host defence inducers and antibiotics, may become a reality in the near future, as they can be produced cheaply in large quantities on an industrial scale, easily separated from the fungal biomass, dried and formulated for spray or drench applications. In the meantime, further experiments should be performed to better understand the mechanisms of action of *Trichoderma* secondary metabolites and their possible synergisms with other compounds used in agriculture.

References

Alfano G, Lewis I, Cakir C, Bos JIB, Miller SA, Madden LV, Kamoun S, Hoitink HAJ. (2007). Systemic modulation of gene expression in tomato by *Trichoderma hamatum* 382. *Phytopathology* 97: 429–437.

Bae YS, Knudsen GR. (2005). Soil microbial biomass influence on growth and biocontrol efficacy of *Trichoderma harzianum*. *Biological Control* 32: 236–242.

Baek JM, Howell CR, Kenerley CM. (1999). The role of an extracellular chitinase from *Trichoderma virens* Gv29-8 in the biocontrol of *Rhizoctonia solani*. *Current genetics* 35: 41–50.

Benytez T, Rincon AM, Limon MC, Codon AC. (2004). Biocontrol mechanisms of *Trichoderma* strains. *International Microbiology* 7: 249–260.

Brenner ML. (1981). Modern methods for plant growth substance analysis. *Annual Review of Plant Physiology* 32: 511–538.

Brunner K, Zeilinger S, Ciliento R, Woo SL, Lorito M, Kubicek CP, Mach RL. (2005). Genetic improvement of a fungal biocontrol agent to enhance both antagonism and induction of plant systemic disease resistance. *Applied Environmental Microbiology* 71: 3959–3965.

Carsolio C, Benhamou N, Haran S, Cortes C, Gutierrez A, Chet I, Herrera-Estrella A. (1999). Role of the *Trichoderma harzianum* endochitinase gene, *ech42*, in mycoparasitism. *Applied Environmental Microbiology* 65: 929–935.

Chet I, Inbar J, Hadar I. (1997). Fungal antagonists and mycoparasites. In: Wicklow, D.T., Soderstrom, B. (Eds.), *The Mycota* IV: *Environmental and Microbial Relationships*. Springer, Berlin, pp. 165–184.

Chet I, Inbar J. (1994). Biological control of fungal pathogens. *Applied Biochemistry and Biotechnology* 48: 37–43.

Claydon N, Allan M, Hanson JR, Avent AG. (1987). Antifungal alkyl pyrones of *Trichoderma harzianum*. *Transactions of the British Mycological Society* 88: 503–513.

Cleland R. (1972). The dosage–response curve for auxin-induced cell elongation: a re-evaluation. *Planta* 104: 1–9.

Cutler HG, Cox RH, Crumley FG, Cole PD. (1986). 6-Pentyl-apyrone from *Trichoderma harzianum*: its plant growth inhibitory and antimicrobial properties. *Agricultural and Biological Chemistry* 50: 2943–2945.

Cutler HG, Himmetsbach DS, Arrendale RF, Cole PD, Cox RH. (1989). Koninginin A: a novel plant regulator from *Trichoderma koningii*. *Agricultural and Biological Chemistry* 53: 2605–2611.

de Boer W, Verheggen P, Klein GPJ, Kowalchuk GA, van Veen JA. (2003). Microbial community composition affects soil fungistasis. *Applied Environmental Microbiology* 69: 835–844.

De Meyer G, Bigirimana J, Elad Y, Hofte M. (1998). Induced systemic resistance in *Trichoderma harzianum* T39 biocontrol of *Botrytis cinerea*. *European Journal of Plant Pathology* 104: 279–286.

Demain AL, Fang A. (2000). The natural functions of secondary metabolites. *Advances in Biochemical Engineering/Biotechnology* 69: 1–39.

Djonovic S, Pozo MJ, Dangott LJ, Howell CR, Kenerley CM. (2006). *Sm1*, a proteinaceous elicitor secreted by the biocontrol fungus *Trichoderma virens* induces plant defense responses and systemic resistance. *Molecular Plant–Microbe Interaction* 19: 838–853.

Fogliano V, Ballio A, Gallo M, Woo SL, Scala F, Lorito M. (2002). Pseudomonas lipodepsipeptides and fungal cell wall-degrading enzymes act synergistically in biological control. *Molecular Plant–Microbe Interaction* 15: 323–333.

Ghisalberti EL, Narbey MJ, Dewan MM, Sivasithamparam K. (1990). Variability among strains of *Trichoderma harzianum* in their ability to reduce take-all and to produce pyrones. *Plant and Soil* 121: 287–291.

Ghisalberti EL, Sivasithamparam K. (1991). Antifungal antibiotics produced by *Trichoderma* spp. *Soil Biology and Biochemistry* 23: 1011–1020.

Gullino ML. (1992). Control of Botrytis rot of grapes and vegetables with *Trichoderma* spp. *In*: Tjamos EC, Papavizas, GC, Cook RJ. (Eds.), *Biological Control of Plant Diseases, Progress and Challenges for the Future*. Plenum Press, New York, pp. 125–132.

Hanson LE, Howell CR. (2004). Elicitors of plant defense responses from biocontrol strains of *Trichoderma virens*. *Phytopathology* 94: 171–176.

Harman GE, Howell CR, Viterbo A, Chet I, Lorito M. (2004). *Trichoderma* species-opportunistic, avirulent plant symbionts. *Nature Review Microbiology* 2: 43–56.

Harman GE, Kubicek CP. (1998). *Trichoderma* and *Gliocladium*. Taylor and Francis, London.

Harman GE. (2000). Myths and dogmas of biocontrol: changes in perceptions derived from research on *Trichoderma harzianum* T-22. *Plant Disease* 84: 377–393.

Harman GE. (2006). Overview of mechanisms and uses of *Trichoderma* spp. *Phytopathology* 96: 190–194.

Hoitink HAJ, Boehm MJ. (1999). Biocontrol within the context of soil microbial communities: a substrate-dependent phenomenon. *Annual Review of Phytopathology* 37: 427–446.

Hoitink HAJ, Madden LV, Dorrance AE. (2006). Systemic resistance induced by *Trichoderma* spp.: interactions between the host, the pathogen, the biocontrol agent, and soil organic matter quality. *Phytopathology* 96: 186–189.

Howell CR, Hanson EL, Stipanovic RD, Puckhaber LS. (2000). Induction of terpenoid synthesis in cotton roots and control of *Rhizoctonia solani* by seed treatment with *Trichoderma virens*. *Phytopathology* 90: 248–252.

Howell CR, Puckhaber LS. (2005). A study of the characteristics of "P" and "Q" strains of *Trichoderma virens* to account for differences in biological control efficacy against cotton seedling diseases. *Biological Control* 33: 217–222.

Howell CR, Stipanovic RD, Lumsden RD. (1993). Antibiotic production by strains of *Gliocladium virens* and its relation to the biocontrol of cotton seedling diseases. *Biocontrol Science and Technology* 3: 435–441.

Howell CR, Stipanovic RD. (1983). Gliovirin, a new antibiotic from *Gliocladium virens*, and its role in the biological control of *Pythium ultimum*. *Canadian Journal of Microbiology* 29: 321–324.

Howell CR. (1998). The role of antibiosis in biocontrol. In: Harman GE. Kubicek CP. (Eds.), *Trichoderma and Gliocladium. Enzymes, Biological Control and Commercial Application*, vol. 2. Taylor and Francis Ltd., London, pp. 173–183.

Howell CR. (2002). Cotton seedling pre-emergence damping-off incited by *Rhizopus oryzae* and *Pythium* spp. and its biological control with *Trichoderma* spp. *Phytopathology* 92: 177–180.

Howell CR. (2003). Mechanisms employed by *Trichoderma* species in the biological control of plant diseases: the history and evolution of current concepts. *Plant Disease* 87: 4–10.

Howell CR. (2006). Understanding the mechanisms employed by *Trichoderma virens* to effect biological control of cotton diseases. *Phytopathology* 96: 178–180.

Khan J, Ooka JJ, Miller SA, Madden LV, Hoitink HAJ. (2004). Systemic resistance induced by *Trichoderma hamatum* 382 in cucumber against *Phytophthora* crown rot and leaf blight. *Plant Disease* 88: 280–286.

Krause MS, Madden LV, Hoitink HAJ. (2001). Effect of potting mix microbial carrying capacity on biological control of *Rhizoctonia* damping-off of radish and *Rhizoctonia* crown and root rot of poinsettia. *Phytopathology* 91: 1116–1123.

Kubicek CP, Mach RL, Peterbauer CK, Lorito M. (2001). *Trichoderma*: from genes to biocontrol. *Journal of Plant Pathology* 83: 11–23.

Kullnig C, Mach RL, Lorito M, Kubicek CP. (2000). Enzyme diffusion from *Trichoderma atroviride* (*T. harzianum* P1) to *Rhizoctonia solani* is a prerequisite for triggering of *Trichoderma ech42* gene expression before mycoparasitic contact. *Applied Environmental Microbiology* 66: 2232–2234.

Le Doan T, El-Hajii M, Rebuffat S, Rajeswari MR, Bodo B. (1986). Fluorescein studies on the interaction of trichorzianine A IIIc with model membranes. *Biochimica et Biophysica Acta* 858: 1–5.

Leandro LFS, Guzman T, Ferguson LM, Fernandez GE, Louws FJ. (2007). Population dynamics of *Trichoderma* in fumigated and compost amended soil and on strawberry roots. *Applied Soil Ecology* 35: 237–246.

Lorito M, Farkas V, Rebuffat S, Bodo B, Kubicek CP. (1996b). Cell wall synthesis is a major target of mycoparasitic antagonism by *Trichoderma harzianum*. *Journal of Bacteriology* 178: 6382–6385.

Lorito M, Harman GE, Hayes CK, Broadway RM, Tronsmo A, Woo SL, Di Pietro A. (1993). Chitinolytic enzymes produced by *Trichoderma harzianum*: antifungal activity of purified endochitinase and chitobiosidase. *Phytopathology* 83: 302–307.

Lorito M, Hayes CK, Di Pietro A, Woo SL, Harman GE. (1994a). Purification, characterization and synergistic activity of a glucan 1,3-b-glucosidase and an N-acetyl-b-glucosaminidase from *Trichoderma harzianum*. *Phytopathology* 84: 398–405.

Lorito M, Peterbauer C, Hayes CK, Harman GE. (1994b). Synergistic interaction between fungal cell wall degrading enzymes and different antifungal compounds enhances inhibition of spore germination. *Microbiology* 140: 623–629.

Lorito M, Scala F. (1999). Microbial genes expressed in transgenic plants to improve disease resistance. *Journal of Plant Pathology* 81: 73–88.

Lorito M, Woo SL, DAmbrosio M, Harman GE, Hayes CK, Kubicek CP, Scala F. (1996a). Synergistic interaction between cell wall degrading enzymes and membrane affecting compounds. *Molecular Plant–Microbe Interaction* 9: 206–213.

Lorito M, Woo SL, Iaccarino M, Scala F. (2006). Microrganismi antagonisti. In: Iaccarino M. (Ed.), *Microrganismi Benefici per le Piante*. Idelson-Gnocchi s.r.l., Napoli, Italia, pp. 146–175.

Lorito M, Woo SL, Scala F. (2004). Le biotecnologie utili alla difesa sostenibile delle piante: i funghi. *Agroindustria* 3: 181–195.

Lorito M. (1998). Chitinolytic enzymes and their genes. In: Harman GE, Kubicek CP. (Eds.), *Trichoderma and Gliocladium*, Vol. 2. Taylor and Francis Ltd., London, pp. 73–99.

Lotan T, Fluhr R. (1990). Xylanase, a novel elicitor of pathogenesisrelated proteins in tobacco, uses a nonethylene pathway for induction. *Plant Physiology* 93: 811–817.

Lu Z, Tombolini R, Woo SL, Zeilinger S, Lorito M, Jansson JK. (2004). *In vivo* study of *Trichoderma*–pathogen–plant interactions with constitutive and inducible *gfp* reporter systems. *Applied Environmental Microbiology* 70: 3073–3081.

Mach RL, Peterbauer CK, Payer K, Jaksits S, Woo SL, Zeilinger S, Kullnig CM, Lorito M, Kubicek CP. (1999). Expression of two major chitinase genes of *Trichoderma* atroviride (*T. harzianum* P1) is triggered by different regulatory signals. *Applied Environmental Microbiology* 65: 1858–1863.

Marra R, Ambrosino P, Carbone V, Vinale F, Woo SL, Ruocco M, Ciliento R, Lanzuise S, Ferraioli S, Soriente I, Gigante S, Turra D, Fogliano V, Scala F, Lorito M. (2006). Study of the three-way interaction between *Trichoderma* atroviride, plant and fungal pathogens by using a proteomic approach. *Current Genetics* 50: 307–321.

Naseby DC, Pascual JA, Lynch JM. (2000). Effect of biocontrol strains of *Trichoderma* on plant growth, *Pythium ultimum* population, soil microbial communities and soil enzyme activities. *Journal of Applied Microbiology* 88: 161–169.

Papavizas GC. (1985). *Trichoderma* and *Gliocladium*: biology, ecology, and potential for biocontrol. *Annual Review Phytopathology* 23: 23–54.

Rebuffat S, El Hajji M, Hennig P, Davoust D, Bodo B. (1989). Isolation, sequence and conformation of seven trichorzianines B from *Trichoderma harzianum*. *International Journal of Peptide and Protein Research* 34: 200–210.

Schirmbock M, Lorito M, Wang YL, Hayes CK, Arisan-Atac I, Scala F, Harman GE, Kubicek CP. (1994). Parallel formation and synergism of hydrolytic enzymes and peptaibol antibiotics, molecular mechanisms involved in the antagonistic action of *Trichoderma harzianum* against phytopathogenic fungi. *Applied Environmental Microbiology* 60: 4364–4370.

Serrano-Carreon L, Hathout Y, Bensoussan M, Belin JM. (1993). Metabolism of linoleic acid and 6-pentyl-a-pyrone biosynthesis by *Trichoderma* species. *Applied and Environmental Microbiology* 59: 2945–2950.

Simon A, Sivasithamparam K. (1989). Pathogen suppression: A case study in biological suppression of *Gaeumannomyces graminis* var. *tritici* in soil. *Soil Biology and Biochemistry* 21: 331–337.

Singh PK, Mishra MK, Vyas D. (2007). Efficacy of *Trichoderma* spp. strains in the control of Fusarium wilt of tomato. *Journal of Mycology and Plant Pathology* 37: 105–107.

Singh PK, Vyas D. (2007). Efficacy of *Trichoderma* sp. in control of wilt of tomato. *Journal of Basic and Applied Mycology* 6: 93–95.

Singh PK, Vyas D. (2008). Effects of chemical fertilizers on the growth of *Trichoderma* spp. in soil. *Journal of Botanical Society of University Sagar*, 42: 82-86.

Sivan A, Chet I. (1989). The possible role of competition between *Trichoderma harzianum* and *Fusarium oxysporum* on rhizosphere colonization. *Phytopathology* 79: 198–203.

Sivasithamparam K, Ghisalberti EL. (1998). Secondary metabolism in *Trichoderma* and *Gliocladium*. In: Harman GE, Kubicek CP. (Eds.), *Trichoderma and Gliocladium*, Vol. 1. Taylor and Francis Ltd., London, pp. 139–191.

Stacey G, Keen NT. (Eds.) 1999). *Plant–Microbe Interactions*, vol. 4. APS Press, St. Paul.

Thimann KV. (1937). On the nature of inhibitions caused by auxin. *American Journal of Botany* 24: 407–412.

Tronsmo A. (1991). Biological and integrated controls of *Botrytis cinerea* on apple with *Trichoderma harzianum*. *Biological Control* 1: 59–62.

van Loon LC, Bakker PAHM, Pieterse CMJ. (1998). Systemic resistance induced by rhizobacteria. *Annual Review of Phytopathology* 36: 453–483.

Vinale F, DAmbrosio G, Abadi K, Scala F, Marra R, Turra D, Woo SL, Lorito M. (2004). Application of *Trichoderma harzianum* (T22) and *Trichoderma atroviride* (P1) as plant growth promoters, and their compatibility with copper oxychloride. *Journal of Zhejiang University Science* 30: 2–8.

Vinale F, Marra R, Scala F, Ghisalberti EL, Lorito M, Sivasithamparam K. (2006). Major secondary metabolites produced by two commercial *Trichoderma* strains active against different phytopathogens. *Letters in Applied Microbiology* 43: 143–148.

Viterbo A, Shoresh M, Brotman Y, Chet I. (2006). Towards understanding the molecular basis for induced resistance in the *Trichoderma*–plant interaction. In: Proceedings of the Ninth International workshop on *Trichoderma* and *Gliocladium*. Vienna, Austria, April 6–8, KS6.

Wakelin SA, Sivasithamparam K, Cole ALJ, Skipp RA. (1999). Saprophytic growth in soil of a strain of *Trichoderma koningii*. *New Zealand Journal of Agricultural Research* 42, 337–345.

Wiest A, Grzegorski D, Xu B, Goulard C, Le Doan S, Ebbole DJ, Bodo B, Kenerley C. (2002). Identification of peptaibols from *Trichoderma virens* and cloning of a peptaibol synthetase. *Journal of Biological Chemistry* 277: 20862–20868.

Woo SL, Donzelli B, Scala F, Mach R, Harman GE, Kubicek CP, Del Sorbo G, Lorito M. (1999). Disruption of the *ech42* (endochitinase encoding) gene affect biocontrol activity in *Trichoderma harzianum* P1. *Molecular Plant–Microbe Interaction* 12: 419–429.

Woo SL, Formisano E, Fogliano V, Cosenza C, Mauro A, Turra D, Soriente I, Ferraioli S, Scala F, Lorito M. (2004). Factors that contribute to the mycoparasitism stimulus in *Trichoderma atroviride* strain P1. *Journal of Zhejiang University Science* 30: 421.

Woo SL, Lorito M. (2007). Exploiting the interactions between fungal antagonists, pathogens and the plant for biocontrol. In: Vurro M, Gressel J. (Eds.), *Novel Biotechnologies for Biocontrol Agent Enhancement and Management*. IOS, Springer Press, Amsterdam, the Netherlands, pp. 107–130.

Woo SL, Scala F, Ruocco M, Lorito M. (2006). The molecular biology of the interactions between *Trichoderma* spp., phytopathogenic fungi, and plants. *Phytopathology* 96: 181–185.

Yedidia I, Benhamou N, Chet I. (1999). Induction of defence responses in cucumber plants (*Cucumis sativus* L.) by the biocontrol agent *Trichoderma harzianum*. *Applied Environmental Microbiology* 65: 1061–1070.

Yedidia I, Shoresh M, Kerem Z, Benhamou N, Kapulnik Y, Chet I. (2003). Concomitant induction of systemic resistance to Pseudomonas syringae pv. lachrymans in cucumber by *Trichoderma asperellum* (T-203) and accumulation of phytoalexins. *Applied Environmental Microbiology* 69: 7343–7353.

Zeilinger S, Galhaup C, Payer K, Woo SL, Mach RL, Fekete C, Lorito M, Kubicek CP. (1999). Chitinase gene expression during mycoparasitic interaction of *Trichoderma harzianum* with its host. *Fungal Genetics and Biology* 26: 131–140.